L.S. MANSFIELD, V.M.D., Ph.D.
DEPARTMENTS OF MICROBIOLOGY AND
LARGE ANIMAL CLINICAL SCIENCE
FOOD SAFETY & TOXICOLOGY, RM. B43
MICHIGAN STATE UNIVERSITY
EAST LANSING, MI. 48824-1234
PHONE: 517-432-6309
FAX: 517-432-2310

Molecular and Cellular Basis
of Inflammation

Current Inflammation Research

Charles N. Serhan, Series Editor

Molecular and Cellular Basis of Inflammation, edited by *Charles N. Serhan and Peter A. Ward*, 1999

Molecular and Cellular Basis of Inflammation

Edited by

Charles N. Serhan

Harvard Medical School, Brigham and Women's Hospital
Boston, MA

and

Peter A. Ward

University of Michigan, Ann Arbor, MI

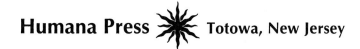

Humana Press ✻ Totowa, New Jersey

Cover design by Patricia F. Cleary.

For additional copies, pricing for bulk purchases, and/or information about other Humana titles, contact Humana at the above address or at any of the following numbers: Tel.: 973-256-1699; Fax: 973-256-8341; E-mail: humana@humanapr.com or visit our Web site: http://humanapress.com

Photocopy Authorization Policy:
Authorization to photocopy items for internal or personal use, or the internal or personal use of specific clients, is granted by Humana Press Inc., provided that the base fee of US $8.00 per copy, plus US $00.25 per page, is paid directly to the Copyright Clearance Center at 222 Rosewood Drive, Danvers, MA 01923. For those organizations that have been granted a photocopy license from the CCC, a separate system of payment has been arranged and is acceptable to Humana Press Inc. The fee code for users of the Transactional Reporting Service is: [0-89603-595-6/98 $8.00 + $00.25].

Printed in the United States of America.   10 9 8 7 6 5 4 3 2 1

Library of Congress Cataloging in Publication Data

Molecular and cellular basis of inflammation/edited by Charles N. Serhan and Peter A. Ward
    p.   cm.
  Includes bibliographical references and index.
  ISBN 0-89603-595-6 (alk. paper)
  1. Inflammation—Mediators.   2.   Inflammation—Immunological aspects.   I. Serhan, Charles N.
II. Ward, Peter A., 1934–   .
  [DNLM: 1. Inflammation—immunology. Immunity, Cellular—physiology.   QW 700 M7175 1999]
RB131.M73   1999
616'.0473—dc21
DNLM/DLC
for Library of Congress   98-47837
                                               CIP

Preface

The study of inflammation has captured the interest of scholars since the earliest recorded history. Symbols identifying the cardinal signs of inflammation were uncovered in both Sanskrit and hieroglyphics *(1)*. Since complete appreciation of the inflammatory process is underscored by the need for knowledge at both the cellular and molecular levels, academic inquiry in the area of inflammation has led, in many respects, the foray of current biomedical research. *Molecular and Cellular Basis of Inflammation* represents research from the cutting edge in the broad view of inflammation. The chapters are written by experts with a multidisciplinary approach to the study of inflammatory and cellular processes, and thus include contributions form the fields of molecular biology, biochemistry, pharmacology, immunology, and pathobiology.

Molecular and Cellular Basis of Inflammation was first conceived during a minisymposium sponsored by the American Society for Investigative Pathology held at FASEB in 1995 entitled "The Role of Reactive Lipids, Oxygen and Nitrogen Metabolites in Inflammation," at which several of the contributing authors delivered lectures. This present, much-extended volume includes leading-front descriptions of both protein and lipid mediators. The chapter devoted to the complement cascade by Ward and colleagues, as well as Chapters 3–7 and 13, provide up-to-date descriptions of the biosynthesis, molecular biology, chemistry, and actions of both protein and lipid mediators. Chapter 3, by Haeggestrom and Serhan, provides an overview and update of eicosanoids, with a particular focus on the biosynthesis and actions of leukotrienes and lipoxins in disease models. An overview of the molecular biology and enzymology of the cascade, including a detailed account of the mutagenesis of the 5-lipoxygenase, an enzyme that plays a central role in leukotriene generation, is given by Dr. Rådmark of the Karolinska Institute, Stockholm, from which much of the work on inflammatory mediators emanated historically.

Chapter 5 focuses on the use of targeted gene disruption models in mice for the elucidation of the role of lipid mediators in inflammation and is contributed by Dr. Colin Funk and colleagues, who generated some of the initial work in this area and now provide an authoritative review of the status of the use of knockout mice.

Another, more recently uncovered series of lipid mediators is termed "isoprostanes." These compounds, which are isomers of the classic prostanoids, appear to play important roles in both vascular disease and as markers of lipid peroxidation. Chapters 6 and 7 have been provided by leaders in this arena. Dr. Garret FitzGerald and colleagues, in addition to giving an update on the role of isoprostanes in vascular disease, provide new results on the role of these compounds in acute respiratory distress syndrome. Dr. Roberts and colleagues, whose laboratory first uncovered the isoprostanes, examine in detail the formation of isoprostanes, the role of free radicals in this process, and their occurrence in atherosclerotic lesions. Chapter 13 focuses on the use of new quantitative methods for the measurement of small molecules and lipid-derived mediators. Dr. Borgeat and colleagues review the important uses of liquid chromatography–electrospray mass spectrometry in product identification, profiling, and quantitation. Moreover, Borgeat et al. also report on the important new role of adenosine in the regulation of endogenous leukotriene biosynthesis by physiologic stimuli. Together these chapters provide us with an update on and overview of the role and novel actions of lipid mediators in inflammatory responses.

One area that has been clearly established to play a key role in leukocyte-mediated tissue injury during inflammation is the formation and release of reactive oxygen species by phagocytic leukocytes. The substantial advances in our knowledge of he assembly of NADPH oxidase components and their signal transduction processes are elegantly reviewed by Dr. Heyworth and colleagues in Chapter 8. The structure and organization of NADPH oxidase and its biochemistry provide not only a cutting-edge look at potential therapeutic opportunities for regulating this system, but also an area of biochemistry that illustrates the complex role of protein–protein interactions in signal transduction and the illuminating lessons this knowledge provides. The activation sequence of leukocytes is examined in biochemical and molecular detail in Chapter 10 by Dr. Jesaitis and colleagues, who have reviewed the structure and transmembrane signaling via the *N*-formyl peptide receptor on phagocytic cells. This is a seven transmembrane-spanning ‚receptor, and study of its signal transduction processes may have wide-reaching implications for the development of novel anti-inflammatory agents. Other cells recently recognized to play an important role in inflammation are the γ/δ T cells as well as other T cell subsets; these are authoritatively reviewed by Dr. Jutila in Chapter 9. Leukocytes also interact with epithelium surfaces of several organs, i.e., lung, gastrointestinal, and immune tissues, and Dr. Masdara and colleagues have provided in Chapter 11 a timely examination of recent studies that evaluate cell–cell interactions between human neutrophils and polarized epithelial cells. The adhesion molecules involved, their regulation by cytokines, and the important role of small molecule mediators as regulators of these cell–cell interactions are reviewed with authority and vision. Neutrophil–epithelial interactions are regulated by both adenosine and lipid mediators, such as lipoxins. Recognition that adenosine can play a novel role as an autocoid inhibiting processes of interest in leukocyte-mediated inflammatory events is presented by an originator of this work, Dr. Bruce Cronstein, in Chapter 12. Description of adenosine, its actions on leukocytes, and the receptors responsible for transducing signaling are reviewed and discussed in this chapter.

Studies at the cellular and molecular level in processes of interest in inflammation culminate with three chapters of wide-ranging scope and implications; these are devoted to our current understanding of the disease mechanisms involved in angiogenesis, autoimmune arthritis, and lupus erythematosus. Drs. Arenberg and Streiter set forth a timely and elegantly presented view of the cellular and molecular events that contribute to angiogenesis. Dr. Kang and colleagues examine the pathogenesis of rheumatoid arthritis and consider the roles and contributions of both cellular and biochemical mediators to the molecular basis for susceptibility to rheumatoid arthritis. In addition, this chapter provides exciting new information regarding the regulation of prostanoid biosynthesis by cyclooxygenase-1 and cyclooxegenase-2, considers the importance of feedback modulation between leukotriene and prostanoid formation, and treats the impact of NSAIDs. The role of matrix metalloproteases in autoimmune arthritis are also considered and reviewed. In addition, an update on lupus erythematosus and the role of adhesion molecules and local mediators is presented by Drs. Abramson and Belmont. Here we learn of the cellular and molecular interactions between the complement systems, selected leukocytes (monocytes, neutrophils), the importance of integrins, platelets, and leukocyte-derived mediators in vascular injury events observed in lupus erythematosus with a consideration of the role of endothelial cell activation in these processes.

Understanding of the molecular and cellular basis of inflammation continues to evolve and grow with the identification of new mediators, feedforward and/or amplification pathways, novel endogenous counterregulatory pathways, and approaches to the study of inflammation in relevant and predictive experimental models. The quest for new anti-inflammatory agents beckons the further elucidation of cellular and molecular mechanisms that are quintessential to both initiating and terminating inflammation. The new and scholarly evaluation of current knowledge by world leaders presented in this book should be of interest to students, medical residents, postdoctoral fellows, practicing physicians, and principal investigators from both academia and industry because of the tour de force in approaches undertaken and discussed here to establish new basic concepts in the elucidation of molecular mechanisms in inflammation. The editors trust that the reader will share our enthusiasm and continued excitement as well as fascination for discoveries in the area of inflammation.

Charles N. Serhan
Peter A. Ward

Reference

1. Manjo, G. (1982) Inflammation and infection: historic highlights, in *Current Topics in Inflammation and Infection* (Manjo, G., Cotran, R. S., and Kaufman, N., eds.), Williams & Wilkins, Baltimore, pp. 1–17.

Contents

Contributors

STEVEN B. ABRAMSON • *Hospital for Joint Diseases, New York University Medical Center, New York, New York, NY*

DOUGLAS A. ARENBERG • *Division of Pulmonary and Critical Care Medicine, Department of Internal Medicine, University of Michigan Medical School, Ann Arbor, MI*

JOHN A. BADWEY • *Harvard Medical School and Boston Biomedical Research Institute, Boston, MA*

LESLIE R. BALLOU • *Departments of Medicine and Biochemistry, University of Tennessee, Memphis, TN, and Department of Veterans Affairs Medical Center, Memphis, TN*

H. MICHAEL BELMONT • *Hospital for Joint Diseases, New York University Medical Center, New York, New York, NY*

PIERRE BORGEAT • *Centre de Recherche du CHUQ, Sainte-Foy, Quebec, Canada*

BRUCE N. CRONSTEIN • *Department of Medicine and Pathology, New York University Medical Center, New York, NY*

JOHN T. CURNUTTE • *Immunology Department, Genentech Inc., South San Francisco, CA*

NANCY DALLAIRE • *Centre de Recherche du CHUQ, Sainte-Foy, Quebec, Canada*

NORMAN DELANTY • *Center for Experimental Therapeutics, Philadelphia, PA*

GARRETT A. FITZGERALD • *Center for Experimental Therapeutics, Philadelphia, PA*

COLIN D. FUNK • *Center for Experimental Therapeutics and Department of Pharmacology, University of Pennsylvania, Philadelphia, PA*

JESPER Z. HAEGGSTRÖM • *Department of Medical Biochemistry and Biophysics, Karolinska Institutet, Stockholm, Sweden*

KAREN A. HASTY • *Department of Anatomy and Neurobiology, University of Tennessee, Memphis, TN, and Department of Veterans Affairs Medical Center, Memphis, TN*

PAUL G. HEYWORTH • *Department of Molecular and Experimental Medicine, The Scripps Research Institute, La Jolla, CA*

ALGIRDAS J. JESAITIS • *Department of Microbiology, Montana State University, Bozeman, MT*

MARK A. JUTILA • *Department of Veterinary Molecular Biology, Montana State University, Bozeman, MT*

ANDREW H. KANG • *Departments of Medicine and Biochemistry, University of Tennessee, Memphis, TN, and Department of Veterans Affairs Medical Center, Memphis, TN*

PAUL LANKEN • *Center for Experimental Therapeutics, Philadelphia, PA*

JOHN LAWSON • *Center for Experimental Therapeutics, Philadelphia, PA*

JAMES L. MADARA • *Department of Pathology and Laboratory Medicine, Emory University School of Medicine, Atlanta, GA*

HEINI M. MIETTINEN • *Department of Microbiology, Montana State University, Bozeman, MT*

JOHN S. MILLS • *Department of Microbiology, Montana State University, Bozeman, MT*

JASON D. MORROW • *Departments of Pharmacology and Medicine, Vanderbilt University, Nashville, TN*

HEDWIG S. MURPHY • *Departmennt of Pathology, University of Michigan Medical School, Ann Arbor, MI*

SERGE PICARD • *Centre de Recherche du CHUQ, Sainte-Foy, Quebec, Canada*

MARC POULIOT • *Centre de Recherche du CHUQ, Sainte-Foy, Quebec, Canada*

OLOF RÅDMARK • *Department of Medical Biochemistry and Biophysics, Karolinska Institutet, Stockholm, Sweden*

RAJENDRA RAGHOW • *Department of Pharmacology, University of Tennessee, Memphis, TN, and Department of Veterans Affairs Medical Center, Memphis, TN*

MUREDACH P. REILLY • *Center for Experimental Therapeutics, Philadelphia, PA*

L. JACKSON ROBERTS II • *Departments of Pharmacology and Medicine, Vanderbilt University, Nashville, TN*

JOSHUA ROCKACH • *Florida Institute of Technology, Claude Pepper Institute for Aging and Therapeutic Research, Melbourne, FL*

EDWARD F. ROSLONIEC • *Department of Veterans Affairs Medical Center, Memphis, TN*

CHARLES N. SERHAN • *Department of Anesthesia, Center for Experimental Therapeutics and Reperfusion Injury, Brigham and Women's Hospital and Harvard Medical School, Boston, MA*

ROBERT M. STREITER • *Division of Pulmonary and Critical Care Medicine, Department of Internal Medicine, University of Michigan Medical School, Ann Arbor, MI*

MARC SURETTE • *Centre de Recherche du CHUQ, Sainte-Foy, Quebec, Canada*

MICHAEL J. VLASES • *Department of Microbiology, Montana State University, Bozeman, MT*

PETER A. WARD • *Department of Pathology, University of Michigan Medical School, Ann Arbor, MI*

1

Role of Complement in Endothelial Cell Activation

Peter A. Ward and Hedwig S. Murphy

Introduction

Complement has long been known to play a key role in the inflammatory response, although the precise mechanisms of its influences are uncertain. Intravascular activation of the complement pathway occurs as a result of the sequential activation of a cascade of proteolytic enzymes. Generation of numerous bioactive complement-derived products in turn evoke a complex series of cardiovascular responses. In vivo and in vitro inflammatory models serve to demonstrate the mechanisms of inflammatory injury, specifically defining complement interaction with vascular endothelial cells, and may provide insights into the central role of complement in the inflammatory response. The contribution of complement activation through an interaction with and activation of vascular endothelial cells is the focus of this chapter.

Activation of vascular endothelial cells is an early critical event in the development of an inflammatory response. Multiple soluble circulating factors, complement and cytokines, as well as bacterial products and toxins, can induce a change in endothelial cell phenotype. Endothelial cell activation results in enhanced expression of surface molecules required for adhesion of circulating inflammatory cells and in release of proinflammatory mediators and vasoactive agents. Sequential expression of adhesion molecules including selectins (E-, P-, and L-selectin) and members of the immuno-globulin superfamily (VCAM-1 and ICAM-1) results in increased adhesiveness of endothelial cells for circulating leukocytes expressing reciprocally recognized adhesion molecules ("counterreceptors"). Soluble mediators released from endothelial cells contribute to the hemodynamic state of vascularized tissue and function as chemotactic factors and cytokines to activate other inflammatory cells. These soluble factors serve

From: *Molecular and Cellular Basis of Inflammation*
Edited by: C. N. Serhan and P. A. Ward © Humana Press Inc., Totowa, NJ

to maintain, regulate, and enhance the continuing process of inflammation, leading ultimately to tissue injury.

Complement activation products have a variety of effects on leukocytes and endothelial cells, promoting leukocyte-endothelial cell interactions and stimulating endothelial cell activation—key events in the early inflammatory process. In vivo and in vitro strategies have been applied to address these issues. Studies using genetic deletion of complement components, complement depletion, or complement blockade have linked complement activation products to neutrophil recruitment and tissue damage in a variety of animal models of injury. Mechanisms of specific endothelial cell responses in inflammation have been investigated in cultured cells, allowing dissection of this complex series of events. Examination of effects of complement activation products on neutrophil–endothelial cell adhesion, regulation of expression of specific adhesion molecules, and secretion of cytokines has allowed some insights into the interactions between complement activation products and endothelial cells.

Complement Activation

Abundant clinical evidence links elevated serum levels of complement activation products with disease states. Sarcoidosis, idiopathic pulmonary fibrosis (IPF), chronic obstructive pulmonary disease, systemic lupus erythematosis, and certain types of glomerulonephritis and ischemia-reperfusion *(1–4)* are states associated with reductions in plasma levels of one or more complement components, indicative of activation of the complement system during periods of disease activity. In preterm infants, elevated C5a levels in tracheobronchial aspirates parallel risk for development of chronic lung disease *(3)*. Sepsis, adult respiratory distress syndrome (ARDS), and, ultimately, multiple organ dysfunction syndrome (MODS), culminating in death, are associated with profound activation of the complement system and with circulating complement activation products *(4–12)*. However, defining the precise role of specific complement activation products in the setting of an inflammatory response has been a challenge.

Intravascular activation of complement is initiated via a variety of agents including antigen–antibody complexes, bacterial products, and toxins; injured endothelial cells as well can activate the complement system *(13)*. Complement consists of multiple components that when activated (and often cleaved), interact to form enzymes or function as binding proteins. Inflammatory cells and cells of the immune system express cell surface receptors not only for specific complement proteins but also for additional regulatory proteins capable of protecting cells from complement attack *(14–19)*. The complement system is organized as two pathways with C3 occupying a central position in both (Fig. 1). Binding of antibody to antigen or to foreign molecules results in activation of the antibody-dependent *classical* pathway whereas the *alternative* pathway is persistently activated in low levels by the spontaneous interaction of C3 with water to yield $C3(H_2O)$ *(20)*. Contact of plasma with bacterial lipopolysaccharide and other nonprotein agents powerfully activates the alternative pathway. C3 is biologically inactive, but cleavage by C3 convertase yields active fragments including C3a and C3b. Deposition of the active cleavage product C3b on the surface of foreign particles or target cells allows recognition by receptors on phagocytic cells whereas C3a is a potent activator of mast cells and basophils and leads to release of histamine from secretory granules. Histamine in turn is a potent endothelial cell activator, inducing vasodilation and vascular permeability as well as P-selectin translocation from Weible-Palade bod-

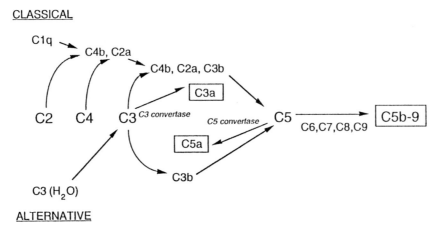

CLASSICAL

ALTERNATIVE

Fig. 1. Molecular organization of the complement pathways. C3 occupies a central position in both pathways, leading to C5 cleavage and formation of the C5b-9 complex.

ies to the endothelial cell surface. Proteolytic cleavage of C5 occurs via both pathways and generates C5a, a potent mediator of inflammation. C5a is the major complement-derived chemotactic agent for neutrophils, eosinophils, monocytes, and macrophages. C5a also has the ability to activate platelets, leading to their aggregation and surface expression of P-selectin. C3 and C5 occupy central positions within the enzyme cascade and allow for amplification of the complement system. Intravascular activation of complement by both pathways leads to generation of the lytic complex C5b-9 (membrane attack complex [MAC]), with C5b as a nidus for assembly of the five complement proteins. The primary direct action of MAC occurs by its cell surface assembly and its insertion into the membrane of the target cell. Interaction of the C7 component of MAC with phospholipid membranes initiates this association and ultimate pore formation. Recently several cytoprotective factors have been identified on surfaces of endothelial cells, including CD59 (protectin) *(14,17,19)*, HRF20 (homologous restriction factor 20) *(18,21)*, DAF (decay-accelerating factor) *(14,21)*, apoA-I and apoA-II *(15,16)*, C1 esterase inhibitor *(22–24)*, MCP (CD46, membrane cofactor protein) *(25)*, and others. These factors provide resistance specifically to complement-mediated cell lysis induced by assembly of the MAC on cell surfaces. Not only is MAC cytotoxic for nucleated cells, red cells, and bacteria, but it is also able to activate phagocytic cells to generate oxidants (e.g., $O_2^{\cdot}$, H_2O) and cytokines. Clearly, blocking of the complement system to prevent generation of these phlogistic products should be tissue protective. A detailed understanding of these events may provide insights into the specific roles of the activation products and direct threrapeutic interventions.

Requirement for Complement in Inflammatory Lung Injury

Experimental animal models of inflammation have focused on complement requirements for the full expression of acute lung injury. In an experimental rat model of lung injury induced by intrapulmonary deposition of IgG immune complexes, the inflammatory reactions are characterized by deposition of immune complexes along the surfaces of alveolar walls, resulting in neutrophil transmigration into tissue. A second model involves a large area (30%) of thermal burn that results in local (skin) and distant (lung) injury; this injury, too, is neutrophil-dependent *(26,27)*. The resulting accumulation of neutrophils and eventual injury is characterized by leakage of albumin into the alveolar compartment along with hemorrhage. The factors associated with production of lung damage include oxidants and proteases. Oxidants, produced by macrophages and neutrophils, derive from NADPH oxidase and inducible nitric oxide synthase. These products can directly injure lung cells and can alter connective tissue matrix by causing cross-binding of glycoproteins, as well as other oxidative damage. Proteinases, including serine proteinases and metalloproteinases, also contribute to tissue injury by bringing about degradation of connective tissue matrix *(28,29)*. It has been recognized that in some forms of injury, this cascade of events leading to injury is complement dependent *(30,31)*.

There are several strategies employed to assess the in vivo requirements for the complement system in acute lung injury, including interference with the generation of specific complement components and blockade or deletion of individual activation products. One method of interfering with complement involves infusion of soluble human recombinant complement receptor-1 (sCR1), which blocks the formation of C3 and C5 convertases, both essential to activation of the complement system and generation of the anaphylatoxins C3a and C5a (Fig. 1). A second method to probe for the role of complement in inflammatory models is to induce complement depletion by serial intraperitoneal injections of purified cobra venom factor (CVF) prior to initiation of the inflammatory responses. CVF interacts with the complement system to bring about activation of the alternative complement pathway, causing consumptive depletion of C3 and the later reactive components. This method of complement depletion reduces plasma protein levels of C3 by >95% and affords effective blockade of the complement activation process for several days. A third method to evaluate the role of specific complement activation products in the animal models involves the use of infusion of specific antibodies directed toward the complement product of interest. The availability of polyclonal antibody that blocks rat C5a but does not react with C5 or affect formation of the C5b-9 complex provides a highly specific agent targeted toward C5a. Additionally, antibody to C5 blocks generation of C5a as well as C5b-9, and both antibodies spare C3 and its bioactive products. A fourth approach has involved the use of animals genetically deficient in components of the complement system, specifically C3 (mice and guinea pigs), C4 (mice and dogs), C5 (mice), and C6 (rabbits and rats).

SCR1 and Depletion of Complement by CVF

Blockade of the complement system, whether by treatment with sCR1 or CVF, has dramatic effects on the inflammatory response *(27,32)*. In the context of the model of IgG immune complex-induced lung injury in rats, which may reflect inflammatory events found in human diseases (rheumatoid arthritis, systemic lupus erythematosis, vasculitis, glomerulonephritis, and so forth), albumin leakage into lung, which is a sensitive indicator of inflammatory damage, is reduced by both methods as is the extent of hemorrhage that is detected by lung accumulation of ^{51}Cr-red blood cells and the lung content of neutrophils compared to lung myeloperoxidase (MPO) or BAL neutrophils. The key to understanding how the complement system plays a role in this inflammatory model is the recognition that depletion results in a greatly diminished accumulation of neutrophils in lung tissue, as reflected by MPO: in the model of immune complex injury, MPO activity was reduced 68% after treatment with sCR1 *(27,33)*.

Clearly, complement activation products are intimately associated not only with the influx of neutrophils but with the development of subsequent tissue injury.

Secondary lung injury, developing after thermal injury to skin, occurs within the context of complement activation. Complement blockade by sCR1 has a striking effect on lung injury following thermal injury to skin. In a manner similar to the immune complex injury, sCR1 treatment reduced hemorrhage by 43% and lung vascular permeability by 64%. MPO content was reduced in lung and skin by 39 and 90%, respectively, again demonstrating an interference with tissue accumulation of neutrophils. In both models, sCR1 blockade of complement provided a high degree of protection against tissue damage.

Complement-Deficient Animals

The availability of animals deficient in specific complement factors has provided new animal models useful for determining the importance of these factors in mediating tissue injury. Disruption of either the C3 or C4 locus by gene targeting resulted in impaired antibody response to T-cell dependent antigens *(34–36)*. Mice deficient in either component were protected against ischemia/reperfusion injury. In this injury model, vascular permeability, as a measure of endothelial cell injury, was reduced by 50% in C3-deficient animals as compared to wild-type animals, an effect that was reversed by administration of sCR1 prior to reperfusion. C4-deficient mice were protected to a similar degree. C3 cleavage occurs by either the classical or alternative pathway (Fig. 1), whereas C4 activation is limited to the antibody-activated classical pathway. The similar findings in mice deficient in either factor indicates that the vascular leakage in this reperfusion model is mediated by the classical pathway, and in both cases, serum immunoglobulin, specifically IgM, was required as well *(37)*.

Early studies in C4-deficient guinea pigs *(38)* and C3-deficient dogs *(39)* indicated a protective role for these components in preventing shock. In the case of endotoxin-induced shock, C3- and C4-deficient mice were significantly more sensitive to injury than wild-type mice (<25% survival in knockout mice compared with >75% survival in wild-type mice), and this sensitivity was reversed by reconstitution with C3. Increased TNF-α and IL1-β production was evident in both knockout mice and was likely owing to the impaired clearance of endotoxin with resulting excess in circulating endotoxin, which was demonstrated in these mice. Replacement of C1 attenuated the endotoxemic shock in the complement-deficient mice, indicating the importance of consumptive depletion of early complement components in the development of this injury *(40)*.

Complement did not appear to play a significant role in three animal models of IgG-triggered inflammation in these same knockout mice *(41)*. In cutaneous immune complex injury, activation and cleavage of C3 occurs via the classical pathway with subsequent release of the chemotactic peptides C3a and C5a and assembly of the C5b-9 membrane attack complex. In experimental autoimmune hemolytic anemia and immune thrombocytopenic purpura, direct activation of complement and formation of C5b-9 results in intravascular hemolysis and platelet clearance. In all three inflammatory injuries, C3- and C4-deficient mice demonstrated edema, hemorrhage, and neutrophil infiltration that was indistinguishable from that in the wild-type controls. In these models, supported by data from Fc receptor-deficient mice *(41)*, it appears that FcγR receptor engagement is necessary and sufficient for antibody-triggered responses, whereas complement is not required.

Studies that have examined the effect of genetic depletion of specific complement components have yielded data that support a critical role for the late complement factors, C5–C9. Mice deficient in C5 have markedly diminished inflammatory lung injury with reduction in neutrophil accumulation, edema and hemorrhage after deposition of IgG immune complexes as compared with C5 sufficient animals *(42)*, and show a four-fold decrease in mortality in a zymosan-induced model of MODS *(43)*. C5-deficient mice are protected from TNF-LPS induced, PAF-mediated shock and tissue injury as well. Reconstitution with normal, C5-sufficient serum resulted in the development of shock and subsequent death *(44,45)*. In this animal model, the availability of C5 appears to be crucial to the full development of inflammatory injury.

The importance of the MAC in acute inflammatory injury was evaluated in animals genetically deficient in the C6 component. In this model, acute lung injury in complement-sufficient rabbits is mediated by intravenous infusion of divalent antibodies to angiotensin-converting enzyme (ACE). The interaction of these antibodies with the enzyme expressed on lung endothelial cells is associated with activation of C3, acute inflammatory capillary lesions, pulmonary edema, respiratory distress, and cardiovascular collapse *(46–48)*. In lung tissue from these animals, deposits of C3 and MAC are found on capillary walls. Animals deficient in C6, which were thus incapable of forming C5b-9, were able to tolerate anti-ACE antibodies without ill effects, and whereas C3 deposits were present on capillary walls, MAC was consistently absent as was the inflammatory cell infiltrate. These animals succumbed to acute pulmonary injury when replenished with C6, which reconstituted the terminal complement pathway, resulting in deposition of MAC on capillary walls. The mechanism of MAC mediation of injury in a second model of antibody-mediated interstitial pneumonitis is less clear. Monovalent anti-ACE Fab fragments, which do not activate complement *(46)*, were used to induce injury that was associated with a fatal interstitial pneumonitis and minimal C3 and MAC deposits. In this model as well, injury was markedly reduced in C6-deficient animals, and both C3 and MAC deposits were absent. In the case of divalent anti-ACE antibodies, the MAC appears to be required for the development of lung injury and neutrophil infiltrate whereas the development of a neutrophil infiltrate is dependent in some fashion on C6 in this second model *(49)*.

Antibody Blockade of C5a

C5a, well known as a chemotactic factor, has been shown to cause pulmonary accumulation of neutrophils when given intratracheally in experimental animal models *(50–52)*, whereas antibody blockade of C5a protects against endotoxin-induced injury in rats *(53)* and in ARDS in septic primates *(54,55)*. Polyclonal antibody directed toward rat C5a was used in two experimental lung inflammatory reactions in rats: CVF and immune complex–induced lung injury. In the case of CVF-induced lung injury, anti-C5a blockade by intravenous injection reduced vascular permeability and lung MPO content (as an indirect measure of neutrophil accumulation in tissue) in a dose-dependent manner such that at a maximum dose of 300 μg, anti-C5a vascular permeability was reduced by 95% and lung MPO content by 39%. In this model, intratracheal administration of antibody had little effect on vascular permeability or MPO content. Conversely, in IgG immune complex lung injury, when C5a antibody was added to the antibovine serum albumin preparation instilled intratracheally, vascular permeability was reduced by 59% and MPO values by 57% whereas intravenous infusion had little effect. C5a is apparently required

Table 1
In Vivo Upregulation of Lung Vascular ICAM-1 is Complement-Dependent

| | % Increase in ICAM-1[a] | | | |
Model	C-intact	C-blocked by sCR1	C-depleted by CVF	C-blocked by C5a antibody
Intrapulmonary deposition of IgG[b] immune complexes	39	13	<5	7
Intrapulmonary deposition of TNF-α[b]	39		<5	
Lung injury secondary to thermal injury[c]	50			<5

[a]Relative to complement-intact negative controls and reflected by binding of ^{125}I-anti-ICAM-1.
[b]Data from refs. *30* and *59*.
[c]Data from ref. *60*.

within the vascular compartment in the CVF model of injury but in the airway compartment in the IgG immune complex model of injury *(56)*.

Complement Requirements for In Vivo Upregulation of Lung Vascular ICAM-1

How might the complement system be functioning to bring about the changes that result in neutrophil recruitment and inflammatory damage in acute lung injury? A multistep process enables neutrophil adhesion to vascular endothelium, extravasation, and ultimate recruitment into tissue. Upregulation of adhesion molecules on vascular tissues during inflammation is an initiating event for leukocyte adhesion and subsequent migration from vascular spaces. Increased expression of these molecules is evident in tissues from patients with IPF *(57)*, ARDS *(58)*, and septic shock *(59)*, with increases in soluble adhesion molecules in the sera of these patients with active disease. In patients with defects in integrin subunits (CD18), the profound reduction in the ability to recruit neutrophils indicates the key role of these adhesion molecules *(60)*. Tissue accumulation of inflammatory cells is markedly attenuated in animals genetically deficient in specific adhesion molecules or in enzymes responsible for the generation of specific glycan components of ligands for these molecules *(61)*. The association of these initial events in recruitment of inflammatory cells with complement components was the focus of a series of in vitro studies.

IgG Immune-Complex Lung Injury

In rats treated with sCR1 or depleted of complement by serial intraperitoneal injections of CVF, it has unexpectedly been found that a key lung vascular adhesion molecule, ICAM-1, was not upregulated after intrapulmonary deposition of IgG immune complexes or after intratracheal instillation of TNF-α, both of which ordinarily cause substantial upregulation of lung vascular ICAM-1. ^{125}I-ICAM-1 monoclonal antibody infused intravenously 4 h after lung deposition of immune complexes binds to the lung vasculature to provide a relative measurement of lung vascular ICAM-1. The use of an irrelevant subclass-matched IgG corrects for "fixation" owing to leakage of protein into damaged lung tissue *(33)*. The results of these findings are summarized in Table 1. Intrapulmonary deposition of IgG immune complexes in rats was associated with a 39% increase in lung vascular ICAM-1. In rats treated with sCR1, there was a significant reduction in this upregulation of lung vascular ICAM-1 to 13%. Much more dramatic effects were seen in complement-depleted rats. Upregulation of lung vascular ICAM-1 was totally suppressed, with the ICAM-1 value falling to <5% of the levels found in complement-intact controls. Thus, complement in some manner is required for upregulation of lung vascular ICAM-1. Murine recombinant TNF-α, which is known to induce upregulation of lung vascular ICAM-1, was delivered into the airways of rats, causing a 30% upregulation in lung vascular ICAM-1. In complement-depleted rats, however, this upregulation was reduced to 5% *(33)*. The inflammatory response to intrapulmonary deposition of IgG immune complexes is known to require TNF-α. Current experiments indicate that upregulation of lung vascular ICAM-1 in response to exogenously administered TNF-α is blocked in the absence of available complement.

As noted previously, when complement is depleted by CVF, ICAM-1 is no longer able to be upregulated by TNF-α, suggesting an absolute requirement for some component of the complement cascade in the development of the full neutrophil-endothelial cell adhesive interaction. It seems possible in the case of airway administration that TNF-α causes an oxidative burst in lung macrophages, resulting in generation of H_2O_2. This oxygen species is known to be able to cause oxidative activation of C5, resulting in formation of MAC. It has recently been shown that MAC acting together with TNFa will cause synergistic upregulation of ICAM-1 *(see below)*, which may explain why, in the absence of complement, TNF-α has greatly reduced ability to induce upregulation of lung vascular ICAM-1.

IgG immune complex–induced lung injury is known to be associated with TNF-α-dependent upregulation of lung vascular ICAM-1 *(62)*. Administration of anti-C5a in this model resulted in an 81% reduction in the binding index of ^{125}I-anti-ICAM-l to lung vasculature, indicating that C5a is necessary for the full upregulation of lung vascular ICAM-1 in this injury (Table 1) *(56)*. Evaluation of TNF-α in BAL fluids in this same model demonstrated that, under conditions of blockade of C5a, TNFa levels were dramatically reduced. It appears then that C5a has an important role in the production of TNFa, possibly in synergism with immune complexes to induce TNF-α generation in lung macrophages. Reduction in upregulation of lung vascular ICAM- 1 by blockade of C5a is likely related to this dramatic reduction in TNF-α.

Lung Injury After Thermal Trauma

A similar requirement for C5a in the upregulation of ICAM-1 was noted in a rat model in which systemic activation of complement occurs following dermal burn injury, and appears to play a significant role in secondary microvascular lung injury. Significant protection against development of lung vascular injury as well as dermal vascular injury is afforded by CVF or sCRI treatment *(27)* (Table 1). Using this same model, blockade of C5a by a polyclonal antibody specific for this complement component resulted in a protective effect such that vascular permeability changes were diminished and MPO content was reduced in lung tissue. Most notably, upregulation of lung vascular ICAM-1 was completely suppressed by pretreatment with the anti-C5a antibody *(63)*. In this model as well, C5a is essential for the development of neutrophil accumulation and vascular permeability increases, and the protective effects of anti-C5a are specifically related to prevention of upregulation of vascular ICAM-1 expression.

In summary, a variety of experimental animal models has demonstrated an important role for complement activation products, especially C5a and MAC in the development of acute lung injury. These factors appear to exert their influence, at least in part, on the accumulation of neutrophils at the site of injury by affecting the expression of vascular endothelial cell adhesion molecules.

Ability of Complement Membrane Attack Complex to Cause Upregulation of Endothelial ICAM-1, VCAM-1, and E-Selectin

Insight into the complex interrelationships among complement, proinflammatory cytokines, and adhesion molecules in acute lung injury can be gained from in vitro studies in which the effects of C5a and the more distal terminal complement components (MAC or C5b-9) on endothelial cells are evaluated. Early in vitro studies have established a role for complement derived products, especially C3b, iC3b, and C5a, in influencing increased neutrophil adhesiveness *(64)*, and this work has been expanded to specifically delineate the role of C5a in activation of endothelial cells.

Increased serum levels of sC5b-9 are correlated with vascular disease; patients with Henoch-Schonlein purpura demonstrate significantly increased serunn levels of sC5b-9 *(65,66)* with no significant change in C3, C4, and CH50 levels as compared to healthy controls. Skin biopsies have revealed leukocytoclastic vasculitis with deposition of the MAC on the vessel walls *(67)*, and ultrastructural examination demonstrated MAC deposits on swollen vascular endothelial cells *(68)*. These findings prompted an examination of the effects of complement on cultured human umbilical vein endothelial cells (HUVEC). Deposition of MAC on cultured endothelial cells at sufficient density resulted in detachment of endothelial cells from underlying substrate and loss of membrane integrity *(69,70)*, correlating with the cytotoxic function of this complement component. There is substantial evidence that in addition to the lytic function of MAC, this complex can alter cell function without causing cell death, a function highly relevant to inflammatory-mediated endothelial cell activation. In vitro studies demonstrated that although MAC at high concentrations (39 µg/mL) was clearly injurious to vascular endothelial cells, deposition of sublytic concentrations (<5 µg/mL) on endothelial cells had a variety of noncytotoxic effects: sublytic MAC–elicited influx of extracellular calcium, plasma membrane vesiculation, secretion of von Willebrand factor *(71)*, release of proslacyclin PGI_2 *(72)*, basic fibroblast growth factor, platelet-derived growth factor *(73)*, and enhanced fibrinolytic activity by expression of plasminogen binding sites *(74)*.

Adhesion Molecule Upregulation by MAC

To further define the noncytolytic effects of MAC on endothelial cells within the context of the inflammatory process, in vitro experiments have employed HUVEC and the assembly of sublytic concentrations of active MAC or cytolytically inactive forms of MAC (iMAC). The active MAC is generated according to the technique developed by Vogt et al. *(75)*, who utilized purified human complement components C5–C9 to assemble the MAC in the absence of other complement-derived products (i.e., iC3b, C3a, C5a). This method allows study of the direct effects of MAC deposition on endothelial cells separate from the influence of other complement components. C5 is oxidized by chloramine T, which specifically attacks the methionine residues in the C5 protein, creating an intact and stable C5b-like molecule with a functional C6 binding

Table 2
In Vitro Upregulation of ICAM-1 and E-Selectin by MAC[a]

Condition[b]	Neutrophil adherence (%) after 4 h				
	No antibody	Anti-ICAM-1	Anti-E-selectin	Anti-ICAM-1+ anti-E-selectin	Anti-P-selectin
Unstimulated HUVEC	8	9	13	11	10
TNF	18	12	13	11	NA
MAC	10	9	12	9	8
TNF followed by MAC assembly	37	20	16	12	30

[a]Data from ref. *73*.

[b]HUVEC monolayers incubated with 10 ng/mL TNF-α (1 h), MAC assembly (30 min), or 10 ng/mL TNF-α (1 h) followed by MAC assembly (30 min).

site that is capable of forming the nucleus for formation of the C5b-9 complex. Under these conditions, C5 behaves like the C5b generated by C5 convertase but is not cleaved, thereby making it a more stable molecule. Since under these special conditions C5a is not generated, the effects of MAC on endothelial cells can be isolated from any effects of C5a. Subsequently, MAC assembly is completed by addition of C7, C8, and C9. This complex, at sufficient density, like its physiological counterpart C5b-9, will cause lysis of nucleated and nonnucleated cells.

Adhesion of peripheral human blood neutrophils to HUVEC was used as a sensitive indicator of adhesion molecule upregulation *(76)*. It is well known that activation of HUVEC by TNF-α results in an increase in neutrophil adhesion that is owing to upregulation of several adhesion molecules, especially ICAM-1 and E-selectin. Assembly of sublytic concentrations of MAC on HUVEC in the absence of other complement-derived components enhanced the TNF-α-induced increase in adherence-promoting factors for neutrophils. Assembly of MAC on quiescent HUVEC resulted in a slight but insignificant increase in adherence (11%), whereas activation of HUVEC for 4 h with a very low concentration of TNF-α alone (1 h) resulted in nearly a twofold increase (18%) in the adherence value (Table 2). The important influence of MAC became apparent when HUVEC were pretreated with TNF-α (1 h) followed by MAC assembly, and the neutrophil adherence increased nearly fourfold over a 4 h time period, dependent on the concentration of both TNF-α and the C5b-like-molecule used to initiate MAC assembly. In the case of exposure of endothelial cells to TNF-α and MAC assembled in the absence of C8 (resulting in an inactive complex), neutrophil adherence values were the same as with TNF-α stimulation alone. These data indicate that treatment of HUVEC with a combination of MAC and TNF-α results in a synergistic upregulation of adhesion-promoting molecules on HUVEC. Of critical necessity is defining the nature of the endothelial adhesion-promoting molecules under these experimental conditions.

TNF-α-induced neutrophil adhesion to endothelial cells is well known to involve endothelial expression of E-selectin and ICAM-1. Monoclonal antibodies to E-selectin and ICAM-1, shown to specifically block neutrophil adherence to endothelial cells stimulated with TNF-α, were used to evaluate the nature of the adhesion molecules involved in MAC-induced adherence *(76)*. Neutrophil adhesion values for non-stimulated HUVEC and HUVEC stimulated with TNF-α followed by MAC assembly were 10% and 37%, respectively. HUVEC, stimulated with both TNF-α and MAC, when subsequently incubated with anti-E-selectin, anti-ICAM-1 or a combination, demonstrated attenuation of neutrophil adhesion values to 16, 20, and 12%, respectively, the last being a nearly complete abolition of the response. By contrast, when anti-P-selectin was employed in this 4-h assay, the adhesion value was 30%, which was not statistically different from the positive control values. Thus, the synergistic increase in neutrophil adherence after dual treatment of HUVEC with TNF-α followed by assembly of MAC is attributable to E-selectin and ICAM-1.

This adhesion molecule response was quantified in a cell-based ELISA in which HUVEC monolayers were stimulated with TNF-α (for 1 h) followed by MAC assembly for 30 min and then incubated in serum-free media for the remainder of the 4 h. Under these conditions, treatment of HUVEC with a constant amount of MAC and increasing amounts of TNF-α revealed that, at the concentration of 3 ng/mL TNF-α, there was a 73% increase in endothelial expression of E-selectin when compared to the effects of TNF-α alone or MAC alone. A similar dose response for upregulation of ICAM-1 indicated that the optimal concentration of TNF-α was 10 ng/mL, which, under the experimental conditions employed, caused a synergistic increase in expression of ICAM-1 by 51%, as compared to TNF-α alone or MAC alone. These data, summrarized in Table 2, demonstrate unequivocally that MAC and TNF-α can interact with endothelial cells to cause enhanced expression of both ICAM-1 and E-selectin, resulting in augmented adhesion of neutrophils to HUVEC. It is possible that, at least in part, these data may explain the in vivo observations described above in which intrapulmonary deposition of TNF-α or IgG immune complexes fail to cause or causes greatly reduced upregulation of ICAM-1 in the absence of available complement *(33)*. Although some studies have suggested that immune complexes may be working through early complement factors, such as C1q, which interacts with endothelial cells *(77)*, the data above suggest that a synergistic relationship exists between TNF-α and distal complement activation products, resulting in upregulation of ICAM-1 and E-selectin.

Adhesion Molecule Upregulation by Inactive MAC (iMAC)

Although the inactive form of MAC has been considered an irrelevant by-product of the complement activation cascade, it may also have an important role in the inflammatory response via its interaction with vascular endothelial cells, as demonstrated by recent in vitro studies. The terminal complex was formed by the assembly of C5b6 and C7–C9. The C7 site required for membrane binding (and subsequent pore-forming activity) rapidly decays so that incubation for 30 min at 37°C followed by 2 h at 25°C ensures loss of cytolytic activity of the complex, resulting in the formation of the inactive MAC (iMAC) *(78,79)*. Assembly of 5–10 μg/mL of iMAC on the endothelial cell surface induced expression of VCAM-1, ICAM-1, and E-selectin. This expression was maximal at 6 h after addition of the complex and persisted up to 12 h in the case of E-selectin, and 24 h in the case of ICAM-1 and VCAM-1. Evaluation by semiquantitative reverse transcriptase PCR (RT-PCR) of RNA for E-selectin and VCAM-1 indicated a clear increase in message for these molecules. These responses were significantly inhibited by addition of antibody directed toward C9, whereas addition of C9 alone (in the absence of the other complement components required for MAC assembly) failed to induce expression of the adhesion molecules *(79)*. In contrast to studies using active MAC, these data demonstrate that binding of the inactive complex to endothelial cells alone can stimulate expression of adhesion molecules, whereas active

Table 3
In Vitro Upregulation of P-Selectin by MAC[a]

	Neutrophil adherence (%) after 30 min		
Condition	No antibody	Anti-ICAM-1[b]	Anti-P-selectin[b]
Unstimulated HUVEC	8	9	8
MAC (30 min)	22	21	10

[a]Kilgore, K.S. University of Michigan, unpublished data.
[b]1 μg/mL antibody added during the last 5 min of incubation with MAC components.

MAC can subserve this function only in a synergistic manner with other pro-inflammatory molecules. Whether such reaction can occur in vivo remains to be determined.

Ability of the MAC and C5a to Cause In Vitro Upregulation of Endothelial P-Selectin

P-selectin is a glycoprotein sequestered in Weibel-Palade granules of endothelial cells, which can be translocated to the endothelial cell surface by a variety of agonists, including histamine and thrombin, resulting in surface expression of this adhesion molecule. Neutrophils contain ligands for P-selectin, including P-selectin glycoprotein ligand-1 and E-selectin ligand-1, the former showing dual binding activity for P- and E-selectin. In addition, it is possible that neutrophil L-selectin contains adequate amounts of the sialylated and fucosylated oligosaccharide sialyl Lewis[x] to facilitate binding with P-selectin, although such a role for L-selectin is debatable *(61)*. Accordingly, upregulation of endothelial P-selectin mediates the early binding of neutrophils to vascular endothelium. There appear to be at least two complement activation products, C5a and C5b-9, that can cause an increase in the adhesive interactions between endothelial cells and neutrophils via P-selectin. These experiments are technically difficult, since constitutive ICAM-1 on endothelial cells could facilitate binding of neutrophils and obscure interpretation of any data. Since both C5a and C5b-9 are known to be potent agonists for neutrophils leading to upregulation of a major ligand for ICAM-1 (namely CDIIb/CD18 on neutrophils), it is important in experiments of this type to determine if complement activation products might be achieving their effects via activation of neutrophils. Nevertheless, accumulating data indicate a clear role for these complement products in regulation of P-selectin expression on endothelial cells.

Upregulation of Endothelial P-Selectin by MAC

Earlier studies have suggested an upregulation of P-selectin on HUVEC in the presence of fresh human serum under conditions in which a rabbit antibody to an unidentified epitope on HUVEC was reactive *(80)*. The response appeared to require deposition of C5b-9 and led to increased P-selectin expression, as determined by binding of ^{125}I-anti-P-selectin to HUVEC. In studies using assembly of active MAC (as described above) on HUVEC, the ability of this complex to cause upregulation of P-selectin on HUVEC has been documented (Table 3). Assembly of the MAC (in the absence of TNF-α) on HUVEC resulted in a rapid (<30 min) increase in P-selectin expression. Parallel studies of neutrophil adhesion to MAC-stimulated HUVEC demonstrated a

Table 4
In Vitro Upregulation of P-Selectin by C5a[a]

Condition	Neutrophil adherence (%)			
	No antibody	Anti-P-selectin	Anti-E-selectin	Anti-ICAM-1
Unstimulated HUVEC	1.5			
C5a (10 min)[b]	10	4	11	11
TNF-α (2 h)[c]	70	72	60	55

[a]Data from ref. 42.

[b]Cells stimulated with 250 nM CSa for 10 min followed by washing and fixation. Neutrophils suspended in media containing blocking antibodies and adhesion measured 30 min later.

[c]Cells stimulated with 25 ng/mL TNF-α for 2 h followed by washing. Neutrophils suspended in media containing blocking antibodies and adhesion measured 30 min later.

concentration and time-dependent increase in neutrophil adhesion. At optimal concentrations of MAC, neutrophil adhesion was increased threefold as compared to adhesion to unstimulated HUVEC (Table 3, 22 vs 8%, respectively). Maximal adhesion was evident at 15–30 min, a time frame consistent with P-selectin upregulation shown previously in response to thrombin and histamine (81). Blocking antibodies to P-selectin and ICAM-1 were utilized to assess the relative contributions of each of these molecules to the early adhesive response. Anti-ICAM-1 failed to alter the degree of neutrophil adhesion, whereas anti-P-selectin reduced neutrophil adhesion from 22 to 10%, a level not significantly different from controls (8%). ICAM-1 appears to play a negligible role in the early adhesion events, whereas the rapid induction of neutrophil adherence in response to MAC deposition is clearly P-selectin dependent. By contrast, as evident in Table 2, in HUVEC stimulated with TNF-α followed by MAC assembly as in the 4-h protocol described above, P-selectin was clearly not involved as an adherence-promoting factor (Table 2).

Upregulation of Endothelial P-Selectin by C5a

C5a generated during activation of the complement cascade is a well recognized, potent neutrophil chemotactic agent (82), which also activates endothelial cells to produce superoxide (83) and to convert endothelial cell xanthine dehydrogenase to xanthine oxidase (84). There is now unequivocal evidence that C5a can also cause upregulation of endothelial cell adhesion molecules as well, specifically P-selectin (Table 4) (85). When assessed by cell-based ELISA, human recombinant C5a, at concentrations from 50 to 500 nM, promoted a dose-dependent upregulation of P-selectin on HUVEC, which paralleled increased neutrophil adhesion and occurred with a time course similar to that seen with thrombin and histamine. The biologically inactive form, C5a des arg, was lacking in this effect.

When C5a-treated monolayers of HUVEC were similarly evaluated for increased expression of E-selectin, no such upregulation was found. In companion experiments, C5a stimulation of HUVEC elicited a fourfold increase in neutrophil adherence (10 vs 1.5% negative control), which was sensitive to anti-P-selectin antibody (a value of 4.0%), and, again, C5a des erg was inactive. The kinetics of C5a-induced expression of P-selectin was similar to the effects of histamine and thrombin: the peak occurred approx 10 min after exposure to C5a and declined gradually over the next 20 min. Under the same conditions, neutrophil adhesion peaked 15 min after addition of C5a and fell gradually thereafter. Although C5a was shown to promote P-selectin expression on HUVEC as well as increased adhesiveness of neutrophils, it also induced one other important endothelial cell response, secretion of von Willebrand factor *(85)*. Thus, in these respects, C5a functions on endothelial cells in a manner similar to thrombin and histamine. In contrast, C3a had a negligible effect on P-selectin, E-selectin, and ICAM-1, as well as on neutrophil adherence to HUVEC *(86)*.

One key aspect of these studies was to determine if any of the increased neutrophil adhesiveness to HUVEC treated with C5a could possibly be attributed to binding of C5a to the endothelial glycocalyx, rather than directly to receptors on the endothelial surface. If this were the case, adherent neutrophils could undergo upregulation of CDIIb/CD18 by contact with endothelial CSa, resulting in adhesion that would be promoted by constitutive endothelial ICAM-1. To assess this possibility, blocking antibodies to P- and E-selectin as well as to ICAM-1 and CD18 were employed. The presence of blocking antibodies to E-selectin, ICAM-1, and CD18 failed to cause any reduction in the number of adhering neutrophils, suggesting that P-selectin is the major mediator responsible for the adhesion of neutrophils to endothelial cells pretreated with C5a.

Complement Requirements for In Vivo Upregulation of Lung Vascular P-Selectin

Companion in vivo studies evaluated the role of vascular P-selectin in CVF-induced lung injury. In this rat injury model, P-selectin antibodies were protective against acute lung injury owing to CVF-induced complement activation, so that neutrophil sequestration and edema formation were inhibited by anti-P-selectin. These findings correlated with reduced MPO content, hemorrhage, and permeability (by 50, 96, and 79%, respectively, when compared to injury in the absence of blocking antibodies) *(87)*. The early appearance of reactivity of endothelial cells with the antibody, beginning 5 min after CVF infusion and persisting for less than 60 min, was consistent with in vitro studies demonstrating early expression of P-selectin on endothelial cells in response to C5a *(85)*. In mice, however, the role of P-selectin in this model of injury has been less clearly defined. In wild-type mice, CVF-induced injury was similar to that demonstrated in rats with the exception of the localization of P-selectin expression: in rats, P-selectin was localized to capillary endothelial cells *(87)* whereas in mice, this adhesion molecule was expressed on noncapillary arterial and venous vessels *(88)*. P-selectin–directed antibodies had similar effects in the two animal models, preventing sequestration of neutrophils and subsequent injury. When CVF injury was induced in P-selectin–deficient mice and compared to injury in wild-type mice, however, no reduction in neutrophil sequestration or lung injury was noted. In these animal models of complement-induced injury, then, the precise role of P-selectin has been unclear, and may be owing to some manner of "adaptation" in the P-selectin–deficient mice.

The in vitro studies described above have defined a role for C5a in the expression of endothelial cell P-selectin. The availability of polyclonal antibody directed toward rat C5a, which blocks this component without affecting C5, has provided a tool to examine the role of C5a in vivo. In CVF-induced, complement-mediated injury in rats, a 70-fold increase in serum C5a levels (as measured by ELISA) occurred within the first 2 min of CVF injection. This same injury was associated with an increase in lung vascular P-selectin as determined quantitatively by measurement of ^{125}I-labeled antibody to P-selectin. Maximal expression of P-selectin (greater than a fivefold increase) occurred

20 min after CVF injection and was unaffected by platelet depletion, indicating that the P-selectin expression occurred on vascular endothelium and not on adherent platelets. When antibody directed toward rat C5a was infused prior to CVF injection, P-selectin expression was reduced 91%. In animals complement depleted by serial CVF injections, P-selectin expression was suppressed by 97% *(89)*. The in vitro studies correlate well with the in vivo data, demonstrating that complement and, specifically, C5a and MAC are necessary for the upregulation of P-selectin in complement-mediated injury.

Ability of Complement Proteins to Induce Endothelial Cell–Derived Chemokines

Soluble inflammatory mediators as well as cell surface molecules can influence events in inflammation. In HUVEC, direct or indirect stimulation by C5a prompts release of a number of molecules active in inflammation, including prostacyclin *(90)*, heparin sulfate *(91)*, and tissue factor *(92)*. MAC deposition on cultured endothelial cells can modulate cell function by inducing release of soluble proinflammatory mediators such as prostacyclin, TNF-α, IL-1, basic fibroblast growth factor, and platelet-derived growth factor *(42,44,72,73,93,94)*. The studies described above demonstrate that C5a and the complement-derived MAC have the capability to activate endothelial cells, inducing a change in their phenotype, with upregulation of adhesion molecules. It is of great interest, then, to determine if these events might also influence recruitment of inflammatory cells indirectly via secretion of soluble factors from endothelial cells.

Assembly of MAC on HUVEC according to the protocol described above resulted in chemotactic activity for neutrophils and monocytes. Neutrophils migrated toward conditioned media from HUVEC placed in a microchemotaxis chamber *(95)*. Media from HUVEC after very short (<5 min) exposure to MAC elicited negligible chemotactic activity, whereas exposure for 2 h resulted in the appearance of neutrophil chemotactic activity, which reached a plateau at 8 h after exposure to sublytic concentrations of MAC. This activity was equivalent to 90% of the chemotactic activity seen in response to 1 μM formyl-met-leu-Phe, which was designated a maximal response. The appearance of monocyte chemotactic activity, on the other hand, was significantly delayed, not occurring until 8 h after MAC assembly on HUVEC, with the maximal response (75% of the maximal chemotactic activity in response to formyl-met-leu-Phe) to media from HUVEC 24 h after exposure to MAC. By comparison, when inactive MAC (devoid of C8) was used to stimulate HUVEC, minimal chemotactic activity was noted.

Employing a strategy for further defining MAC-induced chemokine release, IL-8 and MCP-1 antibody neutralization studies were performed under the assay conditions described above. IL-8, a member of the alpha or CXC subfamily of chemokines, is a powerful neutrophil chemotactic factor. Monocyte chemoattractant protein (MCP-1) is a member of the beta or CC chemokine subfamily, which possesses chemotactic activity for monocytes *(96)*. Both are soluble proinflammatory chemokines known to be secreted by cytokine-activated endothelial cells. Addlition of human IL-8 antibodies to MAC-stimulated HUVEC media decreased neutrophil chemotactic activity by 73%, suggesting IL-8 to be a major contributor to this response. ELISA determination of cytokine secretion from HUVEC indicated that IL-8 release began by 4 h and continued until 24 h following MAC assembly, with a maximal IL-8 concentration of 27 ng/mL. In the case of monocyte chemotaxis, antibodies to MCP-1 significantly decreased chemotaxis (75%) whereas MCP-1 secretion paralleled the pattern of chemotactic activity. Secretion of this chemokine commenced at 8 h, with maximal activity at 24 h following MAC assembly, and reached a maximal MCP-1 concentration of 35 ng/mL, indicating that MCP-1 secretion by HUVEC was responsible for the majority of monocyte chemotaxis. Northern hybridization analysis confirmed that assembly of MAC on HUVEC induced a marked increase in mRNAs for IL-8 and MCP-1 as compared to either unstimulated cells or cells treated with inactive MAC (devoid of C7 or C8) *(95)*. Sequential release of IL-8 and MCP-1 from endothelial cells under the influence of MAC provides an additional mechanism for endothelial cell involvement in the recruitment of specific inflammatory cells. A close relationship is established between complement activation and adhesion molecule expression, and these studies suggest an equally close relationship between complement and cytokine release. MAC, via mediation of IL-8 and MCP-1 release, could augment the chemotactic response to C5a. These data correlate with previous in vivo findings that infusion of antibody to recombinant human IL-8 had significant protective effects in IgG immune complex-induced lung injury in rats and suggest a role for complement activation products in release of IL-8 or its homologs *(97)*.

Signal Transduction Events in Endothelial Cells Stimulated by Complement Activation Products

C5a-Mediated Signal Transduction

Cellular mechanisms by which complement activation products influence endothelial cells to secret chemotactic factors or upregulate expression of adhesion molecules during the inflammatory response remain to be clarified, but initial studies provide some insights. Binding of ^{125}I-C5a to untreated HUVEC has suggested a specific binding pattern consistent with the presence of a C5a receptor *(85)*. The number of binding sites, however, was small, with approx 1000 molecules of C5a bound per cell (approx 1/50 of the number bound to neutrophils). Treatment with TNF-α, bacterial lipopolysaccharide or interferon-γ failed to increase the binding of C5a to HUVEC. RT-PCR-techniques using primers directed against the full open reading frame of mRNA for the C5a receptor on a human neutrophil-like cell line (HL-60) resulted in a product of approx 1000 bp, which is very similar to the cDNA for the neutrophil C5a receptor *(85)*. These data suggest that HUVEC have receptors for C5a, although it remains to be seen whether the mRNA for these receptors can be upregulated or whether, as has been suggested in HL-60 cells, Cos-7 cells, and rat insulinoma cells, regulation of C5a receptors occurs by posttranscriptional mechanisms such as phosphorylation. Supporting data is derived from immunohistochemical studies performed on human brain tissue with six different monoclonal or polyclonal antibodies to the C5a receptor. Although this receptor is minimally expressed on vascular endothelial cells from normal brains, C5a receptor expression was upregulated in a variety of inflammatory disorders *(98)*. In human lung tissue as well, immunostaining has demonstrated C5a receptor expression on endothelial cells *(99)*. This receptor upregulation may provide an additional mechanism for amplification of the inflammatory response.

Signal transduction events in response to C5a were further evaluated in rat pulmonary artery endothelial cells (RPAEC) *(83)*. These cells responded to C5a with formation of D-myo-inositol 1,4,5-trisphosphate [Ins(1,4,5)P$_3$] occurring with a peak activity at 30 s of C5a stimulation in a concentration-dependent manner. The Ins(1,4,5)P$_3$ response was evident at C5a concentrations of 10–200 n*M*, with a 2.7-fold increase over baseline values at 200 nM C5a (72 vs 27 pmol in unstimulated cells). Similarly, C5a at these same concentrations promoted increases in intracellular calcium, assessed with the fluorescent calcium indicator fura-2/AM, with a peak in the first minute after cell stimulation. The fact that C5a induced Ins(1,4,5)P$_3$ formation as well as increases in intracellular calcium suggested that protein kinase C might be involved in this response. Protein kinase C phosphorylation of target proteins is known to be a key event in the mediation of cellular responses. Phosphorylation of protein kinase C specific substrate by cytosolic and particulate fractions of cells was evaluated after stimulation with C5a and compared to bradykinin and the specific protein kinase C agonist phorbol ester (PMA) (Murphy, H. S., unpublished data). In each case, the increment of PKC activity was rapid, occurring by 2 min, and dependent on the concentration of agonist used. Unlike the response to phorbol ester in which reciprocal increase in PKC activity in membrane fraction (165 pmol/5 $\times$ 10^6 cell equivalents) occurred with a decrease in cytosolic fraction (12 pmol/5 $\times$ 10^6 cell equivalents), suggesting translocation, C5a (as well as the inflammatory mediator bradykinin) induced increased activity in both particulate (98 pmol/5 $\times$ 10^6 cell equivalents) and cytosolic fractions (85 pmol/5 $\times$ 10^6 cell equivalents) as compared to unstimulated cells (49 pmol/5 $\times$ 10^6 cell equivalents, particulate; 2 pmol/5 $\times$ 10^6 cell equivalents, cytosolic). Although translocation may have taken place, the coincident increase in total cellular PKC makes translocation difficult to assess. These data, nevertheless, suggest a role for PKC in the signal transduction events in response to C5a.

RPAEC responded to C5a as well as to TNF-α with generation of superoxide (O$_2^{\bullet}$) resulting, at least in part, from the conversion of xanthine dehydrogenase to xanthine oxidase *(84)* and possibly in part from activity of an NADPH oxidase *(100–102)*. This response was used as an end point to determine if, via the effects of various signal transduction inhibitors, additional signal transduction events might be involved in the C5a response *(83)*. Inhibition studies demonstrated that the O$_2^{\bullet}$ response, as well as the increase in Ins(1,4,5)P$_3$, intracellular calcium, and PKC activity, were pertussis toxin (PT)-sensitive (reductions of 90% O$_2^{\bullet}$, 98% Ins(1,4,5)P$_3$, 82% intracellular calcium, 67% PKC activity, respectively), suggesting that C5a binding activates a phospholipase C that is regulated by a PT-sensitive guanine nucleotide binding protein (PT-sensitive G-protein).

MAC-Mediated Signal Transduction

Previous similar studies of a variety of cell types have indicated that MAC, at sublytic concentrations, assembles on the cell surface and initiates a similar signal transduction sequence. Glomerular mesangial cells responded to incubation in the presence of MAC with generation of O$_2^{\bullet}$ and H$_2$O$_2$ *(103)*. In these cells, oxygen radicals served as second messengers for expression of monocyte-directed cytokines—in this case MCP-1 and CSF-1 *(104)*. Membrane assembly of C5b-9 on human platelets as well as on Ehrlich cells initiated activation of protein kinase C and myosin light chain kinase, which in turn was accompanied by formation of inositol phosphates and was dependent on extracellular Ca^{2+} *(105)*. MAC interacted with a PT-sensitive G-protein to stimulate nucleated cells *(106)*, and in these cells as well as in platelets, C5b-8 and C5b-9 stimulated protein kinase C activity that was at least partially mediated by calcium signals and dependent on calcium influx *(80,105,107)*. It is likely that examination of signal transduction events in MAC-stimulated endothelial cells will yield similar results.

Some insights into the molecular mechanisms by which MAC contributes to cytokine secretion come from experiments on redox control of IL-8 and MCP-1 release *(108)*.

The multiprotein complex, nuclear factor κB (NF-κB), after translocation from cytoplasm to nucleus, mediates cytoplasmic signal transduction events that result in gene transcription. Activation of NF-κB requires release of the inhibitory subunit IκB from the heterodimeric DNA binding subunits, p50 and p65 *(109)*. This redoxsensitive reaction is known to be triggered by diverse cytoplasmic signaling events which may all act through a common pathway involving the synthesis of reactive oxygen species *(110)*. As noted above, MAC can elicit production of reactive oxygen intermediates which can influence intracellular redox status and which in turn can affect nuclear factor κB activation. Transcription of messages for ICAM-1, E-selectin and VCAM-1 in endothelial cells are linked to a requirement for NF-κB activation *(111–113)*.

MAC assembly on HUVEC appears to influence the endothelial expression of IL-8 and MCP-1 via the transcriptional regulatory protein NF-κB *(108)*. These studies utilized two NF-κB blocking agents: first, the intracellular antioxidant pyrrolidine dithiocarbamate (PDTC), which reversibly suppresses release of the inhibitory subunit IκB from the cytoplasmic form of NF-κB, potently blocking NF-KB mobilization and subsequent nuclear transcriptional activity *(114)*; and second, SN50, a peptide that specifically inhibits NF-κB entry into nuclei *(115)*. The data in Fig. 2 illustrate that under the same assay conditions described above, pretreatment of HUVEC with PDTC or SN50 effectively reduced subsequent release of MCP-1 (82% with 10 μmol/L PDTC and 95% with 50 μg/mL SN50) and IL-8 (81% with 10 μmol/L PDTC and 86% with 50 μg/mL SN50) from MAC stimulated cells, suggesting a cellular control mechanism by which MAC promotes secretion of these proinflammatory factors. Electrophoretic mobility shift assay analysis of nuclear extracts from HUVEC exposed to sublytic concentrations of MAC or to inactive MAC (devoid of C9) demonstrated NF-κB translocation within 1 h of MAC assembly. By contrast, HUVEC exposed to MAC devoid of C7 demonstrated a markedly reduced band shift. Thus, intact MAC or C5b-8 complex appears to be required for maximal nuclear translocation of NF-κB. In parallel studies, translocation of the p65 component of NF-κB from cytosol to nuclear fractions of HUVEC exposed to intact MAC (but not MAC devoid of C7) was determined by Western blot analysis. Consistent with these data, immunocytochemical analysis detected p65 in cytoplasm of unstimulated cells with little staining in nuclei whereas assembly of intact MAC (but not in the case of MAC devoid of C7) induced marked increase in nuclear staining and a corresponding decrease in cytoplasmic staining *(108)*. NF-κB translocation in endothelial cells exposed to MAC assembly is a mechanism by which these cells are activated to release soluble mediators that can participate in the induction and maintenance of the inflammatory response as described above. Although these studies suggest that release of cytokines is regulated by these intracellular signal transduction events, the mechanism by which MAC assembly on endothelial cells promotes E-selectin, P-selectin, and ICAM-1 upregulation remains to be determined.

Complement Activation of Endothelial Cells During Xenograft Rejection

Shortage of human donor organs has prompted an intensive effort to develop alternative strategies for organ transplantation, including the use of cross-species organs (xenografts). Multiple antigenic differences exist between donor and recipient in xenotransplantation, and "hyperacute" rejection is an immediate and primary obstacle

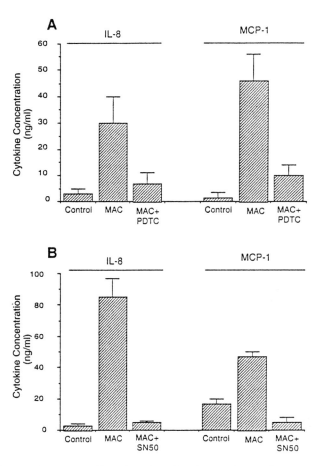

Fig. 2. Inhibition of MAC-mediated IL-8 and MCP-1 release from HUVEC. (A) PDTC (10 µmol/L) for 2 h followed by exposure to MAC for 30 min and media collected at 24 h. (B) Preincubation in media in the presence and absence of SN50 (50 µg/mL) for 15 min followed by exposure to MAC for 30 min and media collected at 24 h. (Data reproduced with permission from ref. *108*.)

to transplantation. Complement as well as naturally occurring xenoreactive antibodies, especially those directed toward alpha 1,3-galactose epitopes (α1,3GT), are two major inciting factors demonstrated to be involved in the development of hyperacute rejection. α1,3GT moieties on N- and O-linked oligosaccharides and glycolipids on the surface of endothelial cells of animal tissues are reactive with a naturally occurring IgM antibody in human serum. Binding of antibodies to these cell surface antigens results in rapid fixation of complement. In vitro comparison of complement-mediated cytotoxicity of murine aortic endothelial cells from α1,3GT-deficient mice and wild-type mice revealed that this epitope, in conjunction with complement, was responsible for cell lysis. Moreover, sera from α1,3GT-deficient mice were able to mediate complement-dependent lysis of wild-type but not null endothelial cells *(116)*. A similar immediate reaction occurs in vascularized xenografts, within minutes to hours *(117–121)*. Delayed xenograft rejection as well appears to involve a vascular component and possibly similar mechanisms of endothelial cell activation, although the role of complement in this reaction remains to be determined *(117)*.

A complete discussion of the role of complement-mediated endothelial cell activation in graft rejection is beyond the scope of this chapter. Several recent reviews have discussed this aspect of xenotransplantation in depth *(117,120,122–124)*. It is likely that many aspects of endothelial cell activation within the context of xeno-transplantation will be determined to be similar to those described above for endothelial cell activation by complement factors in the context of inflammation. For example, deposition of C3 and C5 is associated with P-selectin expression on graft endothelial cells *(125)*; in complement-depleted rats (by CVF), complement deposition in guinea pig xenograft as well as hyperacute rejection was prevented *(126)*; in sCR1-treated rats, significant complement inhibition was associated with reduced inflammatory infiltrate and delayed graft rejection *(127)*; and blockade of complement factors with antibodies directed toward C5 or C8 components attenuated xenograft organ damage *(128)*. Complement regulatory proteins that have been shown to protect endothelial cells from complement- mediated lysis in hyperacute rejection include MCP, DAF, CD59, C1 esterase inhibitor, and sCR1 *(129–133)*. Complement, in the presence of xenoreactive antibodies, appears to contribute to the development of the hyperacute response in transplantation by activation of vascular endothelial cells and leukocytes, leading to serious vascular injury.

Conclusion

Experimental data from in vivo and in vitro studies suggest a mechanism whereby complement activation products interact with endothelial cells within the context of the acute inflammatory process. IgG immune complex-mediated acute injury is dependent on the complex interrelationship among complement activation products, cytokines, and adhesion molecules. MAC, working synergistically with TNF-α, or independently in its iMAC form, facilitates upregulation of ICAM-1 and E-selectin. MAC itself also mediates expression of P-selectin and, indirectly, via transcriptional regulation of NF-κB, release of chemotactic factors IL-8 and MCP-1. C5a, a well-known chemotactic factor itself, also mediates upregulation of P-selectin.

These findings have extended our understanding of the sequence of biological events leading to acute inflammatory injury. Intravascular activation of complement rapidly initiates a series of events that include neutrophil activation, oxidant production, upregulation of adhesion molecules with increased adhesiveness of neutrophils to vascular endothelium, and endothelial cell injury, all of which provide immediate and early augmentation of the inflammatory response. The data here suggest that delayed events in inflammation involving release of cytokines and later recruitment of monocytes are transcriptionally regulated and are also mediated by complement products. Defining these events in the inflammatory process within the context of activation of the complement cascade and interaction of the complement components with vascular endothelial cells will provide novel targets for the development of therapeutic interventions.

References

1. Belmont, H. M., Hopkins, P., Edelson, H. S., Kaplan, H. B., Ludewig, R., Weissman, G., and Abramson, S. (1986) Complement activation during systemic lupus erythematosis: C3a and C5a anaphylatoxins circulate during exacerbations of disease. *Arthritis Rheum.* **29,** 1085–1089.

2. Buyon, J., Tamerius, J., Belmont, H. M., and Abramson, S. (1992) Assessment of disease activity and impending flare in patients with systemic lupus erythematosis: Comparison of the use of complement split products and conventional measurements of complement. *Arthritis Rheum.* **35**, 1028–1037.

3. Groneck, P., Oppermann, M., and Speer, C. P. (1993) Levels of complement anaphylatoxin C5a in pulmonary effluent fluid of infants at risk for chronic lung disease and effects of dexamethasone treatment. *Pediatr. Res.* **34**, 586–590.

4. Solomkin, J. S., Cotta, L. A., Satoh, P. S., Hurst, J. M., and Nelson, R. D. (1985) Complement activation and clearance in acute illness and injury: Evidence for C5a as a cell-directed mediator of the adult respiratory distress syndrome in man. *Surgery* **97**, 668–678.

5. Hammerschmidt, D. E., Weaver, L. J., Hudson, L. D., Craddock, P. R., and Jacob, H. S. (1980) Association of complement activation and elevated plasma-C5a with adult respiratory distress syndrome. Pathophysiological relevance and possible prognostic value. *Lancet* **1**, 947–949.

6. Jones, D. K. (1990) Markers for impending adult respiratory distress syndrome (editorial). *Respir. Med.* **84**, 89–91.

7. Stove, S., Welte, T., Wagner, T. O., Kola, A., Klos, A., Bautsch, W., and Kohl, J. (1996) Circulating complement proteins in patients with sepsis or systemic inflammatory response syndrome. *Clin. Diag. Lab. Immunol.* **3**, 175–183.

8. Kinoshita, M., Uetsuka, N., Wgai, F., Watanabe, H., Uchida, Y., and Kitamura, S. (1986) Measurement of plasma C3a and C5a in patients with various lung diseases and rabbits with endotoxin shock. *Nippon Kyobu Shikkan Gakkai Zasshi* **24**, 145–149.

9. Solomkin, J. S. (1990) Neutrophil disorders in burn injury: complement, cytokines, and organ injury. *J. Trauma* **30**, 580–585.

10. Goya, T., Morisaki, T., and Torisu, M. (1994) Immunologic assessment of host defense impairment in patients with septic multiple organ failure: Relationship between complement activation and changes in neutrophil function. *Surgery* **115**, 145–155.

11. Zilow, G., Joka, T., Obertack, U., Rother, U., and Kirschfink, M. (1992) Generation of anaphylatoxin C3a in plasma and bronchoalveolar lavage fluid in trauma patients at risk of the adult respiratory distress syndrome. *Crit. Care Med.* **20**, 468–473.

12. Michie, H. R. (1996) Metabolism of sepsis and multiple organ failure. *World J. Surg.* **20**, 460–464.

13. Seifert, P. S., Catalfamo, J. L., and Dodds, W. J. (1988) Complement C5a (desArg) generation in serum exposed to damaged aortic endothelium. *Exp. Mol. Pathol.* **48**, 216–225.

14. Charreau, B., Cassard, A., Tesson, L., Mauff, B. L., Navenot, J. M., Blanchard, D., Lublin, D., Soulillou, J. P., and Anegon, I. (1994) Protection of rat endothelial cells from primate complement-mediated lysis by expression of human CD59 and/or decay-accelerating factor. *Transplant* **58**, 1222–1229.

15. Hamilton, K. K. and Sims, P. J. (1991) The terminal complement proteins C5b-9 augment binding of high density lipoprotein and its apolipoproteins A-I and A-II to human endothelial cells. *J. Clin. Invest.* **88**, 1833–1840.

16. Hamilton, K. K., Zhao, J., and Sims, P. J. (1993) Interaction between apolipoproteins A-I and A-II and the membrane attack complex of complement: affinity of the apoproteins for polymeric C9. *J. Biol. Chem.* **268**, 3632–3638.

17. Meri, S., Mattila, P., and Renkonen, R. (1993) Regulation of CD59 expression on the human endothelial cell line EA. hy 926. *Eur. J. Immunol.* **23**, 2511–2516.

18. Nose, M., Katoh, M., Okada, N., Kyogoku, M., and Okada, H. (1990) Tissue distribution of HRF20, a novel factor preventing the membrane attack of homologous complement, and its predominant expression on endothelial cells in vivo. *Immunology* **70**, 145–149.

19. Rautemaa, R. and Meri, S. (1996) Protection of gingival epithelium against complement-mediated damage by strong expression of the membrane attack complex inhibitor protectin (CD59). *J. Dent. Res.* **75**, 568–574.

20. Muller-Eberhard, H. (1988) Molecular organization and function of the complement system. *Ann. Rev. Biochem.* **57**, 321–3n.

21. Hayashi, S., Emi, N., Isobe, K., Yokoyama, I., Okada, H., and Takagi, H. (1996) Inhibitory effect of double transfection to xenoendothelial cells using both decay accelerating factor and homologous restriction factor 20 genes on complement dependent cytolysis. *J. Surg. Res.* **61**, 165–169.

22. Buerke, M., Murohara, T., and Lefer, A. M. (1995) Cardioprotective effects of a C1 esterase inhibitor in myocardial ischemia and reperfusion. *Circulation* **91**, 393–402.

23. Schmaier, A. H., Murray, S. C., Heda, G. D., Farber, A., Kuo, A., McCrae, K., and Cines, D. B. (1989) Synthesis and expression of C1 inhibitor by human umbilical vein endothelial cells. *J. Biol. Chem.* **264,** 18,173–18,179.

24. Kowal-Vern, A., Walenga, J. M., Sharp-Pucci, M., Hoppensteadt, D., and Gamelli, R. L. (1997) Postburn edema and related changes in interleukin-2, leukocytes, platelet activation, endothelin-1, and C1 esterase inhibitor. *J. Burn Care Rehabil.* **18,** 99–103.

25. Goebeler, M., Yoshimura, T., Toksoy, A., Ritter, U., Brocker, E. B., and Gillitzer, R. (1997) The chemokine repertoire of human dermal microvascular endothelial cells and its regulation by inflammatory cytokines. *J. Invest Dermatol.* **108,** 445–451.

26. Friedl, H., Till, G., Trents, O., and Ward, P. (1989) Roles of histamine, complement and xanthine oxidase in thermal injury of skin. *Am. J. Pathol.* **135,** 203.

27. Mulligan, M. S., Yeh, C. G., Rudolph, A. R., and Ward, P. A. (1992) Protective effects of soluble CR1 in complement and neutrophil-mediated tissue injury. *J. Immunol.* **148,** 1479–1485.

28. Till, G. O., Johnson, K. J., Kunkel, R., and Ward, P. A. (1982) Intravascular activation of complement and acute lung injury: dependency on neutrophils and toxic oxygen metabolites. *J. Clin. Invest.* **69,** 1126–1135.

29. Varani, J. and Ward, P. A. (1994) Mechanisms of endothelial cell injury in acute inflammation. *Shock* **2,** 311–319.

30. Ward, P. (1997) Recruitment of inflammatory cells into lung: roles of cytokines, adhesion molecules, and complement. *J. Lab. Clin. Med.* **129,** 400–404.

31. Lukacs, N. W. and Ward, P. A. (1996) Inflammatory mediators, cytokines, and adhesion molecules in pulmonary inflammation and injury. *Adv. Immunol.* **62,** 257–303.

32. Johnson, K. and Ward, P. (1974) Acute immunologic pulmonary alveolitis. *J. Clin. Invest.* **54,** 349–357.

33. Vaporciyan, A. A., Mulligan, M. S., Warren, J. S., Barton, P. A., Miyasaka, M., and Ward, P. O. A. (1995) Upregulation of lung vascular ICAM-1 in rats is complement dependent. *J. Immunol.* **155,** 1442–1429.

34. Fisher, M., Ma, M., Georg, S., Zhou, X., Xia, J., Finco, O., and Han, S. (1996) Regulation of the B cell response to T-dependent antigens by classical pathway complement. *J. Immunol.* **157,** 549–556.

35. Carroll, M. and Fisher, M. B. (1997) Complement and the immune response. *Curr. Opin. Immunol.* **9,** 64–69.

36. Wessels, M., Butko, P., Ma, M., Warren, H., Lage, A., and Carroll, M. (1995) Studies of group C streptococcal infection in mice deficient in complement C3 and C4 demonstrate an essential role for complement in both innate and acquired immunity. *Proc. Natl. Acad. Sci. USA* **92,** 11,490–11,494.

37. Weiser, M., Williams, J., Moore, F., Kobzik, L., Ma, M., Hechtman, H., and Carroll, M. (1996) Reperfusion of ischemic skeletal muscle is mediated by natural antibody and complement. *J. Exp. Med.* **183,** 2343–2348.

38. May, J., Kane, M., and Frank, M. (1972) Host defense against bacerial endotoxemia—contribution of the early and late components of complement to del;oxification. *J. Immunol.* **109,** 893–897.

39. Quezado, Z., Hoffman, W., Winkelstein, J., Yatsiv, I., Koev, C., Elin, L. C. R., Eichacker, P., and Natanson, C. (1994) The third component of complement protects against *Escherichia coli* endotoxin-induced shock and multiple organ failure. *J. Exp. Med.* **179,** 569–579.

40. Fischer, M., Prodeus, A., Nicholson-Weller, A., Ma, M., Murrow, J., Reid, R., Warren, H., Lage, A., Moore, F., Rosen, F. S., and Carroll, M. (1997) Increased susceptibility to endotoxin shock in complement C3- and C4-deficient mice is corrected by C1 inhibitor replacement. *J. Immunol.* **159,** 976–982.

41. Sylvestre, D., Clynes, R., Ma, M., Warren, H., Carroll, M., and Ravetch, J. (1996) Immunoglobulin G-medicated inflammatory responses develop normally in complement-deficient mice. *J. Exp. Med.* **184,** 2385–2392.

42. Larsen, G. L., Mitchell, B. C., and Henson, P. M. (1981) The pulmonary response of C5 sufficient and deficient mice to immune complexes. *Am. Rev. Respir. Dis.* **123,** 4349.

43. Miller, C., Cook, D., and Kotwal, G. (1996) Two chemotactic factors, C5a and MIP 1alpha, dramatically alter mortality from zymosan-induced multiple organ dysfunction syndrome (MODS): C5a contributes to MODS while MIP-1alpha has a protective role. *Mol. Immunol.* **33,** 1135–1137.

44. Sun, X. and Hsueh, W. (1991) Platelet-activating factor produces shock, in vivo complement activation and tissue injury in mice. *J. Immunol.* **147,** 509–514.

45. Hsueh, W., Sun, X., Rioja, N., and Gonzalez Crussi, F. (1990) The role of the complement system in shock and tissue injury induced by tumor necrosis factor and endotoxin. *Immunology* **70,** 309.

46. Caldwell, P., Wigger, H., Fernandez, L., D'Alisa, R., Tse-Eng, D., Butler, V., and Gigli, I. (1981) Lung injury induced by antibody fragments to angiotensin converting enzyme. *Am. J. Pathol.* **105,** 54–63.

47. Barba, L., Caldwell, P., Downie, G., Camussi, G., Brentjens, J., and Andres, G. (1983) Lung injury mediated by antibodies to endothelium. I. In the rabbit a repeated interaction of heterologous anti-angiotensin converting enzyme results in resistance to immune injury through antigenic modulation. *J. Exp. Med.* **158,** 2141–2185.

48. Camussi, G., Caldwell, P., Andres, G., and Brentjens, J. (1987) Lung injury mediated by antibodies to endothelium. II. Study of the effect of repeated antigen–antibody interactions in rabbits tolerant to heterologous antibody. *Am. J. Pathol.* **127,** 216–228.

49. Camussi, G., Biesecker, G., Caldwell, P. R. B., Biancone, L., Andres, G., and Brentjens, J. R. (1993) Role of the membrane attack complex of complement in lung injury mediated by antibodies to endothelium. *Arch. Allergy Immunol.* **102,** 216–223.

50. Desai, U., Kreutzer, D. L., Showell, H., Arroyave, C. V., and Ward, P. A. (1979) Acute inflammatory pulmonary reactions induced by chemotactic factors. *Am. J. Pathol.* **96,** 71–83.

51. Henson, P. M., McCarthy, K., Larsen, G. L., Webster, R. O., Giclas, P. C., Dreisin, R. B., King, T. E., and Shawl, J. O. (1979) Complement fragments, alveolar macrophages, and alveolitis. *Am. J. Pathol.* **97,** 93–110.

52. Larsen, G. L., McCarthy, K., Weber, R. O., Henson, J., and Henson, P. M. (1980) A differential effect of C5a and C5a des Arg in the induction of pulmonary inflammation. *Am. J. Pathol.* **100,** 179–192.

53. Smedegard, G., Cui, L. X., and Hugli, T. E. (1989) Endotoxin-induced shock in the rat. A role for C5a. *Am. J. Pathol.* **135,** 489–497.

54. Stevens, J., O'Hanley, P., Shapiro, J., Mihm, F., Satoh, P., Collins, J., and Raffin, T. (1986) Effects of anti-C5a antibodies on the adult respiratory distress syndrome in septic primates. *J. Clin. Invest.* **77,** 1812–1816.

55. Hangen, D., J. Stevens, Satoh, P., Hall, E., O'Hanley, P., and Raffin, T. (1989) Complement levels in septic primates treated with anti-C5a antibodies. *J. Surg. Res.* **46,** 195–199.

56. Mulligan, M. S., Schmid, E., Beck-Schimmer, B., Till, G. O., Friedl, H. P., Brauer, R. B., Hugli, T. E., Miyasaka, M., Warner, R. L., Johnson, K. J., and Ward, P. A. (1996) Requirment and role of C5a in acute inflammatory injury in rats. *J. Clin. Invest.* **98,** 503–512.

57. Shijubo, N., Imai, K., Aoki, S., Hirasawa, M., Sugawara, H., Koba, H., Tsujisaki, M., Sugiyama, T., Hinoda, Y., and Yachi, A. (1992) Circulating intercellular adhesion molecule-1 (ICAM-1) antigen in sera of patients with idiopathic pulmonary fibrosis. *Clin. Exp. Immunol.* **89,** 58–62.

58. Donnelly, S. C., Haslett, C., Dransfield, I., Robertson, C. E., Carter, D. C., Ross, J. A., Grant, I. S., and Tedder, T. F. (1994) Role of selectins in development of adult respiratory distress syndrome. *Lancet* **344,** 215–219.

59. Newman, W., Beall, L. D., Carson, C. W., Hunder, G. G., Gradben, N., Randhawa, Z. I., Gopal, T. V., Wiener-Kronish, J., and Matthay, M. A. (1993) Soluble E-selectin is found in supernatants of activated endothelial cells and is elevated in the serum of patients with septic shock. *J. Immunol.* **150,** 644–654.

60. Anderson, D. and Springer, T. (1987) Leukocyte adhesion deficiency: An inherited defect in the Mac-1, LFA-1 and pl50,95 glycoproteins. *Annu. Rev. Med.* **38,** 175–194.

61. Lowe, J. B. and Ward, P. (1997) Therapeutic inhibition of carbohydrate-protein interactions in vivo. *J. Clin. Invest.* **99,** 822–826.

62. Mulligan, M. S., Vaporciyan, A. A., Miyasaka, M., Tamatani, T., and Ward, P. A. (1993) Tumor necrosis factor alpha regulated in vivo intrapulmonary expression of ICAM-1. *Am. J. Pathol.* **142,** 1739–1749.

63. Schmid, E., Piccolo, M. S., Fried, H. P., Warner, R. L., Mulligan, M. S., Hugli, T. E., Till, G. O., and Ward, P. A. (1997) Requirement for C5a in lung vascular injury following thermal trauma to rat skin. *Shock* **8,** 119–124.

64. Marks, R. M., Todd, R. F. I., and Ward, P. A. (1989) Rapid induction of neutrophil-endothelial adhesion by endothelial complement fixation. *Nature* **339,** 314–317.

65. Kawana, S. and Nishiyama, S. (1992) Serum SC5b-9 (terminal complement complex) level, a sensitive indicator of disease activity in patients with Henoch-Schonlein purpura. *Dermatology* **184,** 171–176.

66. Kawana, S., Shen, G., Kobayashi, Y., and Nishiyama, S. (1990) Membrane attack complex of complement in Henoch-Schonlein purpura skin and nephritis. *Arch. Dermatol. Res.* **282,** 183–187.

67. Boom, B., Out-Luiting, C., Baldwin, W., Westedt, M. L., Daha, M., and Vermeer, B. (1987) Membrane attack complex of complement in leukocytoclastic vasculitis of the skin. *Arch. Dermatol.* **69,** 477–484.

68. Boom, B., Mommaas, M., Daha, M., and Vermeer, B. (1989) Complement-mediated endothelial cell damage in immune complex vasculitis of the skin: ultrastructural localization of the membrane attack complex. *J. Invest. Dermatol.* **93,** 68S–72S.

69. Kawana, S. (1996) The membrane attack complex of complement alters the membrane integrity of cultured endothelial cells: a possible pathophysiology for immune complex vasculitis. *Act. Derm. Venereol.* **76,** 13–16.

70. Saadi, S. and Platt, J. (1995) Transient perturbation of endothelial integrity induced by natural antibodies and complement. *J. Exp. Med.* **181,** 21–31.

71. Hamilton, K. K., Hattori, R., Esmon, C. T., and Sims, P. J. (1990) Complement proteins C5b-9 induce vesiculation of the endothelial plasma membrane and expose catalytic surface for assembly of the prothrombinase enzyme complex. *J. Biol. Chem.* **265,** 3809–3814.

72. Suttorp, N., Seeger, W., Zinsky, S., and Bhakdi, S. (1987) Complement complex C5b-8 induces PGI_2 formation in cultured endothelial cells. *Am. J. Physiol.* **253,** C13–C21.

73. Benzaquen, L., Nicholson-Weller, A., and Halperin, J. (1994) Terminal complement proteins C5b-9 release basic fibroblast growth factor and platelet-derived growth factor from endothelial cells. *J. Exp. Med.* **179,** 985–992.

74. Christiansen, V. J., Sims, P. J., and Hamilton, K. K. (1997) Complement C5b-9 increases plasminogen binding and activation on human endothelial cells. *Arterioscler. Thromb. Vasc. Biol.* **17,** 164–171.

75. Vogt, W., Zimmerman, B., Hesse, D., and Nolte, R. (1992) Activation of the fifth component of human complement, C5, without cleavage by mc~thionine oxidizing agents. *Mol. Immunol.* **29,** 251–256.

76. Kilgore, K. S., Shen, J. P., Miller, B. F., Ward, P. A., and Warren, J. S. (1995) Enhancment by the complement membrane attack complex of tumor necrosis factor-α-induced endothelial cell expression of E-selectin and ICAM-1. *J. Immunol.* **155,** 1434–1441.

77. Lozada, C., Levin, R. I., Huie, M., Hirschhorn, R., Naime, D., Whitlow, M., Techt, P. A., Golden, B., and Cronstein, B. N. (1995) Identification of Clq as the heat-labile serum cofactor required for immune complexes to stimulate endothelial expression of the adhesion molecules E-selectin and intercellular and vascular cell adhesion molecules 1. *Proc. Natl. Acad. Sci. USA* **92,** 8378–8382.

78. Wang, C., Barbashov, S., Jack, R., Barrett, T., Weller, P., and Nicholson-Weller, A. (1995) Hemolytically inactive C5b67 complex: An agonist of polymorphonuclear leukocytes. *Blood* **85,** 2570–2578.

79. Tedesco, F., Pausa, M., Nardon, E., Introna, M., Mantovani, A., and Dobrina, A. (1997) The cytolytically inactive terminal complement complex activated endothelial cells to express adhesion molecules and tissue factor procoagulant activity. *J. Exp. Med.* **185,** 1619–1627.

80. Hattori, R., Hamilton, K. K., McEver, R. P., and Sims, P. J. (1989) Complement proteins C5b-9 induce secretion of high molecular weight multimers of endothelial von Willebrand factor and translocation of granule membrane protein GMP-140 to the cell surface. *J. Biol. Chem.* **264,** 9053–9060.

81. Zimmerman, G. A., McIntyre, T. M., and Prescott, S. M. (1985) Thrombin stimulates the adherence of neutrophils to human endothelial cells in vitro. *J. Clin. Invest.* **76,** 2235–2246.

82. Gerard, C., Chenoweth, D. E., and Hugli, T. E. (1981) Response of human neutrophils to C5a: a role for the oligosaccharide moiety of human C5a des Arg-74 but not of C5a in biologic activity. *J. Immunol.* **127,** 1978–1982.

83. Murphy, H. S., Shayman, J. A., Till, G. O., Mahrougui, M., Owens, C. B., Ryan, U. S., and Ward, P. A. (1992) Superoxide responses of endothelial cells to C5a and TNFα: divergent signal transduction pathways. *Am. J. Physiol.* **263,** L51–L59.

84. Friedl, H. P., Till, G. O., Ryan, U. S., and Ward, P. A. (1989) Mediator-induced activation of xanthine oxidase in endothelial cells. *FASEB J.* **3,** 2512–2518.

85. Foreman, K. E., Vaporciyan, A. A., Bonish, B. K., Jones, M. L., Johnson, K. J., Glovsky, M. M., Eddy, S. M., and Ward, P. A. (1994) C5a-induced expression of P-selectin in endothelial cells. *J. Clin. Invest.* **94,** 1147–1155.

86. Foreman, K. E., Glovsky, M. M., Warner, R. L., Horvath, S. J., and Ward, P. A. (1995) Does complement activation control tissue trafficking by C3a and C5a? *Int. Arch. Allergy Immunol.* **107,** 394,395.

87. Mulligan, M. S., Polley, M. J., Bayer, R. J., Nunn, M. F., Paulson, J. C., and Ward, P. A. (1992) Neutrophil-dependent acute lung injury: requirement for P-selectin (GMP-140). *J. Clin. Invest.* **90,** 1600–1607.

88. Doerschuk, C. M., Quinlan, W. M., Doyle, N. A., Bullard, D. C., Vestweber, D., Jones, M. L., Takei, F., Ward, P. A., and Beaudet A. L., (1996) The role of P-selectin and ICAM-1 in acute lung injury as determined using blocking antibodies and mutant mice. *J. Immunol.* **157,** 4609–4614.

89. Mulligan, M. S., Schmid, E., Till, G. O., Hugli, T. E., Fried, H. P., Roth, R. A., and Ward, P. A. (1997) C5a-dependent up-regulation in vivo of lung vascular P-selectin. *J. Immunol.* **158,** 1857–1861.

90. Rampart, M., Jose, P. J., and Williams, T. J. (1989) Rabbit leukocytes activated by C5a des arg and N-formyl-methionyl-leucyl-phenylalanine promote endothelial prostacyclin production: Evidence for a role of hydrogen peroxide. *Eicosanoids* **2,** 109–115.

91. Platt, J. L., Dalmasso, A. P., Lindman, B. J., Ihrcke, N. S., and Bach, F. H. (1991) The role of C5a and antibody in the release of heparan sulfate from endothelial cells. *Eur. J. Immunol.* **21,** 2887–2890.

92. Ikeda, K., Nagasawa, K., Horiuchi, T., Tsuru, T., Nishizaka, H., and Niho, Y. (1997) C5a induces tissue factor activity on endothelial cells. *Thromb. Haemost.* **77,** 39–48.

93. Schonermark, M., Deppisch, R., Riedasch, G., Rother, G., and Hansch, G. (1991) Induction of mediator release from human glomerular mesangial cells by the terminal complement components C5b-9. *Int. Arch. Allergy Appl. Immunol.* **96,** 331–337.

94. Lovett, D., Hansch, G., Resch, K., and Gemsa, D. (1987) Activation of glomerular mesangial cells by the terminal membrane attack complex of complement. *J. Immunol.* **138,** 2473–2479.

95. Kilgore, K. S., Flory, C. M., Miller, B. F., Evans, V. M., and Warren, J. S. (1996) The membrane attack complex of complement induces interleukin-8, and monocyte chemoattractant protein-1 secretion from human umbilical vein endothelial cells. *Am. J. Pathol.* **149,** 953–962.

96. Taub, D. and Oppenheim, J. (1993) Review of the chemokine meeting The Third International Symposium of Chemotactic Cytokines. *Cytokine* **5,** 175–179.

97. Mulligan, M. S., Jones, M. L., Bolanowski, M. A., Baganoff, M. P., Deppeler, C. L., Meyers, C. M., Ryan, U. S., and Ward, P. A. (1993) Inhibition of lung inflammatory reaction in rats by an anti-human IL-8 antibody. *J. Immunol.* **150,** 5585.

98. Gasque, P., Singhrao, S. K., Neal, J. W., Gotze, O., and Morgan, B. P. (1997) Expression of the receptor for complement C5a (CD88) is up-regulated on reactive astrocytes, microglia, and endothelial cells in the inflamed human central nervous system. *Am. J. Pathol.* **150,** 31–41.

99. Haviland, D. L., McCoy, R. L., Whitehead, W. T., Akama, H., Molmenti, E. P., Brown, A., Haviland, J. C., Parks, W. C., Perlmutter, D. H., and Wetsel, R. A. (1995) Cellular expression of the C5a anaphylatoxin receptor (C5aR): demonstration of C5aR on nonmyeloid cells of the liver and lung. *J. Immunol.* **154,** 1861–1869.

100. Jones, S. A., O'Donnell, V. B., Wood, J. D., Broughton, J. P., Hughes, E., and Jones, O. T. (1996) Expression of phagocyte NADPH oxidase components in human endothelial cells. *Am. J. Physiol.* **271,** H1626–H1634.

101. Mohassab-h, K. M., Kaminski, P. M., and Wolin, M. S. (1993) NADH oxidoreductase is a major source of superoxide anion in bovine coronary artery endothelium. *Am. J. Physiol.* **266,** H2568–H2572.

102. Zulueta, J. J., Yu, F., Hertig, I. A., Thannickal, V. J., and Hassoun, P. M. (1995) Release of hydrogen peroxide in response to hypoxia-reoxygenation: role of an NADPH oxidase-like enzyme in endothelial cell plasma membrane. *Am. J. Respir. Cell. Mol. Biol.* **12,** 41–49.

103. Adler, S., Baker, P., Johnson, R., Ochi, R., Pritsl, P., and Couser, W. (1986) Complement membrane attack complex stimulates production of reactive oxygen metabolites by cultured rat mesangial cells. *J. Clin. Invest.* **77,** 762–767.

104. Satriano, J., Shuldiner, M., Hora, K., Xing, Y., Zhan, Z., and Schlondorff, D. (1993) Oxygen radicals as second messengers for expression of the monocyte chemoattractant protein, JE/MCP-1 and the monocyte colony-stimulating factor CSF-1, in response to tumor necrosis factor-alpha and immunoglobulin G: Evidence for involvement of reduced nicotinamide adenine dinucleotide phosphate (NADPH)-dependent oxidase. *J. Clin. Invest.* **92,** 1564–1571.

105. Wiedmer, T., Ando, B., and Sims, P. J. (1987) Complement C5b-9-stimulated platelet secretion is associated with a Ca^{2+}-initiated activation of cellular protein kineses. *J. Biol. Chem.* **262,** 13,674–13,681.

106. Niculescu, F., Rus, H., and Shin, M. (1994) Receptor-independent activation of guanine nucleotide-binding regulatory proteins by terminal complement complexes. *J. Biol. Chem.* **269,** 4417–4423.

107. Carney, D. F., Lang, T. J., and Shin, M. L. (1990) Multiple signal messengers generated by terminal complement complexes and their role in terminal complement complex elimination. *J. Immunol.* **145,** 623–629.

108. Kilgore, K., Schmid, E., Shanley, T., Flory, C., Maheswari, V., Tramontini, N., Cohen, H., Ward, P., Friedl, H., and Warren, J. (1997) Sublytic concentration of the membrane attack complex of complement induced endothelial interleukin-β and monocyte chemoattractant protein-1 through nuclear factor-kappa β activation. *Am. J. Pathol.* **150,** 2019–2031.

109. Urban, M. B., Schreck, R., and Baeuerle, P. A. (1991) NF-kappa β contacts DNA by a heterodimer of the p50 and p65 subunit. *EMBO J.* **10,** 1817–1825.

110. Schreck, R., Rieber, P., and Baeuerle, P. A. (1991) Reactive oxygen intermediates as apparently widely used messenger in the activation of the NF-kappa β transcription factor and HIV-1. *EMBO J.* **10,** 2247–2258.

111. Collins, T., Read, M. A., Neish, A. S., Whitley, M. Z., Thanos, D., and Maniatis, T. A. (1995) Transcriptional regulation of endothelial cell adhesion molecules: NF-kappa β and cytokine-inducible enhancers. *FASEB J.* **9,** 899–909.

112. Jahnke, A. and Johnson, J. P. (1994) Synergistic activation of intercellular adhesion molecule 1 (ICAM-1) by TNF-alpha and IFN-gamma is mediated by p65/p50 and p65/c-Rel and interferon-responsive factor Stat 1 alpha (p91) that can be activated by both IFN-gamma and IFN-alpha. *FEBS Lett.* **354,** 220–226.

113. Hou, J., Baichwal, V., and Cao, Z. (1994) Regulatory elements and transcription factors controlling basal and cytokine-induced expression of the gene encoding intercellular adhesion molecule 1. *Proc. Natl. Acad. Sci. USA* **91,** 11,641–11,645.

114. Schreck, R., Meier, B., Mannel, D. N., Croge, W., and Baeuerle, P. A. (1992) Dithiocarbamates as potent inhibitors of nuclear factor kβ activation in intact cells. *J. Exp. Med.* **175,** 1181–1194.

115. Finco, T. S., Beg, A. A., and Baldwin, A. S. J. (1994) Inducible phosphorylation of I kappa β alpha is not sufficient for its dissociation from NF-kappa β and is inhibited by protease inhibitors. *Proc. Natl. Acad. Sci. USA* **91,** 11,884–11,888.

116. Thall, A. D., Murphy, H. S., and Lowe, J. (1996) α1,3-Galactosyltransferase-deficient mice produce naturally occurring cytotoxic anti-gal antibodies. *Transplant Proc.* **28,** 561,562.

117. Bach, F., Robson, S., Ferran, C., Winkler, H., Millan, M., Stuhlmeier, K., Vanhove, B., Blakely, M., Werf, W. J. V., Hofer, E., Marin, R., and Hancock, W. (1994) Endothelial cell activation and thromboregulation during xenograt rejection. *Immunol. Rev.* **141,** 5–29.

118. Artrip, J. H., Itescu, S., Minanov, O. P., Kwiatkowski, P. A., and Michler, R. E. (1997) Cardiac xenotransplantation. *Curr. Opin. Cardiol.* **12,** 172–178.

119. Thall, A., Murphy, H., Homeister, J., Awwad, M., Lowe, J., Gao, L., Buelow, R., and Lussow, A. (1997) Hyperacute rejection of cardiac grafts α1,3-galactosyltransferase "knock-out" mice is analogous to human rejection of xenografts. *Proc. Am. Soc. Transplant. Phys.* May.

120. Sanfilippo, F., and Baldwin, W. M. (1997) Antibody and complement in graft rejection. *Transplant Proc.* **29,** 179,180.

121. Mollnes, T. E. (1997) Biocompatibility: complement as mediator of tissue damage and as indicator of incompatibility. *Exp. Clin. Immunogen.* **14,** 24–29.

122. Bach, F., Dalmasso, G., and Platt, J. (1992) Xenotransplantation: a current perspective. *Transplant. Rev.* **6,** 1.

123. Pattison, J. M., and Krensky, A. M. (1997) New insights into mechanisms of allograft rejection. *Am. J. Med. Sci.* **313,** 257–263.

124. Kaufman, C. L., Gaines, B. A., and Ildstad, S. T. (1995) Xenotransplantation. *Annu. Rev. Immunol.* **13,** 339–367.

125. Coughlan, A., Berndt, M., Dunlop, L., and Hancock, W. (1993) In vivo studies of P-selectin and platelet-activating factor during endotoxemia, accelerated allograft rejection and discordant xenograft rejection. *Transplant Proc.* **25,** 2930.

126. Hancock, W., Barkely, M., Werf, W. V. D., and Bach, F. (1993) Rejection of guinea pig cardiac xenografts post-cobra venom factor therapy is associated with infiltration by mononuclear cells secreting interferon-gamma and diffuse endothelial activation. *Transplant Proc.* **25,** 2932.

127. Pratt, J. R., Hibbs, M. J., Laver, A. J., Smith, R. A., and Sacks, S. H. (1996) Effects of complement inhibition with soluble complement receptor-1 on vascular injury and inflammation during renal allograft rejection in the rat. *Am. J. Pathol.* **149,** 2055–2066.

128. Rollins, S. A., Matis, L. A., Springhorn, J. P., Setter, E., and Wolff, D. W. (1995) Monoclonal antibodies directed against human C5 and C8 block complement-mediated damage of xenogeneic cells and organs. *Transplant* **60,** 1284–1292.

129. Moutabarrik, A., Nakanishi, I., Namiki, M., Hara, T., Matsumoto, M., Ishibashi, M., Okuyama, A., Zaid, D., and Seya, T. (1993) Cytokine-mediated regulation of the surface expression of complement regulatory proteins, CD46 (MCP), CD55 (DAF), and CD59 on human vascular endothelial cells. *Lymphokine Cytokine Res.* **12,** 167–172.

130. Miyagawa, S., Mikata, S., Shirakura, R., Matsudfa, H., Nagasawa, S., Terados, A., Hatanaka, M., Matsumoto, M., and Seya, T. (1996) C5b-8 step lysis of swine endothelial cells by human complement and functional feature of transfected CD59. *Scand. J. Immunol.* **43,** 361–366.

131. Miyagawa, S., Shirakura, R., Iwata, K., Nakata, S., Matsumiya, G., Izutani, H., Matsuda, H., Terado, A., Matsumoto, M., and Nagasawa, S. (1994) Effects of transfected complement regulatory proteins, MCP, DAF, and MCP/DAE hybrid, on complement-mediated swine endothelial cell lysis. *Transplantation* **58,** 834–840.

132. Heckl-Ostreicher, B., Wosnik, A., and Kirschfink, M. (1996) Protection of porcine endothelial cells from complement-mediated cytotoxicity by the human complement regulators CD59, C1 inhibitor, and soluble complement receptor type 1: Analysis in a pig-to-human in vitro model relevant to hyperacute xenograft rejection. *Transplantation* **62,** 1693–1645.

133. Dalmasso, A. P. and Platt, J. L. (1993) Prevention of complement-mediated activation of xenogeneic endothelial cells in an in vitro model of xenograft hyperacute rejection by C1 inhibitor. *Transplantation* **56,** 1171–1176.

2

Angiogenesis

Douglas A. Arenberg and Robert M. Strieter

Introduction

Angiogenesis, defined as the generation of new blood vessels from preexisting vessels, is one of life's essential processes. Without proper angiogenesis, basic life functions, such as embryogenesis, wound repair, and the ovarian/menstrual cycle, would fail. Angiogenesis is distinguished from vasculogenesis, which describes the *de novo* formation of the vascular system during embryogenesis. Development of the heart and great vessels occurs by vasculogenesis, whereas organs that require invasion of blood vessels for development (brain, lung, kidney) are supplied by angiogenesis *(1)*. Neovascularization is a term used interchangeably with angiogenesis, but may be more appropriately reserved for describing aberrant angiogenesis that accompanies pathologic processes, such as tumorigenesis, psoriasis, or fibroproliferative disorders, such as pulmonary fibrosis and rheumatoid arthritis. Inflammation and angiogenesis, although distinct and separable, are closely related processes. One of the histologic hallmarks of chronic inflammation is the presence of "granulation-like" tissue, a prominent feature of which is the presence of neovascularization. Whenever tissue constituents proliferate, repair, or hypertrophy, such change must be accompanied by a proportional increase in capillary blood supply to assure delivery of nutrients, and removal of metabolic waste. This absolute dependence suggests two characteristics of angiogenesis. First, under normal conditions the process must be tightly controlled, able to rapidly up- or downregulate. Second, in the absence of such strict control, abnormal physiology or disease is likely to result. To understand angiogenesis, it is best to start with a description of a "physiologic" condition, such as a wound response (Fig. 1).

Angiogenesis: A Sequence of Overlapping Processes

Although endothelial cells are normally quiescent, during the angiogenic response they become activated. The rate of normal capillary endothelial cell turnover is typi-

From: *Molecular and Cellular Basis of Inflammation*
Edited by: C. N. Serhan and P. A. Ward © Humana Press Inc., Totowa, NJ

The angiogenic response to a wound. Initially there is coagulation due to leakage of plasma proteins, which leads to deposition of a primordial matrix. Many events, including platelet degranulation, macrophage activation, and tissue injury itself can release angiogenic factors. After receiving the angiogenic stimulus, endothelial cells begin to detach from their neighboring cells by altering adherens junctions. In order to maintain the integrity of the circulation, the steps involved in the angiogenic response must occur in a complex and well orchestrated manner.

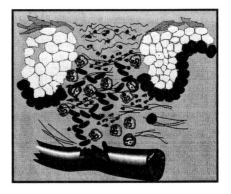

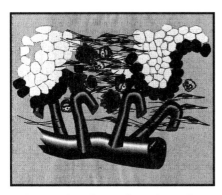

Degradation of basement the membrane requires the action of matrix metalloproteases.
Proteolysis of extracellular matrix occurs by urokinase and tissue type plasminogen activators.
Adhesion to matrix components via $\alpha_V\beta_3$ and $\alpha_V\beta_5$ integrins allows endothelial cell **haptotaxis** through the matrix.
Cell proliferation and DNA synthesis is necessary for continuing the angiogenic response.
Tube formation requires tight cell-cell adhesions via both cadherin 5, and PECAM-1 (CD31).
Collagen synthesis is required for deposition of new basememnt membrane

Regression of newly formed vessels occurs when the expression of angiogenic factors is overcome by expression of angiostatic factors. When this occurs, the new vessels whch formed in response to the wound will regress to the prior steady state level. This process by which this occurs probably involves apoptosis of endothelial cells and subsequent phagocytosis of cellular debris.

Abnormal angiogenesis can result in poor wound healing. However, exaggerated angiogenesis is implicated in chronic inflammatory conditions such as psoriasis, and rheumatoid arthritis, as well as cancer.

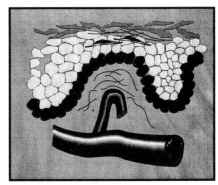

Fig. 1. A schematic example of the sequence of events in tissue undergoing wound repair.

cally measured in months or years *(2,3)*. However, when endothelial cells of the microvasculature are stimulated, they will degrade their basement membrane and proximal extracellular matrix, migrate directionally, divide, and organize into functioning capillaries invested by a new basal lamina, all within a matter of days. These steps are not sequential. Rather, they represent an orchestration of overlapping events necessary to return injured tissue to homeostasis. In each of the steps of angiogenesis, there are gaps in our knowledge of the exact mechanisms. Nevertheless, significant advances in cell and molecular biology have led to a greater understanding of angiogenesis.

The Angiogenic Signal

The signal(s) that initiate this process are not well defined and may be organ-specific *(4)*. The source of the angiogenic signal may be a product of many cells, including tumor cells *(5)*, fibroblasts *(6)*, endothelial cells *(7,8)*, epithelial cells *(9)*, or activated macrophages *(10)*. Tissue injury may lead to the release of angiogenic factors through platelet degranulation *(11)* or proteolytic digestion of extracellular matrix *(12)*. The importance of these latter mechanisms may lie in the fact that they occur rapidly in response to tissue injury because they do not require new protein synthesis *(13)*. Embryonic angiogenesis is activated by genes that are transcribed in response to hypoxia and hypoglycemia in the developing embryonic tissue *(14)*. More importantly, the signal for angiogenesis also may be initiated by a decrease in the presence of an inhibitory signal, rather than simply requiring a positive stimulus *(15)*.

Endothelial Dedifferentiation

Once the endothelial cell receives an angiogenic stimulus, a process of "dedifferentiation" is initiated. For endothelium to invade into the surrounding matrix, cells must first detach from their tight association with neighboring endothelial cells. These cell-cell appositions, called adherens junctions, are composed of proteins of the cadherin family. Vascular endothelial cadherin (VE-cadherin, or cadherin 5) is highly specific for endothelial cells *(16)*, and is associated with the cytoskeleton through other intermediate proteins, β-catenin, and plakoglobin *(17,18)*. One of the earliest events in the angiogenic response is alteration of the adherens junction complexes, leading to increased pericellular permeability, and detachment of the endothelial cell from its neighboring cells *(19)*.

Proteolysis and Cell Migration

To form new vessels, the existing basement membrane must be degraded. Protease activity is necessary to digest the basement membrane, and early in the angiogenic response metalloproteases are expressed *(20)*. Inhibitors of matrix metalloproteases are capable of inhibiting angiogenesis *(21)*. This proteolytic activity also results in the further release of growth factors and angiogenic factors that are sequestered in the basement membrane *(7,12)*.

After proteolysis of the basement membrane, angiogenic endothelial cells must migrate through the extracellular matrix. The structural constituents of extracellular matrix consist of a variety of components, including fibrin, fibronectin, vitronectin, and hyaluronan as well as other glycosaminoglycans *(22)*. Endothelial cells express both urokinase and tissue-type plasminogen activators during angiogenesis that allow invasion into the surrounding matrix *(23)*. Motility through this environment requires cell-matrix adhesion that occurs through cell surface-associated integrins.

In vitro endothelial cell chemotaxis is typically assessed in an aqueous environment. However, endothelial cell migration in vivo occurs in a "solid phase" environment, referred to as haptotaxis. Reversible integrin-mediated binding to matrix components allows haptotaxis of endothelial cells through the extracellular matrix. Since endothelial cells must respond to injury in all organs and tissues of the body, they must be capable of adherence to a variety of matrix components. The $a_v\beta_3$ and $a_v\beta_5$ integrins are important endothelial cell adhesion molecules that display appropriately promiscuous binding profiles, and are both involved in angiogenesis *(24,25)*. The importance of this cell-matrix interaction in angiogenesis is demonstrated by work showing that specific inhibition of integrin binding in angiogenic endothelium leads to apoptosis of the endothelial cells *(24,25)*. Thus, integrin binding not only facilitates adhesive and locomotor functions but also inhibits apoptotic cell death.

Cell Proliferation

Although DNA synthesis occurs early in the angiogenic response, it has been shown both in vitro *(26)* and in vivo *(27)* that vascular sprouting can occur in the absence of endothelial cell proliferation. However, when proliferation is inhibited, the angiogenic response does not progress beyond vascular sprouting, the earliest stage of neovascularization *(27)*. Maintenance of the angiogenic response requires an increase in the number of endothelial cells to provide adequate capillary perfusion to the proliferative and repair processes of wound repair. Although some angiogenic factors are only chemotactic for endothelial cells *(28)*, most are also endothelial cell mitogens *(26,28)*.

The signaling pathways that control cell growth are separable from those that lead to other aspects of the angiogenic response, and may be dependent on the degree of cell-matrix adhesion *(29)*. For example, in vitro studies demonstrate that endothelial cell proliferation occurs in conditions of increased cell-matrix adhesiveness, whereas growth arrest and loss of viability occur in cells plated on poorly adhesive substrates *(29)*. Intermediate levels of adhesiveness promote differentiation into tubelike structures *(29)*. One might hypothesize that these in vitro findings have an in vivo correlate during wound repair. The early primordial matrix of a wound is rich in plasma proteins that provide an abundant source of extracellular matrix to which endothelial cells may adhere, thus promoting cell migration and proliferation. As a wound matures, however, the primordial matrix is altered. Fibroblasts deposit type III collagen, and phagocytic cells remove debris, perhaps leading to reduced adhesiveness of the matrix and promoting capillary tube formation *(10,13,30–32)*.

Additional evidence relating cell adhesion to control of proliferation is seen in studies of cadherin 5, the main component of the endothelial cell adherens junction. Homophilic cell–cell interaction through cadherin 5 inhibits endothelial cell proliferation and motility *(33)*. Similarly, cadherin 5-expressing cells have impaired proliferation when cultured on a cadherin 5-coated substrate *(33)*. Thus, cell–cell contact through the adherens junction and cadherin 5 may impair cell cycle progression. Early alteration of endothelial cell adherens junctions during the angiogenic response allows not only for vascular permeability and motility, but also permits endothelial cell proliferation.

Tube Formation

Once endothelial cells have invaded injured, inflamed, or hypoxic tissue, the integrity of the circulatory system must then be maintained. This critical process requires the formation of functioning capillaries with tight cell–cell adhesion. Investigators are beginning to define the nature of the cellular interactions underlying tube formation. In addition to the importance of cadherin 5 and the adherens junction, tube formation requires the function of CD31 (PECAM-1) *(34)*. PECAM-1 is a 130-kDa membrane glycoprotein and a member of the immunoglobulin supergene family that can mediate both heterotypic and homotypic adhesion *(35)*. The importance of this interaction was demonstrated by a study in which neutralizing antibodies to PECAM-1 inhibited tube formation in vitro, and angiogenesis in vivo *(36)*. In a distinct in vitro model system, other authors have found that a combination of blocking antibodies to both CD31 and cadherin 5 were necessary to inhibit tube formation *(34)*.

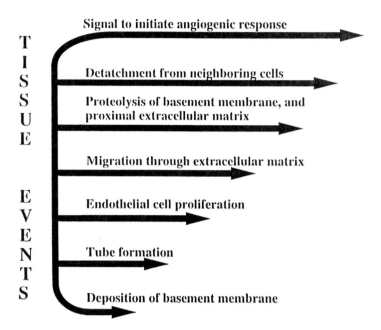

Fig. 2. From a tissue perspective, the events of the angiogenic response occur in an overlapping or parallel fashion. However, on a cellular level, the success of the angiogenic response depends on a complex orchestration of events in a serial fashion.

Subsequent to the formation of a continuous capillary tube, the final step in forming a new blood vessel is the deposition of a basement membrane. Similar to other steps in the sequence of events that occur during angiogenesis, inhibition of collagen biosynthesis both prevents the in vitro formation of capillary-like tubes and inhibits an in vivo model of angiogenesis *(37)*. The inhibition of any of the steps involved in angiogenesis appears to have a profound effect on inhibiting the process as a whole. Thus, whereas on a *tissue* level the events of angiogenesis occur in a parallel fashion, individually interrupting any of these events on a *cellular* level demonstrates the need for a complex orchestration of events in a serial fashion (Fig. 2).

Maintenance of the Angiogenic Response

Persistence of neovascularization requires a proangiogenic environment. This implies that the local expression of angiogenic factors outweighs the expression of angiostatic factors. The events that dictate this imbalance have not been fully defined. Since the number of factors capable of regulating angiogenesis is extensive, it is not possible to discuss all the interactions that might affect this balance. However, there are several potential factors which may be important. First, early in the wound response, tissue injury itself leads to release of angiogenic factors from the extracellular matrix. Second, platelet degranulation releases both angiostatic *(38)* and angiogenic factors *(39)*. Third, activated macrophages release their own angiogenic factors *(10,28,40–42)*, whereas macrophage-derived proteases are probably important in the generation of angiostatic factors such as angiostatin *(43)* and endostatin *(44)*. Finally, other cells that can affect this balance include fibroblasts *(6)*, epithelial cells *(9)*, and endothelial cells

(7). These counterbalancing events that occur simultaneously during a wound response suggest the strict control that is inherent in "physiologic" angiogenesis.

Termination of the Angiogenic Response

Once the balance of angiogenic and angiostatic factors favors angiostasis, the newly formed blood vessels will regress. This process has been studied in the cornea of the rabbit, and the sequence of events was similar whether the vessels formed in response to a wound or to a tumor factor *(45)*. Regression of capillaries begins with morphologic changes of endothelial cells including mitochondrial swelling and development of cytoplasmic projections. This is followed by platelet adherence to vessel walls and platelet degranulation *(45)*. This process is eventually accompanied by degeneration of endothelial cells and removal of debris by mononuclear cells migrating into the area. Regression first occurs in the newest vessels, and proceeds proximally to involve the earliest vessels *(45)*. These morphologic changes described in regressing vessels probably resemble programmed endothelial cell death (apoptosis) *(46)*.

Factors That Regulate Angiogenesis

The paradigm of a balance between angiogenic and angiostatic factors is absolutely essential to understanding net angiogenesis. There is an abundance of factors that can impact on this balance, and the list continues to grow (Table 1). A detailed discussion of each of these is impractical in the context of this chapter, and, therefore, the focus will be on those factors that have been most intensely studied. These include the cytokines, acidic and basic fibroblast growth factor, VEGF, and members of the family of chemotactic cytokines known as CXC chemokines (interleukin-8 [IL-8]; growth-related oncogene [GRO-α], GRO-β, GRO-γ, NH2-terminal truncated forms of platelet basic protein [PBP]: connective tissue activating protein-III [CTAP-III], beta-thromboglobulin [β-TG], neutrophil activating protein-2 [NAP-2]; epithelial neutrophil activating protein-78 [ENA-78]; and granulocyte chemotactic protein-2 [GCP-2]).

Fibroblast Growth Factors

The fibroblast growth factor (FGF) gene family consists of nine members, the prototypes of which are acidic FGF (aFGF) and basic FGF (bFGF). These two members of the FGF family are distinct in that they lack a classic signal peptide to direct their processing in the Golgi apparatus and eventual secretion *(47)*. Consequently, little is known of how aFGF and bFGF become secreted into the extracellular space. Other members of the FGF family that do possess the signal peptide sequence were initially discovered as oncogenic growth factors *(48)*. Transfection of cells with mutants of aFGF that contain a signal peptide leads to cell transformation *(49,50)*. Thus, the lack of signal sequence in aFGF and bFGF is thought to reflect the evolution of a tighter degree of control over their secretion *(49,50)*.

FGFs induce endothelial cell migration, proliferation, and tube formation in vitro *(51,52)*. The involvement of FGFs in pathologic angiogenesis is inferred by studies of tumor associated angiogenesis. Basic FGF may influence angiogenesis associated with Kaposi's sarcoma *(53)*, breast cancer *(54)*, and lung cancer *(55)*. Furthermore, FGFs have been studied in models of myocardial ischemia and may play a therapeutic role in the development of collateral circulation *(56,57)*.

Table 1
Factors That Either Directly or Indirectly Regulate Angiogenesis

Angiogenic	Angiostatic
Proteins and peptides	Proteins and peptides
Angiogenin	Angiopoietin 2
Angiopoietin 1	Angiostatin
Angiotensin II	Endostatin
ELR-CXC chemokines	Eosinophilic major basic protein
Epidermal growth factor	High molecular weight hyaluronan
Fibrin peptide fragments	Interferon-α
Fibroblast growth factors 1 and 2	Interferon-β
Haptoglobin	Interferon-γ
Interleukin 1 (IL-1)	Non-ELR-CXC chemokines
Interleukin 2 (IL-2)	Interleukin-1
Plasminogen activator	Interleukin-4
Polyamines	Interleukin-12
Substance P	Laminin and fibronectin peptides
Scatter factor/hepatocyte growth factor	Placental RNase (angiogenin)
Soluble E-selectin	inhibitor
Transforming growth factor-α	Somatostatin
Transforming growth factor-β	Substance P
Tumor necrosis factor-alpha	Thrombospondin 1
Vascular endothelial growth factor (VEGF)	Tissue inhibitor of
Carbohydrates and lipids	metalloproteinases
12(R)-hydroxyeicosatrienoic acid	Lipids
Hyaluronan fragments	Angiostatic steroids
Platelet activating factor	Retinoids
Monobutyrin	Vitamin A
Prostaglandins E_1 and E_2	Others
Urokinase	Nitric oxide
Others	Vitreous fluids
Adenosine	Prostaglandin synthetase inhibitor
Angiotropin	Protamine
Ceruloplasmin	
Heparin	
Nicotinamide	

FGF Receptors

FGFs bind to glycosaminoglycans *(58)*. Low-affinity heparin binding is necessary for FGFs to bind to their high-affinity cell surface receptors *(59)*. Specific high-affinity FGF receptors have been cloned and exist in three different isoforms (FGFR-1, -2, and -3) that result from alternative splicing of the FGFR gene transcripts. Each receptor has three immunoglobulin (Ig)-like extracellular domains (except for FGFR-2, which has only two Ig domains), a transmembrane domain, and an intracellular tyrosine-kinase domain *(60)*. The alternative extracellular domains confer differing ligand binding specificity for members of the FGF family *(60)*, and these splice variants are distributed in a tissue specific manner *(61)*. There are several inherited disorders of skeletal development associated with mutations of the FGF receptors *(62)*. The multifunctional potential of the FGF family is inferred by the existence of these human disorders.

Vascular Endothelial Cell Growth Factor

Also identified as vascular permeability factor, VEGF is the initial member of a family of proteins with mitogenic and angiogenic activity *(63)*. As its name implies, VEGF also has potent effects on vessel permeability in addition to endothelial cell proliferation and migration. VEGF exists in multiple isoforms, VEGF-189, -165, and -121, distinguished by the amino acid length of the primary structure *(64)*. These different VEGF molecules result from alternative splicing of a single gene transcript *(64)*. VEGF-189 consists of eight exons, with VEGF-165 lacking the amino acids encoded by exon 6, whereas VEGF-121 lacks amino acids encoded by exons 6 and 7. Additionally, the VEGF family consists of two other members, VEGF B *(65)* and C *(66)*, which, while closely related, map to different chromosomes *(67)*. The more recently cloned VEGF B and C are less well characterized, but evidence suggests a critical role for VEGF C in the development of the lymphatic system *(68,69)*. VEGF is biologically active as a dimer *(70)*, and may require downstream activity of nitric oxide synthase and guanylate cyclase to induce angiogenesis *(71)*. Although VEGF was initially thought to be an endothelial cell specific agonist, recent evidence demonstrates expression of specific VEGF receptors on monocytes and that VEGF induces migration of these cells *(72)*.

VEGF-induced angiogenesis is involved in a number of physiologic and pathologic processes. VEGF is expressed in the walls of both normal and atherosclerotic coronary arteries *(73)*, as well as in multiple experimental *(74)* and "naturally occurring" human tumors *(75)*. A recent study has correlated the presence of increased immunostaining for VEGF with a poor prognosis in breast cancer *(76)*. In animal models, neutralizing antibodies to VEGF are effective in inhibiting tumor growth in tumor cell lines expressing VEGF *(77–79)*. In synovia of patients with rheumatoid arthritis, expression of VEGF mRNA is seen in macrophages, fibroblasts, and smooth muscle cells *(80)*. Finally, in a rabbit model of hind-limb ischemia, VEGF and FGF 2 are synergistic in their ability to induce collateral circulation *(81)*.

Perhaps the strongest data demonstrating a role for VEGF-induced angiogenesis is derived from mice with targeted deletion of either the VEGF gene or its receptors. Mouse embryos with a mutation in a single allele of the VEGF gene develop abnormal vessels and die at embryonic d 11–12 *(82,83)*. Similarly, targeted inactivation of either of the two known receptors for VEGF results in embryonic lethality at 8–9 d *(84,85)*. These findings suggest a central role of VEGF in embryonic development.

Among the factors known to regulate expression of VEGF as well as its receptors is hypoxia *(86)*, which induces VEGF from a number of cell types *(86–88)*. Murine embryonic stem cells genetically engineered to lack the gene for the arylhydrocarbon-receptor nuclear translocator (*arnt*) are unable to augment VEGF expression in response to hypoxia. Interestingly, embryos derived from these cells display a developmental phenotype similar to VEGF "knockout" mice *(14)*. This suggests that arnt is a required factor for the hypoxic induction of VEGF gene transcription. Additionally, the expression of VEGF appears to be augmented in the presence of mutant *ras* oncogenes *(89)*. VEGF can form heterodimers with platelet-derived growth factor that have reduced angiogenic activity *(90)*. Through this interaction, angiogenic activity of VEGF may be regulated after secretion.

VEGF Receptors

The two known receptors for VEGF, flk-1/KDR, and flt-1 are both members of the tyrosine kinase family of transmembrane receptors. The receptors probably mediate different actions of VEGF. For example, studies employing VEGF mutants that retain binding to only one of the two receptors reveal that flk-1/KDR mediates VEGF-induced endothelial cell proliferation *(91)*. By contrast, migration of monocytes in response to VEGF occurs via the flt-1 VEGF receptor *(72)*.

Angiostatin and Endostatin

These two recently described molecules are potent inhibitors of angiogenesis *(44,92)*. O'Reilly et al. discovered angiostatin while studying an interesting phenomenon; the growth inhibition of tumor metastases by primary tumors *(92)*. Angiostatin was isolated from the urine of tumor-bearing mice *(92)*. Mice bearing experimental Lewis lung carcinoma tumors typically developed extensive metastases only after removal of the primary tumor. However, when the mice received angiostatin injections, growth of metastases was inhibited, even after removal of the primary tumor *(92)*. Using a similar experimental strategy, O'Reilly et al. subsequently isolated a molecule with similar activity, endostatin *(44)*.

These two molecules also share another property, in that both are internal fragments of larger peptides with neither angiogenic nor angiostatic properties *(44,92)*. Angiostatin is a 38-kDa internal fragment derived from plasminogen *(92)*, and endostatin is a 20-kDa internal fragment of collagen XVIII *(44)*. Subsequent study of angiostatin led to the finding that macrophage metalloelastase is responsible for the proteolytic cleavage of plasminogen to yield angiostatin *(93)*. To date there are no studies to define an analogous mechanism for the generation of endostatin. However, the discovery of these two important inhibitors of angiogenesis will surely lead to a search for similar peptide fragments that are capable of inhibiting angiogenesis. Indeed, one of the more exciting findings about these molecules is their ability to induce and sustain dormancy of micrometastases via suppression of angiogenesis in animal models of cancer *(44,94)*.

The Angiopoietin/Tie Receptor-Ligand System

A recently characterized receptor-ligand system appears to be very important in development of the vascular system, but is not yet widely implicated in pathologic angiogenesis. The Tie receptors (Tie-1 and Tie-2) are protein-tyrosine kinases that are expressed in the embryonic yolk sac and in areas of vascular development. Tie-1 deficient animals develop to birth but die perinatally owing to a defect in vascular integrity, with resulting hemorrhage and generalized edema *(95)*. In contrast, Tie-2 (also known as tek)–deficient embryos die at embryonic d 10–11, with the most prominent abnormalities being failure of development of the endothelial lining of the heart, and failure of the early vascular system to progress beyond its earliest stages of vessel formation *(95)*.

A search for ligands for this receptor system has led to the cloning of angiopoietin-1, which is a specific activating ligand for Tie-2 *(96)*. Expression of angiopoietin-1 in developing embryos is localized predominantly to the myocardial tissue surrounding the endocardium, and later in mesenchymal tissue surrounding the developing vasculature *(96)*. Angiopoietin-1 is not an endothelial cell mitogen, nor does it induce tube formation in vitro, but it plays a vital role in the remodeling of the vascular system during development *(96,97)*, perhaps by facilitating communication between endothelium and the surrounding mesenchymal cells. A naturally occurring antagonist for the Tie-2 receptor exists, termed angiopoietin-2, and is expressed in areas of vascular remodeling in embryonic as well as adult tissues *(98)*.

Table 2
The CXC Chemokines

ELR	Non-ELR
IL-8	Platelet factor-4 (PF4)
ENA-78	Interferon-γ-inducible protein (IP-10)
Growth-related oncogene alpha	Monokine induced by interferon-γ (MIG)
(GRO-α, GRO-β, and GRO-γ)	Stromal cell-derived factor-1 (SDF-1)
GCP-2	
PBP	
CTAP-III	
b-TG	
NAP-2	

Although the Tie/angiopoietin system seems to have a definite role in development, the only pathologic condition in which this receptor-ligand family has thus far been implicated is a familial form of vascular malformations. In this condition, a mutation of the Tie-2 receptor tyrosine kinase domain leads to its constitutive activation *(99)*. However, high levels of mRNA for Tie-2 are found in the endothelium of malignant melanomas *(100)*. Therefore, further study of these novel factors may uncover additional pathologic conditions in which they play a role.

CXC Chemokines

The CXC chemokine family are cytokines that in their monomeric forms are <10-kDa and, like many regulators of angiogenesis, are characteristically basic heparin-binding proteins. This family displays four highly conserved cysteine amino acid residues, with the first two cysteines separated by one nonconserved amino acid, leading to the CXC designation *(101–107)*. In general, these cytokines have specific chemotactic activity for neutrophils. However, PF4 has potent angiostatic and antitumor activity, and was the first member of this family to be identified as a regulator of angiogenesis *(108)*. Subsequently, IL-8, a classic neutrophil chemotactic factor, was identified as a potent inducer of angiogenesis in the absence of inflammation *(109–111)*. A unique aspect of the CXC chemokine family is that they display disparate activity as regulators of angiogenesis *(108,110–115)*. This is the only family of closely related cytokines that is composed of both angiogenic and angiostatic factors. This is especially important when one considers the paradigm that net angiogenic activity reflects a balance of positive and negative regulators of angiogenesis.

The structural feature that appears to distinguish angiogenic and angiostatic CXC chemokines is the presence or absence of three conserved amino acid residues that immediately precede the first cysteine in the primary structure of these cytokines. These are the glutamine-leucine-arginine (ELR) motif *(113)*. CXC chemokines containing the ELR motif are potent angiogenic factors, whereas those CXC chemokines that lack the ELR motif are angiostatic factors *(109–111,113–115)* (Table 2). This disparity may be important in understanding the role of interferons in regulating angiogenesis. IP-10 and MIG are non-ELR CXC chemokines that are angiostatic *(113–116)*. The primary signal leading to expression of IP-10 and MIG is interferon-γ *(117–119)*, and interferons are potent inhibitors of the production of monocyte-derived IL-8, GRO-α, and ENA-78 (all ELR+ angiogenic factors) *(120,121)*. By contrast, the ELR CXC chemokines are primarily induced by TNF-α, and IL-1 *(119,122–125)*. Thus, there appears to be signal specificity for the expression of the angiogenic (ELR) and angiostatic (non-ELR) members of the CXC chemokine family.

This family of molecules may be particularly relevant to the study of angiogenesis in chronic inflammation, given that they are produced by virtually all nucleated cells *(101,107)*. IL-8 is an angiogenic factor in several angiogenesis-dependent chronic inflammatory conditions, including rheumatoid arthritis *(110,126)*, psoriasis *(9,127)* and idiopathic pulmonary fibrosis *(6)*. Additionally, IL-8 is an important source of angiogenic activity in human lung cancer *(55,128)*. The non-ELR CXC chemokines IP-10, PF4, and MIG are potent angiostatic factors that inhibit not only angiogenesis induced by the ELR CXC chemokines, but also by other classic angiogenic factors, such as bFGF and VEGF. For example, IP-10 inhibits in vitro endothelial cell chemotaxis and proliferation, as well as in vivo matrigel invasion in response to basic FGF *(115)*. In the rat corneal model of neovascularization, both IP-10 and MIG inhibit angiogenesis in response to either bFGF or VEGF *(116)*.

A growing body of evidence is supporting the notion that members of the CXC chemokine family regulate net neovascularization in angiogenesis-dependent disorders. For example, in an animal model of human lung cancer, expression of IL-8 correlated directly with tumor size, and inhibition of IL-8 led to inhibition of tumor-derived angiogenic activity and tumor growth *(128)*. Also, IL-8 expression correlates with experimental metastatic activity of some melanoma cell lines *(129)*. Another ELR CXC chemokine, melanoma growth stimulatory activity (GRO-α), is expressed not only in melanomas but also in healing human burn wounds, in areas of neovascularization *(130,131)*. These findings suggest a role for ELR CXC chemokines in a variety of angiogenesis-dependent conditions.

By contrast, the non-ELR CXC chemokines are potent angiostatic factors that may play a role as endogenous inhibitors of angiogenic activity. For example, IP-10 is an endogenous angiostatic factor in human lung cancer *(132)*. Expression of IP-10 had an inverse correlation with tumor size in a mouse model of lung cancer *(132)*, and intratumor administration of IP-10 in this model reduced both tumor growth and metastases *(132)*. IP-10 is probably a major mediator of the antitumor activity of IL-12 *(133,134)*. More recently, MIG, another non-ELR CXC chemokine was found to induce tumor necrosis in vivo *(135)*. These findings suggest that IP-10 and MIG may eventually prove to be useful as therapeutic adjuncts for the treatment of solid tumors. In total, these findings support the hypothesis that net angiogenic activity in many conditions may be dependent, in part, on the balance of expression of ELR and non-ELR CXC chemokines.

Receptors Mediating Angiogenic Activity of CXC Chemokines

The receptor(s) responsible for regulation of angiogenesis by CXC chemokines are currently unknown. However, strong indirect evidence suggests that the CXC chemokine receptor, CXCR2, is the putative receptor that mediates this activity. First, all the ELR CXC chemokines are angiogenic, and all bind to CXCR2 *(136,137)*. Second, expression of CXCR2 has been demonstrated on angiogenic endothelium of human burn wounds, specifically at the advancing edge of the healing wound *(130)*. Interestingly, a recent study has identified a gene encoded by human herpesvirus 8, the virus associated with Kaposi's sarcoma *(138)*, a highly vascular neoplasm characterized by proliferating capillary-like structures. This new gene encodes a G protein-coupled seven transmembrane-domain protein with significant homology to CXCR2 *(138)*. More important, this viral CXCR2 homolog is constitutively activated, perhaps leading to ligand-independent growth signaling in the endothelial-like cells of the Kaposi's sarcoma lesion. This indirect evidence supports the contention that CXCR2 mediates the angiogenic activity of ELR CXC chemokines.

The receptor for the angiostatic activity of non-ELR CXC chemokines is also unknown. IP-10 and PF4 can compete for binding on endothelial cells, and this binding is inhibited by pretreatment of the cells with heparinase *(114)*. There is a specific transmembrane protein receptor for IP-10 and MIG: CXCR3 *(139)*. This receptor has been found in endothelial cells by RT-PCR (Strieter et al., unpublished observations). The role(s) of these receptors in regulating angiostatic activity of non-ELR CXC chemokines remains to be determined. Determining the receptor that mediates this activity will be important in developing antiangiogenic therapy for angiogenesis-dependent disorders.

Conditions Characterized by Abnormal Angiogenesis

Physiologic angiogenesis is rare once the adult stage of development has been achieved. A few situations in which the angiogenic response is appropriate include the ovarian/menstrual cycle in the female reproductive organs, and normal healing of a wound. Other than these examples, angiogenesis in an adult is usually associated with a pathologic condition, such as psoriasis, rheumatoid arthritis, diabetic retinopathy, pulmonary fibrosis, and tumor growth and metastasis.

Psoriasis

Psoriasis is a skin disorder characterized by inflammatory cellular infiltration, abnormal proliferation of keratinocytes, and dermal neovascularization. Although it is not clear that the angiogenesis associated with psoriasis is a primary cause of the pathogenesis of the disease, the angiogenic activity is related to a combination of overproduction of IL-8 and underproduction of the angiogenesis inhibitor, thrombospondin-1 *(9)*. Additionally, the angiostatic factor IP-10 is expressed in psoriatic plaques, with expression being reduced after successful treatment of active lesions *(140)*. The significance of this finding is not clear. However, it highlights the potential importance of endogenous angiostatic factors in angiogenesis-dependent disorders.

Rheumatoid Arthritis

The importance of angiogenesis in the pathogenesis of rheumatoid arthritis has been appreciated for many years *(141)*. The synovial inflammation of rheumatoid arthritis leads to formation of the pannus and eventual destruction of articular cartilage and bone. This tissue destruction may be dependent upon release of proteases and collagenases that are released during the angiogenic response *(142)*. Studies of angiogenic factors have either directly or indirectly implicated IL-8 *(126)*, hepatocyte growth factor *(143)*, and VEGF *(80,144)*, in the angiogenic activity of rheumatoid arthritis. Interestingly, minocycline, an antibiotic with potent angiostatic activity, was found to be beneficial in treating patients with rheumatoid arthritis in a double-blind, placebo-controlled study *(145–147)*.

Pulmonary Fibrosis

As a prototypical fibroproliferative disease, the deposition of extracellular matrix seen in the lungs of patients with pulmonary fibrosis is an example of exaggerated granulation tissue. Indeed, one of the classical early descriptions of the pathology of pulmonary fibrosis included the description of neovascularization *(148)*. Although most studies of this disease have focused on the role of inflammatory cell infiltration and fibroblast function, recent data have suggested a role for CXC chemokines as regulators of angiogenic activity in patients with pulmonary fibrosis *(6)*. Further investigations are needed on the role of angiogenesis in the pathogenesis of pulmonary fibrosis to improve the dismal prognosis associated with this disease.

Tumorigenesis and Metastasis

The dependence of tumor growth on angiogenesis was first noted by Gimbrone et al. in 1972 *(5)*. This is perhaps the most fertile area of research on angiogenesis, and the one in which therapeutic advances are most needed. Early in the pathogenesis of a tumor, and before a tumor can become clinically significant, there must be a switch to an angiogenic phenotype *(149)*. This angiogenic switch can be mediated by either an increase in expression of angiogenic factors *(149,150)*, or a decrease in the expression of angiostatic factors *(15,132,151)*, or both. Many factors have been implicated in the control of tumor-associated angiogenic activity *(152,153)*.

In addition to the growth of a primary tumor, the spread and growth of distant metastases can only be accomplished by individual cells capable of expressing an angiogenic phenotype *(154)*. The population of cells in a primary tumor is heterogeneous, and only those cells that can induce angiogenesis at a distant site will form a clinically evident metastasis *(154)*. One theory that has gained favor in recent studies is that dormant metastases are those which have a balance of proliferation and apoptosis *(5,155)*. Only when the metastatic deposit has made the angiogenic switch will the rate of proliferation surpass the rate of apoptosis, and the metastatic focus become clinically manifest *(94,156)*. An effective inhibitor of tumor-derived angiogenic activity would prevent further growth of a primary tumor and halt the development of metastases. Since tumor endothelium is not genetically abnormal and, therefore, not subject to a high rate of mutation, it is unlikely to develop "drug resistance" to angiostatic therapy. Such an advance could render all other aspects of tumor biology irrelevant. Therefore, some investigators have proposed a two-compartment approach to tumor therapy, one targeted at the malignant cells, and the other at the endothelial cells *(156)*. This is clearly an area in which research into the mechanisms of angiogenesis is potentially beneficial.

Summary

Angiogenesis is a process that is intricately associated with physiologic wound repair and pathologic processes such as chronic inflammation and tumor growth. Given the appropriate signal, dormant endothelial cells can be quickly activated, leading to migration, proliferation, and differentiation into new functioning capillaries to support tissue repair or growth. Whereas angiogenic events in tissue occur in a parallel fashion, on a cellular basis the integrity of the angiogenic response requires that each step be successfully carried out in series. The complex control of angiogenesis is illustrated by the ever increasing number of molecules that can affect the response. Although research has primarily focused on the discovery of angiogenic factors, recent studies have highlighted the importance of endogenous angiostatic factors in many disease states. There has been remarkable progress in the knowledge of angiogenesis in the last three decades.

However, a more thorough understanding of the control of angiogenesis will allow future therapeutic advances that exploit the dependence of chronic inflammation, tumor growth, and wound repair on angiogenesis.

Acknowledgments

This work was supported in part by NIH grants CA66180, HL50057, 1P50HL56402, and CA72543; an American Lung Association Research Grant, and The University of Michigan's Phoenix Memorial Project.

References

1. Risau, W. (1991) Vasculogenesis, angiogenesis and endothelial cell differentiation during embryonic development, in *The Development of the Vascular System* (Feinberg, R. N., Sherer, G. K., and Auerbach, R., eds.) Karger, Basel, Switzerland, pp. 58–68.
2. Engerman, R. L., Pfaffenbach, D., and Davis, M. D. (1967) Cell turnover of capillaries. *Lab. Invest.* **17,** 738–743.
3. Tannock, I. F. and Hayashi, H. S. (1972) The proliferation of capillary and endothelial cells. *Cancer Res.* **32,** 77–82.
4. Auerbach, R. (1991) Vascular endothelial cell differentiation: organ specificity and selective affinities as the basis for developing anticancer strategies. *Int. J. Radiat. Biol.* **60(1–2),** 1–10.
5. Gimbrone, M. A., Leapman, S. B., Cotran, R. S., and Folkman, J. (1972) Tumor dormancy in vivo by prevention of neovascularization. *J. Exp. Med.* **136,** 261–276.
6. Keane, M., Arenberg, D., Lynch, J. P., III, Whyte, R., Iannetoni, M., Burdick, M., Wilke, C., Morris, S., Glass, M., DiGiovive, B., Kunkel, S., and Strieter, R. (1997) The CXC chemokines, IL-8 and IP–10, regulate angiogenic activity in idiopathic pulmonary fibrosis. *J. Immunol.* **159,** 1437–1443.
7. Vlodavski, I., Folkman, J., Sullivan, R., Fridman, R., Ishai-Michaeli, R., Sasse, J., and Klagsbrun, M. (1987) Endothelial cell-derived basic fibroblast growth factor: Synthesis and deposition into subendothelial extracellular matrix. *Proc. Natl. Acad. Sci. USA* **84,** 2292–2296.
8. Strieter, R. M., Kunkel, S. L., Showell, H. J., and Marks, R. M. (1988) Monokine-induced gene expression of human endothelial cell-derived neutrophil chemotactic factor. *Biochem. Biophys. Res. Commun.* **156,** 1340–1345.
9. Nickoloff, B. J., Mitra, R. S., Varani, J., Dixit, V. M., and Polverini, P. J. (1994) Aberrant production of interleukin-8 and thrombospondin-1 by psoriatic keratinocytes mediates angiogenesis. *Am. J. Pathol.* 144 **(4),** 820–828.
10. Leibovich, S. J. and Weisman, D. M. (1988) Macrophages, wound repair and angiogenesis. *Prog. Clin. Biol. Res.* **266,** 131–145.
11. Sato, N., Beitz, J. G., Kato, J., Yamamoto, M., Clark, J. W., Calabresi, P., Raymond, A., and Frackelton, A. R., Jr. (1993) Platelet-derived growth factor indirectly stimulates angiogenesis in vitro. *Am. J. Pathol.* **142(4),** 1119–1130.
12. Vlodavsky, I., Korner, G., Ishai-Michaeli, R., Bashkin, P., Bar-Shavit, R., and Fuks, Z. (1990) Extracellular matrix-resident growth factors and enzymes: Possible involvement in tumor metastases and angiogenesis. *Cancer and Metastases Rev.* **9,** 203–226.
13. Clark, R. A. (1993) Basics of cutaneous wound repair. *J. Dermatol. Surg. Oncol.* **19(8),** 693–706.
14. Maltepe, E., Schmidt, J. V., Baunoch, D., Bradfield, C. A., and Simon, M. C. (1997) Abnormal angiogenesis and responses to glucose and oxygen deprivation in mice lacking the protein ARNT. *Nature* **386,** 403–407.
15. Rastinejad, F., Polverini, P. J., and Bouck, N. P. (1989) Regulation of the activity of a new inhibitor of angiogenesis by a cancer suppressor gene. *Cell* **56(3),** 345–355.
16. Lampugnani, M. G., Resnati, M., Raiteri, M., Pigott, R., Pisacane, A., Houen, G., Ruco, L. P., and Dejana, E. (1992) A novel endothelial-specific membrane protein is a marker of cell-cell contacts. *J. Cell Biol.* **118(6),** 1511–1522.
17. Lampugnani, M. G., Corada, M., Caveda, L., Breviario, F., Ayalon, O., Geiger, B., and Dejana, E. (1995) The molecular organization of endothelial cell to cell junctions: Differential association of plakoglobin, beta-catenin, and alpha-catenin with vascular endothelial cadherin (VE-cadherin). *J. Cell Biol.* **129(1),** 203–217.

18. Tanihara, H., Kido, M., Obata, S., Heimark, R. L., Davidson, M., St. John, T., and Suzuki, S. (1994) Characterization of cadherin-4 and cadherin-5 reveals new aspects of cadherins. *J. Cell Sci.* **107(Pt 6),** 1697–1704.

19. Dejana, E. (1996) Endothelial adherens junctions: Implications in the control of vascular permeability and angiogenesis. *J. Clin. Invest.* **98(9),** 1949–1953.

20. Pepper, M. S., Vassaui, J. D., Orci, L., and Montesano, R. (1992) Proteolytic balance and capillary morphogenesis in vitro, in *Angiogenesis: Key Principles* (Steiner, R., Weisz, P. B., and Langer, R., eds.), Birkhauser Verlag, Basel, Switzerland, pp. 137–145.

21. Takigawa, M., Nishida, Y., Suzuki, F., Kishi, J., Yamashita, K., and Hayakawa, T. (1990) Induction of angiogenesis in chick yolk-sac membrane by polyamines and its inhibition by tissue inhibitors of metalloproteinases (TIMP and TIMP-2). *Biochem. Biophys. Res. Commun.* **171(3),** 1264–1271.

22. Arnold, F. and West, D. C. (1991) Angiogenesis in wound healing. *Pharmacol. Ther.* **52(3),** 407–422.

23. Gross, J. L., Moscatelli, D., and Rifkin, D. B. (1983) Increased capillary endothelial cell protease activity in response to angiogenic stimuli in vitro. *Proc. Natl. Acad. Sci. USA* **80(9),** 2623–2627.

24. Brooks, P. C., Montgomery, A. M., Rosenfeld, M., Reisfeld, R. A., Hu, T., Klier, G., and Cheresh, D. A. (1994) Integrin alpha v beta 3 antagonists promote tumor regression by inducing apoptosis of angiogenic blood vessels. *Cell* **79(7),** 1157–1164.

25. Brooks, P. C., Clark, R. A., and Cheresh, D. A. (1994) Requirement of vascular integrin alpha v beta 3 for angiogenesis. *Science* **264(5158),** 569–571.

26. Koolwijk, P., van Erck, M. G., de Vree, W. J., Vermeer, M. A., Weich, H. A., Hanemaaijer, R., and van Hinsbergh, V. W. (1996) Cooperative effect of TNF-alpha, bFGF, and VEGF on the formation of tubular structures of human microvascular endothelial cells in a fibrin matrix. Role of urokinase activity. *J. Cell Biol.* **132(6),** 1177–1188.

27. Sholly, M. M., Fergusen, G. P., Seibel, H. R., Montour, J. L., and Wilson, J. D. (1984) Mechanisms of neovascularization: Vascular sprouting can occur without proliferation of endothelial cells. *Lab. Invest.* **51,** 624–634.

28. Sunderkotter, C., Goebeler, M., Schulze-Osthoff, K., Bhardwaj, R., and Sorg, C. (1991) Macrophage-derived angiogenesis factors. *Pharmacol. Ther.* **51(2),** 195–216.

29. Ingber, D. E. and Folkman, J. (1989) Mechanochemical switching between growth and differentiation during fibroblast growth factor-stimulated angiogenesis in vitro: Role of extracellular matrix. *J. Cell Biol.* **109(1),** 317–330.

30. Davidson, J. M. (1992) Wound repair, in *Inflammation: Basic Principles and Clinical Correlates* (Gallin, J. I., Goldstein, I. M., and Snyderman, R., eds.), Raven, New York.

31. French-Constant, C., Van, D. W. L., Dvorak, H. F., and Hynes, R. O. (1989) Reappearance of an embryonic pattern of fibronectin splicing during wound healing in the adult rat. *J. Cell Biol.* **109,** 903–914.

32. Kurkinen, M., Vaheri, A., Roberts, P. J., and Stenan, S. (1980) Sequential appearance of fibronectin and collagen in experimental granulation tissue. *Lab. Invest.* **43,** 47–51.

33. Caveda, L., Martin-Padura, I., Navarro, P., Breviario, F., Corada, M., Gulino, D., Lampugnani, M. G., and Dejana, E. (1996) Inhibition of cultured cell growth by vascular endothelial cadherin (cadherin-5/VE-cadherin). *J. Clin. Invest.* **98(4),** 886–893.

34. Matsumura, T., Wolff, K., and Petzelbauer, P. (1997) Endothelial cell tube formation depends on cadherin 5 and CD31 interactions with filamentous actin. *J. Immunol.* **158(7),** 3408–3416.

35. DeLisser, H. M., Chilkotowski, J., Yan, H. C., Daise, M. L., Buck, C. A., and Albelda, S. M. (1994) Deletions in the cytoplasmic domain of platelet-endothelial cell adhesion molecule-1 (PECAM-1, CD31) result in changes in ligand binding properties. *J. Cell. Biol.* **124(1–2),** 195–203.

36. Delisser, H. M., Christofidou-Solomidou, M., Strieter, R. M., Burdick, M. D., Robinson, C. S., Wexler, R. S., Kerr, J. S., Garlanda, C., Merwin, J. R., and Albelda, S. M. (1997) Involvement of endothelial PECAM–1/CD31 in angiogenesis. *Am. J. Pathol.*, **151(3),** 671–677.

37. Haralabopoulos, G. C., Grant, D. S., Kleinman, H. K., Lelkes, P. I., Papaioannou, S. P., and Maragoudakis, M. E. (1994) Inhibitors of basement membrane collagen synthesis prevent endothelial cell alignment in matrigel in vitro and angiogenesis in vivo. *Lab. Invest.* **71(4),** 575–582.

38. Hansell, P., Maione, T. E., and Borgstrom, P. (1995) Selective binding of platelet factor 4 to regions of active angiogenesis in vivo. *Am. J. Physiol.* **269(3 Pt. 2),** H829–H836.
39. Walz, A. and Baggiolini, M. (1990) Generation of the neutrophil-activating peptide NAP-2 from platelet basic protein or connective tissue-activating peptide III through monocyte proteases. *Exp. Med.* **171,** 449–454.
40. Koch, A. E., Leibovich, S. J., and Polverini, P. J. (1989) Stimulation of neovascularization by human rheumatoid synovial tissue macrophages. *Arthritis Rheum.* **29(4),** 471–479.
41. Polverini, P. J., Cotran, P. S., Gimbrone, M. A., and Unanue, E. R. (1977) Activated macrophages induce vascular proliferation. *Nature (Lond.)* **269(5631),** 804–806.
42. Polverini, P. J. (1996) How the extracellular matrix and macrophages contribute to angiogenesis-dependent diseases. *Eur. J. Cancer.* **32A(14),** 2430–2437.
43. Dong, Z., Kumar, R., Yang, X., and Fidler, I. J. (1997) Macrophage-derived metalloelastase is responsible for the generation of angiostatin in Lewis lung carcinoma. *Cell* **88,** 801–810.
44. O'Reilly, M., Boehm, T., Shing, Y., Fukai, N., Vasios, G., Lane, W., Flynn, E., Birkhead, J., Olsen, B., and Folkman, J. (1997) Endostatin: an endogenous inhibitor of angiogenesis and tumor growth. *Cell* **88(2),** 277–285.
45. Ausprunk, D. H. and Folkman, J. (1978) The sequence of events in the regression of corneal capillaries. *Lab. Invest.* **38,** 284–296.
46. Robaye, B., Mosselmans, R., Fiers, W., Dumont, J. E., and Galand, P. (1991) Tumor necrosis factor induces apoptosis (programmed cell death) in normal endothelial cells in vitro. *Am. J. Pathol.* **138(2),** 447–453.
47. Burgess, W. H. and Maciag, T. (1989) The heparin-binding (fibroblast) growth factor family of proteins. *Annu. Rev. Biochem.* **58,** 575–606.
48. Talarico, D. and Basilico, C. (1991) The K-fgf/hst oncogene induces transformation through an autocrine mechanism that requires extracellular stimulation of the mitogenic pathway. *Mol. Cell Biol.* **11(2),** 1138–1145.
49. Forough, R., Xi, Z., MacPhee, M., Friedman, S., Engleka, K. A., Sayers, T., Wiltrout, R. H., and Maciag, T. (1993) Differential transforming abilities of nonsecreted and secreted forms of human fibroblast growth factor-1. *J. Biol. Chem.* **268(4),** 2960–2968.
50. Rogelj, S., Weinberg, R. A., Fanning, P., and Klagsbrun, M. (1988) Basic fibroblast growth factor fused to a signal peptide transforms cells. *Nature* **331(6152),** 173–175.
51. Connolly, D. T., Stoddard, B. L., Harakas, N. K., and Feder, J. (1987) Human fibroblast-derived growth factor is a mitogen and chemoattractant for endothelial cells. *Biochem. Biophys. Res. Commun.* **144(2),** 705–712.
52. Montesano, R., Vassalli, J. D., Baird, A., Guillemin, R., and Orci, L. (1986) Basic fibroblast growth factor induces angiogenesis in vitro. *Proc. Natl. Acad. Sci. USA* **83(19),** 7297–7301.
53. Ensoli, B., Markham, P., Kao, V., Barillari, G., Fiorelli, V., Gendelman, R., Raffeld, M., Zon, G., and Gallo, R. C. (1994) Block of AIDS-Kaposi's sarcoma (KS) cell growth, angiogenesis, and lesion formation in nude mice by antisense oligonucleotide targeting basic fibroblast growth factor: a novel strategy for the therapy of KS. *J. Clin. Invest.* **94(5),** 1736–1746.
54. Lewis, C. E., Leek, R., Harris, A., and McGee, J. O. (1995) Cytokine regulation of angiogenesis in breast cancer: The role of tumor-associated macrophages. *J. Leukoc Biol.* **57(5),** 747–751.
55. Smith, D. R., Polverini, P. J., Kunkel, S. L., Orringer, M. B., Whyte, R. I., Burdick, M. D., Wilke, C. A., and Strieter, R. M. (1994) Inhibition of IL-8 attenuates angiogenesis in bronchogenic carcinoma. *J. Exp. Med.* **179,** 1409–1415.
56. Sellke, F. W., Li, J., Stamler, A., Lopez, J. J., Thomas, K. A., and Simons, M. (1996) Angiogenesis induced by acidic fibroblast growth factor as an alternative method of revascularization for chronic myocardial ischemia. *Surgery* **120(2),** 182–188.
57. Isner, J. M. (1996) The role of angiogenic cytokines in cardiovascular disease. *Clin. Immunol. Immunopathol.* **80(3 Pt. 2),** S82–S91.
58. Friesel, R. E. and Maciag, T. (1995) Molecular mechanisms of angiogenesis: fibroblast growth factor signal transduction. *FASEB J.* **9(10),** 919–925.
59. Yayon, A., Klagsbrun, M., Esko, J. D., Leder, P., and Ornitz, D. M. (1991) Cell surface, heparin-like molecules are required for binding of basic fibroblast growth factor to its high affinity receptor. *Cell* **64(4),** 841–848.
60. Johnson, D. E. and Williams, L. T. (1993) Structural and functional diversity in the FGF receptor multigene family. *Adv. Cancer Res.* **60,** 1–40.

61. Orr-Urtreger, A., Bedford, M. T., Burakova, T., Arman, E., Zimmer, Y., Yayon, A., Givol, D., and Lonai, P. (1993) Developmental localization of the splicing alternatives of fibroblast growth factor receptor 2 (FGFR2). *Dev. Biol.* **158,** 475–486.

62. Muenke, M. and Schell, U. (1995) Fibroblast-growth-factor receptor mutations in human skeletal disorders. *Trends Genet.* **11(8),** 308–313.

63. Tischer, E., Gospodarowicz, D., Mitchell, R., Silva, M., Schilling, J., Lau, K., Crisp, T., Fiddes, J. C., and Abraham, J. A. (1989) Vascular endothelial growth factor: A new member of the platelet-derived growth factor gene family. *Biochem. Biophys. Res. Commun.* **165(3),** 1198–1206.

64. Tischer, E., Mitchell, R., Hartman, T., Silva, M., Gospodarowicz, D., Fiddes, J. C., and Abraham, J. A. (1991) The human gene for vascular endothelial growth factor: Multiple protein forms are encoded through alternative exon splicing. *J. Biol. Chem.* **266(18),** 11,947–11,954.

65. Olofsson, B., Pajusola, K., Kaipainen, A., von Euler, G., Joukov, V., Saksela, O., Orpana, A., Pettersson, R. F., Alitalo, K., and Eriksson, U. (1996) Vascular endothelial growth factor B, a novel growth factor for endothelial cells. *Proc. Natl. Acad. Sci. USA* **93(6),** 2576–2581.

66. Joukov, V., Pajusola, K., Kaipainen, A., Chilov, D., Lahtinen, I., Kukk, E., Saksela, O., Kalkkinen, N., and Alitalo, K. (1996) A novel vascular endothelial growth factor, VEGF-C, is a ligand for the Flt4 (VEGFR-3) and KDR (VEGFR-2) receptor tyrosine kinases. *EMBO J.* **15(2),** 290–298. (published erratum appears in *EMBO J.* (1996) **15[7],** 1751)

67. Wei, M. H., Popescu, N. C., Lerman, M. I., Merrill, M. J., and Zimonjic, D. B. (1996) Localization of the human vascular endothelial growth factor gene, VEGF, at chromosome 6p12. *Hum. Genet.* **97(6),** 794–797.

68. Kukk, E., Lymboussaki, A., Taira, S., Kaipainen, A., Jeltsch, M., Joukov, V., and Alitalo, K. (1996) VEGF-C receptor binding and pattern of expression with VEGFR-3 suggests a role in lymphatic vascular development. *Development* **122(12),** 3829–3837.

69. Jeltsch, M., Kaipainen, A., Joukov, V., Meng, X., Lakso, M., Rauvala, H., Swartz, M., Fukumura, D., Jain, R. K., and Alitalo, K. (1997) Hyperplasia of lymphatic vessels in VEGF-C transgenic mice. *Science* **276(5317),** 1423–1425.

70. Claffey, K. P., Senger, D. R., and Spiegelman, B. M. (1995) Structural requirements for dimerization, glycosylation, secretion, and biological function of VPF/VEGF. *Biochim. Biophys. Acta* **1246(1),** 1–9.

71. Ziche, M., Morbidelli, L., Choudhuri, R., Zhang, H.-T., Donnini, S., and Granger, H. J. (1997) Nitric oxide synthase lies downstream from vascular endothelial growth factor-induced, but not basic fibroblast growth factor-induced angiogenesis. *J. Clin. Invest.* **99,** 2626–2634.

72. Barleon, B., Sozzani, S., Zhou, D., Weich, H. A., Mantovani, A., and Marme, D. (1996) Migration of human monocytes in response to vascular endothelial growth factor (VEGF) is mediated via the VEGF receptor flt-1. *Blood* **87(8),** 3336–3343.

73. Couffinhal, T., Kearney, M., Witzenbichler, B., Chen, D., Murohara, T., Losordo, D. W., Symes, J., and Isner, J. M. (1997) Vascular endothelial growth factor/vascular permeability factor (VEGF/VPF) in normal and atherosclerotic human arteries. *Am. J. Pathol.* **150(5),** 1673–1685.

74. Warren, R. S., Yuan, H., Matli, M. R., Gillett, N. A., and Ferrara, N. (1995) Regulation by vascular endothelial growth factor of human colon cancer tumorigenesis in a mouse model of experimental liver metastasis. *J. Clin. Invest.* **95(4),** 1789–1797.

75. Takahashi, Y., Kitadai, Y., Bucana, C. D., Cleary, K. R., and Ellis, L. M. (1995) Expression of vascular endothelial growth factor and its receptor, KDR, correlates with vascularity, metastasis, and proliferation of human colon cancer. *Cancer Res.* **55(18),** 3964–3968.

76. Toi, M., Hoshina, S., Takayanagi, T., and Tominaga, T. (1994) Association of vascular endothelial growth factor expression with tumor angiogenesis and with early relapse in primary breast cancer. *Jpn. J. Cancer Res.* **85(10),** 1045–1049.

77. Claffey, K. P., Brown, L. F., del Aguila, L. F., Tognazzi, K., Yeo, K. T., Manseau, E. J., and Dvorak, H. F. (1996) Expression of vascular permeability factor/vascular endothelial growth factor by melanoma cells increases tumor growth, angiogenesis, and experimental metastasis. *Cancer Res.* **56(1),** 172–181.

78. Borgstrom, P., Hillan, K. J., Sriramarao, P., and Ferrara, N. (1996) Complete inhibition of angiogenesis and growth of microtumors by anti-vascular endothelial growth factor neutralizing antibody: Novel concepts of angiostatic therapy from intravital videomicroscopy. *Cancer Res.* **56(17),** 4032–4039.

79. Kim, J. K., Li, B., Winer, J., Armanini, M., Gillett, N., Phillips, H. S., and Ferrara, N. (1993) Inhibition of vascular endothelial growth factor-induced angiogenesis suppresses tumor growth in vivo. *Nature* **362**, 841–844.

80. Nagashima, M., Yoshino, S., Ishiwata, T., and Asano, G. (1995) Role of vascular endothelial growth factor in angiogenesis of rheumatoid arthritis. *J. Rheumatol.* **22(9)**, 1624–1630.

81. Asahara, T., Bauters, C., Zheng, L. P., Takeshita, S., Bunting, S., Ferrara, N., Symes, J. F., and Isner, J. M. (1995) Synergistic effect of vascular endothelial growth factor and basic fibroblast growth factor on angiogenesis in vivo. *Circulation* **92(9 Suppl. II)**, 365–371.

82. Ferrara, N., Carver-Moore, K., Chen, H., Dowd, M., Lu, L., O'Shea, K. S., Powell-Braxton, L., Hillan, K. J., and Moore, M. W. (1996) Heterozygous embryonic lethality induced by targeted inactivation of the VEGF gene. *Nature* **380(6573)**, 439–442.

83. Carmeliet, P., Ferreira, V., Breier, G., Pollefeyt, S., Kieckens, L., Gertsenstein, M., Fahrig, M., Vandenhoeck, A., Harpal, K., Eberhardt, C., Declercq, C., Pawling, J., Moons, L., Collen, D., Risau, W., and Nagy, A. (1996) Abnormal blood vessel development and lethality in embryos lacking a single VEGF allele. *Nature* **380(6573)**, 435–439.

84. Fong, G. H., Rossant, J., Gertsenstein, M., and Breitman, M. L. (1995) Role of the Flt-1 receptor tyrosine kinase in regulating the assembly of vascular endothelium. *Nature* **376(6535)**, 66–70.

85. Shalaby, F., Rossant, J., Yamaguchi, T. P., Gertsenstein, M., Wu, X. F., Breitman, M. L., and Schuh, A. C. (1995) Failure of blood-island formation and vasculogenesis in Flk-1-deficient mice. *Nature* **376(6535)**, 62–66.

86. Detmar, M., Brown, L. F., Berse, B., Jackman, R. W., Elicker, B. M., Dvorak, H. F., and Claffey, K. P. (1997) Hypoxia regulates the expression of vascular permeability factor/vascular endothelial growth factor (VPF/VEGF) and its receptors in human skin. *J. Invest. Dermatol.* **108(3)**, 263–268.

87. Freeman, M. R., Schneck, F. X., Gagnon, M. L., Corless, C., Soker, S., Niknejad, K., Peoples, G. E., and Klagsbrun, M. (1995) Peripheral blood T lymphocytes and lymphocytes infiltrating human cancers express vascular endothelial growth factor: A potential role for T cells in angiogenesis. *Cancer Res.* **55(18)**, 4140–4145.

88. Brogi, E., Wu, T., Namiki, A., and Isner, J. M. (1994) Indirect angiogenic cytokines upregulate VEGF and bFGF gene expression in vascular smooth muscle cells, whereas hypoxia upregulates VEGF expression only. *Circulation* **90(2)**, 649–652.

89. Rak, J., Mitsuhashi, Y., Bayko, L., Filmus, J., Shirasawa, S., Sasazuki, T., and Kerbel, R. S. (1995) Mutant ras oncogenes upregulate VEGF/VPF expression: Implications for induction and inhibition of tumor angiogenesis. *Cancer Res.* **55(20)**, 4575–4580.

90. Cao, Y., Chen, H., Zhou, L., Chiang, M. K., Anand-Apte, B., Weatherbee, J. A., Wang, Y., Fang, F., Flanagan, J. G., and Tsang, M. L. (1996) Heterodimers of placenta growth factor/vascular endothelial growth factor: Endothelial activity, tumor cell expression, and high affinity binding to Flk–1/KDR. *J. Biol. Chem.* **271(6)**, 3154–3162.

91. Keyt, B. A., Nguyen, H. V., Berleau, L. T., Duarte, C. M., Park, J., Chen, H., and Ferrara, N. (1996) Identification of vascular endothelial growth factor determinants for binding KDR and FLT–1 receptors: Generation of receptor-selective VEGF variants by site-directed mutagenesis. *J. Biol. Chem.* **271(10)**, 5638–5646.

92. O'Reilly, M. S., Holmgren, L., Shing, Y., Chen, C., Rosenthal, R. A., Moses, M., Lane, W. S., Cao, Y., Sage, E. H., and Folkman, J. (1994) Angiostatin: A novel angiogenesis inhibitor that mediates suppression of metastases by a Lewis lung carcinoma. *Cell* **79(2)**, 315–328.

93. Dong, Z., Kumar, R., Yang, X., and Fidler, I. J. (1997) Macrophage-derived metalloelastase is responsible for the generation of angiostatin in Lewis lung carcinoma. *Cell.* **88(6)**, 801–810.

94. O'Reilly, M. S., Holmgren, L., Chen, C., and Folkman, J. (1996) Angiostatin induces and sustains dormancy of human primary tumors in mice. *Nat. Med.* **2(6)**, 689–692.

95. Sato, T. N., Tozawa, Y., Deutsch, U., Wolburg-Buchholz, K., Fujiwara, Y., Gendron-Maguire, M., Gridley, T., Wolburg, H., Risau, W., and Qin, Y. (1995) Distinct roles of the receptor tyrosine kinases Tie-1 and Tie-2 in blood vessel formation. *Nature* **376(6535)**, 70–74.

96. Davis, S., Aldrich, T. H., Jones, P. F., Acheson, A., Compton, D. L., Jain, V., Ryan, T. E., Bruno, J., Radziejewski, C., Maisonpierre, P. C., and Yancopoulos, G. D. (1996) Isolation of angiopoietin-1, a ligand for the TIE2 receptor, by secretion-trap expression cloning. *Cell* **87(7)**, 1161–1169 (see comments).

97. Suri, C., Jones, P. F., Patan, S., Bartunkova, S., Maisonpierre, P. C., Davis, S., Sato, T. N., and Yancopoulos, G. D. (1996) Requisite role of angiopoietin-1, a ligand for the TIE2 receptor, during embryonic angiogenesis. *Cell* **87(7)**, 1171–1180 (see comments).

98. Maisonpierre, P. C., Suri, C., Jones, P. F., Bartunkova, S., Wiegand, S. J., Radziejewski, C., Compton, D., McClain, J., Aldrich, T. H., Papadopoulos, N., Daly, T. J., Davis, S., Sato, T. N., and Yancopoulos, G. D. (1997) Angiopoietin-2, a natural antagonist for Tie2 that disrupts in vivo angiogenesis. *Science* **277(5322)**, 55–60 (see comments).

99. Vikkula, M., Boon, L. M., Carraway K. L., III, Diamonti, A. J., Goumnerov, B., Warman, M. L., Cantley, L. C., Mulliken, J. B., and Olsen, B. R. (1996) Vascular dysmorphogenesis caused by an activating mutation in the receptor tyrosine kinase TIE2. *Cell* **87**, 1181–1190.

100. Kaipainen, A., Vlaykova, T., Hatva, E., Bohling, T., Jekunen, A., Pyrhonen, S., and Alitalo, K. (1994) Enhanced expression of the tie receptor tyrosine kinase mesenger RNA in the vascular endothelium of metastatic melanomas. *Cancer Res.* **54(24)**, 6571–6577.

101. Walz, A., Kunkel, S. L., and Strieter, R. M. (1996) CXC chemokines-an overview, in *Chemokines in Disease* (Koch, A. E., and Strieter, R. M., eds.) R. G. Landes, Austin, TX, pp. 1–26.

102. Strieter, R. M. and Kunkel, S. L. (1997) Chemokines and the lung, in *Lung: Scientific Foundations*, 2nd edition. (Crystal, R., West, J., Weibel, E., and Barnes, P., eds.), Raven, NY. 155–186.

103. Strieter, R. M., Lukacs, N. W., Standiford, T. J., and Kunkel, S. L. (1993) Cytokines and lung inflammation. *Thorax* **48**, 765–769.

104. Baggiolini, M., Walz, A., and Kunkel, S. L. (1989) Neutrophil-activating peptide-1/interleukin 8, a novel cytokine that activates neutrophils. *J. Clin. Invest.* **84**, 1045–1049.

105. Baggiolini, M., Dewald, B., and Walz, A. (1992) Interleukin-8 and related chemotactic cytokines, in *Inflammation: Basic Principles and Clinical Correlates* (Gallin, J. I., Goldstein, I. M., and Snyderman, R., eds.), Raven, New York.

106. Matsushima, K. and Oppenheim, J. J. (1989) Interleukin 8 and MCAF: Novel inflammatory cytokines inducible by IL–1 and TNF. *Cytokine* **1**, 2–13.

107. Miller, M. D. and Krangel, M. S. (1992) Biology and biochemistry of the chemokines: A family of chemotactic and inflammatory cytokines. *Crit. Rev. Immunol.* **12**, 17–46.

108. Maione, T. E., Gray, G. S., Petro, J., Hunt, A. J., Donner, A. L., Bauer, S. I., Carson, H. F., and Sharpe, R. J. (1990) Inhibition of angiogenesis by recombinant human platelet factor-4 and related peptides. *Science* **247(4938)**, 77–79.

109. Strieter, R. M., Kunkel, S. L., Elner, V. M., Martonyl, C. L., Koch, A. E., Polverini, P. J., and Elner, S. G. (1992) Interleukin-8: A corneal factor that induces neovascularization. *Am. J. Pathol.* **141**, 1279–1284.

110. Koch, A. E., Polverini, P. J., Kunkel, S. L., Harlow, L. A., DiPietro, L. A., Elner, V. M., Elner, S. G., and Strieter, R. M. (1992) Interleukin-8 (IL-8) as a macrophage-derived mediator of angiogenesis. *Science* **258**, 1798–1801.

111. Hu, D. E., Hori, Y., and Fan, T. P. D. (1993) Interleukin-8 stimulates angiogenesis in rats. *Inflammation* **17**, 135–143.

112. Strieter, R. M., Kunkel, S. L., Shanafelt, A. B., Arenberg, D. A., Koch, A. E., and Polverini, P. J. (1996) CXC chemokines in regulation of angiogenesis, in *Chemokines in Disease*. (Koch, A. E. and Strieter, R. M., eds.), R. G. Landes, Austin, TX, pp. 195–210.

113. Strieter, R. M., Polverini, P. J., Kunkel, S. L., Arenberg, D. A., Burdick, M. D., Kasper, J., Dzuiba, J., Van Damme, J., Walz, A., Marriott, D., Chan, S., Roczniak, S., and Shanafelt, A. (1995) The functional role of the ELR motif in CXC chemokine-mediated angiogenesis. *J. Biol. Chem.* **270(45)**, 27,348–27,357.

114. Luster, A. D., Greenberg, S. M., and Leder, P. (1995) The IP–10 chemokine binds to a specific cell surface heparan sulfate shared with platelet factor 4 and inhibits endothelial cell proliferation. *J. Exp. Med.* **182**, 219–232.

115. Angiolillo, A. L., Sgadari, C., Taub, D. T., Liao, F., Farber, J. M., Maheshwari, S., Kleinman, H. K., Reaman, G. H., and Tosato, G. (1995) Human interferon-inducible protein 10 is a potent inhibitor of angiogenesis in vivo. *J. Exp. Med.* **158**, 155–162.

116. Strieter, R. M., Kunkel, S. L., Arenberg, D. A., Burdick, M. D., and Polverini, P. J. (1995) Interferon gamma-inducible protein 10 (IP-10), a member of the C-X-C chemokine family, is an inhibitor of angiogenesis. *Biochem. Biophys. Res. Commun.* **210(1)**, 51–57.

117. Farber, J. M. (1993) HuMIG: a new member of the chemokine family of cytokines. *Biochem. Biophys. Res. Commun.* **192**, 223–230.

118. Farber, J. M. (1990) A macrophage mRNA selectively induced by gamma-interferon encodes a member of the platelet factor 4 family of cytokines. *Proc. Natl. Acad. Sci. USA* **87(14),** 5238–5242.

119. Boorsma, D. M., de Haan, P., Willemze, R., and Stoof, T. J. (1994) Human growth factor (huGRO), interleukin-8 (IL-8) and interferon-gamma-inducible protein (gamma-IP-10) gene expression in cultured normal human keratinocytes. *Arch. Dermatol. Res.* **286(8),** 471–475.

120. Gusella, G. L., Musso, T., Bosco, M. C., Espinoza-Delgado, I., Matsushima, K., and Varesio, L. (1993) IL-2 up-regulates but IFN-g suppresses IL-8 expression in human monocytes. *J. Immunol.* **151,** 2725–2732.

121. Schnyder-Candrian, S., Strieter, R. M., Kunkel, S. L., and Walz, A. (1995) Interferon-α and interferon-γ downregulate the production of interleukin-8 and ENA-78 in human monocytes. *J. Leuk. Biol.,* **57(6),** 929–935.

122. Strieter, R. M., Phan, S. H., Showell, H. J., Remick, D. G., Lynch, J. P., Genord, M., Raiford, C., Eskandari, M., Marks, R. M., and Kunkel, S. L. (1989) Monokine-induced neutrophil chemotactic factor gene expression in human fibroblasts. *J. Biol. Chem.* **264,** 10,621–10,626.

123. Standiford, T. J., Kunkel, S. L., Basha, M. A., Chensue, S. W., Lynch, J. P., III, Toews, G. B., Westwick, J., and Strieter, R. M. (1990) Interleukin-8 gene expression by a pulmonary epithelial cell line: A model for cytokine networks in the lung. *J. Clin. Invest.* **86,** 1945–1953.

124. Strieter, R. M., Kunkel, S. L., Showell, H., Phan, D. G. R. H., Ward, P. A., and Marks, R. M. (1989) Endothelial cell gene expression of a neutrophil chemotactic factor by TNF-a, LPS, and IL-1b. *Science* **243,** 1467–1469.

125. Kasahara, T., Mukaido, N., Yamashita, K., Yagisawa, H., Akahoshi, T., and Matsushima, K. (1991) IL-1 and TNF-alpha induction of IL-8 and monocyte chemotactic and activating factor (MCAF) mRNA expression in a human astrocytoma cell line. *Immunol.* **74,** 60–67.

126. Koch, A. E., Kunkel, S. L., Burrows, J. L., Evanoff, H. L., Haines, G. K., Pope, R. M., and Strieter, R. M. (1991) The synovial tissue macrophage as a source of the chemotactic cytokine interleukin-8. *J. Immunol.* **147,** 2187–2195.

127. Nickoloff, B. J., Karabin, G. D., Barker, J. W. C. N., Griffiths, C. E., Sarma, V., Mitra, R., Elder, J. T., Kunkel, S. L., and Dixit, V. M. (1991) Cellular localization of interleukin-8 and its inducer, tumor necrosis factor-alpha in psoriasis. *Am. J. Pathol.* **138,** 129–140.

128. Arenberg, D. A., Kunkel, S. L., Polverini, P. J., Glass, M., Burdick, M. D., and Strieter, R. M. (1996) Inhibition of interleukin-8 reduces tumorigenesis of human nonsmall cell lung cancer in SCID mice. *J. Clin. Invest.* **97(12),** 2792–2802.

129. Singh, R. K., Gutman, M., Radinsky, R., Bucana, C. D., and Fidler, I. J. (1994) Expression of interleukin 8 correlates with the metastatic potential of human melanoma cells in nude mice. *Cancer Res.* **54(12),** 3242–3247.

130. Nanney, L. B., Mueller, S. G., Bueno, R., Peiper, S. C., and Richmond, A. (1995) Distributions of melanoma growth stimulatory activity or growth-related gene and the interleukin-8 receptor type B in human wound repair. *Am. J. Pathol.* **147(5),** 1248–1260.

131. Richmond, A. and Thomas, H. G. (1988) Melanoma growth stimulatory activity: isolation from human melanoma tumors and characterization of tissue distribution. *J. Cell. Biochem.* **36,** 185–198.

132. Arenberg, D. A., Kunkel, S. L., Polverini, P. J., Morris, S. B., Burdick, M. D., Glass, M., Taub, D. T., Iannetoni, M. D., Whyte, R. I., and Strieter, R. M. (1996) Interferon-γ-inducible protein 10 (IP–10) is an angiostatic factor that inhibits human non-small cell lung cancer (NSCLC) tumorigenesis and spontaneous metastases. *J. Exp. Med.* **184(3),** 981–992.

133. Angiolillo, A. L., Sgadari, C., and Tosato, G. (1996) A role for the interferon-inducible protein 10 in inhibition of angiogenesis by interleukin-12. *Ann. NY Acad. Sci.* **795,** 158–167.

134. Sgadari, C., Angiolillo, A. L., and Tosato, G. (1996) Inhibition of angiogenesis by interleukin-12 is mediated by the interferon-inducible protein 10. *Blood* **87(9),** 3877–3882.

135. Sgadari, C., Farber, J. M., Angiolillo, A. L., Liao, F., Teruya-Feldstein, J., Burd, P. R., Yao, L., Gupta, G., Kanegane, C., and Tosato, G. (1997) Mig, the monokine induced by interferon-gamma, promotes tumor necrosis in vivo. *Blood* **89(8),** 2635–2643.

136. Moser, B., Schumacher, von Tschamer, V., Clark-Lewis, I., and Baggiolini, M. (1991) Neutrophil-activating peptide 2 and gro/melanoma growth-stimulatory activity interact with neutrophil-activating peptide 1/interleukin 8 receptors on human neutrophils. *J. Biol. Chem.* **266,** 10,666–10,671.

137. Lee, J., Horuk, R., Rice, G. C., Bennett, G. L., Camerato, T., and Wood, W. I. (1992) Characterization of two high affinity human interleukin-8 receptors. *J. Biol. Chem.* **267,** 16,283–16,287.

138. Arvanitakis, L., Geras-Raaka, E., Varma, A., Gershengorn, M. C., and Cesarman, E. (1997) Human herpesvirus KSHV encodes a constitutively active G-protein- coupled receptor linked to cell proliferation. *Nature* **385(6614),** 347–350 (see comments).

139. Loetscher, M., Gerber, B., Loetscher, P., Jones, S. A., Piali, L., Clark-Lewis, I., Baggiolini, M., and Moser, B. (1996) Chemokine receptor specific for IP-10 and Mig: structure, function, and expression in activated T-lymphocytes. *J. Exp. Med.* **184,** 963–969.

140. Gottlieb, A. B., Luster, A. D., Posnett, D. N., and Carter, D. M. (1988) Detection of a gamma interferon-induced protein IP-10 in psoriatic plaques. *J. Exp. Med.* **168(3),** 941–948.

141. Harris, E. D. (1976) Recent insights into the pathogenesis of the proliferative lesion in rheumatoid arthritis. *Arthritis Rheum.* **19,** 68.

142. Kimball, E. S. and Gross, J. L. (1991) Angiogenesis in pannus formation. *Agents Actions* **34(3–4),** 329–331.

143. Koch, A. E., Halloran, M. M., Hosaka, S., Shah, M. R., Haskell, C. J., Baker, S. K., Panos, R. J., Haines, G. K., Bennett, G. L., Pope, R. M., and Ferrara, N. (1996) Hepatocyte growth factor: a cytokine mediating endothelial migration in inflammatory arthritis. *Arthritis Rheum.* **39(9),** 1566–1575.

144. Koch, A. E., Harlow, L. A., Haines, G. K., Amento, E. P., Unemori, E. N., Wong, W. L., Pope, R. M., and Ferrara, N. (1994) Vascular endothelial growth factor. A cytokine modulating endothelial function in rheumatoid arthritis. *J. Immunol.* **152(8),** 4149–4156.

145. Tamargo, R. J., Bok, R. A., and Brem, H. (1991) Angiogenesis inhibition by minocycline. *Cancer Res.* **51(2),** 672–675.

146. Gilbertson-Beadling, S., Powers, E. A., Stamp-Cole, M., Scott, P. S., Wallace, T. L., Copeland, J., Petzold, G., Mitchell, M., Ledbetter, S., and Poorman, R. (1995) The tetracycline analogs minocycline and doxycycline inhibit angiogenesis in vitro by a nonmetalloproteinase-dependent mechanism. *Cancer Chemother. Pharmacol.* **36(5),** 418–424. (published erratum appears in *Cancer Chemother. Pharmacol.* (1995) **37(1–2),** 194.)

147. Tilley, B. C., Alarcon, G. S., Heyse, S. P., Trentham, D. E., Neuner, R., Kaplan, D. A., Clegg, D. O., Leisen, J. C., Buckley, L., Cooper, S. M. (1995) Minocycline in rheumatoid arthritis: A 48–week, double-blind, placebo- controlled trial. MIRA Trial Group. *Ann. Intern. Med.* **122(2),** 81–89 (see comments).

148. Turner-Warwick, M. (1963) Precapillary systemic-pulmonary anastomoses. *Thorax* **18,** 225–237.

149. Folkman, J., Watson, K., Ingber, D., and Hanahan, D. (1989) Induction of angiogenesis during the transition from hyperplasia to neoplasia. *Nature* **339,** 58–61.

150. Hanahan, D., Christofori, G., Naik, P., and Arbeit, J. (1996) Transgenic mouse models of tumour angiogenesis: The angiogenic switch, its molecular controls, and prospects for preclinical therapeutic models. *Eur. J. Cancer* **32A(14),** 2386–2393.

151. Good, D. J., Polverini, P. J., Rastinejad, F., Le Beau, M. M., Lemons, R. S., Frazier, W. A., and Bouck, N. P. (1990) A tumor suppressor-dependent inhibitor of angiogenesis is immunologically and functionally indistinguishable from a fragment of thrombospondin. *Proc. Natl. Acad. Sci. USA* **87(17),** 6624–6628.

152. Folkman, J. (1993) Tumor angiogenesis, in *Cancer Medicine,* vol. 1 (Holland, J. F., Kufe, D. W., Morton, D. L., and Weischelbaum, R. R., eds.), Lea & Febiger, Philadelphia, PA, pp. 153–170.

153. Folkman, J. and Klagsbrun, M. (1987) Angiogenic factors. *Science* **235,** 442–447.

154. Fidler, I. J. (1990) Critical factors in the biology of human cancer metastasis: Twenty-Eighth G. H. A. Clowes Memorial Award Lecture. *Cancer Res.* **50,** 6130–6138.

155. Holmgren, L., O'Reilly, M. S., and Folkman, J. (1995) Dormancy of micrometastases: Balanced proliferation and apoptosis in the presence of angiogenesis suppression. *Nat. Med.* **1(2),** 149–153 (see comments).

156. Folkman, J. (1995) Clinical applications of research on angiogenesis. *N. Engl. J. Med.* **333(26),** 1757–1763.

3

Update on Arachidonic Acid Cascade

Leukotrienes and Lipoxins in Disease Models

Jesper Z. Haeggström and Charles N. Serhan

Introduction

Biomembranes act as barriers to cellular compartments and serve as storage sites for precursors of rapidly generated, structurally diverse lipid-derived mediators (LMs). Cellular responses are accompanied by the rapid remodeling of membrane lipids, by activated lipases, with concomitant generation of bioactive lipids that can serve as both intra- and/or extracellular mediators. To qualify as an LM, the product of these pathways must act in a stereoselective fashion and be generated by cells and tissues in quantities that are commensurate with their potency and range of actions in vivo. The generation and release of extracellular LMs are generally cell-type specific as is the case with individual classes of eicosanoids, whereas the biosynthesis of key intracellular LMs such as diacylglycerol (DAG) or ceramide appear to be ubiquitous in signal transduction. Given the profile of bioactions of individual LMs and the cell types presently known to be involved in their formation, they are held to play essential roles in a wide range of processes involving cell–cell communication, including host defense, inflammation, ischemia-reperfusion, hemostasis, and other vascular events.

Activation of specific phospholipases within individual cell types via extracellular signals (i.e., autacoids including peptides, cytokines, and eicosanoids) during these multicellular processes is a critical early step in the biosynthesis of several structurally diverse LMs. These lipases include PLA_2, PLD, and PLC, which are each pivotal in signaling pathways. They can be activated either by specific cell surface (i.e., cytokine and/or seven transmembrane-spanning) receptors or by membrane perturbations such as in trauma or reperfusion injury. The LMs produced include free fatty acids and their oxygenated products (e.g., eicosanoids), lysophospholipids, platelet-activating factor (PAF), DAGs, phosphatidic acid (PtdOH), and ceramide. These individual groups of

From: *Molecular and Cellular Basis of Inflammation*
Edited by: C. N. Serhan and P. A. Ward © Humana Press Inc., Totowa, NJ

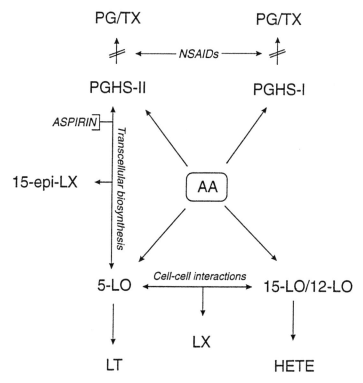

Fig. 1. Novel concepts in eicosanoid circuitry. Arachidonic acid, the central precursor molecule in eicosanoid formation, can be oxidized by PGHS-I or PGHS-II and further converted into pro- and anti-inflammatory PGs and TXs, reactions that can be blocked by nonsteroidal antiinflammatory drugs (NSAIDs). Alternatively, arachidonic acid can be oxidized by individual 5-, 12-, or 15-lipoxygenases (LO) to generate hydroxy fatty acids (HETE) and the proinflammatory LTs. In addition, 5-LO in conjunction with 15-/12-LO can produce anti-inflammatory LXs via cell–cell interactions. Finally, 15-epi-LX, which possess even stronger antiinflammatory properties, can be formed via the action of aspirin-treated PGHS-II.

LMs, some of which have extensive molecular diversity within their class, are each implicated as essential mediators in a variety of tissue and cell functions.

Generation of eicosanoids, which as a family include prostaglandins (PGs), thromboxanes (TXs), leukotrienes (LTs), and lipoxins (LXs), remains the focus of rational drug design targets, given their established roles in cell–cell communication and as mediators in inflammation and pathophysiologic events (Fig. 1). Key enzymes in these pathways were cloned and sequenced, and their subcellular organization was investigated. Unexpected findings implicate involvement of the nuclear membrane at the functional level and, perhaps, intracellular as well as nuclear roles for products of these enzymes. Several LM receptors were identified and cloned including those for PG, TX, LTB, and LXA, and results from transgenic and gene-deficient animals have provided intriguing new insights for several key enzymes and receptors. In addition, novel bioactive eicosanoids were discovered including the aspirin-triggered 15-epi-LXs and isoprostanes, which give new concepts to consider in the formation of and roles for

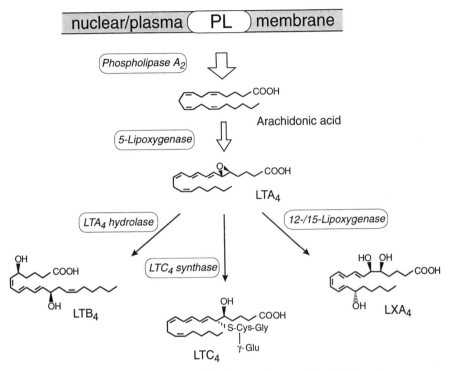

Fig. 2. Key enzymes, intermediates, and major products of the 5-LO pathway: generation of LTs and LXs. PL = phospholipids.

eicosanoids and the therapeutic actions of traditional NSAIDs. When combined, these findings indicate that LMs such as eicosanoids play critical and essential roles in both intracellular signal transduction and cell–cell communication within the microenvironment, and continue to be important biosynthetic pathways to be considered in rational development for novel therapeutic agents (Figs. 1 and 2).

Cytokines exert a dramatic multilevel impact in both regulating enzymes in individual LM pathways as well as in generating LM essential for their actions. Thus, there are many interrelationships between the bioprocesses evoked by cytokine and LM networks that can be relevant within the cellular microenvironment. For example, cytokines (1) stimulate *de novo* biosynthesis of LM; (2) induce the enzymes that regulate LM biosynthesis, degradation (inactivation), or actions (e.g., appearance of receptors); and (3) act synergistically with a given LM to exert bioactions. In addition *individual* or *groups* of certain eicosanoids can likewise display a similar multilevel impact in the biosynthesis and actions of cytokines. It follows that, depending on the class of eicosanoid generated, they can initiate "stimulatory or inhibitory" circuits that translate to either pro- or anti-inflammatory programs at the tissue level. Detailed knowledge of the cellular and biochemical pathways involved in the eicosanoid cascade and its cellular networks is evolving and, in many settings, is unknown since new members are still being discovered in each class of bioactive molecules. Here, the authors provide an overview and update of progress in elucidating molecular mechanisms in eicosanoid formation and actions with emphasis on the cellular events in inflammation.

Major Phospholipases Involved in Eicosanoid Production

The precursors of eicosanoids are stored in cell membranes and must be released and enzymatically transformed to generate bioactive molecules. Phospholipase A_2 plays a major role in this signaling event in most tissues and cell types studied to date. Each major group of phospholipase contains multiple family members that carry out a similar reaction but are differentially regulated and can act on different substrates, thus providing alternative pathways for the highly controlled process of phospholipid degradation and metabolism. The properties and regulation of PLC isozymes have recently been reviewed and will not be covered (*see* refs. *1* and *2*). The initial products of PLA_2, free fatty acid and lysophospholipid, are also regulatory molecules, and are precursors of eicosanoids and PAF *(3)*. Mammalian cells contain multiple structurally diverse PLA_2 enzymes *(4)*. The most extensively characterized are the secretory (also termed low molecular weight) PLA_2 enzymes ($sPLA_2$). These enzymes are structurally related to the two groups of $sPLA_2$ present in snake venoms *(4)*. The two groups are distinguished by differences in primary structure as well as distribution of disulfide bonds. Mammalian pancreatic $sPLA_2$ is a Group I enzyme, whereas Group II $sPLA_2$, which was first identified in synovial fluid and platelets, is now known to be present in a wide range of cell types. $sPLA_2$s require millimolar Ca^{2+} for catalytic activity and show no specificity for acyl chains. There is considerable interest in Group II $sPLA_2$ because its levels are found to be increased in serum and inflammatory exudates in diseases such as septic shock and rheumatoid arthritis *(4)*. Group II PLA_2 is implicated as an acute phase protein and may play a role in host defense. Cytokines, such as IL-1, TNF, and IL-6, induce increased expression of Group II $sPLA_2$ in a variety of cells that correlates with increased PG production, both of which can be suppressed by glucocorticoids *(4)*. Group II $sPLA_2$ plays a role in mediating arachidonic acid release and PG production in a $P388D_1$ macrophage line treated with lipopolysaccharide (LPS) and PAF *(5)*. The mechanism whereby Group II $sPLA_2$ mediates arachidonic acid release is not fully elucidated *(4)*.

Cytosolic PLA_2 ($cPLA_2$) is the first arachidonic acid-selective PLA_2 identified, and it is now recognized as an important enzyme (85 kDa) for mediating agonist-induced arachidonic acid release *(6)*. In addition to PLA_2 activity, $cPLA_2$ exhibits relatively high lysophospholipase activity and can completely deacylate diacylphospholipids, thus preventing accumulation of potentially toxic lysophospholipids *(7)*. The active site Ser-228 of $cPLA_2$ is essential for both PLA_2 and lysophospholipase catalytic activities *(8)*. $cPLA_2$ contains an N-terminal, Ca^{2+}, and phospholipid binding (CaLB) domain that is responsible for Ca^{2+}-dependent membrane association. $cPLA_2$ requires micromolar levels of Ca^{2+} for PLA_2 activity *(6)*.

Mammalian cells also contain calcium-independent forms of PLA_2 ($iPLA_2$) *(9)*. Myocardium is rich in $iPLA_2$, and the purified enzyme is a 40-kDa protein that exhibits specificity for plasmalogen substrates, the predominant form of phospholipid in myocardium *(9)*. This $iPLA_2$ exists as a high-mol-wt complex composed of the 40-kDa catalytic subunit and an 85-kDa regulatory subunit homologous to phosphofructokinase. ATP enhances PLA_2 activity of the complex, but has no effect on the purified 40-kDa subunit *(9)*. Bromoenol lactone, a cell permeant mechanism-based inhibitor for $iPLA_2$, was used to suggest that $iPLA_2$ is responsible for arachidonic acid release in smooth muscle and pancreatic islet cells. An 80-kDa $iPLA_2$ was purified from the $P388D_1$ macrophage line *(9)*. This $iPLA_2$ is also inhibited by bromoenol lactone, and exists as a

Table 1
Molecular Properties of Enzymes in Eicosanoid Biosynthesis[a]

	Protein size (no. of amino acids)[b]	Prosthetic group	Gene size (kb)	Exon no.	Potential *cis*-elements of promoter region	Chromosomal location	KO[d] mice
PGHS-1	598 [576][c]	Heme	≈22	11	Sp1, AP-2, GATA-1	9	+
PGHS-2	603 [587][c]	Heme	>8.3	10	TATA, CRE, NF-κB, Sp1, AP-2	1	+
5-LO	673	Fe	>82	14	Sp1, AP-2, NF-kB	10	+
12-LO	662	Fe	≈17	14	Sp1, AP-2, GRE	17	—
15-LO (I)	661	Fe	—	—	—	17	
15-LO (II)	675	Fe	—	—	—	—	—
FLAP	160	—	>31	5	TATA, AP-2, GRE	13	+
LTA$_4$ hydrolase	610	Zn	>35	19	XRE, AP-2	12	—
LTC$_4$ synthase	149	—	≈2.5	5	Sp1, AP-1, AP-2	5	—

[a]Biochemical data refers to human enzymes and have been collected from refs. *11, 15, 16, 26, 27, 29–31, 33, 35, 36, 43, 47* and references therein.

[b]The number of amino acids in the polypeptide chain, excluding the initial methionine. Values within parenthesis represent processed proteins after removal of signal peptides.

[c]The native enzyme is glycosylated, which causes an increase in M_r in SDS-PAGE.

[d]KO = so called knockout mice generated by targeted gene disruption.

370-kDa oligomer, but does not appear to contain phosphofructokinase. Unlike the 40 kDa iPLA$_2$, purified P388D$_1$ enzyme retains the ability to be regulated by ATP. The iPLA$_2$ in P388D$_1$ cells is suggested to function in resting cells to regulate basal acyl group turnover. Thus, this enzyme provides the lysophospholipid acceptor needed for basal esterification of arachidonic acid into phospholipid *(9)*.

Molecular Biology of Enzymes in the Arachidonic Acid Cascade

Key enzymes involved in the formation of PGs, TXs, LTs, and LXs (*see* Figs. 1 and 2) are cloned and sequenced. For some of them, the complete gene structure and promoter are characterized (Table 1). This section highlights advances in the understanding of the expression, regulation, and mechanism of key enzymes in eicosanoid biosynthesis.

Prostaglandin Endoperoxide Synthases

Prostaglandin endoperoxide synthase (PGHS), the well-known target of NSAIDs, exists in two isoforms that are quite similar in terms of overall amino acid identities (~60%), catalytic properties, and substrate specificity *(10)*. PGHS-I is currently regarded as a constitutive enzyme, required for basal formation of PGs whereas PGHS-II can be induced by a variety of agents, such as cytokines, growth factors, and tumor promoters. Glucocorticoids can reverse induction of PGHS-II. PGHS-I is expressed in gastric mucosa, and the gastric lesions frequently accompanying the use of NSAIDs are believed to result from reduced formation of cytoprotective PGs. The current explosion of new information on these two enzymes is reviewed in ref. *11*. Interestingly, PGHS-I and PGHS-II exhibit different profiles of inhibition when tested in vitro against a wide range of NSAIDs. The possibility of finding a selective PGHS-II inhibitor with all the beneficial analgesic and antipyretic properties of classical NSAIDs, such as aspirin, but without their negative side effects, has focused attention on this area of eicosanoid research. Indeed, several pharmaceutical companies have already presented compounds with promising inhibitory profiles and biological properties *(12)*. Furthermore, the possible involvement of PGHS-I or PGHS-II in the development of various intestinal neoplasias and the well-documented preventive effects of NSAIDs on colon cancer have extended the interest in NSAIDs and their potential use in cancer therapy or prevention *(13)*.

Enzymes in LT Biosynthesis

In the LT cascade, all key enzymes are purified, cloned, and sequenced (Fig. 2, Table 1). Computer-assisted sequence comparisons have identified segments conserved among isoenzymes and also established unexpected relationships among proteins with a low degree of overall homology. Several conserved segments, including six histidines, have been identified among LOs, and a so-called Src homology-3 *(SH3)* motif is present in the primary structure of 5-LO *(14)* (*see below*). Another striking example is the discovery of a zinc binding motif in LTA_4 hydrolase, similar to those present in certain zinc metalloproteases and aminopeptidases *(15)*. As a result, LTA_4 hydrolase was found to contain 1 mol zinc/mol protein and also to exhibit a previously unknown peptide cleaving activity (Fig. 3). In addition, significant sequence similarities are present between LTC_4 synthase and FLAP, both of which are membrane proteins of similar molecular mass *(16)*. Interestingly, it was recently shown that both of these proteins are members of a superfamily of microsomal glutathione S-transferases (MGST) *(17)*. One member of this family, MGST-II, is expressed in endothelial cells, exhibits significant LTC_4 synthase activity, and probably accounts for most of the cysteinyl LTs formed during transcellular metabolism of LTA_4 along the PMNL/endothelial cell axis *(18)*.

Using site-directed mutagenesis, some molecular properties of the respective active sites have been unraveled. For instance, three out of six conserved histidines in 5-LO, namely, His-367, His-372, and His-550, are required for 5-LO activity, and only the latter two appear to bind iron. From the crystal structure of soybean LO-1, the C-terminal Ile, conserved among LOs including 5-LO, was also identified as an iron ligand. Glu-376 and Asn-554 are critical for 5-LO activity, although their precise role in catalysis is unknown *(19)*.

Concerning LTA_4 hydrolase, mutagenetic replacements demonstrate that the catalytic zinc is complexed to His-295, His-299, and Glu-318 (Fig. 3). Exchange of the conserved Glu-296 abrogates its peptidase activity but spares the epoxide hydrolase activity, indicating a critical role of Glu-296, presumably as a general base in peptidolysis *(15)*. These data also demonstrated that the two enzyme activities are exerted via overlapping active sites (Fig. 3). Sequence comparisons followed by mutational analysis of conserved residues/regions also identified Tyr-383 as a possible proton donor in the peptidase reaction *(20)*. Interestingly, Tyr-383 was also present in a heneicosapeptide spanning Leu-365 to Lys-385, which was shown to specifically bind LTA_4 during catalysis and suicide inactivation *(21)* (Fig. 3). However, amino acid sequence analysis of a modified form of this peptide indicated that the LT epoxide reacts with Tyr-378, rather than with Tyr-383. Further mutational analysis of residues within this region demonstrated that Tyr-378 is indeed a major structural determinant for binding of LTA_4 to the protein during suicide inactivation. Thus, exchange of Tyr-378 for a Phe yielded a recombinant enzyme that was resistant to inactivation and displayed a 2.5-fold increase in substrate turnover *(22)*. In addition, the mutant converted

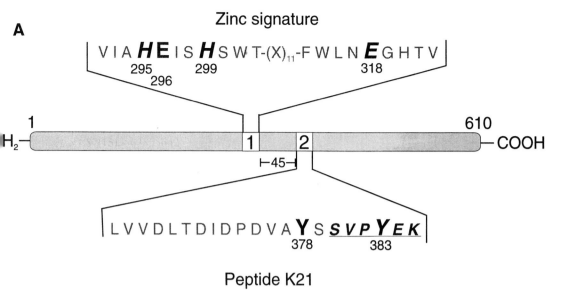

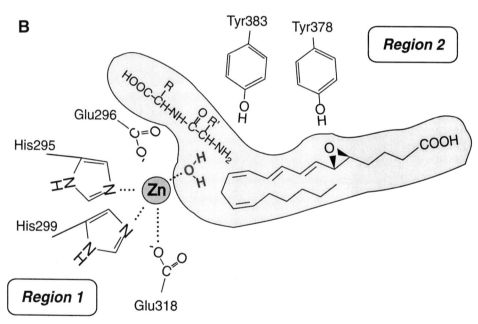

Fig. 3. Structure-function relationships in LTA$_4$ hydrolase. **(A)** Two catalytic domains are present in the central portion of the polypeptide chain. The first domain is represented by the zinc binding signature with the metal ligands His-295, His-299, and Glu-318, as well as Glu-296, which is essential for the peptidase activity. The second domain corresponds to the proteolytic fragment peptide K21 and appears to be functionally centered around Tyr-378 and Tyr-383, primarily involved in the enzyme's suicide inactivation and peptidase activity, respectively. Tyr-383 may act as a proton donor and is located within a putative proton donor motif (italics and underlined). For details, *see text*. **(B)** Model for the active-site structure of LTA$_4$ hydrolase.

LTA$_4$, not only into LTB$_4$ but also into the isomer Δ^6-*trans*-Δ^8-*cis*-LTB$_4$, which in turn suggests that Tyr-378 may play a role in the formation of the correct double-bond geometry during the conversion of LTA$_4$ into LTB$_4$ *(23)*. A careful analysis of the catalytic properties of three mutants of LTA$_4$ hydrolase in which Tyr-383 (the potential proton donor in Fig. 3) has been exchanged for Phe, His, or Gln unexpectedly revealed that they all could produce large quantities of $5(S),6(S)$-7,9-*trans*-11,14-*cis*-eicosatetraenoic acid [$5(S),6(S)$-DHETE], in addition to the expected product LTB$_4$ *(24)*. The stereochemical configuration of the vicinal diol indicates an S$_N$1 type of reaction in its formation, which, by definition, involves a carbocation intermediate. Since the mutants could make both $5(S),6(S)$-DHETE and LTB$_4$, it appears very likely that hydrolysis of LTA$_4$ into LTB$_4$, catalyzed by LTA$_4$ hydrolase, proceeds according to the same mechanism. Moreover, previous work in the author's laboratory has shown that xenobiotic soluble epoxide hydrolase (sEH) utilizes LTA$_4$ as substrate to produce $5(S),6(R)$-DHETE, an epimer at C-6 to the product formed by the mutants of Tyr-383. Hence, the authors' results also suggest a functional and structural relationship between LTA$_4$ hydrolase and xenobiotic epoxide hydrolases.

Sequence comparisons among various members of the LTC$_4$ synthase/FLAP/MGST-II gene family (*vide supra*) have identified conserved residues of potential functional importance. Further mutational analysis has suggested that Arg-51 and Tyr-93 in human LTC$_4$ synthase are both essential for catalysis. The guanidinium moiety of Arg-51 is thus believed to open the epoxide, whereas Tyr-93 will act as a base to generate a GSH thiolate anion for attack at C-6 of LTA$_4$ *(25)*.

Gene Structures and Promoters of Enzymes in Eicosanoid Biosynthesis

Several genes and corresponding promoters are characterized (Table 1). PGHS-I and PGHS-II genes are divided into 11 and 10 exons, respectively. In agreement with the presumed functional dichotomy between PGHS-I and PGHS-II, the genes are located on different chromosomes (1 and 9) and the promoters exhibit distinct features *(26)*. The promoter of human PGHS-I lacks a canonical TATA box, but instead is rich in GC, typical of a so-called house keeping gene. By contrast, the PGHS-II promoter contained a TATA box and several potential regulatory elements, including CRE, NF-κB, Sp1, and AP2 sites.

The gene for human 5-LO spans more than 82 kb of DNA, consists of 14 exons, and is located next to chromosome 10 *(27)*. Regarding PGHS-I, the promoter region lacks a TATA or a CCAT box but contains multiple GC boxes (potential Sp1 sites) typical for housekeeping genes, which is surprising since 5-LO appears to be expressed exclusively in bone-marrow–derived cells. In the region –176 to –146 bp upstream of the ATG translation start site, the promoter contains five Sp1 sites in tandem. Interestingly, a naturally occurring polymorphism has been demonstrated in this region consisting of +1, –1, and –2 Sp1/Egr-1 sites, variants that may be accompanied by differences in gene transcription in vivo *(28)*. The FLAP gene spans >31 kb on chromosome 13 and is divided into 5 exons *(29)*. Its 5'-flanking region contains a TATA box and a possible GRE and AP2 binding site. The LTC$_4$ synthase gene, on the other hand, is located on chromosome 5 and spans only approx 2.5 kb, but its structure is quite similar to that of the FLAP gene in that it contains five exons of similar sizes and exon–intron borders *(30)*. The promoter region of the LTC$_4$ synthase gene contains several potential *cis*-elements including Sp1, AP1, and AP2. Like the 5-LO and FLAP genes, the gene for LTA$_4$ hydrolase is large (>35 kb) and contains 19 exons, the smallest of which consists of only 24 bp *(31)*. Surprisingly, components of the zinc-binding motif are split between exons 10 and 11. An alternatively spliced short form of LTA_4 hydrolase mRNA has been identified in several different cell types *(32)*. This mRNA was formed by deletion of exon 17 (83 bp), leading to a shift in the reading frame and a preterminal stop after 22 amino acids. The short message predicts the expression of an enzyme with a truncated carboxy terminus and a calculated molecular mass of 59 kDa. The presence of this short LTA_4 hydrolase in vivo has not yet been reported, and its biochemical properties remain to be determined. The complete gene encoding LTA_4 hydrolase is located on chromosome 12, and the 5'-flanking region contains two XRE, potential *cis*-elements in the regulation of transcription. It is clear that a more detailed gene promoter analysis is required to gain a better understanding of constitutive, induced, and cell-specific expression not only of LTA_4 hydrolase but of all enzymes in eicosanoid biosynthesis.

A Second Human 15S-Lipoxygenase

Three major types of LOs exist in mammals, classified on the basis of their positional specificity for incorporation of oxygen in the substrate arachidonic acid, i.e., 5-, 12-, and 15-LO (*see* Table 1). In certain species, two types of 12-LO have been described, usually referred to as the "platelet" and "leukocyte" type, respectively. In humans, only the platelet type of 12-LO has been identified and, thus, according to the current dogma, only three human LOs have been thought to exist (i.e., 5-, 12-, and 15-LO). However, in a recent study by Brash et al., a previously unrecognized human 15-LO was described *(33)*. It was expressed in certain epithelial cells of prostate, hair follicles, lung, and cornea but not in several other cell types, e.g., peripheral blood leukocytes, which typically express 15-LO activity. The cDNA encodes a protein comprised of 676 amino acids with a calculated molecular mass of 76 kDa. Surprisingly, the primary structure is only about 40% identical with the amino acid sequences of the known 5-, 12-, and 15-LO. In addition, the enzyme converts arachidonic acid exclusively into 15S-HPETE, as opposed to the regular 15-LO, which also makes small amounts of 12S-HPETE. The unique structure, pattern of expression, and catalytic properties of this 15-LO strongly indicate that it has distinct physiological functions that are yet to be determined. Most likely the presence of another isoform of 15-LO will result in intense efforts to find analogous isoenzymes corresponding to other LO (12- and 5-LO) activities. Given the diversity of products within the eicosanoid cascade and their wide range of functions, it is not surprising that additional isoenzymes of LOs will be uncovered that display distinct physiological roles.

Eicosanoids in Cell Function

Two Functionally Different Prostanoid Biosynthetic Systems

PGHS-I and PGHS-II are membrane-bound enzymes; however, in murine 3T3 cells and in human and bovine endothelial cells, PGHS-II is twice as abundant in the nuclear envelope as compared to the endoplasmic reticulum, whereas PGHS-I is in equal amounts in the two compartments *(34)*. PGHS-I is mostly functional in the endoplasmic reticulum whereas PGHS-II activity is mainly detected in the nucleus. These findings, in conjunction with the differences in gene expression and earlier observations that PGHS-I and PGHS-II utilize different subcellular sources of arachidonate, suggest that the two isozymes represent separate and independently operating PG biosynthetic systems. According to this hypothesis, PGHS-I produces PG constitutively for secretion as extracellular mediators, and PGHS-II would be active only under certain circumstances to produce PG at, or within, the nucleus to possibly influence processes such as cell division, growth, and differentiation.

Mouse lines that do not express either PGHS-I or PGHS-II were developed by targeted gene disruption *(35,36)*. PGHS-I (–/–) mice exhibit reduced fertility, platelet aggregability, and sensitivity to arachidonic acid–induced ear inflammation, but no apparent gastric or kidney pathology. Interestingly, PGHS-II–deficient mice give normal inflammatory responses with phorbol ester or exogenous arachidonic acid, but exhibit marked pathological changes in their kidneys and an increased incidence of suppurative peritonitis. Although some of these exciting results should be interpreted with caution, they do agree with the view that PGHS-I and PGHS-II are two distinct prostanoid biosynthetic systems with separate biological functions for their products. Further studies with these "knockout" animals will help clarify the role of these enzymes in a number of physiological and pathological processes.

Leukotriene Biosynthesis via a Complex Assembled at the Nuclear Membrane

In intact leukocytes, 5-LO becomes activated and translocates from cytosol to membranes in response to calcium, a process accompanied by catalysis and enzyme inactivation *(29)*. Cellular 5-LO activity is dependent on the small membrane protein FLAP, which presumably transfers arachidonic acid to 5-LO. Unexpectedly, it was discovered that FLAP is localized to the nuclear envelope of resting and activated human neutrophils and that 5-LO, on cell activation, translocated from cytosol to the same compartment. Further analysis revealed that 5-LO can also be present in the nucleus of resting cells associated with the nuclear euchromatin, a site from which it translocates to the nuclear envelope *(37)*. In a recent report, 5-LO translocation was associated with leukocyte functional responses such as activation and adherence *(38)*. However, the subcellular distribution of 5-LO and its directional migration in response to activation and Ca^{2+} mobilization appears to differ among species and cell types *(39)*. 5-LO has been shown to associate with growth factor receptor-binding protein 2 (Grb2), an "adaptor" protein for tyrosine kinase–mediated cell signaling, through SH3 domain interactions. SH3 interactions regulate the assembly of protein complexes involved in cell signaling and cytoskeletal organization, and may form the molecular basis for 5-LO translocation and compartmentalization. Cytosolic PLA_2 also translocates to the nuclear membrane on cell stimulation, and LTC_4 synthase apparently resides at the same site *(39–41)*.

Together these findings imply that LT biosynthesis is executed by a complex of enzymes assembled at the nuclear membrane. This conclusion, in turn, suggests that these enzymes and their products may have additional, intracellular/intranuclear functions, perhaps related to signal transduction or gene regulation. Moreover, a complex network of transport mechanisms must exist to make possible the intracellular trafficking of these lipids and proteins. In this context, it is of interest to note that LTB_4 has been shown to act as a ligand to PPARα, a subclass of the nuclear hormone receptor family. Since these receptors signal upregulation of peroxisomal enzymes and are believed to participate in the regulation of fatty acid metabolism, coupling of LTB_4 to PPARα may increase the catabolism and thereby reduce the bioavailability of this potent lipid mediator *(42)*.

5-LO was also inactivated by gene targeting *(43)*. 5-LO–deficient mice are more resistant to lethal effects of shock induced by PAF and also show a marked reduction in the ear inflammatory response to exogenous arachidonic acid but not to phorbol ester. Interestingly, the inflammatory response induced by arachidonic acid could be virtually eliminated by the PGHS-inhibitor indomethacin in 5-LO–deficient mice, but not in normal animals, suggesting links between the PGHS systems and 5-LO pathways during inflammatory reactions *(44)*. It has also been shown that 5-LO null mice are more susceptible to infections with *Klebsiella pneumoniae* in line with a role for 5-LO and its products in antimicrobial host defense *(45)*. Moreover, 5-LO–deficient mice exhibited a reduced airway reactivity in response to methacholine and produced lower levels of serum immunoglobulins *(46)*.

The role of LTs as inflammatory mediators has also been corroborated from studies of FLAP-deficient mice. Like the 5-LO–deficient mice, these animals showed a blunted response to topical arachidonic acid, had increased resistance to PAF-induced shock, and responded with less edema in zymosan-induced peritonitis *(47)*. Interestingly, the severity of collagen-induced arthritis was substantially reduced in FLAP (−/−) mice, indicating a role for LTs in this model of inflammation *(48)*.

Cytokines That Regulate LT and LX Biosynthesis

A complex and functionally redundant signaling array of cytokines is generated in vivo at sites of inflammation that exert a regulatory action in the biosynthetic eicosanoid routes, particularly within the local milieu. These involve crosstalk between cells and crosstalk within the signaling pathways they evoke. A well-known example is IL-1 stimulation of PGE_2 formation. IL-1 and TNF each induce $sPLA_2$, $cPLA_2$, and PGHS-II in a wide range of cell types. GM-CSF and IL-3 induce 5-LO in human monocytes *(49)*, and GM-CSF *primes* neutrophils for the generation of both PAF and 5-LO products. In pre-B-lymphocytes, several factors, which may prove to be related to cytokines, regulate the expression of $cPLA_2$, PGHS-II, 5-LO, and FLAP *(50)*. IL-4 and IL-13 each induce 15-LO in monocytes *(51)*. At the functional level, LTs and LXs (at subnanomolar concentrations) modulate growth of human myeloid progenitors in the presence of GM-CSF *(52)*. Thus, an individual cytokine can change the profile of intracellular LMs and eicosanoids released by a specific cell type or those formed during transcellular biosynthesis. Only limited information is available for cytokines *(49–54)* that specifically induce key LM enzymes in vitro. It is likely that cells in vivo are exposed to several cytokines simultaneously, which together can alter a profile of LMs that in themselves represents a different constellation in acute vs chronic events. The greatest portion of these interactions between cytokines and LMs remains to be elucidated.

Molecular Characterization of PG and LT Seven-Transmembrane Spanning Receptors

Eicosanoids are autacoids and act on other cells in the immediate environment to produce a variety of biological responses. These bioactivities are elicited via specific cell surface receptors coupled to different signaling pathways, depending on the agonist and cell type in question. For prostanoids, i.e., PGs, TXs, and prostacyclins, our current understanding of the receptor biology has increased tremendously over the past decade, owing to the pioneering work by Narumiya et al. In 1989 they purified the TXA_2 receptor from human platelets *(55)* and later cloned it from human placenta *(56)*, which revealed that this receptor is G-protein coupled, contains seven transmembrane domains, and belongs to the rhodopsin-type superfamily of receptors. These initial studies paved the way for detailed molecular investigations of prostanoid receptors. Within only a few years, no less than eight types and subtypes of mouse prostanoid receptors had been cloned and characterized. By homology cloning, the corresponding human receptors were cloned and characterized as well *(57)*. From studies of the molecular properties and structure-function relationships, it was revealed that receptor isoforms may be created through alternative splicing *(58)*. Thus, variants may differ only at their intracellular carboxyl tail, in the region after the seventh transmembrane domain, which in turn may lead to important functional consequences. For instance, it was shown that such splice variants may couple to different G-proteins and utilize different signal transduction pathways *(58)*. These isoforms may also differ in their efficacy to bind G proteins or in their sensitivity to agonist-induced desensitization *(59,60)*. Moreover, in a recent study, construction of chimeric receptors was used to identify domain(s) that confer ligand-binding specificity *(61)*.

More recently, receptor-deficient mice have been produced by targeted gene disruption. The biological properties of such "knockout" animals have provided new insights into the role of prostanoids, and their cognate receptors, in several physiological as well as pathophysiological conditions. Thus, female mice lacking the $PGF_{2\alpha}$ receptor showed impaired parturition owing to a lack of response to oxytocin *(62)*. Apparently signaling via the $PGF_{2\alpha}$ receptor induces luteolysis and cessation of progesterone formation, which in turn upregulates the levels of mRNA for the oxytocin receptor, a prerequisite for oxytocin sensitivity. Whether this endocrine loop also plays the same role in species other than the mouse remains to be determined. The phenotype of mice lacking the TXA_2 receptor included reduced platelet aggregation in response to low-dose thrombin or collagen and prolonged bleeding times *(63)*. Furthermore, aortic rings from these animals did not contract when exposed to a TXA_2 agonist. The homozygous (–/–) animals were also resistant to arachidonic acid-induced platelet aggregation and exhibited reduced mortality following challenge with this agent. Taken together these biological properties corroborate the authors' previous notion that TXA_2 is an important mediator of vasoconstriction, platelet aggregation, and hemostasis. On the other hand, mice lacking the PGI_2 receptor exhibited an increased susceptibility to thrombosis *(64)*, as one would expect from the known ability of PGI_2 to counteract the effects of TXA_2 and to inhibit platelet aggregation. Interestingly several inflammatory and pain responses were blunted in these animals, and were in fact equal to those of wild-type animals treated with indomethacin. Hence, in addition to its established role as an antithrombotic agent, PGI_2 appears to be an important, hitherto unrecognized, mediator of inflammation and pain. Moreover, inhibition of its biosynthesis may, at least in part, explain the antiphlogistic and analgesic properties of NSAIDs.

Much less is known about the surface receptors for LTs, and only recently the receptor for LTB_4 was cloned and characterized *(65)*. Like the prostanoid receptors, the LTB_4 receptor is G protein coupled and contains seven transmembrane domains. Receptor mRNA is expressed particularly in leukocytes but also in bone marrow, lymph nodes, thymus, and spleen *(66)*. Computer-assisted sequence comparisons showed that the LTB_4 receptor is distantly related to certain somatostatin receptors as well as some of the chemoattractant and chemokine receptors, e.g., those that bind and respond to *f*MLP, LXA_4 (vide infra; Fig. 8), and C5a *(65,66)*. The LTB_4 receptor was obtained from the retinoic acid-differentiated HL-60 cells that were also used to obtain the human myeloid

LXA$_4$ receptor *(67–69)*. Note that this LTB$_4$ receptor was originally an orphan receptor and was later shown to respond as a purinoreceptor *(65)*. Evidently, we are just beginning to understand the biology of the LT receptors, and in the near future we will probably see a rapid development in their molecular characterization, which, among many things, will help delineate the physiological as well as pathophysiological role of LTs.

Transcellular Biosynthesis and Cell–Cell Interactions

In addition to cell-specific biosynthesis, eicosanoids can be formed via transcellular pathways, which may amplify the formation of a given compound or result in products that neither of the participating cell types can generate alone. LTA$_4$, e.g., is exported from activated leukocytes for conversion to LTB$_4$, cysLTs, and LX by a variety of cell types *(70)*. Interestingly, not only intact cells but also cell fragments may participate in transcellular biosynthesis of eicosanoids. Thus, platelet microparticles, formed by microvesicular shedding, were recently shown to influence the local environment via bioactive eicosanoids formed by transcellular metabolism of arachidonic acid *(71)*.

Recruitment of circulating phagocytes to a site of inflammation involves a series of cell–cell interactions and a complex interplay of factors including adhesion molecules, cytokines, lipid mediators, nitric oxide, and chemotactic peptides. Some of the interrelationships in this network have been dissected, especially concerning the triad eicosanoids—cytokines—adhesion molecules, and their role is illustrated here in kidney autoimmune and inflammatory diseases.

Actions of Leukotrienes in Acute Glomerulonephritis

In the kidney, LTB$_4$ stimulates adhesion of PMN to glomerular EC, apparently via a CD11/CD18-dependent mechanism, and this response is augmented if neutrophils are primed with GM-CSF and if EC are activated with TNF-α *(70)*. Cysteinyl LTs exert a number of pathophysiological effects on renal function, such as proteinuria and glomerular hemodynamic abnormalities. Translated to the pathogenesis of glomerulonephritis, LTB$_4$ appears to be involved in leukocyte infiltration and cysLTs in the hemodynamic and functional impairments *(72)*.

Cell Adhesion Promotes Transcellular Biosynthesis

In the kidney, the principal source of LTs and LXs appears to be activated leukocytes, both directly and via transcellular routes. Costimulation of PMN and glomerular EC leads to increased biosynthesis of LTC$_4$, an effect more pronounced if PMN are primed with GM-CSF. Likewise, transcellular biosynthesis of LXs, involving platelet-PMN interactions, is demonstrable in immune complex glomerulonephritis *(70)*.

Cell adhesion via selectins and integrins in conjunction with their respective cognate carbohydrate and immunoglobulin-like receptors strongly influences transcellular biosynthesis of eicosanoids. For example, biosynthesis of LTC$_4$ in coincubations of PMN and glomerular EC is inhibited by monoclonal antibodies against leukocyte L-selectin and the integrin β$_2$-chain CD18. Also, LX biosynthesis via platelet-PMN interactions during immune complex glomerulonephritis is disrupted by antibodies against P-selectin, an important component of platelet-neutrophil adhesion *(70)*. Hence, leukocyte adhesion promotes transcellular biosynthesis of both LTs and LXs, probably by approximating lipid bilayers and facilitating transfer of the epoxide intermediate LTA_4 during cell–cell interactions.

Clinical Impact and Drug Development

Pharmacological intervention in LT biosynthesis and action is now possible at several levels, and some compounds are already marketed as antiasthmatic drugs. To date the most promising are 5-LO inhibitors and LT-receptor antagonists. Direct inhibitors of 5-LO may be iron chelators, exemplified by Zileuton (Abbott) or competitive inhibitors such as ICI D2138 (Zeneca), whereas Montelukast (Merck) and Accolate (Zeneca), are $CysLT_1$ receptor antagonists. Alternatively, inhibitors may be targeted against FLAP and 5-LO translocation, e.g., MK886, MK0591 (Merck), and Bay X1005 (Bayer). Attempts to develop inhibitors of distal enzymes in the LT cascade has just begun. Thus, LTA_4 hydrolase can be inhibited by bestatin and captopril, and more potent and selective compounds, effective as inhibitors of LTB_4 biosynthesis in intact human PMNL, have recently been synthesized. In particular, an α-keto-β-amino ester, thiolamine, and amino hydroxamic acid have proven effective against both purified enzyme and whole cells *(73,74)*. Perhaps the most interesting and promising inhibitors of LTA_4 hydrolase were recently presented by Searle. In particular, SC-57461, *N*-methyl-*N*-[3-[4-(phenylmethyl)-phenoxy]propyl]-β-alanine, blocked ionophore-induced LTB_4 production in human whole blood with an IC_{50} of only 49 n*M* *(75)*. Notably, this compound was orally active and showed very promising results in an animal model of colitis *(76)*.

Introduction to LX

It is now well established that two classes of eicosanoids, namely LTs and PGs, constitute mediators with important actions relevant to pathobiology of human airway inflammation as well as vascular events, and may play new physiologic roles as regulators of human myelopoiesis *(52, 77)*. There is increasing evidence that administration of pharmacologic agents that inhibit LT biosynthesis or LT receptor antagonists have a salutary impact in asthma *(78)*. Although the evidence for proinflammatory roles of LT are established, there is also new evidence that other eicosanoids, such as LXs *(79–81)* and the recently uncovered aspirin-triggered LXs (ATL), namely, 15-epi-LX *(82)* (Fig. 4), possess potent counterregulatory actions. Recent findings raise the very likely possibility that the integrated response of the host, recognized as human diseases such as vasculitis and arthritis, in part reflects an overall balance as well as temporal orchestration between "proinflammatory" and "antiinflammatory" signals. Among such signals, the role of lipid-derived mediators, in particular select eicosanoids, remains unclear, likely because these products are rapidly generated, often through transcellular biosynthesis, exist ephemerally, and act within the local microenvironment. In this regard, the LXs and the recently identified aspirin-triggered 15-epi-LXs are of particular interest.

These eicosanoids are derived from lipid precursors through the sequential action of two LOs (Figs. 1 and 2). Given the requirement for two lipoxygenation steps, it seemed likely that these compounds were formed via *transcellular* biosynthesis. Indeed, the potential requirement for transcellular mechanisms originally led to questions as to whether LXs could be formed in vivo (*vide infra*). In this regard, LX formation involves

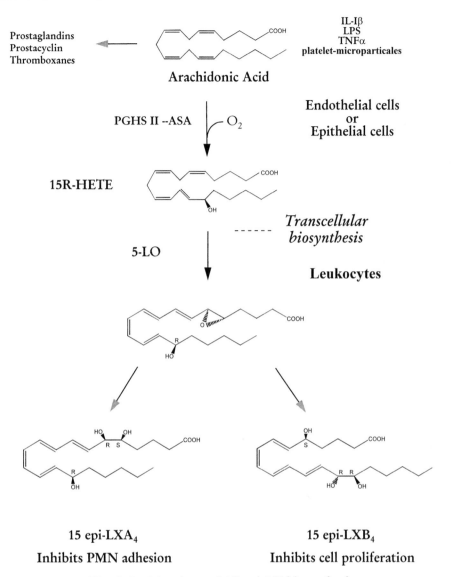

Fig. 4. Aspirin-triggered 15-epi-LX biosynthesis.

two main enzymatic steps and subsequent reactions similar to that of PGs, which also require the insertion of molecular oxygen at two sites within arachidonate to produce the prostanoid structure, at carbon 9 and 11 of arachidonate. Since there was a requirement for two lipoxygenation steps in LX biosynthesis to generate two of the alcohol groups and the third from water (carbon 6 position in LXA$_4$ and carbon 14 position alcohol in LXB$_4$ are derived from H$_2$O), it seemed likely that these eicosanoids were formed via transcellular biosynthetic routes, as illustrated in Figs. 1 and 2. It is clear from the results of numerous studies that LXs are not only formed in vitro from endogenous sources of arachidonate in isolated cells, but are also formed in vivo and across many species, from fish to humans *(83)*. The next four sections will focus on the following: (1) What are the major routes and bioactions of the LXs?; and

(2) Is knowledge of their formation and actions of value for new approaches to regulate acute inflammatory events?

Overview of LX Biosynthesis

Biosynthesis of eicosanoids by *transcellular* and *cell–cell interactions* is now recognized as an important means of amplifying as well as generating new lipid-derived mediators, particularly those produced by LOs *(79,84,85)*. In humans LX biosynthesis is an example of LO-LO interactions (Fig. 1) via transcellular mechanisms *(79–81)*. Thus, LXs can be generated by two LO routes: the first involves initial lipoxygenation by 15-LO (insertion of O_2 predominantly in the S configuration) followed by 5-LO and generation of a 5(6)-epoxytetraene. The authors also established a second route, initiated by 5-LO from leukocytes with formation of LTA_4, which unexpectedly is converted by platelet 12-LO into the epoxide intermediate (Fig. 1). This platelet-PMN model exemplifies the pivotal role of LTA_4 released by activated PMN that can be converted to either LTC_4 or LX by platelets *(80,85,86)*. Results with recombinant platelet 12-LO confirmed this and revealed that it also serves as an LX-synthase producing both LXA_4 and LXB_4 *(87)* (Figs. 1 and 2). Recently, a third unexpected pathway was uncovered (Fig. 4), which is triggered by ASA acetylation of PGHS II in endothelial cells. The modified enzyme generates 15R-HETE from arachidonic acid, which is rapidly transformed by leukocytes in a transcellular biosynthetic route involving leukocytes and either vascular endothelial cells or epithelial cells *(82,88)*.

Formation of 15-epi-LXs can also be initiated from products generated by cytochrome P450 oxygenation of arachidonate, known to occur in certain tissues, and subsequent 5-LO oxygenation in leukocytes *(88)*. ATLs or 15-epi-LXs show intriguing bioactions that include anti-inflammatory and antiproliferative actions in vitro *(88–90)*, which may be relevant when considering some of ASA's new-found beneficial impact in reducing vascular disease and protecting against certain cancers, including breast, lung, and colon cancer *(13,91,92)*. This novel action of ASA and generation of 15-epi-LX as potential endogenous mediators (Figs. 1 and 4) will be considered as well as recent results from the laboratory of one of the authors that indicate that the bioavailability and biohalf-life of ATL can be increased and exploited for pharmacologic use in in vivo models of inflammation *(89,90)*.

15-Lipoxygenase-Initiated Pathway

The first LX biosynthetic route reported in 1984 rationalized the generation of tetraene-containing structures that are now known as LXs by reactions involving insertion of molecular oxygen into the carbon (C) 15 position of arachidonic acid, predominantly in the S configuration. The pathway implicated the involvement of a 15-LO in the generation of bioactive molecules *(93)*, and was of interest because the role of the 15-LO was not known (for review, *see* ref. *94*). It is now clear that the human 15-LO, which has been subsequently found to be abundant in human eosinophils, alveolar macrophages, monocytes, and epithelial cells, is controlled by cytokines and regulated primarily by IL-4 and IL-13 *(51,95–97)*. These two cytokines are implicated as negative regulators of the inflammatory response or anti-inflammatory cytokines *(98)*. This is intriguing and perhaps more than a coincidence because recent studies on the actions of LX implicate both LXA_4 and B_4 as potential anti-inflammatory compounds (*vide infra*). Also, Brash et al. cloned a new human 15-LO that is selective for AA and generates 15S-HETE in a stereoselective fashion *(33)*. It will be of considerable interest to determine the role and contribution of this new second 15-LO to the biosynthesis of LX. It is highly expressed in human epithelial cells and shows a clear difference in substrate specificity compared to the well-known form of the enzyme present in blood cells.

Oxygenation of arachidonic acid at the C-15 position generates 15-HPETE. The 15S-hydroperoxy form, and/or 15S-HETE, the reduced alcohol form, can each serve as a substrate for 5-LO in leukocytes. These transformations can occur within the cell type of origin or via transcellular routes in humans. The product of the 5-LO's action on 15-HPETE is a 5S,15S-dihydroperoxy eicosatetraenoic acid (5S,15S-DHPETE), which is then rapidly converted to a 5,6-epoxytetraene. The 5-LO is also regulated by cytokines, such as GM-CSF and IL-3 *(49,99,100)*, and 5-LO is highly expressed in human neutrophils and monocytes.

Once produced, the 5(6)-epoxytetraene is rapidly converted by hydrolases to either 5S,6R,15S-trihydroxy-7,9,13-*trans*-11-*cis*-eicosatetraenoic acid, termed LXA$_4$, or, via LXB$_4$ hydrolase, to 5S,14R,15S-trihydroxy-6,10,12-*trans*-8-*cis*-eicosatetraenoic acid, termed LXB$_4$. LXA$_4$ and B$_4$ are each vasoactive; primarily vasodilatory in most isolated organs and in vivo models tested *(101,102)*, and they both regulate leukocyte functions *(90,103,104)*, perhaps serving as down regulatory molecules.

Concomitant with the biosynthesis of LXs by the 15-LO-initiated route, LT biosynthesis is blocked at the level of the 5-LO *(81,88)*, resulting in an inverse relationship between LT and LX formation. Therefore, when LXs are generated by human neutrophils from conversion of 15-HETE carrying its alcohol in either the *R* or *S* configuration, LT formation is dramatically reduced, whereas LXs and 15-epi-LX are released.

Recent evidence indicates that primed leukocytes from patients with inflammatory disorders, such as asthma, that are exposed in vivo to various cytokines and other inflammatory stimuli generate LXs entirely from endogenous sources of arachidonic acid from a single cell type without the aid of platelets. The finding that primed cells *(86,105–107)* and cells from peripheral blood of individuals with various diseases can generate LXs from endogenous sources of arachidonic acid raises questions with respect to the current understanding of the generation of eicosanoids in inflammatory diseases, namely, what is the temporal relationship between each of the classes of eicosanoids during the progression of an inflammatory response from acute to chronic phase in vivo? Information along these lines will help in understanding the biological impact of each individual class of eicosanoid because in experimental models they each regulate key responses during multicellular events. This is particularly evident in view of findings with transgenic rabbits that express classic human 15-LO in a macrophage-specific fashion *(108)*. When the 15-LO overexpressing rabbits were fed an atherogenic diet, the expression of 15-LO was found to have a protective impact on the development of atherosclerosis. This was an unexpected finding for the authors and it is likely that this action of 15-LO is causally related to biosynthesis and local anti-inflammatory mediators that may include LX.

5-LO–Initiated Pathway: LTA$_4$-Dependent LX Biosynthetic Route

The second route recognized for LX biosynthesis occurs among cell types within the vasculature. These intraluminal sources of LO products sharply contrast interstitial or mucosal origins. This pathway is best studied with the interaction of human neutrophils with platelets (*see* Fig. 2). The key insertion of molecular oxygen in this biosynthetic scheme involves 5-LO within human neutrophils and 12-LO that is present in high levels in human platelets *(80,85,86,109)*. Platelet–leukocyte interactions in the biosynthesis of LXs and other eicosanoids serve as a model of cell–cell interactions in other tissues and cell types because of the ease with which one is able to obtain sufficient numbers of neutrophils and platelets to carry out experiments in vitro. Unprimed neutrophils apparently do not generate appreciable quantities of LXs on their own *(85,86)*, and >50% of their LTA_4 formed from the 5-LO is released to the extracellular milieu *(110)*.

Platelets that are adherent to PMN pick up LTA_4 and convert it via the 12-LO to a carbocation intermediate in a reaction mechanism that is similar to that of 15-LO *(85,111)*. In this reaction, the platelet 12-LO abstracts hydrogen at C-13 and inserts molecular oxygen into the C-15 position of LTA_4, and converts it into a cation intermediate that opens to either LXB_4 when attacked by water at the C-14 position or LXA_4 when attacked by water at the C-6 position *(87,112,113)*. The formation of both LXB_4 and LXA_4 is unique to the 12-LO; 15-LO does convert LTA_4 to the 5(6) epoxytetraene and then nonenzymatically opens to LXA_4 and its isomers *without* a high yield generation of LXB_4. This new activity of 12-LO, for which a functional role of the enzyme in platelets had remained elusive, indicates that the 12-LO serves as a LX synthase in platelets *(85)*. Observations with isolated intact platelets from human peripheral blood were confirmed using recombinant 12-LO. 12-LO converts LTA_4 to both LXA_4 and LXB_4 *(87)*. The enzyme undergoes suicide inactivation with LTA_4 as substrate for LXB_4 but continues to produce LXA_4. This catalytic regulatory mechanism has implications for the separate biological actions of LXA_4 and LXB_4 when generated within the vasculature, which is the likely place for platelets and leukocytes to adhere and interact *(114,115)*. Thus, cell–cell interactions as exemplified here with platelets-leukocytes result in the formation of new molecules by transcellular communication, which in turn regulate cell function. This type of cell interaction may be illustrative of the self-limiting nature of intravascular adhesion events that permit the resolution of multicellular traffic jams within vessels.

Aspirin-Triggered 15-Epi-Lipoxin Circuit

A new major route to tetraene-containing eicosanoids was recently uncovered *(82,88)* (*see* Figs. 1 and 4). In this transcellular biosynthetic scheme (illustrated in Fig. 4), PGHS-II expressed in either endothelial cells or epithelial cells after exposure to proinflammatory cytokines such as IL-1β, LPS, or TNF switches its catalytic activity in the presence of aspirin, generating 15R-HETE instead of PG intermediates. In this setting, aspirin inhibits PG biosynthesis by both PGHS-I and PGHS-II (reviewed in ref. *11*). PGHS-II, when acetylated in endothelial or epithelial cells, is not enzymatically inactive. Instead, this isozyme converts endogenous arachidonic acid to 15R-HETE, which is released and transformed via transcellular routes to form 15-epi-LXs by leukocytes in close proximity. The activated and, in most instances, adherent leukocytes in this scenario possess 5-LO and transform 15R-HETE to a 5(6)-epoxytetraene within leukocytes, which carries its C-15 position alcohol in the R configuration. This proposed common intermediate leads to the formation of both 15-epi-LXA_4 and 15-epi-LXB_4, which each carry the *R* configuration at C-15. 15-epi-LXA_4 proves to be more potent than native LXA_4 in inhibiting neutrophil adhesion *(82,90)*, and 15-epi-LXB_4 inhibits cell proliferation *(88)*. The R configuration at C-15 increases their bioactivity in both molecules.

Recombinant PGHS-II, when acetylated by ASA, switches its substrate binding to an altered conformer that favors the generation of 15R-HETE *(116,117)*. The well-known in vivo inhibition of PGHS-II by ASA is readily demonstrable with recombinant enzyme with the appearance of 15R-generating activity within minutes that drops sharply with time. The interest in the ASA-triggered pathway outlined in Fig. 4 is that PGHS-II is present in abundance in inflammatory reactions and in disease states, including colon cancer *(11,13)*, and is in place when individuals take aspirin for its therapeutic benefit. Thus, not only is PGHS-II likely to be in place in vivo when ASA is taken, but it is more than likely that inflammatory cell types are adhering and in position in these scenarios.

One is accustomed to thinking of aspirin as an inhibitor of eicosanoid biosynthesis, and these new results clearly establish that aspirin can trigger the biosynthesis of novel compounds, namely, the ATL, which can serve as potential endogenous anti-inflammatory signals or mediators of some of aspirin's newly recognized beneficial actions. These new actions of ASA include prevention of myocardial infarction *(118,119)* and protection from colorectal adenoma, as well as other forms of cancer *(13,120)*. The mechanism of ASA's beneficial actions is likely to include the biosynthesis of 15-epi-LX and related compounds and could represent a novel mechanism for this drug for which a wealth of toxicology data is available worldwide. Because of ASA's widespread use and absence of a clear mechanism to explain its newly appreciated actions, it is important to gain a more complete understanding of its cellular impact and site of its therapeutic actions. These new findings suggest that ASA, in addition to inhibiting PGs, can actively fight inflammation in vivo by triggering the biosynthesis of 15-epi-LXs that reduce cell–cell interactions.

LX Circuits and Local Bioimpact

Three major routes lead to the formation of trihydroxytetraene-containing eicosanoids and each can be operative independently or in concert within the vasculature. GM-CSF-primed neutrophils, e.g., recruited to an inflammatory site, can interact with platelets. When platelets adhere to neutrophil surfaces *(85,114,115,121)*, activated PMN generate LTA$_4$ that is released and transformed via the 12-LO in platelets to generate LXs (Figs. 1 and 2). These routes are not inhibited by ASA or other NSAIDs, and both LT and LX biosynthesis persist with these drugs on board *(113)*. Also, within the vasculature, the ATL pathway can be operative with cytokine-activated endothelial cells with adherent neutrophils generating 15-epi-LX.

Leukocytes interacting with epithelial surfaces, as in the case of respiratory, renal, or gastrointestinal inflammation, can also generate LXs via bidirectional routes, in which both 15S- and 15R-HETE are released by the epithelial cell and converted to LX or 15-epi-LX by neutrophils. The other component of this bidirectional interaction can involve neutrophil-released LTA$_4$ *(122)* that is converted by the abundant 15-LO in epithelial cells *(123)*, particularly tracheal epithelial cells, to generate LXs via a LTA$_4$-dependent mechanism. Of interest, LTA$_4$ is also a newly appreciated substrate for the soybean 15-LO and can be converted to LX *(85,123)*. A less prominent route to LX formation can involve 5,6-dihydroxyeicosanoids, which have also been shown to be substrates for LX production *(124)*. These reactions may include either 15-LO– or 12-LO–based conversion of 5,6-dihydroxyeicosanoid substrates to produce LX *(124)*.

Cytokines and Priming in LX Generation

Cytokines enhance the appearance of the enzymes required as well as prime for LX formation, suggesting that there is a close association between the local cytokines within the site of generation of LXs and the site of LX action. Another recognized source of LX biosynthesis involves a new form of "priming" that involves the esterification of 15-HETE in inositol-containing phospholipids within the membranes of human neutrophils *(125)*. Cells rapidly esterify 15-HETE into their inositol-containing lipids, which, on subsequent agonist stimulation, release 15-HETE from this source that is further enzymatically transformed. In this case, the deacylated mono-HETEs are released and transformed, to LX, or perhaps to other eicosanoids that have yet to be identified. This discovery suggests that precursors of LX biosynthesis can be stored within membranes of inflammatory cells and then released by stimuli-activating PLA_2 *(125)*. This form of membrane priming to generate bioactive lipid-derived signals has implications in second messengers generated, such as 15-hydroxy-PIP_2 and diglyceride, which contain 15-HETE that may alter their intracellular signaling activities. As is the case with 15*S*-HETE, 15*R*-HETE is also rapidly esterified into membrane phospholipids and thus is likely to serve as a reservoir for 15-epi-LX formation *(88)*. GM-CSF and IL-3 regulate expression of 5-LO, and IL-4 and IL-13 specifically regulate the gene expression of 15-LO *(49,51,95,96,99)*. Of interest, IL-10 and IL-4 were recently shown to induce cyclooxygenase (COX)-2 in human PMN *(126)*. The generation of PGs by peripheral blood PMN has been debated for some years. This new finding with cytokine-inducible COX-2 may explain many reported differences and inconsistencies among eicosanoid product profiles generated by human PMN in vitro. Specific cytokines that can regulate the expression of 12-LO in human megakaryocytes have not been observed *(112)*. Functional integration of these pathways and their regulation by cytokines requires further study but clearly provide cells and tissues with diverse routes to generate LX. This redundant biosynthetic capacity to produce LX in human tissues is orchestrated by cell–cell interactions of diverse cell types and is likely to reflect the basic functional requirements for these compounds in regulating essential tissue responses.

Current understanding of cell–cell interactions, namely, that PMN-platelet microaggregates do indeed form in vivo *(114,115)* and that key eicosanoid biosynthetic enzymes are regulated by specific cytokines *(51,95)* provides new concepts for appreciating the signaling networks involved in LX formation *(127)* and actions. GM-CSF enhances LX generation during receptor-mediated PMN and platelet interactions *(86)*, and T_H2 cells can produce the 15-LO–regulating cytokines IL-4 and IL-13, which are in the local milieu *(51,95,98)*. Thus, an in vivo microenvironment, particularly in a specific disease state, is highly likely to contain specific cytokines that can enhance production of LXs and other novel bioactive lipid mediators.

Cell Adhesion in Transcellular Biosynthesis In Vivo

This type of cellular LX circuit is demonstrated in an animal model of glomerular nephritis in which platelet-leukocyte interactions lead to the generation of LXs in vivo *(121)*. Antibodies against P-selectin, a mediator of platelet-leukocyte adhesion, block transcellular LX biosynthesis both in vitro and during ConA-F glomerular nephritis in vivo *(128)*. Neutrophil infiltration was unexpectedly more pronounced during acute nephrotoxic serum nephritis in P-selectin knockout mice than in wild-type mice because it was anticipated that infiltration of PMN in the P-selectin–deficient mouse would be reduced, not enhanced as observed. Consistent with this notion, P-selectin–deficient mice show a reduced efficiency of transcellular LX generation *(121)*. LXA_4 levels are restored and the difference in neutrophil infiltration is eliminated when the P-selectin-deficient mice are infused with wild-type platelets. These observations raise the possibility that platelet-neutrophil adherence and transcellular biosynthesis are important inflammatory events that regulate neutrophil recruitment via initiating the formation of lipid mediators that suppress pro-inflammatory responses. Thus, LX generation by platelets may have an important impact in regulating the entry of recruiting and infiltrating neutrophils.

Transcellular biosynthetic circuits and networks such as those illustrated by the model of platelet-neutrophil interactions can yield both LXs and LTs (*see* Figs. 1 and 2). If LXs act as a "braking signal" or as an endogenous "stop signal" for the recruitment of leukocytes, it is likely that molecular switches are thrown that direct eicosanoid product profiles from a pro-inflammatory to an anti-inflammatory phenotype. In this regard, cytokines, as well as the local redox potential of the inflammatory microenvironment, play important roles in the generation of LXs, particularly in platelets. Agents that reduce the intracellular platelet level of glutathione such as nitroprusside enhance LX generation by platelets and block the formation of cysteinyl-containing LT *(86)*.

LXs: Conserved Structures

LXs are evolutionary conserved molecules in that they are generated in large quantities (i.e., microgram amounts/incubation) by a variety of fish tissues including leukocytes and brain *(83)*. The levels generated by isolated fish cells are ~10–100 times greater than the amount generated by human cells in coincubation, suggesting that they possess important roles in fish. Their role in fish brain is not known, but LXs inhibit proliferation of fish lymphocytes *(83)*. Phylogenetic analysis shows that LXs are also generated by frog leukocytes and thrombocytes *(129)*. LXA_4 stimulates chemotaxis of trout macrophages *(83)*, a response that is shared by human monocytes *(130)*, but not by human neutrophils *(89)*. Produced in human marrow, LXs are implicated in regulating myelopoiesis *(52)*. Thus, it appears that LXs have a primitive physiological role that has evolved and changed in humans but that has held the LX structure tightly conserved.

Tissues and Diseases: LX Generation In Vivo

LXs are generated within organs and are associated with a variety of human inflammatory events, with the first demonstration in bronchial lavage *(131)*. LXA_4 and LXB_4 are formed in nasal polyps *(123)* and, of interest, LXA_4 is generated in nasal lavage from aspirin (ASA)-sensitive asthmatics *(132)* and in experimental nephritis *(128)*. Along these lines, Chavis et al. *(105)* proposed that LXs are useful biomarkers of asthma, and Thomas et al. *(107)* proposed that LXs are biomarkers of long-term clinical improvement in arthritic patients. The list of diseases and tissues in Table 2 is not exhaustive, and it is likely to represent examples of in vivo scenarios in which cell–cell interaction is accelerated and the generation of LXs is detected because of the abundance of cytokines and cell–cell interactions in these settings. Rupture of the atherosclerotic plaque leads to rapid generation of LXA_4 in the intracoronary artery *(133)*. LXs are also generated by normal human bone marrow *(52,134)*. During chronic myelocytic leukemia, platelets lose 12-LO. They also lose

Table 2
LT and LX Formation In Vivo

• Asthma	• Glomerulonephritis
• Aspirin-sensitive asthmatics	• Sarcoidosis
• Angioplasty-induced plaque rupture	• Pneumonia
• Bone marrow generation	• Nasal polyps
• Alterations in both LT and LX	• Rheumatoid arthritis
biosynthesis—(defect in LX generation	
in chronic myeloid leukemia)	

their ability to generate LX, and this finding may be related to blast crisis observed in chronic myelocytic leukemia *(52)*.

LX and ATL Actions

LX Bioactions: Vasoactive and Anti-Inflammatory

LXs show vasodilatory as well as counterregulatory roles in both in vivo and in vitro experimental models (for further details, *see* refs. *81,102*). Both LXA_4 and LXB_4 promote vasorelaxation and relax aorta and pulmonary arteries. LXA_4 reverses pre-contraction of the pulmonary artery induced by $PGF_{2\alpha}$ as well as the potent vaso-constrictor enzyme endothelin (ET-1). The mechanisms underlying LXA_4- and LXB_4-induced vasodilation involve endothelium-dependent vasorelaxation and both PG-dependent and independent pathways *(102)*. In certain tissues, LXs can stimulate the formation of, e.g., prostacyclin, by endothelial cells *(135)*, which can contribute to vasodilation. Prostanoid-dependent actions of LXs are inhibitable by COX inhibitors *(102)* indicating that LXs can stimulate in certain cell types the biosynthesis of a second set of mediators, i.e., PGs. These also include LX-stimulated generation of nitric oxide *(136)*, which may mediate a component of LX-regulated vascular tone. LXA_4 stimula-tion of NO has been shown to regulate cholinergic neurotransmission and reduces vagal nerve-mediated contraction of airway smooth muscle *(137)*.

LX bioactions, shown to date, are in sharp contrast to those of most other lipid mediators that are primarily proinflammatory; these include LTs, PAFs, and TXs. LXA_4 displays human leukocyte-selective actions (Table 3). LXs inhibit both neutrophil and eosinophil chemotaxis in the nanomolar range *(138,139)*. LXA_4 inhibits PMN transmi-gration across both endothelial and epithelial cells *(140)*, blocks PMN diapedesis from postcapillary venules *(141)*, and inhibits PMN entry into inflamed tissues in animal models *(72,128)*.

In human PMN, LXA_4 and LXB_4 block at nanomolar concentrations the transmigra-tion and chemotaxis of PMN by a mechanism that regulates CD11/CD18 *(142,143)* and also blocks agonist-induced generation of IP_3 *(144)*. In contrast to PMN and eosino-phils *(139,144)*, LXs are potent chemoattractants for monocytes *(145)*. LXA_4 and LXB_4 each stimulate monocyte chemotaxis and adherence, which may be related to the recruitment of monocytes to sites of wound injury. Of interest, monocytes do not gen-erate superoxide anions or degranulate in response to LX, suggesting that their actions on these cells are selective and relate to locomotion. LXs stimulate myeloid progenitors in the subnanomolar concentration range *(52)*. The selective actions of LXs on leuko-cytes are of interest, given the finding that LXs are not further transformed by neutro-

Table 3
Human Leukocyte Selective Actions of Lipoxins

Cell type	Lipoxin	Activity	Reference
PMN	LXA_4 and LXB_4	• Block emigration in microcirculation	*141*
		• Inhibits chemotaxis	*138*
		• Downregulate CD11/18	*142*
		• Downregulates intracellular IP_3, Ca^{2+}	*144*
		• Inhibit PMN-endothelial cell and epithelial cell transmigration	*140,143*
Eosinophils	LXA_4	• Inhibits chemotaxis to PAF and *f*MLP	*139*
Monocytes	LXA_4 and LXB_4	• Stimulate chemotaxis and adherence	*145,160*
		• Stimulate myeloid bone marrow-derived progenitors	*161*

phils, but are rapidly converted by human monocytes via dehydrogenation to inactive compounds *(90)*. The biohalf-life of LX is regulated by PBM, which, like other autacoids, are rapidly formed and inactivated by specific metabolic routes. These results also raise the likelihood that LXs can play a role in wound healing, given the central role of monocytes and macrophages in this process.

In human subjects, a potentially important role for LXA_4 is underscored by the finding that inhalation of LXA_4 blocks airway constriction in asthmatics *(146)*. Also demonstrable in vivo, LXs inhibit diapedesis of PMN from postcapillary venules *(141)* and inhibit the entry of leukocytes into inflamed tissues *(143)*. LXA_4 downregulates LTB_4-mediated delayed hypersensitivity reactions *(147)*, and both antagonizes the actions of LTD_4 in renal hemodynamics and competes at the receptor for LTD_4 *(104)*. LXB_4, which has not yet been studied extensively in vivo, induces sleep, a finding that has also been shown for PGD_2. In this respect LXB_4 is less potent than PGD_2 *(148)*. Thus, not only do LXs serve counterregulatory roles in the physiologic events of interest in inflammation, but enantiomerically modified LXs, as generated in the case of aspirin (Fig. 4), may also be actual effectors of well-established anti-inflammatory therapies (*vide infra*).

LX In Vivo and Disease Models

LXs are also generated in vivo in humans and in experimental animals (reviewed in ref. *149*) and are associated with diseases (*see* Table 2). LXA_4 and LXB_4 are also both formed in ischemic rat brain *(150)*, and LXA_4 is generated in mouse kidneys with glomerulonephritis in a P-selectin–dependent fashion, predominantly via interactions between platelets and neutrophils *(121)*. In rats the infiltration of neutrophils to glomerulonephritic kidneys is markedly inhibited by prior exposure of neutrophils to LXA_4 *(128)*. LXA_4 has recently been found to regulate LTB_4-mediated delayed hypersensitivity reactions in guinea pigs *(147)*. Interest in the actions of LXA_4 is also heightened by findings with animal models and in human subjects (Tables 2 and 3).

LXA_4 Mechanism of Action

The actions of LXA_4 are not mediated by competition at the LTB_4 receptor *(67)*, but LXA_4 is reported to antagonize the formation of intracellular signals such as IP_3 *(144)*.

In addition to its selective actions with leukocytes, LXA_4 also modulates the vasoconstrictor actions of LTD_4 in renal hemodynamics and is vasodilatory *(104)*. These actions of LXA_4 are mediated by a receptor distinct from that of the myeloid LXA_4R and are consistent with LXA_4 acting on a subtype of the peptidoleukotriene receptors, competing for LTC_4 and LTD_4 high-affinity sites that are present on both mesangial *(104)* and endothelial cells *(68)*.

LX Stable Analogs: LX Inactivation Pathways
Do ATLs Act as Endogenous LX Stable Analogs?

Eicosanoids and other bioactive lipids are rapidly generated within seconds, act locally, and are quickly inactivated. Most LO-derived products are inactivated by ω-oxidation *(81)*. PGs and other products of PGHS-I or II are, in general, rapidly inactivated by dehydrogenation at C-15 by a specific enzyme termed PG dehydrogenase. LXs undergo both ω-oxidation and dehydrogenation *(90,145)*. Dehydrogenation vs ω-oxidation of LXs is both organ- and cell type-specific. The major route of LX inactivation is via dehydrogenation by monocytes that convert LXA_4 to 15-oxo-LXA_4 and LXB_4 to 5-oxo-LXB_4 followed by specific reduction of the double bond adjacent to the ketone. These specific enzymatic steps, namely, dehydrogenation followed by reduction of LX-derived intermediates, resemble the inactivation of PGs *(145)*. Since the LXs and ATLs appear to serve as downregulating autacoids, a series of analogs was designed and prepared by total organic synthesis that was intended to increase the biohalf-life of the LX, as well as to enhance their bioavailability to further test the notion that these LX pathways and bioactions are antiinflammatory in vivo.

To this end LXA_4 analogs were constructed with bulky groups placed at both the C-15 and the ω-end (Fig. 4) *(90)*. LXB_4 analogs were designed with bulky groups at C-5 to disrupt the dehydrogenation step at this site. Placement of these specific groups within the LXA_4 structure template not only prevents oxidation and LX inactivation, but also proves to be modest enough to retain their native bioactivities. In some cases, the analogs were equally or more potent than the native LX structures. Their potencies depend on the tissues and routes of inactivation effected. For example, LXA_4 stable analogs are potent inhibitors of both PMN adherence to endothelial cells and PMN transmigration across endothelial cell surfaces *(90)*. During coincubations of PMN with endothelial cells, native LXA_4 is not further metabolized in appreciable quantities or inactivated. Thus, LXA_4 and its analogs are essentially equipotent, with a rank order of $LXA_4 \approx$ 15-(*R/S*)-methyl-LXA_4-ME $\approx$ 15-cyclohexyl-LXA_4-ME $\approx$ 16-phenoxy-LXA_4-ME, with an apparent EC_{50} of $\approx$1 n*M*. PMN coincubations of epithelial cells, by contrast, show a sharp difference in rank order and potency of the LX analogs because epithelial cells can degrade LX in vitro. Therefore, in these cell–cell interactions, 15-(*R/S*)-methyl-LXA_4-ME and 16-phenoxy-LXA_4-ME proved to be more potent than native LXA_4, with inhibition of PMN transmigration observed at concentrations of the LX analogs as low as picomolar levels. Of interest, the ATL (15-epi-LXA_4) is less effectively converted in vitro to its 15-oxo-metabolite than LXA_4 is converted by recombinant PG dehydrogenase *(90)*. This not only indicates that the dehydrogenation step is highly stereospecific, but also suggests that when ATLs are generated in vivo, their biohalf-life is increased by approximately twofold as compared to native LXA_4, thereby enhancing their ability to evoke bioactions. These LXA_4 stable analogs not only prove to inhibit PMN adhesion and transmigration but also act as potent stimuli for monocyte migration as the native LXA_4 *(130)*. Therefore, biologically stable analogs of LX and ATL can be engineered to enhance the bioactions, suggesting that they are useful tools and potential leads for therapeutic modalities.

LX-Specific Receptors: Anti-Inflammatory Signaling?

LX actions are cell type–, species-, and organ-specific. These actions can be assigned to one or a combination of three mechanisms as follows: (1) LXs act at their own specific cell surface receptors *(67)* (LXA_4 specific and separate LXB_4 receptor); (2) LXA_4 interacts with a subclass of LTD_4 receptors (pharmacologically defined) that also binds LXA_4 *(102,104)*; and (3) LXs can act at *intracellular* targets after LX transport/uptake or within its cell of origin *(67,151)*.

LXA_4 and LXB_4 each act at two distinct sites and in some cell types they evoke similar responses, whereas in others their actions differ. The profile of LXA_4 activities relevant to inflammation (Table 3) suggested that its actions as an autacoid are mediated by a cell surface receptor, whereas in its cell of origin, LX could evoke responses by acting on specific enzyme systems *(67,81)*. Labeled LXA_4 was prepared, which facilitated the identification of specific LXA_4 receptors on leukocytes *(67,89)*. These receptors are inducible in HL-60 cells, and specific binding of the ^3H-labeled LXA_4 correlated with the appearance of function in these cells. The temporal appearance of surface binding and functional responses led to the identification of orphan cDNA clones of a seven-transmembrane-spanning G-protein–coupled receptor that specifically binds LXA_4 and transmits its signal in transfected cells. The LXA_4 receptors are expressed on PMN, monocytes, and endothelial cells and evoke actions in each cell type *(68)*. Of interest, the human LXA_4-R identified from HL-60 cells also showed regions of homology to the recently identified LTB_4 receptor that was also identified by using the HL-60 cell line *(65)*. The monocyte and PMN LXA_4 receptors proved to be identical at the cDNA level yet evoked different responses in these cell types. The endothelial site that binds LXA_4 appears to be a structurally distinct form of the LXAR (*vide infra*).

Cloning of the Mouse LXA_4R

The authors first sought the identification and distribution of the murine LXA_4 receptor to evaluate the role(s) and actions of LX and ATL stable analogs in an in vivo model. The mouse LXA_4 receptor was obtained from a mouse spleen cDNA library using the human LXA_4R as a probe *(69,142)*. Since this initial clone lacked the amino terminus, a full-length clone was obtained using the rapid amplification of cDNA ends (RACE) technique *(89)*. The resulting full-length clone had an open reading frame encoding 351 amino acids (Fig. 5). To confirm this clone obtained by the RACE technique, the authors amplified the coding region of mouse LXA_4R by RT-PCR from RNA obtained from isolated mouse neutrophils. When the PCR product was sequenced, five independent clones were obtained that were each identical to the clone isolated from spleen. Therefore, the authors concluded that this LXA_4R cDNA is indeed present not only in the mouse cDNA spleen library, but also in mouse neutrophils.

Hydrophobicity analysis showed, as expected, the presence of a putative seven-transmembrane domain characteristic of the G-protein–coupled receptor superfamily *(89,152)*. The mouse LXA_4R has two *N*-glycosylation sites in the *N*-terminal extracel-

```
                                                                    TM1
mouse   MESNYSIHLNGSEVVVYDSTISRVLWILSMVVVSITFFLGVLGNGLVIWV
human   METNFSTPLNEYEEVSYESAGYTVLRILPLVVLGVTFVLGVLGNGLVIWV      50
                        TM2
mouse   AGFRMPHTVTTIWYLNLALADFSFTATLPFLLVEMAMKEKWPFGWFLCKL
human   AGFRMTRTVTTICYLNLALADFSFTATLPFLIVSMAMGEKWPFGWFLCKL     100
            TM3
mouse   VHIAVDVNLFGSVFLIAVIALDRCICVLHPVWAQNHRTVSLARNVVVGSW
human   IHIVVDINLFGSVFLIGFIALDRCICVLHPVWAQNHRTVSLAMKVIVGPW     150
                TM4
mouse   IFALILTLPLFLFLTTVRDARGDVHCRLSFVSWGNSVEERLNTAITFVTT
human   ILALVLTLPVFLFLTTVTIPNGDTYCTFNFASWGGTPEERLKVAITMLTA     200
                    TM5
mouse   RGIIRFIVSFSLPMSFVAICYGLITTKIHKKAFVNSSRPFRVLTGVVASF
human   RGIIRFVIGFSLPMSIVAICYGLIAAKIHKKGMIKSSRPLRVLTAVVASF     250
            TM6                                         TM7
mouse   FICWFPFQLVALLGTVWLKEMQFSGSYKIIGRLVNPTSSLAFFNSCLNPI
human   FICWFPFQLVALLGTVWLKEMLFYGKYKIIDILVNPTSSLAFFNSCLNPM     300
                    #   #         #   #         #       #
mouse   LYVFMGQDFQERLIHSLSSRLQRALSEDSGHISDTRTNLASLPEDIEIKAI   351
human   LYVFVGQDFRERLIHSLPTSLERALSEDSAPTNDTAANSASPPAETELQAM
```

Fig. 5. Alignment of human and mouse LXA_4R. The amino acid sequence of human LXA_4R was aligned to the mouse homologue. Their amino acid sequences were 73% identical. Both putative glycosylation (*) and phosphorylation sites (#) are conserved. The mouse LXA_4R sequence data are available from GenBank under the accession number U78299.

lular domain, which are also conserved in human LXA_4R *(69,153)*. The carboxyl terminus or cytoplasmic tail of the mouse LXA_4R had nine serine or threonine residues, among which six were also conserved in human LXA_4R (Fig. 5). The overall homology between human and mouse LXA_4Rs was 76% at the nucleotide level and 73% at the amino acid level. A high degree of homology was noted in the sixth transmembrane domain and second intracellular loop (i.e., 89% and 100%, respectively), suggesting important roles for these regions in ligand recognition and signal transduction.

Specific ³H-LXA₄ Binding of Mouse LXA₄R

Human LXA_4R displays both specific and stereoselective binding and activation with LXA_4; K_d ~ 0.5 nM in human PMN and ~1.7 nM with transfected CHO cells *(67,69,142)*. We next tested the ability of this mouse LXA_4R to bind LXA_4. CHO cells were transfected with mouse LXA_4R cDNA and tested for their ability to specifically bind ³H-LXA_4. Mouse LXA_4R showed specific binding to ³H-LXA_4. When performed at 4°C, the binding saturated after 5 min. Scatchard analysis gave a K_d of 1.5 ± 0.6 nM, which was obtained with four separate concentrations of unlabeled LXA_4 (mean ± SEM, n = 4), a value similar to that of the human receptor (K_d 1.7 nM) *(69)*, suggesting that this mouse clone encodes the high-affinity LXA_4 receptor *(89)*.

Mouse LXA4R Stable Transformant

A stable transformant of the mouse LXA_4R was established in CHO cells to further evaluate the ability of mouse LXA_4R to transmit signals. One clone (designated P4-5) gave the highest mRNA expression of mouse LXA_4R when examined by northern hybridization. The authors examined GTP hydrolysis activity using the stable cell line P4–5 to test whether the mouse LXA_4R transmits signal when exposed to LXA_4. Treatment of CHO cells expressing human LXA_4R with LXA_4 stimulates GTPase activation (*see* ref. *69*). The mouse LXA_4R stable transformant activated GTPase approximately twofold when compared to vehicle alone (vehicle 0.07 ± 0.01 vs LXA_4 0.15 ± 0.03 pmol/min/10^6 cells, mean $\pm$ SEM, $n = 5$, $p < 0.05$) when exposed to 10^{-8} M LXA_4. This activation was stereoselective because equimolar amounts of the positional isomer of LXA_4, namely LXB_4, did not elicit this activation (vehicle 0.07 ± 0.01 vs 0.06 ± 0.01 pmol/10^6 cells, mean $\pm$ SEM, $n = 5$ and 4, respectively). Mock transfected CHO cells did not respond to LXA_4. Thus, the authors concluded that they had identified a functional LXA_4R of mouse.

Tissue Distribution of Mouse and Human LXA4R

Northern hybridization of mouse and human multiple tissue blot was performed to obtain the tissue distribution of mouse LXA_4R mRNA and to compare it to that of human. In mouse there was one major band of ~1.4 kb under high-stringency conditions. LXA_4R mRNA was most abundant in neutrophils, followed by spleen and lung, organs known to carry contaminants for leukocytes *(89)*. When the blots were exposed longer (for 14 d), there were faint bands associated with heart and liver. In humans the authors have previously found that LXA_4R mRNA is abundant in lung tissue *(69)*. LXA_4R mRNA was also abundant in peripheral leukocytes, followed by spleen. In these two organs, in addition to a major band of ~1.4 kb, another band of ~2.4 kb was also observed. In testis there was a single band of ~1.7 kb, which was not present in mouse. These bands of different sizes suggest the possibility of alternative splicing in human tissues, but by comparison they are lacking in mouse tissues.

LXA4 and 15-Epi-LXA4–Stable Analogs Mimic LXA4 and Compete for 3H-LXA4

LXA_4 is rapidly converted within seconds to minutes in the microenvironment to inactive LX metabolites, involving dehydrogenation at the C-15 position as the predominant route. To evaluate the action of LXs in vivo, LXA_4 stable analogs were designed and prepared by total organic synthesis, which resist dehydrogenation and ω-oxidation and retain bioactivity *(90)*. Both 15(R/S)-methyl-LXA_4 and 16-phenoxy-LXA_4 were more resistant to dehydrogenation by recombinant 15-hydroxy PG dehydrogenase (15-PGDH) than LXA_4, were also resistant to conversion by differentiated HL-60 cells, and were potent inhibitors of neutrophil transmigration and adhesion with IC_{50} ranging from 1 to 50 nM. 15-epi-LXA_4 (carrying a C-15 alcohol in the R configuration; Fig. 4), one of the new eicosanoids triggered by aspirin treatment, also displays a slower rate of conversion by recombinant enzyme, suggesting that it may display a longer in vivo biohalf-life than native LXA_4 with its C-15 alcohol in the S configuration.

Human Neutrophils

With these LXA_4 stable analogs in hand, the authors next examined whether they compete at the same site as native LXA_4. ^3H-LXA_4 binds to its specific receptor on human neutrophils *(67)*, and, therefore, human cells were used for the purpose of direct comparison with previous findings. Moreover, it was not possible to obtain mouse peripheral blood neutrophils in the amounts that would permit specific binding experiments and parallel evaluation of each of the synthetic LX analogs. Each of these bioactive LXA_4 analogs competitively displaced ^3H-LXA_4 binding in the following rank order: homoligand $LXA_4 \approx$ 15-epi-$LXA_4 >$ 15(R/S)-methyl-$LXA_4 >$ 16-phenoxy-LXA_4 *(89)*. The K_i values for LXA_4 in the present experiments (~2.0 nM) were comparable to previously reported values for human neutrophils *(67)* and CHO cells expressing human LXA_4R *(69)*. Thus, LXA_4 stable analogs compete at the same myeloid receptor as native LXA_4 on human PMN.

Human Endothelial Cells

LXA_4 also carries a vasodilatory action and is known to modulate the specific binding of LTD_4 on endothelial cells *(68)* and glomerular mesangial cells *(104)*. Thus, in addition to acting at the myeloid LXA_4R, LXA_4 also competes at a receptor subtype that also recognizes and responds to the peptidoLT LTD_4. LXA_4 also inhibits peptidoLT (LTC_4 and LTD_4)-induced upregulation of P-selectin in endothelial cells *(143)*. In view of these findings, the authors examined whether these LXA_4 stable analogs could compete for ^3H-LTD_4 specific binding to endothelial cells. Both native LXA_4 and 15-epi-LXA_4 competed with ^3H-LTD_4 as effectively as the homoligand LTD_4 and the well-characterized LTD_4 receptor antagonist SKF-104353. The LX stable analogs 15-(R/S)-methyl-LXA_4 and 16-phenoxy-LXA_4 each gave K_i values within the same range as the LTD_4 antagonist SKF-104353. These results suggest that these LXA_4 stable analogs and 15-epi-LXA_4 recognize the same receptors present on both neutrophils and endothelial cells as LXA_4, although it is clear that the endothelial receptors and neutrophil receptors are physiologically and pharmacologically distinct forms of the LXA_4R.

Human Monocytes

LXA_4 and LXB_4 both activate human monocytes, in contrast to their inhibitory actions on other human leukocytes *(145)*. LXA_4 is rapidly converted by monocytes to inactive products, and to resist metabolism, synthetic analogs of LXA_4 were designed. Recently, the authors examined the bioactivity of several LXA_4 analogs with monocytes and found, for chemotaxis, 15(R/S)-methyl-LXA_4 and 15-epi-LXA_4 were equal in activity, and that 16-phenoxy-LXA_4 was more potent than native LXA_4. Both 15*(R/S)*-methyl-LXA_4 and 16-phenoxy-LXA_4 were approximately one log order of magnitude more potent than LXA_4 in stimulating THP-1 cell adherence ($EC_{50} \approx 1 \times 10^{-10}$ M). Dimethylamide derivatives of the LXA_4 analogs also possessed agonist, rather than antagonist, properties for monocytes. Neither LXA_4 nor 16-phenoxy-LXA_4 affected monocyte-mediated cytotoxicity. Also, the authors cloned an LXA_4 receptor from THP-1 cells identical to that found in PMN *(130)*.

Evidence of receptor-mediated function of LXA_4 and the stable analogs in monocytes, to date, includes desensitization of intracellular calcium mobilization to a second challenge by equimolar concentrations of these analogs, but not to LTB_4. Increases in $[Ca^{2+}]_i$ by LXA_4 and the analogs were specifically inhibited by an antipeptide antibody to the LXA_4 receptor; and both LXA_4- and analog-induced adherence and increments in Ca^{2+} were sensitive to pertussis toxin. These findings indicate that the LXA_4 stable analogs are potent monocyte chemoattractants and are more potent than native LXA_4 in stimulating THP-1 cell adherence, at subnanomolar concentrations. Moreover, they provide additional evidence that the LXA_4 stable analogs retain selective bioactivity in monocytes, in which these LX analogs act as potent LX mimetics. Thus, it is possible that endogenous LXs recruit monocytes for wound-healing events and their own inactivation.

Analogs of LXA₄ and Aspirin-Triggered 15-Epi-LXA₄ Inhibit Mouse Ear Inflammation

LXA_4 inhibits neutrophil adhesion and transmigration in vitro *(143)*, and causes downregulation of CD11b/CD18 on human neutrophils *(142)*. To evaluate this potential antiinflammatory action of LXA_4 and to test whether these compounds do indeed carry this action in established in vivo models, the authors induced skin inflammation in mouse ears and examined the impact of several new LXA_4 stable analogs. After topical application of LTB_4 on mouse ear, time-dependent increase of myeloperoxidase (MPO) activity in ear skin was observed (Fig. 6, A–C). MPO is well established as a marker of neutrophil infiltration *(154)*; thus, the authors calibrated the degree of MPO activity and the number of neutrophils using standard curves obtained from neutrophils isolated after peritoneal lavage (Fig. 6A, inset). At equimolar concentrations, neither *f*MLP nor PAF induced PMN infiltration when applied topically in acetone (Fig. 6A). In contrast to the chemotactic ability of LTB_4, the same amounts of LTD_4 did not stimulate neutrophil infiltration into this tissue (Fig. 6B).

16-phenoxy-LXA_4, applied alone to the ear, had no direct effect on neutrophil infiltration (0–8 h; Fig. 6B). Also, no neutrophil influx was noted at intervals up to 48 h. When mouse ears were exposed to 16-phenoxy-LXA_4 just prior to the application of LTB_4, neutrophil infiltration was markedly attenuated at each time point and the percent inhibition observed at 24 h was approx 85%. Hematoxylin and eosin staining of ear biopsies and light microscopy confirmed these biochemical results and established that 16-phenoxy-LXA_4 applied alone did not alter the tissue architecture. Ears exposed to LTB_4 exhibited prominent PMN infiltration in perivascular regions (Fig. 6B), and this PMN infiltration was markedly attenuated when the ear was exposed to topical 16-phenoxy-LXA_4 *(89)*.

The inhibitory actions of 16-phenoxy-LXA_4 were concentration dependent (Fig. 6D), and an IC_{50} was estimated from the results of these experiments to be approx 120 nmol/cm². When its potency was directly compared in the same model to a known anti-inflammatory agent, dexamethasone, 16-phenoxy-LXA_4 was as potent as dexamethasone at the equivalent concentrations.

In the case of native LXA_4, its stereoisomer 15-epi-LXA_4, which is generated with aspirin treatment, carries its C-15 alcohol in the *R* configuration and is known to be more potent than native LXA_4 in vitro *(82)*. To address the importance of chirality at C-15 position in vivo, the authors prepared and examined the actions of 15-epi-16-phenoxy-LXA_4 that carries its C-15 alcohol in the *R* configuration. This analog, like 16-phenoxy-LXA_4, was designed to resist inactivation *(90)* and is an analog of the aspirin-triggered 15-epi-LXA_4 from this series of LXA_4 mimetics (For structure, see Fig. 4). 15-epi-16-phenoxy-LXA_4 was as potent as, or more potent than, 16-phenoxy-LXA_4 (Fig. 7), a finding that supports the notion

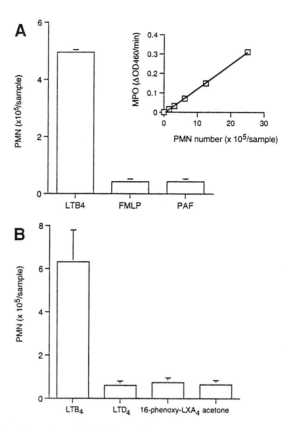

Fig. 6. Topical application of LXA$_4$ and 15-epi-LXA$_4$ analogs inhibits neutrophil infiltration in vivo. **(A)** Mouse ears were topically treated with equimolar amounts of LTB$_4$ (1 µg), *f*MLP (1.3 µg), or PAF (1.6 µg) in 20 µL of acetone. After 24 h, punch biopsy samples (6 mm diameter) were obtained from each ear, and MPO activity was measured as described in ref. *89*). MPO activity was further converted into number of neutrophils using the standard curve obtained using peritoneal neutrophils (*inset*). Results are mean ± SEM of $n = 3$–5. **(B)** Mouse ears were treated topically with vehicle alone (acetone) or vehicle containing 16-phenoxy-LXA$_4$ (240 nmol), LTB$_4$ (5 µg), or LTD$_4$ (5 µg). PMN infiltration was determined after 8 h. Results are mean ± SEM of $n = 4$ (vehicle, LTB$_4$), $n = 3$ (LTD$_4$), or $n = 2$ (16-phenoxy-LXA$_4$). *(continued on next page)*

Summary and Conclusions

These results demonstrate (Figs. 5–7), for the first time, cloning of the mouse myeloid LXA$_4$R and an anti-inflammatory action for both LXA$_4$ and novel aspirin-triggered LXA$_4$ stable analogs in vivo, namely, that topical application of these analogs and association with the murine receptor inhibits neutrophil infiltration in skin. The mouse LXA$_4$R isolated from a spleen cDNA library had a characteristic sequence of seven-transmembrane-spanning G protein-coupled receptors *(152)*, and its homology to the human LXA$_4$R *(69)* was 73% at the amino acid level (Fig. 5). Mouse LXA$_4$R gave high-affinity binding to 3H-LXA$_4$ (K_d 1.5 nM), with values similar to those obtained with the

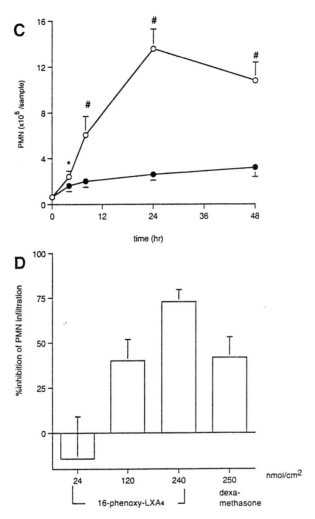

Fig. 6. **(C)** Ears were treated topically with either vehicle (○) or 16-phenoxy-LXA$_4$ (240 nmol) (●) and then 5 μg of LTB$_4$ was added. Results represent mean ± SEM of $n = 4$. *, $p < 0.01$; #, $p < 0.05$ vs 16-phenoxy-LXA$_4$ treatment. **(D)** Mouse ears were exposed topically to either vehicle or the indicated amounts of 16-phenoxy-LXA$_4$ or dexamethasone and then stimulated by 5 μg of LTB$_4$ for 8 h. Percent inhibition of PMN infiltration was calculated with vehicle treated ear as 100% after background levels (MPO activity of ear treated with acetone alone) were subtracted. Results are mean ± SEM of $n = 3$ or 4.

human LXA$_4$R (1.7 nM) expressed in CHO cells *(69)*. CHO cells stably transfected with mouse LXA$_4$R and exposed to LXA$_4$ selectively hydrolyzed GTP, indicating that LXA$_4$ stimulates functional coupling of LXA$_4$R and G protein. Tissue distribution of mouse LXA$_4$R mRNA paralleled the appearance of human LXA$_4$R mRNA, and this mRNA was most abundant in mouse neutrophils, followed by spleen and lung. Bioactive LXA$_4$ stable analogs effectively displaced both ^{3}H-LXA$_4$ and ^{3}H-LTD$_4$ binding to human neutrophils and endothelial cells, respectively, results that are consistent with those obtained with native LXA$_4$ *(67,68)*. These LXA$_4$ and ATL analogs inhibited

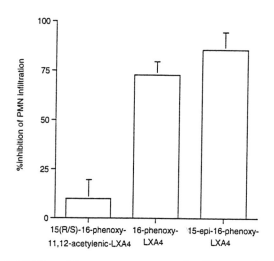

Fig. 7. Selective inhibition. Mouse ears were topically treated with either vehicle or 15(*R*/*S*)-16-phenoxy-11,12-acetylenic-LXA$_4$ (120 nmol); 16-phenoxy-LXA$_4$ (240 nmol); or 15-epi-16-phenoxy-LXA$_4$ (240 nmol), and then exposed to LTB$_4$ (5 mg) for 8 h. Results represent the mean ± SEM of n = 3–6.

neutrophil infiltration in the mouse ear inflammation model, and the level of inhibition was as potent as the well-established antiinflammatory steroid dexamethasone (Fig. 6D). The inhibitory actions of LXA$_4$ stable analogs were stereoselective, with the *R* epimer (i.e., 15-epi-16-phenoxy-LXA$_4$: aspirin-triggered 15-epi-LXA$_4$ analog) showing a trend for greater potency in this model (Figs. 6 and 7).

In the phylogenetic tree, mouse and human LXA$_4$R are closely related and belong to the chemokine receptor family (*see* dendogram in Fig. 8), rather than having an association with members of the family of prostanoid receptors *(155)*. The receptor for LTB$_4$ was recently cloned and characterized *(65)*. As one would perhaps expect, it was distantly related to certain chemokine receptors including the LXA$_4$R. The homology between LXA$_4$R and LTB$_4$R is greatest in the second and seventh TM regions. Although the LXA$_4$ receptors are highly analogous to the FMLP receptor in humans and mice, mouse leukocytes do not show a potent response to FMLP, and no endogenous ligands are known for these receptors in the mouse. The chemokine receptor group also includes both the Fusin (CXCR-4) receptor and RANTES receptor, which have recently been shown to serve as cofactors for HIV-1 infection *(156,157)*. LXA$_4$ is indeed generated during HIV infection by monocytes and astrocytes interacting in vitro *(158)*, but whether there is a connection between these and the authors' present results with LXA$_4$ actions remains to be determined.

Results reviewed here are also the first direct demonstration of the ability of both LXA$_4$ and novel aspirin-triggered LXA$_4$ stable analogs to inhibit neutrophil migration in vivo. 16-phenoxy-LXA$_4$, which resists enzymatic degradation and is a potent inhibitor of neutrophil adhesion and transmigration in vitro *(90)*, applied topically to mouse ear skin just prior to induction of inflammation clearly blocks neutrophil infiltration in a concentration-dependent fashion. LXA$_4$ analog-induced inhibition of neutrophil infiltration into the ear skin was as potent as topical applications of dexamethasone and required the tetraene structure, since the 11,12-acetylenic–containing analog was

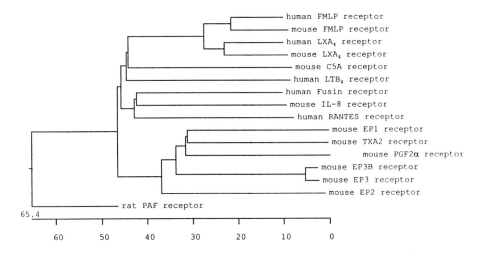

Fig. 8. Dendogram: phylogenetic relationship for the LXA_4R (mouse and human) compared to other known receptors. LXA_4 and LTB_4 receptors are more closely related to each other than to PG receptors.

essentially not effective within this concentration range (Fig. 7). It is of particular interest to point out that other eicosanoid stable analogs such as the analog of PGI_2, Iloprost, significantly enhanced LTB_4-induced leukocyte infiltration in this mouse ear model *(159)*. Thus, the inhibitory actions of LXA_4 and 15-epi-LXA_4 stable analogs established here, for the first time, in an in vivo model provide evidence for the ability of LXA_4 to block neutrophil migration, which appears to be a unique action of LXs when compared to other eicosanoids that either initiate (i.e., LTB_4) or enhance (PGE_2, PGI_2) this response in vivo *(141,159)*.

The inhibitory actions of LXA_4 and 15-epi-LXA_4 analog reviewed here are not 5likely to be the result of blocking LTB_4 binding to its receptor on neutrophils, because LXA_4 does not compete for the specific binding of ^3H-LTB_4 (4°C) to neutrophils or differentiated HL-60 cells expressing LTB_4 receptors *(68)*. One possible cellular basis for this in vivo inhibitory action of these analogs is the downregulation of neutrophil CD11b/CD18 as the authors have recently demonstrated for native LXA_4 in vitro, which requires the engagement of LXA_4R *(142)*. Since these LXA_4 and 15-epi-LXA_4 analogs, which stereoselectively inhibit neutrophil migration, also effectively displace specific binding of ^3H-LXA_4 to its myeloid receptor on neutrophils, it is likely that these LXA_4 analogs interact with the LXA_4R in vivo. This notion is supported by the finding that the mouse receptor is primarily associated with mouse neutrophils, which appear to be the target for their in vivo actions. To address a possible systemic action of the LX analogs applied topically, the authors added 15-epi-16-phenoxy-LXA_4 to one ear, and LTB_4 was applied to the other ear. In this setting, the LXA_4 analog did not inhibit LTB_4-induced PMN infiltration, suggesting that the action of these analogs was local. Together these findings indicate that activation of the LXA_4R in vivo results in an anti-inflammatory outcome counteracting the actions of proinflammatory signals, such as LTB_4 in vivo. Moreover, the findings reviewed here provide the first evidence for anti-inflammatory seven transmembrane spanning receptors and pathways.

Addition of aspirin to various cell types in vitro enhances native LX production during cell–cell interactions and triggers the generation of 15-epi-LXs by a separate biosynthetic pathway (reviewed in ref. *149*). These novel LX *R* epimers appear to mediate some of the beneficial actions of aspirin, in particular, 15-epi-LXA$_4$, which blocks neutrophil adhesion to endothelial cells *(82)*. Therefore, it is of interest that 15-epi-16-phenoxy-LXA$_4$, an analog of 15-epi-LXA$_4$, was the most potent inhibitor of neutrophil infiltration in vivo of this series of LXA$_4$ and 15-epi-LXA$_4$ analogs (Fig. 7). Aspirin has both beneficial and deleterious actions in humans. It is possible that certain of aspirin's beneficial actions might now be open to further experimentation using analogs of 15-epi-LXs. Taken together, the present findings provide direct further evidence that LXA$_4$ and novel aspirin-triggered 15-epi-LXA$_4$ stable analogs, as well as mouse LXA$_4$R cDNA, serve as useful tools to investigate the actions and role of LXA$_4$ and aspirin-triggered 15-epi-LXA$_4$ in in vivo models.

Acknowledgments

The authors thank Mary Halm Small for expert assistance in preparation of this chapter. The authors are also grateful to Dr. N. Petasis and V. Fokin (Department of Chemistry, University of Southern California, Los Angeles, CA 90089) for their collaborative efforts in the total synthesis of LXA$_4$ analogs used in the experiments reviewed here, and Tomoko Takano, MD, PhD and Jane Maddox, DVM, PhD for their efforts in the studies reviewed here from the C.N.S. laboratory. Thanks are also extended to Martin Mueller, Martina Blomster Andberg, Anders Wetterholm, Mats Hamberg, Eva Ohlson, Hans Jörnvall, and Bengt Samuelsson for their contributions to the work reviewed from the J.Z.H. laboratory.

Studies in the laboratory were supported in part by National Institutes of Health grant nos. GM-38765 and P01-DK50305 (C.N.S.), the Swedish Medical Research Council grant no. O3X-10350, Vårdalstiftelsen, and European Union grant no. BMH4-CT960229 (J.Z.H.).

References

1. Rhee, S. G., and Choi, K. D. (1992) Regulation of inositol phospholipid-specific phospholipase C isozymes. *J. Biol. Chem.* **267,** 12,393–12,396.
2. Serhan, C. N., Haeggström, J. Z., and Leslie, C. C. (1996) Lipid mediator networks in cell signaling: Update and impact of cytokines. *FASEB J.* **10,** 1147–1158.
3. Venable, M. E., Zimmerman, G. A., McIntyre, T. M., and Prescott, S. M. (1993) Platelet-activating factor: a phospholipid autacoid with diverse actions. *J. Lipid Res.* **34,** 691–702.
4. Kudo, I., Murakami, M., Hara, S., and Inoue, K. (1993) Mammalian nonpancreatic phospholipases A$_2$. *Biochim. Biophys. Acta* **177,** 217–231.
5. Barbour, S. E. and Dennis, E. A. (1993) Antisense inhibition of group II phospholipase A$_2$ expression blocks the production of prostaglandin E$_2$ by P388D$_1$ cells. *J. Biol. Chem.* **268,** 21,875–21,882.
6. Clark, J. D., Schievella, A. R., Nalefski, E. A., and Lin, L.-L. (1995) Cytosolic phospholipase A$_2$. *J. Lipid Med. Cell Signal.* **12,** 83–117.
7. De Carvalho, M., Garritano, J., and Leslie, C. (1995) Regulation of lysophospholipase activity of the 85 kDa phospholipase A$_2$ and activation in mouse peritoneal macrophages. *J. Biol. Chem.* **35,** 20,439–20,446.
8. Sharp, J. C., Pickard, R. T., Chiou, X. G., Manetta, J. V., Kovacevic, S., Miller, J. R., Varshavsky, A. D., Roberts, E. F., Strifler, B. A., Brems, D. N., and Kramer, R. M. (1994) Serine 228 is essential for catalytic activities of 85-kDa cytosolic phospholipase A$_2$. *J. Biol. Chem.* **269,** 23,250–23,254.

9. Ackermann, E. J. and Dennis, E. A. (1995) Mammalian calcium-independent phospholipase A_2. *Biochim. Biophys. Acta* **1259,** 125–136.
10. Smith, W. L., and DeWitt, D. L. (1995) Biochemistry of prostaglandin endoperoxide H synthase-1 and synthase-2 and their differential susceptibility to nonsteroidal anti-inflammatory drugs. *Semin. Nephrol.* **15,** 179–194.
11. Herschman, H. R. (1996) Prostaglandin synthase 2. *Biochim. Biophys. Acta* **1299,** 125–140.
12. Riendeau, D., Percival, M. D., Boyce, S., Brideau, C., Charleson, S., Cromlish, W., Ethier, D., Evans, J., Falgueyret, J. P., Ford-Hutchinson, A. W., Gordon, R., Greig, G., Gresser, M., Guay, J., Kargman, S., Leger, S., Mancini, J. A., Oneill, G., Ouellet, M., Rodger, I. W., Therien, M., Wang, Z., Webb, J. K., Wong, E., Xu, L., et al. (1997) Biochemical and pharmacological profile of a tetrasubstituted furanone as a highly selective COX-2 inhibitor. *Br. J. Pharmacol.* **121,** 105–117.
13. Levy, G. N. (1997) Prostaglandin H synthases, nonsteroidal anti-inflammatory drugs, and colon cancer. *FASEB J.* **11,** 234–247.
14. Lepley, R. A. and Fitzpatrick, F. A. (1994) 5–Lipoxygenase contains a functional Src homology 3–binding motif that interacts with the Src homology 3 domain of Grb2 and cytoskeletal proteins. *J. Biol. Chem.* **269,** 24,163–24,168.
15. Haeggström, J. Z., Wetterholm, A., Medina, J. F., and Samuelsson, B. (1993) Leukotriene A_4 hydrolase: Structural and functional properties of the active center. *J. Lipid Med.* **6,** 1–13.
16. Lam, B. K., Penrose, J. F., Freeman, G. J., and Austen, K. F. (1994) Expression cloning of a cDNA for human leukotriene C_4 synthase, an integral membrane protein conjugating reduced glutathione to leukotriene A_4. *Proc. Natl. Acad. Sci. USA* **91,** 7663–7667.
17. Jakobsson, P. J., Mancini, J. A., and Ford-Hutchinson, A. W. (1996) Identification and Characterization of a novel human microsomal glutathione s-transferase with leukotriene C_4 synthase activity and significant sequence identity to 5-lipoxygenase-activating protein and leukotriene C_4 synthase. *J. Biol. Chem.* **271,** 22,203–22,210.
18. Scoggan, K. A., Jakobsson, P.-J., and Ford-Hutchinson, A. W. (1997) Production of leukotriene C_4 in different human tissues is attributable to distinct membrane bound biosynthetic enzymes. *J. Biol. Chem.*, **272,** 10,182–10,187.
19. Hammarberg, T., Zhang, Y. Y., Lind, B., Rådmark, O., and Samuelsson, B. (1995) Mutations at the C-terminal isoleucine and other potential iron ligands of 5-lipoxygenase. *Eur. J. Biochem.* **230,** 401–407.
20. Blomster, M., Wetterholm, A., Mueller, M. J., and Haeggström, J. Z. (1995) Evidence for a catalytic role of tyrosine 383 in the peptidase reaction of leukotriene A_4 hydrolase. *Eur. J. Biochem.* **231,** 528–534.
21. Mueller, M. J., Wetterholm, A., Blomster, M., Jörnvall, H., Samuelsson, B., and Haeggström, J. Z. (1995) Leukotriene A_4 hydrolase: Mapping of a henicosapeptide involved in mechanism-based inactivation. *Proc. Natl. Acad. Sci. USA* **92,** 8383–8387.
22. Mueller, M. J., Blomster, M., Oppermann, U. C. T., Jornvall, H., Samuelsson, B., and Haeggstrom, J. Z. (1996) Leukotriene A_4 hydrolase—protection from mechanism-based inactivation by mutation of tyrosine-378. *Proc. Natl. Acad. Sci. USA* **93,** 5931–5935.
23. Mueller, M. J., Blomster, M., Samuelsson, B., and Haeggström, J. Z. (1996) Leukotriene A_4 hydrolase: Mutation of tyrosine-383 allows conversion of leukotriene A_4 into an isomer of leukotriene B_4. *J. Biol. Chem.* **271,** 24,345–24,348.
24. Blomster Andberg, M., Hamberg, M., and Haeggström, J. Z. (1997) Mutation of tyrosine 383 in leukotriene A_4 hydrolase allows formation of 5S,6S-dihydroxy-7,9-*trans*-11,14-*cis*-eicosatetraenoic acid: Implications for the epoxide hydrolase mechanism. *J. Biol. Chem.* **272,** 23,057–23,063.
25. Lam, B. K., Penrose, J. F., Xu, K. Y., Baldasaro, M. H., and Austen, K. F. (1997) Site-directed mutagenesis of human leukotriene C_4 synthase. *J. Biol. Chem.* **272,** 13,923–13,928.
26. Wang, L. H., Hajibeigi, A., Xu, X. M., Loose-Mitchell, D., and Wu, K. K. (1993) Characterization of the promoter of human prostaglandin H synthase-1 gene. *Biochem. Biophys. Res. Commun.* **190,** 406–411.
27. Funk, C. D. (1993) Molecular biology in the eicosanoid field. *Prog. Nucleic Acid Res. Mol. Biol.* **45,** 67–98.
28. In, K. H., Asano, K., Beier, D., Grobholz, J., Finn, P. W., Silverman, E. K., Silverman, E. S., Collins, T., Fischer, A. R., Keith, T. P., Serino, K., Kim, S. W., Desanctis, G. T., Yandava, C.,

Pillari, A., Rubin, P., Kemp, J., Israel, E., Busse, W., Ledford, D., Murray, J. J., Segal, A., Tinkleman, D., and Drazen, J. M. (1997) Naturally occurring mutations in the human 5-lipoxygenase gene promoter that modify transcription factor binding and reporter gene transcription. *J. Clin. Invest.* **99,** 1130–1137.

29. Ford-Hutchinson, A. W., Gresser, M., and Young, R. N. (1994) 5-lipoxygenase. *Ann. Rev. Biochem.* **63,** 383–417.

30. Penrose, J. F., Spector, J., Baldasaro, M., Xu, K. Y., Boyce, J., Arm, J. P., Austen, K. F., and Lam, B. K. (1996) Molecular cloning of the gene for human leukotriene C_4 synthase—organization, nucleotide sequence, and chromosomal localization to 5q35. *J. Biol. Chem.* **271,** 11,356–11,361.

31. Mancini, J. A. and Evans, J. F. (1995) Cloning and characterization of the human leukotriene A4 hydrolase gene. *Eur. J. Biochem.* **231,** 65–71.

32. Jendraschak, E., Kaminski, W. E., Kiefl, R., and von Schacky, C. (1996) The human leukotriene A_4 hydrolase gene is expressed in two alternatively spliced mRNA forms. *Biochem. J.* **314,** 733–737.

33. Brash, A. R., Boeglin, W. E., and Chang, M. S. (1997) Discovery of a second 15*S*-lipoxygenase in humans. *Proc. Natl. Acad. Sci. USA* **94,** 6148–6152.

34. Morita, I., Schindler, M., Regier, M. K., Otto, J. C., Hori, T., DeWitt, D. L., and Smith, W. L. (1995) Different intracellular locations for prostaglandin endoperoxide H synthase-1 and -2. *J. Biol. Chem.* **270,** 10,902–10,908.

35. Morham, S. G., Langenbach, R., Loftin, C. D., Tiano, H. F., Vouloumanos, N., Jennette, J. C., Mahler, J. F., Kluckman, K. D., Ledford, A., Lee, C. A., and Smithies, O. (1995) Prostaglandin synthase 2 gene disruption causes severe renal pathology in the mouse. *Cell* **83,** 473–482.

36. Langenbach, R., Morham, S. G., Tiano, H. F., Loftin, C. D., Ghanayem, B. I., Chulada, P. C., Mahler, J. F., Lee, C. A., Goulding, E. H., Kluckman, K. D., Kim, H. S., and Smithies, O. (1995) Prostaglandin synthase 1 gene disruption in mice reduces arachidonic acid-induced inflammation and indomethacin-induced gastric ulceration. *Cell* **83,** 483–492.

37. Woods, J. W., Coffey, M. J., Brock, T. G., Singer, I. I., and Peters-Golden, M. (1995) 5-Lipoxygenase is located in the euchromatin of the nucleus in resting human alveolar macrophages and translocates to the nuclear envelope upon cell activation. *J. Clin. Invest.* **95,** 2035–2046.

38. Brock, T. G., McNish, R. W., Bailie, M. B., and Peters-Golden, M. (1997) Rapid import of cytosolic 5-lipoxygenase into the nucleus of neutrophils after in vivo recruitment and in vitro adherence. *J. Biol. Chem.* **272,** 8276–8280.

39. Brock, T. G., McNish, R. W., and Peters-Golden, M. (1995) Translocation and leukotriene synthetic capacity of nuclear 5-lipoxygenase in rat basophilic leukemia cells and alveolar macrophages. *J. Biol. Chem.* **270,** 21,652–21,658.

40. Schievella, A. R., Regier, M. K., Smith, W. L., and Lin, L.-L. (1995) Calcium-mediated translocation of cytosolic phospholipase A_2 to the nuclear envelope and endoplasmic reticulum. *J. Biol. Chem.* **270,** 30,749–30,754.

41. Glover, S., de Carvalho, M. S., Bayburt, T., Jonas, M., Chi, E., Leslie, C. C., and Gelb, M. H. (1995) Translocation of the 85-kDa phospholipase A_2 from cytosol to the nuclear envelope in rat basophilic leukemia cells stimulated with calcium ionophore or IgE/antigen. *J. Biol. Chem.* **270,** 15,359–15,367.

42. Devchand, P. R., Keller, H., Peters, J. M., Vazquez, M., Gonzalez, F. J., and Wahli, W. (1996) The PPARα—leukotriene B_4 pathway to inflammation control. *Nature* **384,** 39–43.

43. Chen, X. S., Sheller, J. R., Johnson, E. N., and Funk, C. D. (1994) Role of leukotrienes revealed by targeted disruption of the 5-lipoxygenase gene. *Nature* **372,** 179–182.

44. Goulet, J. L., Snouwaert, J. N., Latour, A. M., Coffman, T. M., and Koller, B. H. (1994) Altered inflammatory responses in leukotriene-deficient mice. *Proc. Natl. Acad. Sci. USA* **91,** 12,852–12,856.

45. Bailie, M. B., Standiford, T. J., Laichalk, L. L., Coffey, M. J., Strieter, R., and Peters-Golden, M. (1996) Leukotriene-deficient mice manifest enhanced lethality from *Klebsiella* pneumonia in association with decreased alveolar macrophage phagocytic and bactericidal activities. *J. Immunol.* **157,** 5221–5224.

46. Irvin, C. G., Tu, Y. P., Sheller, J. R., and Funk, C. D. (1997) 5-lipoxygenase products are necessary for ovalbumin-induced airway responsiveness in mice. *Am. J. Physiol.* **16,** L1053–L1058.

47. Byrum, R. S., Goulet, J. L., Griffiths, R. J., and Koller, B. H. (1997) Role of the 5-lipoxygenase-activating protein (FLAP) in murine acute inflammatory responses. *J. Exp. Med.* **185,** 1065–1075.

48. Griffiths, R. J., Smith, M. A., Roach, M. L., Stock, J. L., Stam, E. J., Milici, A. J., Scampoli, D. N., Eskra, J. D., Byrum, R. S., Koller, B. H., and McNeish, J. D. (1997) Collagen-induced arthritis is reduced in 5-lipoxygenase-activating protein-deficient mice. *J. Exp. Med.* **185,** 1123–1129.

49. Ring, W. L., Riddick, C. A., Baker, J. R., Munafo, D. A., and Bigby, T. D. (1996) Lymphocytes stimulate expression of 5-lipoxygenase and its activating protein in monocytes in vitro via granulocyte-macrophage colony stimulating factor and interleukin-3. *J. Clin. Invest.* **97,** 1293–1301.

50. Feltenmark, S., Runarsson, G., Larsson, P., Jakobsson, P.-J., Björkholm, M., and Claesson, H.-E. (1995) Diverse expression of cytosolic phospholipase A_2, 5-lipoxygenase and prostaglandin H synthase 2 in acute pre-B-lymphocytic leukaemia cells. *Br. J. Haematol.* **90,** 585–594.

51. Nassar, G. M., Morrow, J. D., Roberts, L. J. II, Lakkis, F. G., and Badr, K. F. (1994) Induction of 15-lipoxygenase by interleukin-13 in human blood monocytes. *J. Biol. Chem.* **269,** 27,631–27,634.

52. Stenke, L., Reizenstein, P., and Lindgren, J. A. (1994) Leukotrienes and lipoxins—new potential performers in the regulation of human myelopoiesis. *Leukemia Res.* **18,** 727–732.

53. Hannun, Y. A. and Obeid, L. M. (1995) Ceramide: An intracellular signal for apoptosis. *Trends Biol. Sci.* **20,** 73–77.

54. Ballou, L. R., Laulederkind, S. J. F., Rosloniec, E. F., and Raghow, R. (1996) Ceramide signalling and the immune response. *Biochim. Biophys. Acta* **1301,** 273–287.

55. Ushikubi, F., Nakajima, M., Hirata, M., Okuma, M., Fujiwara, M., and Narumiya, S. (1989) Purification of the thromboxane A_2/prostaglandin H2 receptor from human blood platelets. *J. Biol. Chem.* **264,** 16,496–16,501.

56. Hirata, M., Hayashi, Y., Ushikubi, F., Yokota, Y., Kageyama, R., Nakanishi, S., and Narumiya, S. (1991) Cloning and expression of cDNA for a human thromboxane A_2 receptor. *Nature* **349,** 617–620.

57. Ushikubi, F., Hirata, M., and Narumiya, S. (1995) Molecular biology of prostanoid receptors; an overview. *J. Lipid Mediators & Cell Signalling* **12,** 343–359.

58. Namba, T., Sugimoto, Y., Negishi, M., Irie, A., Ushikubi, F., Kakizuka, A., Ito, S., Ichikawa, A., and Narumiya, S. (1993) Alternative splicing of C-terminal tail of prostaglandin E receptor subtype EP3 determines G-protein specificity. *Nature* **365,** 166–170 (see comments).

59. Sugimoto, Y., Negishi, M., Hayashi, Y., Namba, T., Honda, A., Watabe, A., Hirata, M., Narumiya, S., and Ichikawa, A. (1993) Two isoforms of the EP3 receptor with different carboxyl-terminal domains: Identical ligand binding properties and different coupling properties with Gi proteins. *J. Biol. Chem.* **268,** 2712–2718.

60. Negishi, M., Sugimoto, Y., Irie, A., Narumiya, S., and Ichikawa, A. (1993) Two isoforms of prostaglandin E receptor EP3 subtype. Different COOH-terminal domains determine sensitivity to agonist-induced desensitization. *J. Biol. Chem.* **268,** 9517–9521.

61. Kobayashi, T., Kiriyama, M., Hirata, T., Hirata, M., Ushikubi, F., and Narumiya, S. (1997) Identification of domains conferring ligand binding specificity to the prostanoid receptor—studies on chimeric prostacyclin/prostaglandin d receptors. *J. Biol. Chem.* **272,** 15,154–15,160.

62. Sugimoto, Y., Yamasaki, A., Segi, E., Tsuboi, K., Aze, Y., Nishimura, T., Oida, H., Yoshida, N., Tanaka, T., Katsuyama, M., Hasumoto, K., Murata, T., Hirata, M., Ushikubi, F., Negishi, M., Ichikawa, A., and Narumiya, S. (1997) Failure of parturition in mice lacking the prostaglandin f receptor. *Science* **277,** 681–683.

63. Matsuoka, T., Murata, T., Hirata, M., Ushikubi, F., Yoshida, N., and Narumiya, S. (1997) Analyses of TP-receptor deficient mice. Abstract at the Keystone symposia, Lipid Mediators: Recent Advances in Molecular Biology, Understanding of Regulation and Pharmacology, Keystone, CO., Jan. 26–31, Abstract no. 209, p. 16.

64. Murata, T., Ushikubi, F., Matsuoka, T., Hirata, M., Yamasaki, A., Sugimoto, Y., Ichikawa, A., Aze, Y., Tanaka, T., Yoshida, N., Ueno, A., Ohishi, S., and Narumiya, S. (1997) Altered pain perception and inflammatory response in mice lacking prostacyclin receptor. *Nature* **388,** 678–682.

65. Yokomizo, T., Izumi, T., Chang, K., Takuwa, T., and Shimizu, T. (1997) A G-protein-coupled receptor for leukotriene B_4 that mediates chemotaxis. *Nature* **387,** 620–624.

66. Owman, C., Nilsson, C., and Lolait, S. J. (1996) Cloning of cDNA encoding a putative chemoattractant receptor. *Genomics* **37,** 187–194.

67. Fiore, S., Ryeom, S. W., Weller, P. F., and Serhan, C. N. (1992) Lipoxin recognition sites. Specific binding of labeled lipoxin A_4 with human neutrophils. *J. Biol. Chem.* **267**, 16,168–16,176.

68. Fiore, S., Romano, M., Reardon, E. M., and Serhan, C. N. (1993) Induction of functional lipoxin A_4 receptors in HL-60 cells. *Blood* **81**, 3395–3403.

69. Fiore, S., Maddox, J. F., Perez, H. D., and Serhan, C. N. (1994) Identification of a human cDNA encoding a functional high affinity lipoxin A_4 receptor. *J. Exp. Med.* **180**, 253–260.

70. Brady, H. R., Papayianni, A., and Serhan, C. N. (1995) Potential vascular roles for lipoxins in the "stop programs" of host defense and inflammation. *Trends Cardiovasc. Med.* **5**, 186–192.

71. Barry, O. P., Pratico, D., Lawson, J. A., and FitzGerald, G. A. (1997) Transcellular activation of platelets and endothelial cells by bioactive lipids in platelet microparticles. *J. Clin. Invest.* **99**, 2118–2127.

72. O'Meara, Y. M., and Brady, H. R. (1997) Lipoxins, leukocyte recruitment and the resolution phase of acute glomerulonephritis. *Kidney Intl.* **51(Suppl. 58)**, S56–S61.

73. Hogg, J. H., Ollmann, I. R., Haeggström, J. Z., Wetterholm, A., Samuelsson, B., and Wong, C.-H. (1995) Amino hydroxamic acids as potent inhibitors of LTA_4 hydrolase. *Bioorg. Med. Chem.* **3**, 1405–1415.

74. Wetterholm, A., Haeggström, J. Z., Samuelsson, B., Yuan, W., Munoz, B., and Wong, C.-H. (1995) Potent and selective inhibitors of leukotriene A_4 hydrolase: Effects on purified enzyme and human polymorphonuclear leukocytes. *J. Pharmacol. Exp. Ther.* **275**, 31–37.

75. Yuan, J. H., Birkmeier, J., Yang, D. C., Hribar, J. D., Liu, N., Bible, R., Hajdu, E., Rock, M., and Schoenhard, G. (1996) Isolation and identification of metabolites of leukotriene A_4 hydrolase inhibitor SC-57461 in rats. *Drug Metab. Dispos.* **24**, 1124–1133.

76. Smith, W. G., Russell, M. A., Liang, C.-D., Askonas, L. A., Kachur, J. F., Kim, S., Souresrafil, N., Price, D. V., and Clapp, N. K. (1996) Pharmacological characterization of selective inhibitors of leukotriene A_4 hydrolase. *Prostaglandins Leukotrienes Essential Fatty Acids* **55(Suppl. 1)**, 13.

77. Dahlén, S.-E., Dahlén, B., Kumlin, M., Björck, T., Ihre, E., and Zetterström, O. (1994) Clinical and experimental studies of leukotrienes as mediators of airway obstruction in humans. *Adv. Prostaglandin Thromboxane Leukotriene Res.* **22**, 155–166.

78. Israel, E., Dermarkarian, R., Rosenberg, M., Sperling, R., Taylor, G., Rubin, P., and Drazen, J. M. (1990) The effects of a 5-lipoxygenase inhibitor on asthma induced by cold, dry air. *N. Engl. J. Med.* **323**, 1740–1744.

79. Samuelsson, B., Dahlén, S. E., Lindgren, J. Å., Rouzer, C. A., and Serhan, C. N. (1987) Leukotrienes and lipoxins: Structures, biosynthesis, and biological effects. *Science* **237**, 1171–1176.

80. Lindgren, J. A., and Edenius, C. (1993) Transcellular biosynthesis of leukotrienes and lipoxins via leukotriene A_4 transfer. *Trends Pharmacol. Sci.* **14**, 351–354.

81. Serhan, C. N. (1994) Lipoxin biosynthesis and its impact in inflammatory and vascular events. *Biochim. Biophys. Acta* **1212**, 1–25.

82. Clària, J., and Serhan, C. N. (1995) Aspirin triggers previously undescribed bioactive eicosanoids by human endothelial cell-leukocyte interactions. *Proc. Natl. Acad. Sci. USA* **92**, 9475–9479.

83. Rowley, A. F., Hill, D. J., Ray, C. E., and Munro, R. (1997) Haemostasis in fish—an evolutionary perspective. *Thromb. Haemost.* **77**, 227–233.

84. Marcus, A. J., Broekman, M. J., Safier, L. B., Ullman, H. L., Islam, N., Serhan, C. N., Rutherford, L. E., Korchak, H. M., and Weissmann, G. (1982) Formation of leukotrienes and other hydroxy acids during platelet-neutrophil interactions in vitro. *Biochem. Biophys. Res. Commun.* **109**, 130–137.

85. Serhan, C. N., and Sheppard, K. A. (1990) Lipoxin formation during human neutrophil-platelet interactions. Evidence for the transformation of leukotriene A_4 by platelet 12-lipoxygenase in vitro. *J. Clin. Invest.* **85**, 772–780.

86. Fiore, S., and Serhan, C. N. (1990) Formation of lipoxins and leukotrienes during receptor-mediated interactions of human platelets and recombinant human granulocyte/macrophage colony-stimulating factor-primed neutrophils. *J. Exp. Med.* **172**, 1451–1457.

87. Romano, M., Chen, X. S., Takahashi, Y., Yamamoto, S., Funk, C. D., and Serhan, C. N. (1993) Lipoxin synthase activity of human platelet 12-lipoxygenase. *Biochem. J.* **296**, 127–133.

88. Clària, J., Lee, M. H., and Serhan, C. N. (1996) Aspirin-triggered lipoxins (15-epi-LX) are generated by the human lung adenocarcinoma cell line (A549)-neutrophil interactions and are potent inhibitors of cell proliferation. *Mol. Med.* **2**, 583–596.

89. Takano, T., Fiore, S., Maddox, J. F., Brady, H. R., Petasis, N. A., and Serhan, C. N. (1997) Aspirin-triggered 15-epi-lipoxin A$_4$ and LXA$_4$ stable analogs are potent inhibitors of acute inflammation: Evidence for anti-inflammatory receptors. *J. Exp. Med.* **185**, 1693–1704.

90. Serhan, C. N., Maddox, J. F., Petasis, N. A., Akritopoulou-Zanze, I., Papayianni, A., Brady, H. R., Colgan, S. P., and Madara, J. L. (1995) Design of lipoxin A$_4$ stable analogs that block transmigration and adhesion of human neutrophils. *Biochemistry* **34**, 14,609–14,615.

91. Marcus, A. J. (1995) Aspirin as prophylaxis against colorectal cancer. *N. Engl. J. Med.* **333**, 656–658.

92. Giovannucci, E., Rimm, E. B., Stampfer, M. J., Colditz, G. A., Ascherio, A., and Willett, W. C. (1994) Aspirin use and the risk for colorectal cancer and adenoma in male health professionals. *Ann. Intern. Med.* **121**, 241–246.

93. Serhan, C. N., Hamberg, M., and Samuelsson, B. (1984) Lipoxins: novel series of biologically active compounds formed from arachidonic acid in human leukocytes. *Proc. Natl. Acad. Sci. USA* **81**, 5335–5339.

94. Ford-Hutchinson, A. W. (1991) Arachidonate 15-lipoxygenase; characteristics and potential biological significance. *Eicosanoids* **4**, 65–74.

95. Levy, B. D., Romano, M., Chapman, H. A., Reilly, J. J., Drazen, J., and Serhan, C. N. (1993) Human alveolar macrophages have 15-lipoxygenase and generate 15(*S*)-hydroxy-5,8,11-*cis*-13-*trans*-eicosatetraenoic acid and lipoxins. *J. Clin. Invest.* **92**, 1572–1579.

96. Sigal, E., and Conrad, D. J. (1994) Human 15-lipoxygenase: A potential effector molecule for interleukin-4. *Adv. Prostaglandin Thromboxane Leukotriene Res.* **22**, 309–316.

97. Katoh, T., Lakkis, F. G., Makita, N., and Badr, K. F. (1994) Co-regulated expression of glomerular 12/15–lipoxygenase and interleukin-4 mRNA in rat nephrotoxic nephritis. *Kidney Int.* **46**, 341–349.

98. Anderson, G. P. and Coyle, A. J. (1994) TH$_2$ and 'TH$_2$-like' cells in allergy and asthma: pharmacological perspectives. *Trends Pharmacol. Sci.* **15**, 324.

99. Pouliot, M., McDonald, P. P., Borgeat, P., and McColl, S. R. (1994) Granulocyte/macrophage colony-stimulating factor stimulates the expression of the 5-lipoxygenase-activating protein (FLAP) in human neutrophils. *J. Exp. Med.* **179**, 1225–1232.

100. L'Heureux, G. P., Bourgoin, S., Jean, N., McColl, S. R., and Naccache, P. H. (1995) Diverging signal transduction pathways activated by interleukin-8 and related chemokines in human neutrophils: Interleukin-8, but not NAP-2 or GROAα, stimulates phospholipase D activity. *Blood* **85**, 522–531.

101. Lefer, A. M., Stahl, G. L., Lefer, D. J., Brezinski, M. E., Nicolaou, K. C., Veale, C. A., Abe, Y., and Smith, J. B. (1988) Lipoxins A$_4$ and B$_4$: comparison of icosanoids having bronchoconstrictor and vasodilator actions but lacking platelet aggregatory activity. *Proc. Natl. Acad. Sci. USA* **85**, 8340–8344.

102. Dahlén, S.-E. and Serhan, C. N. (1991) Lipoxins: bioactive lipoxygenase interaction products, in *Lipoxygenases and Their Products* (Wong, A. and Crooke, S. T., eds.), Academic, San Diego, pp. 235–276.

103. Lee, T. H., Lympany, P., Crea, A. E., and Spur, B. W. (1991) Inhibition of leukotriene B$_4$–induced neutrophil migration by lipoxin A$_4$: Structure-function relationships. *Biochem. Biophys. Res. Commun.* **180**, 1416–1421.

104. Badr, K. F., DeBoer, D. K., Schwartzberg, M., and Serhan, C. N. (1989) Lipoxin A$_4$ antagonizes cellular and in vivo actions of leukotriene D$_4$ in rat glomerular mesangial cells: Evidence for competition at a common receptor. *Proc. Natl. Acad. Sci. USA* **86**, 3438–3442.

105. Chavis, C., Chanez, P., Vachier, I., Bousquet, J., Michel, F. B., and Godard, P. (1995) 5-15-diHETE and lipoxins generated by neutrophils from endogenous arachidonic acid as asthma biomarkers. *Biochem. Biophys. Res. Commun.* **207**, 273–279.

106. Chavis, C., Vachier, I., Chanez, P., Bousquet, J., and Godard, P. (1996) 5(S),15(S)-Dihydroxy-eicosatetraenoic acid and lipoxin generation in human polymorphonuclear cells: Dual specificity of 5-lipoxygenase towards endogenous and exogenous precursors. *J. Exp. Med.* **183**, 1633–1643.

107. Thomas, E., Leroux, J. L., Blotman, F., and Chavis, C. (1995) Conversion of endogenous arachidonic acid to 5,15–diHETE and lipoxins by polymorphonuclear cells from patients with rheumatoid arthritis. *Inflamm. Res.* **44**, 121–124.

108. Shen, J., Herderick, E., Cornhill, J. F., Zsigmond, E., Kim, H.-S., Kühn, H., Guevara, N. V., and Chan, L. (1996) Macrophage-mediated 15-lipoxygenase expression protects against atherosclerosis development. *J. Clin. Invest.* **98**, 2201–2208.

109. Edenius, C., Haeggström, J., and Lindgren, J. A. (1988) Transcellular conversion of endogenous arachidonic acid to lipoxins in mixed human platelet-granulocyte suspensions. *Biochem. Biophys. Res. Commun.* **157**, 801–807. (published erratum appears in *Biochem. Biophys. Res. Commun.* (1989) **159(1)**, 370.)

110. Fiore, S. and Serhan, C. N. (1989) Phospholipid bilayers enhance the stability of leukotriene A_4 and epoxytetraenes: Stabilization of eicosanoids by liposomes. *Biochem. Biophys. Res. Commun.* **159**, 477–481.

111. Corey, E. J. and Mehrotra, M. M. (1986) A stereoselective and practical synthesis of 5,6(S,S)-epoxy-15(S)-hydroxy-7(E), 9(E), 11(Z), 13(E)-eicosatetraenoic acid (4), possible precursor of the lipoxins. *Tetrahedron Lett.* **27**, 5173–5176.

112. Sheppard, K. A., Greenberg, S. M., Funk, C. D., Romano, M., and Serhan, C. N. (1992) Lipoxin generation by human megakaryocyte-induced 12-lipoxygenase. *Biochim. Biophys. Acta* **1133**, 223–234.

113. Romano, M. and Serhan, C. N. (1992) Lipoxin generation by permeabilized human platelets. *Biochemistry* **31**, 8269–8277.

114. Lehr, H.-A., Olofsson, A. M., Carew, T. E., Vajkoczy, P., von Andrian, U. H., Hübner, C., Berndt, M. C., Steinberg, D., Messmer, K., and Arfors, K. E. (1994) P-selectin mediates the interaction of circulating leukocytes with platelets and microvascular endothelium in response to oxidized lipoprotein in vivo. *Lab. Invest.* **71**, 380–386.

115. Lehr, H.-A., Frei, B., and Arfors, K.-E. (1994) Vitamin C prevents cigarette smoke-induced leukocyte aggregation and adhesion to endothelium in vivo. *Proc. Natl. Acad. Sci. USA* **91**, 7688–7692.

116. Xiao, G., Tsai, A.-L., Palmer, G., Boyar, W. C., Marshall, P. J., and Kulmacz, R. J. (1997) Analysis of hydroperoxide-induced tyrosyl radicals and lipoxygenase activity in aspirin-treated human prostaglandin H synthase-2. *Biochemistry* **36**, 1836–1845.

117. Mancini, J. A., Vickers, P. J., O'Neill, G. P., Boily, C., Falgueyret, J.-P., and Riendeau, D. (1997) Altered sensitivity of aspirin-acetylated prostaglandin G/H synthase-2 inhibition by nonsteroidal anti-inflammatory drugs. *Mol. Pharmacol.* **51**, 52–60.

118. Savage, M. P., Goldberg, S., Bove, A. A., Deutsch, E., Vetrovec, G., Macdonald, R. G., Bass, T., Margolis, J. R., Whitworth, H. B., Taussig, A., Hirshfeld, J. W., Cowley, M., Hill, J. A., Marks, R. G., Fischman, D. L., Handberg, E., Herrmann, H., and Pepine, C. J. (1995) Effect of thromboxane A_2 blockade on clinical outcome and restenosis after successful coronary angioplasty. *Circulation* **92**, 3194–3200.

119. Hennekens, C., Jonas, M., and Buring, J. (1994) The benefits of aspirin in acute myocardial infarction: Still a well-kept secret in the United States. *Arch. Intern. Med.* **154**, 37–39.

120. Giovannucci, E., Egan, K. M., Hunter, D. J., Stampfer, M. J., Colditz, G. A., Willett, W. C., and Speizer, F. E. (1995) Aspirin and the risk of colorectal cancer in women. *N. Engl. J. Med.* **333**, 609–614.

121. Mayadas, T. N., Mendrick, D. L., Brady, H. R., Tang, T., Papayianni, A., Assmann, K. J. M., Wagner, D. D., Hynes, R. O., and Cotran, R. S. (1996) Acute passive anti-glomerular basement membrane nephritis in P-selectin-deficient mice. *Kidney Int.* **49**, 1342–1349.

122. Garrick, R. and Wong, P. Y. (1991) Enzymatic formation and regulatory function of lipoxins and leukotriene B_4 in rat kidney mesangial cells. *Adv. Exp. Med. Biol.* **314**, 361–369.

123. Edenius, C., Kumlin, M., Björk, T., Anggard, A., and Lindgren, J. A. (1990) Lipoxin formation in human nasal polyps and bronchial tissue. *FEBS Lett.* **272**, 25–28.

124. Tornhamre, S., Gigou, A., Edenius, C., Lellouche, J. P., and Lindgren, J. A. (1992) Conversion of 5,6–dihydroxyeicosatetraenoic acids: a novel pathway for lipoxin formation by human platelets. *FEBS Lett.* **304**, 78–82.

125. Brezinski, M. E. and Serhan, C. N. (1990) Selective incorporation of (15S)-hydroxyeicosatetraenoic acid in phosphatidylinositol of human neutrophils: agonist-induced deacylation and transformation of stored hydroxyeicosanoids. *Proc. Natl. Acad. Sci. USA* **87**, 6248–6252.

126. Niiro, H., Otsuka, T., Izuhara, K., Yamaoka, K., Ohshima, K., Tanabe, T., Hara, S., Nemoto, Y., Tanaka, Y., Nakashima, H., and Niho, Y. (1997) Regulation by interleukin-10 and interleukin-4 of cyclooxygenase-2 expression in human neutrophils. *Blood* **89**, 1621–1628.

127. Brady, H. R. and Serhan, C. N. (1992) Adhesion promotes transcellular leukotriene biosynthesis during neutrophil-glomerular endothelial cell interactions: Inhibition by antibodies against CD18 and L-selectin. *Biochem. Biophys. Res. Commun.* **186**, 1307–1314.

128. Papayianni, A., Serhan, C. N., Phillips, M. L., Rennke, H. G., and Brady, H. R. (1995) Transcellular biosynthesis of lipoxin A_4 during adhesion of platelets and neutrophils in experimental immune complex glomerulonephritis. *Kidney Int.* **47,** 1295–1302.

129. Gronert, K., Virk, S. M., and Herman, C. A. (1995) Thrombocytes are the predominant source of endogenous sulfidopeptide leukotrienes in the bullfrog (*Rana catesbeiana*). *Biochim. Biophys. Acta* **1255,** 311–319.

130. Maddox, J. F., Hachicha, M., Takano, T., Petasis, N. A., Fokin, V. V., and Serhan, C. N. (1997) Lipoxin A_4 stable analogs are potent mimetics that stimulate human monocytes and THP-1 cells via a G-protein linked lipoxin A_4 receptor. *J. Biol. Chem.* **272,** 6972–6978.

131. Lee, T. H., Crea, A. E., Gant, V., Spur, B. W., Marron, B. E., Nicolaou, K. C., Reardon, E., Brezinski, M., and Serhan, C. N. (1990) Identification of lipoxin A_4 and its relationship to the sulfidopeptide leukotrienes C_4, D_4, and E_4 in the bronchoalveolar lavage fluids obtained from patients with selected pulmonary diseases. *Am. Rev. Respir. Dis.* **141,** 1453–1458.

132. Levy, B. D., Bertram, S., Tai, H. H., Israel, E., Fischer, A., Drazen, J. M., and Serhan, C. N. (1993) Agonist-induced lipoxin A_4 generation: detection by a novel lipoxin A_4-ELISA. *Lipids* **28,** 1047–1053.

133. Brezinski, D. A., Nesto, R. W., and Serhan, C. N. (1992) Angioplasty triggers intracoronary leukotrienes and lipoxin A_4: impact of aspirin therapy. *Circulation* **86,** 56–63.

134. Stenke, L., Näsman-Glaser, B., Edenius, C., Samuelsson, J., Palmblad, J., and Lindgren, J. Å. (1990) Lipoxygenase products in myeloproliferative disorders: Increased leukotriene C_4 and decreased lipoxin formation in chronic myeloid leukemia. *Adv. Prostaglandin Thromboxane Leukotriene Res.* **21B,** 883–886.

135. Leszczynski, D. and Ustinov, J. (1990) Protein kinase C-regulated production of prostacyclin by rat endothelium is increased in the presence of lipoxin A_4. *FEBS Lett.* **263,** 117–120.

136. Bratt, J. and Gyllenhammar, H. (1995) The role of nitric oxide in lipoxin A_4-induced polymorphonuclear neutrophil-dependent cytotoxicity to human vascular endothelium in vitro. *Arthritis Rheum.* **38,** 768–776.

137. Tamaoki, J., Tagaya, E., Yamawaki, I., and Konno, K. (1995) Lipoxin A_4 inhibits cholinergic neurotransmission through nitric oxide generation in the rabbit trachea. *Eur. J. Pharmacol.* **287,** 233–236.

138. Lee, T. H., Horton, C. E., Kyan-Aung, U., Haskard, D., Crea, A. E., and Spur, B. W. (1989) Lipoxin A_4 and lipoxin B_4 inhibit chemotactic responses of human neutrophils stimulated by leukotriene B_4 and N-formyl-L-methionyl-L-leucyl-L-phenylalanine. *Clin. Sci.* **77,** 195–203.

139. Soyombo, O., Spur, B. W., and Lee, T. H. (1994) Effects of lipoxin A_4 on chemotaxis and degranulation of human eosinophils stimulated by platelet-activating factor and N-formyl-L-methionyl-L-leucyl-L-phenylalanine. *Allergy* **49,** 230–234.

140. Colgan, S. P., Serhan, C. N., Parkos, C. A., Delp-Archer, C., and Madara, J. L. (1993) Lipoxin A_4 modulates transmigration of human neutrophils across intestinal epithelial monolayers. *J. Clin. Invest.* **92,** 75–82.

141. Raud, J., Palmertz, U., Dahlén, S. E., and Hedqvist, P. (1991) Lipoxins inhibit microvascular inflammatory actions of leukotriene B_4. *Adv. Exp. Med. Biol.* **314,** 185–192.

142. Fiore, S. and Serhan, C. N. (1995) Lipoxin A_4 receptor activation is distinct from that of the formyl peptide receptor in myeloid cells: inhibition of CD11/18 expression by lipoxin A_4-lipoxin A_4 receptor interaction. *Biochemistry* **34,** 16,678–16,686.

143. Papayianni, A., Serhan, C. N., and Brady, H. R. (1996) Lipoxin A_4 and B_4 inhibit leukotriene-stimulated interactions of human neutrophils and endothelial cells. *J. Immunol.* **156,** 2264–2272.

144. Grandordy, B. M., Lacroix, H., Mavoungou, E., Krilis, S., Crea, A. E., Spur, B. W., and Lee, T. H. (1990) Lipoxin A_4 inhibits phosphoinositide hydrolysis in human neutrophils. *Biochem. Biophys. Res. Commun.* **167,** 1022–1029.

145. Maddox, J. F. and Serhan, C. N. (1996) Lipoxin A_4 and B_4 are potent stimuli for human monocyte migration and adhesion: selective inactivation by dehydrogenation and reduction. *J. Exp. Med.* **183,** 137–146.

146. Christie, P. E., Spur, B. W., and Lee, T. H. (1992) The effects of lipoxin A_4 on airway responses in asthmatic subjects. *Am. Rev. Respir. Dis.* **145,** 1281–1284.

147. Feng, Z., Godfrey, H. P., Mandy, S., Strudwick, S., Lin, K.-T., Heilman, E., and Wong, P. Y.-K. (1996) Leukotriene B_4 modulates *in vivo* expression of delayed-type hypersensitivity by a receptor-mediated mechanism: Regulation by lipoxin A_4. *J. Pharmacol. Exp. Ther.* **278,** 950–956.

148. Kantha, S. S., Matsumura, H., Kubo, E., Kawase, K., Takahata, R., Serhan, C. N., and Hayaishi, O. (1994) Effect of prostaglandin D_2, lipoxins and leukotrienes on sleep and brain temperature of rats. *Prostaglandins Leukotrienes Essential Fatty Acids* **51**, 87–93.
149. Serhan, C. N. (1997) Lipoxins and novel aspirin-triggered 15-epi-lipoxins (ATL): a jungle of cell–cell interactions or a therapeutic opportunity? *Prostaglandins* **53**, 107–137.
150. Kim, S. J. and Tominaga, T. (1989) Formation of lipoxins by the brain. *Ann. NY Acad. Sci.* **559**, 461–464.
151. Simchowitz, L., Fiore, S., and Serhan, C. N. (1994) Carrier-mediated transport of lipoxin A_4 in human neutrophils. *Am. J. Physiol.* **267**, C1525–1534.
152. Strader, C. D., Fong, T. M., Tota, M. R., Underwood, D., and Dixon, R. A. (1994) Structure and function of G protein-coupled receptors. *Annu. Rev. Biochem.* **63**, 101–132.
153. Perez, H. D., Holmes, R., Kelly, E., McClary, J., and Andrews, W. H. (1992) Cloning of a cDNA encoding a receptor related to the formyl peptide receptor of human neutrophils. *Gene (Amst.)* **118**, 303,304.
154. Bradley, P. P., Priebat, D. A., Christensen, R. D., and Rothstein, G. (1982) Measurement of cutaneous inflammation: estimation of neutrophil content with an enzyme marker. *J. Invest. Dermatol.* **78**, 206–209.
155. Toh, H., Ichikawa, A., and Narumiya, S. (1995) Molecular evolution of receptors for eicosanoids. *FEBS Lett.* **361**, 17–21.
156. Feng, Y., Broder, C. C., Kennedy, P. E., and Berger, E. A. (1996) HIV–1 entry cofactor: functional cDNA cloning of a seven-transmembrane, G protein-coupled receptor. *Science* **272(5263)**, 872–877.
157. Oravecz, T., Pall, M., and Norcross, M. A. (1996) β-chemokine inhibition of monocytotropic HIV-1 infection: Interference with a postbinding fusion step. *J. Immunol.* **157**, 1329–1332.
158. Genis, P., Jett, M., Bernton, E. W., Boyle, T., Gelbard, H. A., Dzenko, K., Keane, R. W., Resnick, L., Mizrachi, Y., Volsky, D. J., Epstein, L. G., and Gendelman, H. E. (1992) Cytokines and arachidonic metabolites produced during human immunodeficiency virus (HIV)-infected macrophage-astroglia interactions: Implications for the neuropathogenesis of HIV disease. *J. Exp. Med.* **176**, 1703–1718.
159. Ekerdt, R. and Müller, B. (1992) Role of prostanoids in the inflammatory reaction and their therapeutic potential in the skin. *Arch. Dermatol. Res.* **284**, S18–21.
160. Romano, M., Maddox, J. F., and Serhan, C. N. (1996) Activation of human monocytes and the acute monocytic leukemia cell line (THP-1) by lipoxins involves unique signaling pathways for lipoxin A_4 versus lipoxin B_4. *J. Immunol.* **157**, 2149–2154.
161. Stenke, L., Mansour, M., Edenius, C., Reizenstein, P., and Lindgren, J. A. (1991) Formation and proliferative effects of lipoxins in human bone marrow. *Biochem. Biophys. Res. Commun.* **180**, 255–261.

4

Mutagenesis Studies
of Mammalian Lipoxygenases

Olof Rådmark

Introduction

A widely used assay in studies of lipoxygenases (LOs) is the oxygenation of arachidonic acid, and, to date, mammalian enzymes that introduce oxygen at C-5, C-8, C-12, and C-15 of the arachidonic acid backbone have been described. Oxygenation of arachidonic acid is a physiological function, e.g., for 5-LO in leukotriene biosynthesis. However, it is possible that these enzymes also have other roles, one indication is the low activity of mouse epidermal 12-LO regarding oxygenation of free fatty acids (1).

Several recent reviews cover data regarding mammalian LOs (2–6). This chapter focuses mainly on mutagenesis studies concerning two topics: the ligands to iron in LOs and the positional specificity of 12/15-LOs.

Mammalian LO cDNAs

Complementary DNAs encoding mammalian LOs are summarized in Table 1. Sequences describing the same protein have been grouped together, although there are occasional differences in the deduced amino acid sequences, as indicated. The open reading frames encode proteins 662 to 677 amino acids long (including initiation methionines). Thus, the mature proteins vary between 661 and 662 amino acids for almost all the 12/15-LOs, the 5-LOs are somewhat longer (672 or 673 amino acids), and the longest are the novel second human 15-LO (675 amino acids) and the mouse 8-LO (676 amino acids). Using the program PileUp in the Wisconsin Package (27), the dendrogram in Fig. 1 was generated. It shows similarities among almost all 12/15-LOs, gathering these in one group, whereas the 5-LOs appear in another group. Interestingly,

From: *Molecular and Cellular Basis of Inflammation*
Edited by: C. N. Serhan and P. A. Ward © Humana Press Inc., Totowa, NJ

Table 1
Mammalian LO cDNAs[a]

Species, length excluding initation Met	Accesion no., references, ambiguities
Human 12-LO, 662	m35418 *(7)*; m38792 *(8)*; m62982 *(9)*; four differences
Mouse platelet type 12-LO, 662	u04334 *(10)*; s80446 *(11)*; one difference
Rat 12-LO, 662	l06040 *(10)*; s69383 *(13)*; two differences
Mouse leukocyte type 12-LO, 662	u04331 *(10)*; 134570 *(14)*; three differences
Rabbit 15-LO, 662	m27214 *(15)*
Rabbit 12-LO, 662	z97654 *(71)*
Human 15-LO type 1, 661	m23892 *(16)*
Porcine leukocyte 12-LO, 662	m31417 *(17)*
Bovine trachea 12-LO, 662	s96247 *(18)*
Mouse epidermis 12-LO, 661	u39200 *(1)*; x99252 *(19)*
Rat 5-LO, 673	j03960 *(20)*
Mouse 5-LO, 673	l42198 *(21)*
Hamster 5-LO, 672	u43333 *(22)*
Human 5-LO, 673	j03571 *(23)*; j03600 *(24)*
Human 15-LO type 2, 675	u78294 *(25)*
Mouse 8-LO, 676	u93277 *(26)*

[a]In order of similarity according to the program PileUp, compare to Figs. 1 and 2. Ambiguities regarding deduced amino acid sequences are indicated (number of differences).

the novel second human 15-LO and the mouse 8-LO constitute a separate pair, which has the most resemblance to the 5-LOs.

For all cDNA sequences except rat 5-LO, the deduced C-terminal amino acid is isoleucine. However, it was suggested that this could be owing to a cloning artifact regarding the rat 5-LO cDNA *(28,29)*. Thus, if a nucleotide A is inserted before T at position 2090 of the original sequence *(20)*, the C-terminal amino acid sequence becomes identical to the other 5-LOs. If this assumption is true, rat 5-LO consists of 673 amino acids and terminates with an isoleucine.

Comparisons

The crystal structure of soybean lipoxygeanse-1 *(28,30)*, which was also one of the first LOs cloned *(31)*, has had a substantial impact on the studies of mammalian LOs. Different parts and residues of the sequences have been connected with various functionalities, and in many cases this has been made possible by molecular modeling of mammalian LOs, with soybean LO-1 as template. However, before the crystal structure appeared, six conserved histidine residues, which are present in almost all LOs, were recognized. Three of these conserved His-residues appear to function as iron ligands in all LOs (*see* sections on mutagenesis studies). In soybean LO-1, two of the histidine iron ligands reside in the longest helix (nr 9), whereas the third His-ligand resides in helix nr 18. Modeling of the human LO sequences *(29)* also indicated that in the mammalian proteins, four regions of conserved residues are present. Three of these regions should anchor the two long helices in the enzyme structures, and the fourth should be involved in stabilization of the loop ending with the fourth iron ligand, i.e., the C-terminus. Thus, one would assume that this infers that similar helices, and a C-

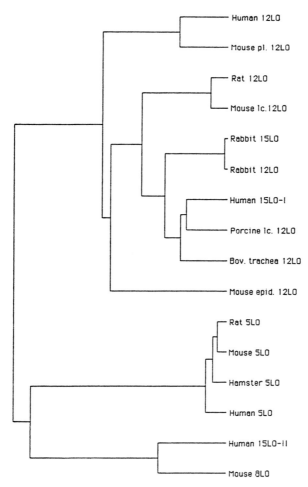

Human 12LO

Mouse pl. 12LO

Rat 12LO

Mouse lc. 12LO

Rabbit 15LO

Rabbit 12LO

Human 15LO-I

Porcine lc. 12LO

Bov. trachea 12LO

Mouse epid. 12LO

Rat 5LO

Mouse 5LO

Hamster 5LO

Human 5LO

Human 15LO-II

Mouse 8LO

Fig. 1. Dendrogram of 16 mammalian LOs, generated by the program PileUp *(27)*. Distance along the horizontal axis is proportional to the difference between sequences.

terminal loop, could also be present in mammalian LOs. An additional feature of the soybean LO structure is the presence of two cavities, connecting the surface with the prosthetic iron *(30)*. One of these is believed to be the channel for oxygen entry, connecting a position opposite to one of the His iron ligands (the third conserved His) with the surface. The other should accommodate the fatty acid substrate; it faces the C-terminus and two His ligands (the second and third conserved His). Comparisons regarding residues lining the wall of the substrate tunnel have been important for mutagenesis studies concerning positional specificity and substrate binding in 12/15-LOs (*see below*).

In addition, simple sequence comparisons give some indications; thus five short parts of the mammalian amino acid sequences are identical or very similar. The first and second (in human 5-LO) are Phe-97 to Trp-102, and Phe-232 to Gly-239. The third and fourth (Trp-347 to Lys-351, Trp-353 to Phe-359) overlap with Prigge et al.'s conserved region 1 *(29)*. The fifth is Thr-427 to His-432, which contains four gly-

```
Human 12LO      330 LFLPSDPPLA WLLAKSWVRN SDFQLHEIQY HLLNTHLVAE VIAVATMRCL
Mouse pl. 12LO  330 LFLPSDPPLA WLLAKIWVRN SDFQLQELQF HLLNTHLVAE VIAVATMRCL
Rat 12LO        331 IFTPSDPPMD WLLAKCWVRS SDLQLHELQA HLLRGHLMAE LFAVATMRCL
Mouse lc. 12LO  331 IFTPLDPPMD WLLAKCWVRS SDLQLHELQA HLLRGHLVAE VFAVATMRCL
Rabbit 15LO     331 LFLPTDPPMV WLLAKCWVRS SDFQVHELNS HLLRGHLMAE VFTVATMRCL
Rabbit 12LO     331 LFLPTDPPMV WLLAKCWVRS SDLQVHELNS HLLRGHLMAE VFTVATMRCL
Human 15LO-I    330 LFLPTDPPMA WLLAKCWVRS SDFQLHELQS HLLRGHLMAE VIVVATMRCL
Porc. lc. 12LO  331 LFLPTDPPMV WLLAKCWVRS SDFQLHELHS HLLRGHLMAE VIAVATMRCL
Bov. tr. 12LO   331 LFLPTDPPMT WLLAKCWVRS SDFQLHELHS HLLRGHLVAE VIAVATMRCL
Mouse ep. 12LO  330 LFLPSDPPMA WLLAKIWVRS SDFQLHQLQS HLLRGHLMAE VISVATMRSL
Rat 5LO         336 IFLPTDSKYD WLLAKIWVRS SDFHIHQTIT HLLRTHLVSE VFGIAMYRQL
Mouse 5LO       337 IFLPTDSKYD WLLAKIWVRS SDFHVHQTIT HLLRTHLVSE VFGIAMYRQL
Hamster 5LO     336 IFLPSDAKYD WLLAKIWVRS SDFHVHQTIT HLLCTHLVSE VFGIAMYRQL
Human 5LO       337 IFLPSDAKYD WLLAKIWVRS SDFHVHQTIT HLLRTHLVSE VFGIAMYRQL
Human 15LO-II   343 IFLPTDDKWD WLLAKTWVRN AEFSFHEALT HLLHSHLLPE VFTLATLRQL
Mouse 8LO       344 IFLPSDDTWD WLLAKTWVRN SEFYIHEAVT HLLHAHLIPE VFALATLRQL


Human 12LO      380 PGLHPIFKFP IPHIRYTMEI NTRARTQLIS DGGIFDKAVS TGGGGHVQLL
Mouse pl. 12LO  380 PGLHPIFKLL VPHIRYTMEI NTRTRTQLIS DGGIFDQVVS TGGGGHVQLL
Rat 12LO        381 PSVHPVFKLL VPHLLYTMEI NVRARSDLIS ERGFFDKAMS TGGGGHLDLL
Mouse lc. 12LO  381 PSVHPVFKLL VPHLLYTMEI NVRARSDLIS ERGFFDKVMS TGGGGHLDLL
Rabbit 15LO     381 PSIHPVFKLI VPHLRYTLEI NVRARNGLVS DFGIFDQIMS TGGGGHVQLL
Rabbit 12LO     381 PSIHPVFKLI VPHLRYTLEI NVRARNGLVS DFGIFDQIMS TGGGGHVQLL
Human 15LO-I    380 PSIHPIFKLI IPHLRYTLEI NVRARTGLVS DMGIFDQIMS TGGGGHVQLL
Porc. lc. 12LO  381 PSIHPIFKLL IPHFRYTMEI NVRARNGLVS DLGIFDQVVS TGGGGHVELL
Bov. tr. 12LO   381 PSIHPMFKLL IPHLRYTMEI NIRARTGLVS DSGVFDQVVS TGGGGHVELL
Mouse ep. 12LO  380 PSLHPIYKLL APHFRYTMEI NTLARNNLVS EWGIFDLVVS TGSGGHVDIL
Rat 5LO         386 PAVHPLFKLL VAHVRFTIAI NTKAREQLNC EYGLFDKANA TGGGGHVQMV
Mouse 5LO       387 PAVHPLFKLL VAHVRFTIAI NTKAREQLIC EYGLFDKANA TGGGGHVQMV
Hamster 5LO     386 PAVHPIFKLL VAHVRFTIAI NTKAREQLIC EYGLFDKANA TGGGGHVQMV
Human 5LO       387 PAVHPIFKLL VAHVRFTIAI NTKAREQLIC ECGLFDKANA TGGGGHVQMV
Human 15LO-II   393 PHCHPLFKLL IPHTRYTLHI NTLARELLIV PGQVVDRSTG IGIEGFSELI
Mouse 8LO       394 PRCHPLFKLL IPHIRYTLHI NTLARELLVA PGKLIDKSTG LGTGGFSDLI


Human 12LO      525 LC HFLTMCVFTC TAQHAAINQG QLDWYAWVPN APCTMRMPPP TTK
Mouse pl. 12LO  525 LC HFLTMCVFTC TAQHAAINQG QLDWYGWVPN APCTMRMPPP TSK
Rat 12LO        526 AC YFITMCIFTC TAQHSSVHLG QLDWFYWVPN APCTMRLPPP TTK
Mouse lc. 12LO  526 AC HFITMCIFTC TAQHSSIHLG QLDWFYWVPN APCTMRLPPP KTK
Rabbit 15LO     526 AC HFVTMCIFTC TGQHSSIHLG QLDWFTWVPN APCTMRLPPP TTK
Rabbit 12LO     526 AC HFVTMCIFTC TGQHSSIHLG QLDWFTWVPN APCTMRLPPP TTK
Human 15LO-I    525 VC HFVTMCIFTC TGQHASVHLG QLDWYSWVPN APCTMRLPPP TTK
Porc. lc. 12LO  526 LC HFVTMCIFTC TGQHSSNHLG QLDWYTWVPN APCTMRLPPP TTK
Bov. tr. 12LO   526 LC HFVTMCIFTC TGQHSSTHLG QLDWYSWVPN APCTMRLPPP TTK
Mouse ep. 12LO  525 LC RFVAMCIFTC TGQHASTHLG QLDWYAWIPN GPCTMRKPPP ISK
Rat 5LO         534 LS EYLTVVIFTA SAQHAAVNFG QYDWCSWIPN APPTMRAPPP TAK
Mouse 5LO       535 LS EYLTVVIFTA SAQHAAVNFG QYDWCSWIPN APPTMRAPPP TAK
Hamster 5LO     534 LS EYLTVVIFTA SAQHAAVNFG QYDWCSWIPN APPTMRAPPA TAK
Human 5LO       535 LS EYLTVVIFTA SAQHAAVNFG QYDWCSWIPN APPTMRAPPP TAK
Human 15LO-II   538 LV QYVTMVIFTC SAKHAAVSAG QFDSCAWMPN LPPSMQLPPP TSK
Mouse 8LO       539 LV QYITMVIFTC SAKHAAVSSG QFDSCVWMPN LPPTMQLPPP TSK
```

Fig. 2. Sequence alignment of parts of 16 mammalian LO sequences. Six conserved histidine residues are shown in bold for orientation. Mutated residues are underlined.

cines in sequence. Interestingly, the fourth and fifth stretches include (or are close to) residues determining positional specificity for the 12/15-LOs (in human 15-LO: F353, I417, and M418) (compare Fig. 2). However, the recently cloned human 15-LO type 2 and mouse 8-LO diverge regarding these similarities. For these only 21:22 of the total 32 residues in the five short parts are identical to the other mammalian LOs.

A sixth conserved histidine (His-550) constitutes one of the iron ligands. This residue is always preceded by a stretch of hydrophobic residues, and in the following sequence (to Lys-579 in 5-LO), the similarity between the mammalian enzymes is notable and several features appear. These are the suggested fifth iron ligand (Asn-554 in 5-LO [28]), residues taking part in stabilizing hydrogen bonds (Val-553, Gln-557 [29]), and the proline residues that are part of the Src homology 3 (SH3)–binding motif in 5-LO (32). Regarding this region, the recently cloned human 15-LO type 2 and mouse 8-LO are also similar to the other mammalian LOs. For example, they contain all the proline residues present in 5-LOs, and could thus be candidates for interaction with other proteins (e.g., Grb2) via a SH3-binding motif. However, at the position of the putative fifth iron ligand, both human 15-LO type 2 and mouse 8-LO display Ser residues (Asn or His in all other mammalian LOs) (*see* Fig. 2).

5-LO is activated by calcium and adenosine triphosphate (ATP), but strict homologies to well-defined calcium- or ATP-binding domains have not been found. However, two stretches in the 5-LOs (Gly-16 to Ser-28; Lys-579 to Arg-594) showed weak similarity to a 17 amino acid consensus sequence reported for the annexins (a group of calcium binding proteins). Also, a sequence similar to the interface lipid-binding domain, e.g., in human lipoprotein lipase, is present in the 5-LOs (His-367 to Ala-381). This was suggested to be important for the enzyme-substrate interaction (20,34). These features of 5-LO are valid also for the more recently cloned mouse and hamster enzymes. One of the six proline residues in the region of the SH3-binding motif is absent in hamster 5-LO. However, this particular Pro does not seem crucial, compared to a SH3-binding motif consensus sequence (33).

Comparisons of secondary structure predictions reveal some additional similarities among the mammalian LOs. Using the program Peptidestructure in the Wisconsin package (27), secondary structures were generated for the 16 mammalian LOs (Table 1). When these are compared, conserved hydrophilic/hydrophobic regions are observed (compare to Fig. 1 in ref. 5). All proteins contain a hydrophilic region (for 5-LO between residues 120 and 143), and a hydrophobic region just upstream of the sixth conserved histidine (for 5-LO between residues 539 and 548). The region 120–143 does not overlap with conserved primary structure, whereas this is the case for the region 539–548.

Mutagenesis of Ligands to the Prosthetic Iron in Mammalian LOs

One of the soybean LOs was the first LO shown to contain iron (34–36). Subsequently this was found also for recombinant human 5-LO, expressed in insect cells (37). The role of iron in the generally accepted scheme for the LO reaction is to act as electron acceptor and donor, during hydrogen abstraction and peroxide formation. In this reaction mechanism, the LO is first converted from the resting ferrous state to the ferric form. It then cycles between the ferric form and the substrate reduced ferrous form (38).

Heme or iron-sulfur clusters were not found in soybean LO, and it was suggested that the iron should be bound directly to functional groups in the protein (39). Soybean LO was analyzed by extended X-ray absorption fine structure, which indicated that the iron was bound by 4 ± 1 nitrogen ligands (imidazole) and 2 ± 1 oxygen ligands *(40)*. The iron center is believed to be similar among the LOs, and six histidines are conserved in almost all cloned LOs. Thus, the involvement of histidine residues as iron ligands in LO was strongly inferred, and the conserved histidine residues were among the initial targets in the mutagenesis of LOs.

Mutagenesis of Putative Iron Ligands in 5-LO: Studies of Crude Recombinant Proteins

In five studies, effects of mutations regarding enzyme activity of crude recombinant protein were presented *(21,41–44)*. The results are summarized in Table 2.

Most of the data were obtained after expression in *Escherichia coli*, which has given reproducible yields of nonmutated 5-LO. However, mutants of His-390 and -399 have been difficult to express in *E. coli*. Thus, Zhang et al. *(44)* found that for the mutants H390Q and H399Q, low expression temperature (18°C) was essential to obtain activity. Ishii et al. *(42)* obtained small amounts of the mutants H390A, H390N, and H399A, after expression at 26°C. Nguyen et al. *(43)* found that after expression of mutants regarding His-372, -390, and -399 (at 37°C), almost all recombinant protein was insoluble. Nguyen et al. *(43)* therefore turned to insect cells for expression of serine mutants of His-362, -367, -372, -390, and -399. However, for those mutants that have been expressed in both *E. coli* and insect cells (H362S, H372S), the results were the same.

The data collected in Table 2 give a reasonably uniform message, i.e., that His-367, -372, -550, Glu-376, and the C-terminus are required for 5-LO activity, whereas His-362, -390, and -399 are not. In one study, not only the oxygenase activity of 5-LO was determined, but also the further conversion of arachidonic acid to LTA_4, as well as the 8-LO activity *(44)*. The results indicated that His-367, 372, 550, and the C-terminus were crucial both for the oxygenase and the LTA_4 synthase activities, supporting that they coincide in one active site.

Mutagenesis of Iron Ligands in 5-LO: Studies Involving Purification of Mutated Proteins, Iron Analysis, and Enzyme Assays

To determine the importance of various residues as ligands to iron in 5-LO, mutated proteins were purified, and assayed for iron content and specific activity. During these studies, crystal structures for the resting ferrous form of soybean LO-1 were presented by two groups *(28,30)*, confirming the function of three of the conserved His as ligands. The crystal structures also gave additional suggestions regarding possible iron ligands in 5-LO. Both groups thus found that the carboxyl group of the C-terminal isoleucine was a ligand in the resting ferrous form of soybean LO. In addition, Minor et al. *(28)* presented that Asn-694 (corresponds to Asn-554 in 5-LO) should be a ligand in soybean LO. However, Boyington et al. *(30)* suggested an alternative function for this residue, i.e., that Asn-694 is part of a network that stabilizes the iron center by hydrogen bonds.

In the author's laboratory, 5-LO mutants were expressed in *E. coli* at 27°C and purified by ATP-agarose affinity chromatography, and iron content was determined by graphite furnace atomic absorption spectrophotometry. Data from two papers are compiled in Table 3 *(45,46)*. For nonmutated 5-LO, the iron content was 0.94 ± 0.26 mol/mol (mean $\pm$ SD, data from 17 preparations). The specific activity in a 5-min assay was 23 ± 4.5 μmol of product per mg (mean $\pm$ SD, data from nine preparations).

For most of the 14 mutated proteins, yields and behavior on the ATP-agarose column were practically the same as for nonmutated 5-LO. However, the mutated protein

Table 2
Mutations of Six Conserved Histidines, Glu-376, and the C-Terminus in Recombinant 5-LO[a]

Residue	Exchanges leading to retained activity[b]	Exchanges leading to undetectable activity
His-362	Asn[c], Cys[d], Gln[e], Ser[c,d,f]	Lys[d]
His-367		Ala[c], Asn[c], Cys[d], Gln[e], Lys[d], Ser[d]
His-372		Asn[c], Gln[e], Ser[c–e]
Glu-376		Gln[c]
His-390	Asn[c], Gln[e], Ser[d]	Ala[c]
His-399	Asn[c], Gln[e], Ser[d]	Ala[c]
His-550		Ala[c], Leu[e], Asn[c], Gln[e]
Val-671		Met[g]
Pro-668 to Ile-673		Deletion[e]

[a]Crude preparations were used for determinations of enzyme activity.
[b]Retained activity means that activity was 1–100% of control.
[c]See ref. *42*.
[d]See ref. *43*.
[e]See ref. *44*.
[f]See ref. *41*.
[g]See ref. *21*.

Table 3
Iron Contents and Specific Activities of 5-LO and Mutated Proteins

	Fe-content (mol/mol)	Enzyme activity (μmol/mg)
Nonmutated control	0.94 ± 0.26	23 ± 4.5
Mutation		
His-372 Gln	0	0
His-550 Gln	0	0
Ile-673 deleted	0	0
His-367 Gln/Asn/Ser/Ala	0.5/0.2/0.5/0.4	0/0/0/0
Glu-376 Gln	0.7	0
Asn-554 Gln/Asp/Ala	0.7/1/1.1	0/0.3/0.2
His-362 Gln	0.9	2
His-390 Gln	0.8	13
His-399 Gln	0.9	12

[a]For nonmutated 5-LO, mean ± SD are given; for mutated proteins mean values of at least two determinations.

H362Q was found to be unstable during the purification on ATP-agarose. Thus, when compared to nonmutated control, H362Q appeared less active after purification than in the crude stage *(44)*. Also, the protein H390Q (and on some occasions H399Q) was obtained in low amounts. The three mutated proteins H362Q, H390Q, and H399Q are certain to contain iron, but owing to the low protein yield the iron content of H390Q (Table 3) is approximate.

In the study carried out at Merck, recombinant 5-LO was expressed in Sf9 insect cells and purified by ATP-agarose affinity chromatography, and iron was routinely determined by a colorimetric method. The iron content of the nonmutated 5-LO purified from the insect cells has varied between 0 and 1.1 mol/mol, in direct proportion to the enzyme activity *(37)*. It was suggested that this depends on the degree of iron release and inactivation, occurring during growth and preparation. Also, deliberate inactivation, by exposure to oxygen, resulted in loss of iron.

Five mutated 5-LO proteins, in which histidines 362, 367, 372, 390, and 399 had been exchanged to serine, were purified in the absence of dithiotheitol (to prevent formation of hydrogen peroxide) *(47)*. The specific activity of nonmutated purified 5-LO was 18 µmol/min/mg. Iron was not detected for the mutated protein H372S, but was present in H367S, H362S, H390S, and H399S. The oxygenase and LTA$_4$ synthase activities were assayed and found to vary in parallell for the various mutants. In addition, two hydroperoxidase activities were determined. The results can be summarized as follows. Mutation of His-372 to Ser gave complete loss of iron and all activities. Mutation of His-367 to Ser gave retention of iron, combined with loss of the activities that would depend on association with an eicosanoid (oxygenase, LTA$_4$ synthase, and arachidonate-dependent hydroperoxidase activity). However, there was still a significant reducing agent–dependent hydroperoxidase activity (approx 20% of control). It was thus suggested that His-367 could be involved in the binding of arachidonic acid, or in the oxidation and hydrogen abstraction step *(47)*. Finally, exchanges of either of the three histidines 362, 390, or 399 (to serine) gave mutated proteins with iron content and enzyme activities similar to that of the control.

The mutagenesis data presented above have been discussed in detail *(5)*. Briefly, certain spectroscopic studies regarding soybean LO *(38,48–50)* support the concept that one of the ligands to iron is replaced during the catalytic cycle. Thus, the putative ligands to iron in 5-LO were considered as permanent or replaceable ligands. It was suggested that His-372, His-550, and Ile-673 can be regarded as permanent ligands to iron in 5-LO (*see* Table 3). Not only His-367 but also Glu-376 or Asn-554 were suggested as possible replaceable ligands (*see* middle group in Table 3). However, based on several observations, His-367 in 5-LO (the second of the six conserved histidines) appears most plausible as a replaceable iron ligand. The remaining three conserved histidine residues (His-362, -390, and -399) should not function as ligands, permanent or replaceable (*see* bottom group in Table 3). Interestingly, in murine platelet 12-LO, the first conserved histidine (corresponding to His-362) was absent; a glutamine residue appeared at this position *(10)*.

Mutagenesis of Iron Ligands in Other LOs

Putative ligands to iron in other LOs have also been subjected to mutagenesis. Most results, but not all, are similar to those obtained for 5-LO. In particular, studies of other LOs have not indicated that the second of the conserved histidine residues should function as a replaceable ligand to iron.

Soybean LO-1 was expressed in *E. coli* (expression temperature 15°C) and purified to a high specific activity (193 µmol/min/mg) *(51)*. The six conserved histidines (at positions 494, 499, 504, 522, 531, and 690) were exchanged. The mutants H494Q, H494S, H522Q, and H531Q retained enzyme activity, whereas the mutants H499Q, H504Q, H504S, and H690Q were inactive *(52)*. None of the inactive mutants contained iron, as determined by autoradiography of electrophoresis gels after culture in the presence of ^{59}Fe *(52)*. The active mutants were not analyzed for iron content. Thus, the findings regarding enzyme activity are compatible with the 5-LO model, and the second, third, and sixth conserved histidines are crucial for oxygenase activity. However, after mutation of the second conserved histidine, the iron content differed from the findings for 5-LO. Specifically, the soybean LO-1 mutant H499Q was reported not to contain iron, whereas 5-LO mutants H367Q, H367S, H367N, and H367A all contained iron (*see above*).

The molecular basis of a naturally occurring null mutation in soybean LO-2 was determined *(53)*. It was found that the third conserved histidine (His-532) had been exchanged to glutamine. This mutation led to loss of enzyme activity and apparent instability; LO-2 was not detectable in mature soybean seeds. Also, in 5-LO, the third conserved histidine was essential for activity.

Porcine leukocyte 12-LO was expressed in *E. coli* (expression temperature 20°C) and nonmutated 12-LO, and mutated proteins were purified *(54)*. Possibly the purification method (immunoaffinity chromatography *[55]*) was the reason for the seemingly low specific activity, 1–2 μmol/min/mg for nonmutated purified enzyme. The six conserved histidines (at positions 356, 361, 366, 384, 393, and 541) were subject to exchange. The mutants H356L and H384L retained enzyme activity, whereas the mutants H361L, H361Q, H366L, and H541L were inactive. For the mutated protein H393L, no activity was detectable; however, this was probably owing to instability. Thus, the findings regarding enzyme activity are compatible with the 5-LO model, in the sense that the second, third, and sixth conserved histidines are crucial for oxygenase activity. The iron content for nonmutated 12-LO, analyzed by atomic absorption spectrometry, was 0.53 mol/mol. The inactive mutated proteins had reduced iron contents (H361L, 0.10 mol/mol; H361Q, 0.01 mol/mol; H366L, 0.06 mol/mol; H541L, 0.06 mol/mol). Regarding the second conserved histidine (His-361), exchange to Gln thus led to practically complete loss of iron, whereas after exchange to Leu the iron content was still approx 20% of control. The author concluded that His-361 is an important iron-binding site in porcine 12-LO. Apparently, for porcine leukocyte 12-LO, mutation of the second conserved histidine resulted in more severe loss of iron than found for 5-LO.

Human platelet type 12-LO was expressed in human embryonal kidney 293 cells *(56)*. Also, for this LO, mutations regarding the second, third, and sixth conserved histidines (His-360, -365, or -540) led to loss of oxygenase activity, whereas mutants of the remaining conserved histidines (at positions 355, 383, and 392) retained activity. Subsequently, both mouse platelet type 12-LO and mouse leukocyte type 12-LO were expressed in HEK 293 cells. Deletions of the C-terminal isoleucines led to complete loss of activity for both enzymes *(10)*. These findings are compatible with the 5-LO model. In addition, for mouse platelet type 12-LO, the C-terminal Ile was exchanged to a number of residues *(10)*. The mutant I663V was as active as the nonmutated positive control and exchanges to charged amino acids (Asp, Arg, Lys) or the small Gly gave nearly undetectable activity, whereas exchanges to Ser, Asn, or Leu gave activities that were 8–15% of control. In this context, it is of interest that in the recently cloned 8*R*-LO from the coral *Plexaura homomalla*, the C-terminal amino acid is threonine *(57)*.

Positional Specificity of 12/15-LOs

Three amino acid residues of importance for positional specificity in 12/15-LOs have been found. In human 15-LO, they are Phe-353, Ile-417, and Met-418.

Comparisons of the sequences of human and rabbit 15-LOs, human platelet 12-LO, porcine leukocyte 12-LO, and bovine trachea 12-LO, and subsequent mutagenesis and expression in *E. coli* identified Met-418 as a determinant of positional specificity regarding hydrogen abstraction and introduction of oxygen in human 15-LO *(58)*. Exchange of Met-418 to Val (which is present in the corresponding position of the three compared 12-LOs) gave a 15/12-HETE product ratio of 1:1, instead of 9:1 for the native 15-LO. Also, when two adjacent residues were converted to imitate the sequence of human platelet 12-LO (Q416K/I417A/M418V) the resulting 15/12-HETE product ratio was 1:15. Thus, it was apparent that a part of 15-LO important to positional specificity had been found. Subsequently, human 15-LO was mutated to imitate the sequence of bovine trachea 12-LO (I417V/M418V), which also resulted in conversion to a 12-LO *(59)*.

These findings were interpreted to mean that the bulk of the side chain at residues 417 and 418 determined positional specificity. Thus, the bulk of Ile-417 and Met-418, presumably close to the bottom of the substrate pocket of 15-LO, would position arachidonic acid suitably for hydrogen abstraction at C-13, and oxygenation at C-15. Decreased bulk at the bottom of the substrate pocket (after mutations as described above) would allow for deeper insertion of the fatty acid methyl terminus, compatible with hydrogen abstraction at C-10, and oxygenation at C-12. When the crystal structure of soybean LO was presented, amino acids lining the putative substrate pocket were identified *(30)*. Sequence alignment showed that Ile-417 and Met-418 in human 15-LO correspond to two of the residues in soybean LO that line the pocket (Thr-556 and Phe-557), favoring their role for positional specificity *(60)*.

Subsequently, when the sequences of more 12-LOs were determined, the picture became less clear-cut. Particularly rat 12-LO, mouse leukocyte 12-LO, and rabbit 12-LO all have a Met at the position corresponding to Met-418 in 15-LO (Fig. 2). In addition, attempts to convert 12-LOs to 15-LO, by exchanges introducing the IleMet sequence typical for 15-LO, gave mixed results. For rat 12-LO, there was practically no change in the positional specificity *(12,13)*. For human platelet and bovine trachea 12-LOs, the 15/12-HETE ratio increased, but remained below 1:3 *(56,59)*. However, for porcine leukocyte 12-LO, there was a drastic change, to a 15/12-HETE ratio of 5.7:1 *(54)*. Thus, the relevance of residues in 12-LO, at the positions corresponding to 15-LO Ile-417 and Met-418, vary for the different 12-LOs. In turn, this indicates that other parts of the proteins could be more important for positional specificity, at least for some of the 12-LOs.

Additional mutations were performed regarding Met-418 in human 15-LO, and the mutants were expressed in *E. coli (60)*. It was found that the nonpolar Met could be changed to polar Asn, and also to charged Lys, with retained activity. The positional specificities for these mutants were 15/12-HETE 1:1 for M418Q, and 1:9 for M418K. Because such drastic changes of the polarity of the residue 418 side-chain were well tolerated, it was concluded that the side chain is probably not in direct contact with the substrate, but that it defines positional specificity in a less direct way. Also in this study *(60)*, one mutated protein (I417V,M418V) was expressed in insect cells and purified. The yield of recombinant protein was high (approx 15% of the soluble protein), and 20–30 mg of pure enzyme could be obtained from 1 L of cell culture; however, with quite low specific activity. Apparent K_M and V_{max} were determined for the purified mutated protein I417V,M418V with arachidonic acid as substrate. There were either no or only small changes as compared to unmutated 15-LO, indicating that the important energetic interactions between enzyme and substrate were unaffected by the mutations. The mutated protein I417V,M418V was also tested with a variety of other fatty acid substrates. The observed substrate preference, as well as the dual positional specificity on arachidonic acid, indicated that this 15-LO mutant is more similar to leukocyte type

12-LO than to platelet type 12-LO (which is in accordance with the dendrogram in Fig. 1). It was also attempted to replace the residues 416-419 in 15-LO (QIMS) with the corresponding sequence from 5-LO (KANA); no activity could be detected. In this context, it should be mentioned that two residues putatively situated in the substrate tunnel wall of 5-LO *(30)* have been mutated. When Asp-358 was converted to Asn, activity was almost the same as for control *(42,45)*. When Gln-557 was mutated to Glu, activity was reduced to 3% of control *(44)*. Gln-557 may also be part of a hydrogen bond network, supporting one of the iron ligands (His-367 in 5-LO) *(30)*.

The importance of Phe-353 for positional specificity was suggested after molecular modeling of mammalian 15-LO sequences *(29)*. A series of chimeras, in which pieces of 12-LOs and 15-LOs were mixed, provided information strengthening this proposition *(61)*. A construct mainly consisting of rabbit 15-LO, but in which an 86-residue fragment had been replaced with sequence from murine macrophage 12-LO, was particularly informative. This construct retained the original Ile-417 and Met-418 of 15-LO; nevertheless, after expression in *E. coli*, it had a 15/12-HETE ratio of 24:76. On the other hand, an analogous chimera with 86 residues from porcine leukocyte 12-LO, was still a 15-LO (15/12-HETE ratio 94:6). Modeling of 3D-structure and sequence comparisons (performed also by Borngräber et al.) indicated that Phe-353 in the wall of the putative substrate cavity should be the residue responsible for these effects. Phe-353 is present in 15-LO and in porcine leukocyte 12-LO, but in murine macrophage 12-LO (and also in rat 12-LO) a Leu is found at this position (compare to Fig. 2). This was confirmed by site-directed mutagenesis; the 15-LO mutant F353L had a 15/12-HETE ratio of 22:78. The study by Borngräber et al. *(61)* also shows that LO chimeras can provide information, when sequences from closely related LOs are mixed. Previously tested LO chimeras were not expressed or were inactive *(56)*.

A model for the effect of Phe-353 was presented *(61)*. It was suggested that the presence of a bulky Phe-353 in the wall of the substrate-binding pocket would lead to a bent substrate, in turn leading to contact between the methyl terminus of the substrate and the residues at positions 417 and 418. Thus, if Phe-353 is present, the bulk of Ile-417 and Met-418 influence positional specificity. On the other hand, if the smaller Leu is present at position 353, the fatty acid can be in a straight form, avoiding contact with the side chains of residues 417 and 418 (bulky or not).

The recently cloned second human 15-LO displays Phe-365 at the position corresponding to Phe-353, but the residues corresponding to the positions 417 and 418 are Ser-430 and Thr-431 (*see* Fig. 2). In addition, mouse 8-LO, but none of the other mammalian LOs, has Ser and Thr at these positions. Human 15-LO type 2 is a "clean" 15-LO *(25)*; it does not display any detectable 12-LO activity (as does human 15-LO type 1). However, a mutant of 15-LO type 1 (M418T) showed a modestly decreased 15/12-HETE ratio (3:1) *(60)*. Possibly, there is still more to find regarding determination of positional specificity, at least for human 15-LO type 2.

Further modeling of the putative substrate-binding pocket in human 15-LO indicated two additional residues that should be of importance for binding of the fatty acid (albeit not primary determinants of positional specificity): Arg-402 and Phe-414 *(62)*. The positively charged Arg-402 was suggested to interact with the negative charge of the substrate carboxylate, and the aromatic Phe-414 was suggested to interact with the *cis* double bonds of the substrate. After mutagenesis, R402L, R402K, F414I, and F414Trp were expressed in insect cells and purified. However, the specific activity of purified nonmutated recombinant human 15-LO was only 1.2 µmol/min/mg. This is substantially lower than the activity obtained previously utilizing the same expression system and purification procedure *(63)*, and less than 10% of the activity of native purified human 15-LO *(64,65)*. The properties of the mutated proteins (K_m, V_{max}, specific activity with various substrates, positional specificity) supported the roles proposed for these residues.

Methionines and Inactivation

It was reported that stoichiometric amounts of 13-HPODE could inactivate native rabbit reticulocyte 15-LO *(66)* and that this was correlated to oxygenation of a methionine residue to methionine sulfoxide *(67)*. This was the basis for mutagenesis studies aiming to identify the involved Met residue. 15-LOs, both from rabbit reticulocytes and from insect cells expressing recombinant human enzyme, were purified. Reactions with 13-HPODE, followed by tryptic digestions, peptide separations, and mass spectrometry identified the modified Met residues as Met-590 in human 15-LO and Met-591 in rabbit 15-LO *(68)*. The human 15-LO mutant M590L was expressed in *E. coli* and purified. It was found that the mutated 15-LO could still be inactivated by 13-HPODE, although there was no accompanying modification of the protein. Also, 15-HPETE could inactivate nonmutated 15-LO, without oxidation of Met-590. A partial loss of iron was observed, and it was suggested that this could explain part of the inactivation. It was concluded that inactivation of 15-LO by lipid hydroperoxide is separate from methionine oxidation. The specific activity also of 15-LO expressed in *E. coli* was low (1.1 µmol/min/mg).

Methionine residues in porcine leukocyte 12-LO were also mutated, to investigate the effects on turnover-dependent inactivation, and the inhibition by ETYA *(69)*. Porcine leukocyte 12-LO was expressed in *E. coli* and purified 109-fold (recovery 56%) to give an enzyme with good specific activity (12 µmol/min/mg). In this study, the recombinant 12-LO was purified by anion exchange and chromatofocusing chromatographies, thereby appearing to give an enzyme with higher specific activity than purification by immunoaffinity chromatography. On the basis of sequence comparisons between mammalian 12-LOs and 15-LOs, three Met residues were selected for mutagenesis. Three mutants (M338L, M367V, M562L) were expressed and purified. However, there were no appreciable effects regarding enzyme kinetics, or inactivation processes.

Acknowledgments

Studies in the author's laboratory were supported by grants from the Swedish Medical Research Council (03X-217), the Vårdal foundation (A95 067), and the Verum foundation.

References

1. Funk, C. D., Keeney, D. S., Oliw, E. H., Boeglin, W. E., and Brash, A. R. (1996) Functional expression and cellular localization of a mouse epidermal lipoxygenase. *J. Biol. Chem.* **271(38),** 23,338–23,344.
2. Ford-Hutchinson, A. W. (1994) 5-Lipoxygenase. *Ann. Rev. Biochem.* **63,** 383–417 (review, 164 refs.).
3. Funk, C. D. (1993) Molecular biology in the eicosanoid field. *Prog. Nucleic Acid Res. Mol. Biol.* **45(67),** 67–98 (review, 176 refs.).
4. Kuhn, H. and Thiele, B. J. (1995) Arachidonate 15-lipoxygenase. *J. Lipid Mediators Cell Signal.* **12(2–3),** 157–170 (review, 72 refs.).

5. Radmark, O. (1995) Arachidonate 5-lipoxygenase. *J. Lipid Mediators Cell Signal* **12(2–3)**, 171–184 (review, 59 refs.).

6. Yoshimoto, T. and Yamamoto, S. (1995) Arachidonate 12-lipoxygenase. *J. Lipid Mediators Cell Signal.* **12(2–3)**, 195–212 (review, 128 refs.).

7. Funk, C. D., Furci, L., and FitzGerald, G. A. (1990) Molecular cloning, primary structure, and expression of the human platelet/erythroleukemia cell 12-lipoxygenase. *Proc. Natl. Acad. Sci. USA* **87(15)**, 5638–5642.

8. Izumi, T., Hoshiko, S., Rådmark, O., and Samuelsson, B. (1990) Cloning of the cDNA for human 12-lipoxygenase. *Proc. Natl. Acad. Sci. USA* **87(19)**, 7477–7481.

9. Yoshimoto, T., Yamamoto, Y., Arakawa, T., Suzuki, H., Yamamoto, S., Yokoyama, C., Tanabe, T., and Toh, H. (1990) Molecular cloning and expression of human arachidonate 12-lipoxygenase. *Biochem. Biophys. Res. Commun.* **172(3)**, 1230–1235.

10. Chen, X. S., Kurre, U., Jenkins, N. A., Copeland, N. G., and Funk, C. D. (1994) cDNA cloning, expression, mutagenesis of C-terminal isoleucine, genomic structure, and chromosomal localizations of murine 12-lipoxygenases. *J. Biol. Chem.* **269(19)**, 13,979–13,987.

11. Krieg, P., Kinzig, A., Ress, L. M., Vogel, S., Vanlandingham, B., Stephan, M., Lehmann, W. D., Marks, F., and Furstenberger, G. (1995) 12-Lipoxygenase isoenzymes in mouse skin tumor development. *Mol. Carcinog.* **14(2)**, 118–129.

12. Watanabe, T. and Haeggstrom, J. Z. (1993) Rat 12-Lipoxygenase—mutations of amino acids implicated in the positional specificity of 15-lipoxygenase and 12-lipoxygenase. *Biochem. Biophys. Res. Commun.* **192(3)**, 1023–1029.

13. Hada, T., Hagiya, H., Suzuki, H., Arakawa, T., Nakamura, M., Matsuda, S., Yoshimoto, T., Yamamoto, S., Azekawa, T., Morita, Y., Ishimura, K., and Kim, H. Y. (1994) Arachidonate 12-lipoxygenase of rat pineal glands—catalytic properties and primary structure deduced from its cDNA. *Bba-Lipid Lipid Metab.* **1211(2)**, 221–228.

14. Freire-Moar, J., Alavinassab, A., Ng, M., Mulkins, M., and Sigal, E. (1995) Cloning and characterization of a murine macrophage lipoxygenase. *Bba-Lipid Lipid Metab.* **1254(1)**, 112–116.

15. Fleming, J., Thiele, B. J., Chester, J., O'Prey, J., Janetzki, S., Aitken, A., Anton, I. A., Rapoport, S. M., and Harrison, P. R. (1989) The complete sequence of the rabbit erythroid cell-specific 15-lipoxygenase mRNA: Comparison of the predicted amino acid sequence of the erythrocyte lipoxygenase with other lipoxygenases. *Gene* **79(1)**, 181–188.

16. Sigal, E., Craik, C. S., Highland, E., Grunberger, D., Costello, L. L., Dixon, R. A., and Nadel, J. A. (1988) Molecular cloning and primary structure of human 15-lipoxygenase. *Biochem. Biophys. Res. Commun.* **157(2)**, 457–464.

17. Yoshimoto, T., Suzuki, H., Yamamoto, S., Takai, T., Yokoyama, C., and Tanabe, T. (1990) Cloning and sequence analysis of the cDNA for arachidonate 12-lipoxygenase of porcine leukocytes. *Proc. Natl. Acad. Sci. USA* **87(6)**, 2142–2146.

18. Demarzo, N., Sloane, D. L., Dicharry, S., Highland, E., and Sigal, E. (1992) Cloning and expression of an airway epithelial 12-lipoxygenase. *Am. J. Physiol.* **262(2)**, L198–L207.

19. Kinzig, A., Furstenberger, G., Burger, F., Vogel, S., MullerDecker, K., Mincheva, A., Lichter, P., Marks, F., and Krieg, P. (1997) Murine epidermal lipoxygenase (Aloxe) encodes a 12-lipoxygenase isoform. *FEBS Lett.* **402(2–3)**, 162–166.

20 Balcarek, J. M., Theisen, T. W., Cook, M. N., Varrichio, A., Hwang, S. M., Strohsacker, M. W., and Crooke, S. T. (1988) Isolation and characterization of a cDNA clone encoding rat 5-lipoxygenase. *J. Biol. Chem.* **263(27)**, 13,937–13,941.

21. Chen, X. S., Naumann, T. A., Kurre, U., Jenkins, N. A., Copeland, N. G., and Funk, C. D. (1995) cDNA cloning, expression, mutagenesis, intracellular localization, and gene chromosomal assignment of mouse 5-lipoxygenase. *J. Biol. Chem.* **270(30)**, 17,993–17,999.

22. Kitzler, J. W. and Eling, T. E. (1996) Cloning, sequencing and expression of a 5-lipoxygenase from Syrian hamster embryo fibroblasts. *Prostaglandins Leukotrienes & Essential Fatty Acids* **55(4)**, 269–277.

23. Matsumoto, T., Funk, C. D., Rådmark, O., Höög, J. O., Jörnvall, H., and Samuelsson, B. (1988) Molecular cloning and amino acid sequence of human 5-lipoxygenase. *Proc. Natl. Acad. Sci. USA* **85(1)**, 26–30 (published erratum appears in *Proc. Natl. Acad. Sci. USA* [1988] **85(10)**, 3406).

24. Dixon, R. A., Jones, R. E., Diehl, R. E., Bennett, C. D., Kargman, S., and Rouzer, C. A. (1988) Cloning of the cDNA for human 5-lipoxygenase. *Proc. Natl. Acad. Sci. USA* **85(2)**, 416–420.

25. Brash, A. R., Boeglin, W. E., and Chang, M. S. (1997) Discovery of a second 15S-lipoxygenase in humans. *Proc. Natl. Acad. Sci. USA* **94(12),** 6148–6152.

26. Jisaka, M., Kim, R. B., Boeglin, W. E., Nanney, L. B., and Brash, A. R. (1997) Molecular cloning and functional expression of a phorbol ester-inducible 8s-lipoxygenase from mouse skin. *J. Biol. Chem.* **272(39),** 24,410–24,416.

27. Devereux, J., Haeberli, P., and Smithies, O. (1984) A comprehensive set of sequence analysis programs for the VAX. *Nucleic Acids Res.* **12(1),** 387–395.

28. Minor, W., Steczko, J., Bolin, J. T., Otwinowski, Z., and Axelrod, B. (1993) Crystallographic Determination of the active site iron and its ligands in soybean lipoxygenase L-1. *Biochemistry* **32(25),** 6320–6323.

29. Prigge, S. T., Boyington, J. C., Gaffney, B. J., and Amzel, L. M. (1996) Structure conservation in lipoxygenases: structural analysis of soybean lipoxygenase-1 and modeling of human lipoxygenases. *Protein-Struct. Funct. Genet.* **24(3),** 275–291.

30. Boyington, J. C., Gaffney, B. J., and Amzel, L. M. (1993) The 3-dimensional structure of an arachidonic acid 15-lipoxygenase. *Science* **260(5113),** 1482–1486.

31. Shibata, D., Steczko, J., Dixon, J. E., Hermodson, M., Yazdanparast, R., and Axelrod, B. (1987) Primary structure of soybean lipoxygenase-1. *J. Biol. Chem.* **262(21),** 10,080–10,085.

32. Lepley, R. A. and Fitzpatrick, F. A. (1994) 5-lipoxygenase contains a functional Src homology 3–binding motif that interacts with the Src homology 3 domain of Grb2 and cytoskeletal proteins. *J. Biol. Chem.* **269(39),** 24,163–24,168.

33. Yu, H., Chen, J. K., Feng, S., Dalgarno, D. C., Brauer, A. W., and Schreiber, S. L. (1994) Structural basis for the binding of proline-rich peptides to SH3 domains. *Cell* **76(5),** 933–945.

34. Chan, H. W. (1973) Soya-bean lipoxygenase: An iron-containing dioxygenase. *Biochim. Biophys. Acta* **327(1),** 32–35.

35. Pistorius, E. K. and Axelrod, B. (1974) Iron, an essential component of lipoxygenase. *J. Biol. Chem.* **249(10),** 3183–3186.

36. Roza, M. and Francke, A. (1973) Soyabean lipoxygenase: an iron-containing enzyme. *Biochim. Biophys. Acta* **327(1),** 24–31.

37. Percival, M. D. (1991) Human 5-lipoxygenase contains an essential iron. *J. Biol. Chem.* **266(16),** 10,058–10,061.

38. Van der Heijdt, L. M., Feiters, M. C., Navaratnam, S., Nolting, H. F., Hermes, C., Veldink, G. A., and Vliegenthart, J. F. G. (1992) X-ray absorption spectroscopy of soybean lipoxygenase-1— influence of lipid hydroperoxide activation and lyophilization on the structure of the non-heme iron active site. *Eur. J. Biochem.* **207(2),** 793–802.

39. Veldink, G. A. and Vliegenthart, J. F. (1984) Lipoxygenases, nonheme iron-containing enzymes. *Adv. Inorg. Biochem.* **6(139),** 139–161.

40. Navaratnam, S., Feiters, M. C., Al, H. M., Allen, J. C., Veldink, G. A., and Vliegenthart, J. F. (1988) Iron environment in soybean lipoxygenase–1. *Biochim. Biophys. Acta,* **956(1),** 70–76.

41. Funk, C. D., Gunne, H., Steiner, H., Izumi, T., and Samuelsson, B. (1989) Native and mutant 5-lipoxygenase expression in a baculovirus/insect cell system. *Proc. Natl. Acad. Sci. USA* **86(8),** 2592–2596.

42. Ishii, S., Noguchi, M., Miyano, M., Matsumoto, T., and Noma, M. (1992) Mutagenesis studies on the amino acid residues involved in the iron-binding and the activity of human 5-lipoxygenase. *Biochem. Biophys. Res. Commun.* **182(3),** 1482–1490.

43. Nguyen, T., Falgueyret, J. P., Abramovitz, M., and Riendeau, D. (1991) Evaluation of the role of conserved his and met residues among lipoxygenases by site-directed mutagenesis of recombinant human 5-lipoxygenase. *J. Biol. Chem.* **266(32),** 22,057–22,062.

44. Zhang, Y. Y., Radmark, O., and Samuelsson, B. (1992) Mutagenesis of some conserved residues in human 5-lipoxygenase—effects on enzyme activity. *Proc. Natl. Acad. Sci. USA* **89(2),** 485–489.

45. Hammarberg, T., Zhang, Y. Y., Lind, B., Radmark, O., and Samuelsson, B. (1995) Mutations at the C-terminal isoleucine and other potential iron ligands of 5-lipoxygenase. *Eur. J. Biochem.* **230(2),** 401–407.

46. Zhang, Y. Y., Lind, B., Radmark, O., and Samuelsson, B. (1993) Iron content of human 5-lipoxygenase, effects of mutations regarding conserved histidine residues. *J. Biol. Chem.* **268(4),** 2535–2541.

47. Percival, M. D. and Ouellet, M. (1992) The characterization of 5 histidine-serine mutants of human 5-lipoxygenase. *Biochem. Biophys. Res. Commun.,* **186(3),** 1265–1270.

48. Funk, M. O., Carroll, R. T., Thompson, J. F., Sands, R. H., and Dunham, W. R. (1990) Role of iron in lipoxygenase catalysis. *J. Am. Chem. Soc.* **112,** 5375–5376.

49. Zang, Y., Elgren, T. E., Dong, Y. H., and Que, L. (1993) A high-potential ferrous complex and its conversion to an alkylperoxoiron(III) intermediate—a lipoxygenase model. *J. Am. Chem. Soc.* **115(2),** 811–813.

50. Zhang, Y., Gebhard, M. S., and Solomon, E. I. (1991) Spectroscopic studies of the non-heme ferric active site in soybean lipoxygenase—magnetic circular dichroism as a probe of electronic and geometric structure—ligand-field origin of zero-field splitting. *Am. Chem. Soc.* **113(14),** 5162–5175.

51. Steczko, J., Donoho, G. A., Dixon, J. E., Sugimoto, T., and Axelrod, B. (1991) Effect of ethanol and low-temperature culture on expression of soybean lipoxygenase L-1 in Escherichia coli. *Protein Express. Purif.* **2(2–3),** 221–227.

52. Steczko, J., Donoho, G. P., Clemens, J. C., Dixon, J. E., and Axelrod, B. (1992) Conserved histidine residues in soybean lipoxygenase—functional consequences of their replacement. *Biochemistry* **31(16),** 4053–4057.

53. Wang, W. H., Takano, T., Shibata, D., Kitamura, K., and Takeda, G. (1994) Molecular basis of a null mutation in soybean lipoxygenase 2, Substitution of glutamine for an iron-ligand histidine. *Proc. Natl. Acad. Sci. USA* **91(13),** 5828–5832.

54. Suzuki, H., Kishimoto, K., Yoshimoto, T., Yamamoto, S., Kanai, F., Ebina, Y., Miyatake, A., and Tanabe, T. (1994) Site-directed mutagenesis studies on the iron-binding domain and the determinant for the substrate oxygenation site of porcine leukocyte arachidonate 12-lipoxygenase. *Bba-Lipid Lipid Metab* **1210(3),** 308–316.

55. Yokoyama, C., Shinjo, F., Yoshimoto, T., Yamamoto, S., Oates, J. A., and Brash, A. R. (1986) Arachidonate 12-lipoxygenase purified from porcine leukocytes by immunoaffinity chromatography and its reactivity with hydroperoxyeicosatetraenoic acids. *J. Biol. Chem.* **261(35),** 16,714–16,721.

56. Chen, X. S. and Funk, C. D. (1993) Structure-function properties of human platelet 12-lipoxygenase—chimeric enzyme and in vitro mutagenesis studies. *FASEB J.* **7(8),** 694–701.

57. Brash, A. R., Boeglin, W. E., Chang, M. S., and Shieh, B. H. (1996) Purification and molecular cloning of an 8R-lipoxygenase from the coral Plexaura homomalla reveal the related primary structures of R- and S-lipoxygenases. *J. Biol. Chem.* **271(34),** 20,949–20,957.

58. Sloane, D. L., Leung, R., Craik, C. S., and Sigal, E. (1991) A primary determinant for lipoxygenase positional specificity. *Nature* **354(6349),** 149–152.

59. Sloane, D. L. and Sigal, E. (1994) On the positional specificity of 15-lipoxygenase. *Ann. NY Acad. Sci.* **744(99),** 99–106 (review, 24 refs).

60. Sloane, D. L., Leung, R., Barnett, J., Craik, C. S., and Sigal, E. (1995) Conversion of human 15-lipoxygenase to an efficient 12-lipoxygenase: the side-chain geometry of amino acids 417 and 418 determine positional specificity. *Protein Eng.* **8(3),** 275–282.

61. Borngraber, S., Kuban, R. J., Anton, M., and Kuhn, H. (1996) Phenylalanine 353 is a primary determinant for the positional specificity of mammalian 15-lipoxygenases. *J. Mol. Biol.* **264(5),** 1145–1153.

62. Gan, Q. F., Browner, M. F., Sloane, D. L., and Sigal, E. (1996) Defining the arachidonic acid binding site of human 15-lipoxygenase—molecular modeling and mutagenesis. *J. Biol. Chem.* **271(41),** 25,412–25,418.

63. Kuhn, H., Barnett, J., Grunberger, D., Baecker, P., Chow, J., Nguyen, B., Bursztyn, P. H., Chan, H., and Sigal, E. (1993) Overexpression, purification and characterization of human recombinant 15-lipoxygenase. *Biochim. Biophys. Acta* **1169(1),** 80–89.

64. Izumi, T., Radmark, O., Jornvall, H., and Samuelsson, B. (1991) Purification of two forms of arachidonate 15-lipoxygenase from human leukocytes. *Eur. J. Biochem.* **202(3),** 1231–1238.

65. Sigal, E., Grunberger, D., Craik, C. S., Caughey, G. H., and Nadel, J. A. (1988) Arachidonate 15-lipoxygenase (omega-6 lipoxygenase) from human leukocytes: Purification and structural homology to other mammalian lipoxygenases. *J. Biol. Chem.* **263(11),** 5328–5332.

66. Hartel, B., Ludwig, P., Schewe, T., and Rapoport, S. M. (1982) Self-inactivation by 13–hydroperoxylinoleic acid and lipohydroperoxidase activity of the reticulocyte lipoxygenase. *Eur. J. Biochem.* **126(2),** 353–357.

67. Rapoport, S., Hartel, B., and Hausdorf, G. (1984) Methionine sulfoxide formation: The cause of self-inactivation of reticulocyte lipoxygenase. *Eur. J. Biochem.* **139(3),** 573–576.

68. Gan, Q. F., Witkop, G. L., Sloane, D. L., Straub, K. M., and Sigal, E. (1995) Identification of a specific methionine in mammalian 15-lipoxygenase which is oxygenated by the enzyme product 13-HPODE: Dissociation of sulfoxide formation from self-inactivation. *Biochemistry* **34(21),** 7069–7079.

69. Richards, K. M. and Marnett, L. J. (1997) Leukocyte 12 lipoxygenase: Expression, purification, and investigation of the role of methionine residues in turnover-dependent inactivation and 5,8,11,14-eicosatetraynoic acid inhibition. *Biochemistry* **36(22),** 6692–6699.

70. Wantanabe, T., Medina, J. F., Haeggström, J. Z., Rådmark, O., and Samuelsson, B. (1993) Molecular cloning of a 12-lipoxygenase cDNA from rat brain. *Eur. J. Biochem.* **212(2),** 605–612.

71. Berger, M., Schuarz, K., Thiele, H., Reimann, I., Huth, A., Borngraeber, S., Kuehn, H., and Thiele, B. J. (1998) Simultaneous expression of leukocyte-type 12-lipoxygenase and reticulocyte-type 5-lipoxygenase in rabbits. *J. Mol. Biol.* **278,** 935–948.

5

Lipid-Mediator-Deficient Mice in Models of Inflammation

Colin D. Funk

Introduction

Prostaglandins (PGs) and leukotrienes (LTs) have long been known to be important endogenous mediators of inflammation (for reviews *see* refs. *1,2*). The pathways for PG formation were elucidated first in the early 1960s by Bergström et al. *(3)*, and by van Dorp et al. *(4)*, and those for the LTs in 1979–1980 *(5,6)*. Their biological actions were assessed by classical pharmacological experiments involving bioassays and addition of cyclooxygenase (COX) or lipoxygenase (LO) inhibitors or receptor antagonists. The early discovery of nonsteroidal antiinflammatory drugs (NSAID), like aspirin and indomethacin which specifically inhibit COX enzyme activity *(7,8)*, greatly simplified the task of ascertaining the role of PGs in inflammation. Progress in defining specific inhibitors and receptor antagonists for the LT pathway was relatively slow in comparison.

PGs, synthesized by the initial action of PG H synthase (commonly referred to as COX), are known to mediate a significant proportion of the pain and hyperemia associated with inflammation. These potent bioactive lipids are made by nearly every cell in the body including macrophages, mast cells, and lymphocytes. An important discovery in the early 1990s by several groups indicated that in addition to the "classical" COX, there was a second form of the enzyme that was highly inducible, especially by common inflammatory signals *(9–12)*. This second COX, or COX-2, has been the target for intensive development of a new generation of specific anti-inflammatory compounds.

LTs are synthesized by neutrophils, mast cells, eosinophils, and macrophages. Leukotriene B_4 (LTB_4) was found to be a potent agent capable of inducing neutrophil chemotaxis *(13)*, soon after its structural elucidation. The other class of LTs, the cysteinyl-containing LTs, LTC_4, LTD_4, and $LTDE_4$, were discovered to be the active

From: *Molecular and Cellular Basis of Inflammation*
Edited by: C. N. Serhan and P. A. Ward © Humana Press Inc., Totowa, NJ

components of the "slow-reacting substance of anaphylaxis" *(2,14)*. As such, these compounds were found to promote vascular leakage, induce airway smooth muscle contraction, and increase mucus secretion *(2,14–16)*.

A wealth of information about the actions of PGs and LTs in various inflammatory and injurious settings has been gleaned over the past 20–30 yr. It is beyond the scope of this chapter to review this material here. Instead, an attempt will be made to draw out the potentially important contributions that can be made by the use of lipid mediator "knockout" mice in models of inflammation and the data that has been accumulated in this field to date, which is still in its infancy. The generation of knockout mice to study PG or LT function can be approached by several different strategies. First, one can make mice that are lipid mediator deficient by knocking out the first enzyme in the respective biosynthetic pathways (i.e., COX for the PG pathway, and 5-LO for the LT pathway). A second approach would be to inactivate an important accessory factor, or enzyme. For instance, FLAP (5-LO–activating protein) involved in LT biosynthesis or one of the phospholipase enzymes that releases the substrate for use by either COX or 5-LO could be inactivated by disruption of their respective genes. A third alternative would be to leave the lipid mediators intact but to ablate expression of specific eicosanoid receptors.

One of the major advantages of knockout technology over standard pharmacological manipulation is its ability to specifically and completely ablate the gene product. Thus, mice totally deficient in LT synthesis have been generated *(17,18)*. It should be emphasized that in some of these strategies it may not be possible to abolish completely all lipid mediators in a single knockout (e.g., phospholipase or COX-2) because there are multiple members of the same enzyme family. Potential drawbacks of targeted gene inactivation techniques include the chance for shunting of substrate arachidonic acid to other eicosanoid pathways, developmental abnormalities, or compensatory mechanisms that are not easy to ascertain.

Targeted gene inactivation technology is currently only in routine use in mice. The mouse has a long history of use as a key biological tool for inflammation research. It has its advantages and disadvantages. Advantages include its well-studied genetics, short generation cycle, eicosanoid biosynthetic pathways common to humans, and well-characterized models. The ear inflammation model *(19,20)* is a standard assay used by the pharmaceutical industry in screening for anti-inflammatory drugs. Peritonitis models and reactions to infection with various microorganisms can be performed easily in mice. Drawbacks relate to the small size of mice for some physiological testing and sample preparations, variability in susceptibility to inflammatory stimuli owing to genetic strain differences, and some differences to humans with respect to biological activity of lipid mediators. Nonetheless, significant strides in the understanding of inflammation can be gained with the use of knockout mice. The next section will deal with the generation of the various lipid mediator–deficient mice.

Generation of Gene Knockout Mice

5-LO–Deficient Mice

The complete mouse 5-LO gene has not been cloned; only partial clones have been obtained. This gene is situated in the central region of mouse chromosome 6 *(21)*. Based on the human 5-LO gene, which was previously isolated and found to encompass more than 80 kb *(22)*, targeting vectors were constructed with mouse genomic clones to inactivate this gene. Funk et al. *(17)* inactivated the gene in exon 6 by insertion of a resistance cassette for neomycin, whereas Goulet et al. *(18)* deleted a portion of exon 10 and the upstream intron. Since all LOs have a catalytically essential nonheme iron atom that is liganded by three histidine residues encoded by exons 8 and 9, and the C-terminal isoleucine encoded by exon 14 *(23)*, any disruption of these sites would be expected to lead to a nonfunctional protein. Both gene-targeting vectors were successful in producing null alleles. 5-LO–deficient mice were generated according to Mendelian ratios during interbreeding of heterozygous mice *(17,18)*. The knockout mice were incapable of LT biosynthesis from either exogenous or endogenous substrate when macrophages or mast cells were stimulated with calcium ionophore or antigen/IgE, respectively.

FLAP-Deficient Mice

A fragment of the mouse FLAP gene was isolated and an 800-bp segment containing a 130-bp exon encoding the C-terminal amino acids 108–151 was eliminated in a targeting vector *(24,25)*. Targeted embryonic stem (ES) cell clones were obtained at high frequency with this construct, and chimeric mice were generated from two different cell lines. As for the 5-LO–deficient mice, homozygous-deficient mice were present in the expected numbers based on Mendelian ratios for heterozygous matings. There were no outward abnormalities in these mice *(24,25)*. FLAP mRNA was absent in the homozygous mice, and macrophages from these mice were unable to synthesize LTs. These observations indicated that the C-terminal tail of FLAP is critical for its function and message stability. Moreover, the results are indicative of the essential role FLAP plays in LT biosynthesis.

COX-1–Deficient Mice

The mouse COX-1 gene is 22 kb in length *(26)* and resides on chromosome 2 *(27)*. The gene consists of 11 exons and 10 introns *(26)*. The strategy chosen for inactivation of this gene was based on the premise that serine-530, the site acetylated by aspirin, is an important residue *(28)*. Thus, the gene was disrupted prior to the codon for this amino acid, by deletion of 1 kb of intron 10 along with the first part of exon 11, and insertion of a neomycin resistance cassette in its place. Although this residue, in fact, is not critical for enzyme activity (only when it is acetylated by aspirin does this residue block access of the substrate to the active site), this disruption would be expected to give rise to a truncated protein. However, analysis of macrophage message and protein for COX-1 revealed no evidence for a truncated or altered transcript, and absence of COX-1 protein. Thus, the gene disruption in exon 11 resulted in a null allele. COX-1–deficient mice were obtained in normal ratios from interbreeding of heterozygous siblings and appeared outwardly normal *(28)*, which was surprising because PGs have been implicated in so many physiological homeostatic mechanisms.

COX-2–Deficient Mice

The COX-2 gene is similar in structure to the COX-1 gene, with 10 exons and 9 introns, lacking only a small 5' initial exon that encodes mainly for untranslated sequence *(29)*. However, this gene is much smaller (8 kb) and is situated on chromosome 1, not 2 *(27,29)*. This gene was disrupted by two separate groups. Morham et al. *(30)* chose to disrupt the gene in exon 8 by deleting a region that encodes two amino acid residues that are essential for catalytic activity (Tyr-371 and His-374). Dinchuk et al. *(31)* removed the transcription and translation start sites and all of exon 1 in their construct. Both groups observed abnormalities in obtaining homozygous null animals. In one case, approx 35% of the expected number of animals was obtained *(31)*. In the other case, females were obtained at normal ratios, but males were significantly underrepresented *(30)*. COX-2–deficient mice have significant renal abnormalities and, in some cases, cardiac fibrosis. Adult COX-2–deficient mice succumb to the progressive chronic renal failure of developmental origin.

12/15-LO–Deficient Mice

The mouse leukocyte-type 12-LO gene (also known as 12/15-LO gene) was cloned and found to reside on midchromosome 11 *(32)*. The gene is about 7.5 kb in length and a targeting vector was constructed with a fragment containing the first eight exons *(33)*. Exon 3 was disrupted with two neomycin resistance cassettes, and several gene-targeted clones were obtained. Homozygous-deficient mice were generated at the expected ratios. Although no 12/15-LO sequence was deleted in the targeted construct, no mRNA was detected in peritoneal macrophages by Northern blot analysis, nor was 12/15-LO protein or enzyme activity present in these cells. Nonfunctional transcripts in other tissues have been detected by PCR and Northern analysis (unpublished observations). Macrophages from homozygous mice under certain conditions synthesize more 5-LO products than wild-type mice *(33)*. However, under normal physiological conditions these mice showed no evidence for overt abnormalities.

Platelet-Type 12-LO–Deficient Mice

The mouse platelet-type 12-LO gene is 15–17 kb in size and resides near the leukocyte-type 12-LO gene on chromosome 11 *(32)*. This gene proved quite difficult for generating homologous recombinant gene-targeted ES cell clones. On the fourth attempt, a vector with a deletion of exon 8 yielded properly targeted clones that were injected into host blastocysts *(34)*. One male chimera transmitted the disruption to the germline, and homozygous mice were subsequently generated at the predicted numbers. Platelet 12-LO activity was absent in these mice, but the COX/thromboxane pathway remained intact. Platelet-type 12-LO–deficient platelets exhibited a selective hyperreactivity to the platelet agonist ADP but not to other well-known agonists *(34)*.

PG F$_{2\alpha}$ (FP) Receptor–Deficient Mice

To generate a FP receptor deficient mouse line, Narumiya et al. *(35)* removed a 1.3-kb fragment containing exon 2 of the FP gene that encodes most of the protein (up to amino acid 266 in the sixth transmembrane domain) from a 9.8-kb genomic fragment and replaced it with *LacZ* and neomycin resistance cassettes. Two lines of ES cells were obtained with the gene disruption and were injected into host blastocysts. Mice lacking the FP receptor develop normally and are obtained in normal ratios from heterozygous crosses. However, FP-receptor–deficient females are unable to initiate normal parturition *(35)*.

Prostacyclin-Receptor–Deficient Mice

A prostacyclin receptor gene-targeted ES cell line was created by replacement of a 2.4-kb segment including exons 2 and 3 with a neomycin resistance cassette in the targeting vector *(36)*. This deletion would disrupt the sixth transmembrane domain to the C-terminus of the protein. Chimeric mice were generated from two separate lines and were backcrossed to C57BL/6 mice. Surprisingly, there were significant aberrations from Mendelian ratios in heterozygous cross-matings. Males were obtained only at 62% of the expected values, whereas females were generated at 80% normal. These results are similar to those obtained in COX-2–deficient mice and suggest that there is some form of prenatal mortality as a result of prostacyclin receptor deficiency. Of the homozygous mice that did survive, they grew normally, were fertile, and showed no signs of abnormal blood pressure *(36)*.

Mouse Models of Inflammation

Acute inflammation is characterized by hyperemia, edema, leukocyte infiltration, and pain responses. Eicosanoids may participate in each, or some, of these events. For instance, PGs can cause peripheral vasodilatation and can sensitize primary afferents to harmful stimuli.

Ear Inflammation Model

One of the most commonly used standard inflammatory models in mice involves topical administration of either arachidonic acid or tetradecanoylphorbol acetate (TPA) to the ear *(19,20)*; vehicle (acetone) is administered to the opposite ear. Indices of inflammation are usually measured as increase in ear thickness over the vehicle-treated ear, or increase in ear weight of punch biopsies. In general, the arachidonic acid model shows maximal swelling at 1 h postapplication, whereas the TPA model exhibits inflammation over a longer time course (4–24 h) and is associated with an influx of neutrophils *(19,20,37)*. Arachidonic acid–induced ear edema probably results from the rapid production of LTC_4/LTD_4 and PGE_2, in which these mediators act to promote vasodilatation and enhanced vascular permeability. Most likely they interact synergistically to promote edema. The TPA model, based on inhibitor studies, is the result of PG production and other mediators, which include histamine, bradykinin, and serotonin.

5-LO–deficient mice show a statistically significant reduction in ear inflammation in the arachidonic acid ear model when compared to littermate controls *(17,25)*. This difference was observed by measurement of ear swelling, biopsy weight, and plasma extravasation (Fig. 1). The differences were observed both on a "pure" 129 Sv genetic background and on a hybrid C57BL/6 × 129 Sv background *(17,25)*. Additionally, at a later time point (7 h), neutrophil influx was markedly reduced as measured by myeloperoxidase activity. Similar results were also seen with FLAP-deficient mice, although the increment was slightly lower in the edema assays *(25)*. A cocktail of LTs injected into 5-LO–deficient mouse ears just prior to the arachidonic acid phlogistic was able to rescue the phenotype to that of wild-type mice *(17)*. 5-LO–deficient mice demonstrated no alterations in their response to TPA, as observed in previous studies that employed LO inhibitors *(17)*.

Interestingly, and perhaps unexpectedly, COX-1–deficient mice, but not COX-2–deficient mice, had a reduced response in the arachidonic acid edema model, and neither showed an altered response to TPA *(28,30,31)*. The COX-1 homozygous-deficient response was approx 30% of the control response in the arachidonic acid model, whereas the 5-LO–deficient response ranged between 30 and 50% of that observed in wild-type mice (Fig. 1A). Thus, it is likely that LTs (probably LTC_4 or LTD_4) and COX-1–derived PGE_2 account for all the edema in this model, which would agree totally with the early inhibitor studies. In fact, preliminary data have

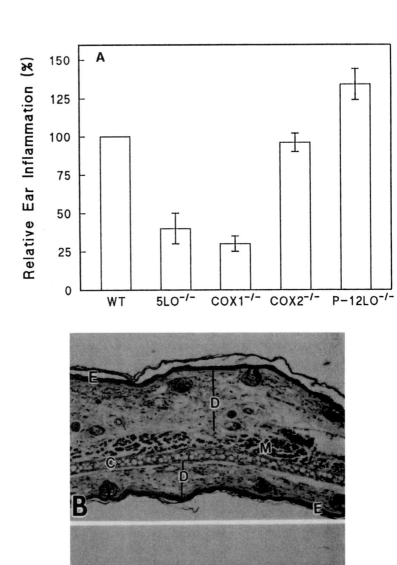

Fig. 1. Ear inflammation in lipid mediator–deficient mice. **(A)** Relative ear inflammatory responses in the arachidonic acid-induced edema model. Inflammation response in wild-type mice has been set to 100%. Data are representative of that presented in refs. *17* and *25* for 5-LO–deficient (5-LO$^{-/-}$), ref. *28* for COX-1–deficient, refs. *30* and *31* for COX-2 deficient, and unpublished data for platelet-type 12-LO–deficient (P-12-LO$^{-/-}$) mice. **(B,C)** Photomicrographs of mouse ear sections through a 5-LO–deficient (C) and wild-type (B) ear 1 h after topical administration of arachidonic acid (2 mg in 20 µL acetone). The edema-

shown that double knockout 5-LO/COX-1 mice show no swelling in the arachidonic acid model (unpublished observations).

12/15-LO–deficient mice did not respond differently than wild-type mice in the two inflammation models, but preliminary evidence indicates that platelet-type 12-LO–deficient mice actually have an enhanced edematous response (ref. *33* and unpublished observations). The mechanism for this enhanced inflammation has not been determined yet, but it could be caused by an increased availability of substrate to be converted to LTs or PGs. Platelet-type 12-LO is expressed in skin *(38,39)*, and its absence at this site, where 12-HETE is a major metabolite, could also be a reason for enhanced inflammation.

Carrageenan-Induced Paw Edema and Pleurisy

Carrageenan, a gelatin isolated from various seaweeds, has been used extensively in inflammation studies because it elicits a robust nonimmunological edematous response when injected into the footpad of rodents *(40)*. Carrageenan causes a time-dependent increase in paw volume in normal mice. This increase was suppressed by approx 50% in mice deficient for the prostacyclin receptor *(36)*. A similar suppression was observed in indomethacin-pretreated wild-type mice. These data demonstrated that endogenous prostacyclin is a key prostanoid that governs the inflammatory response in this model. In further studies, a significant reduction of exudate volume was recovered from the pleural cavity of prostacyclin receptor knockout mice that had been injected 3 h previously with carrageenan when compared to wild-type injected mice *(36)*.

Both COX-1– and COX-2–deficient mice can mount an inflammatory response to carrageenan, but these responses are apparently different than those seen in wild-type mice regarding macrophage recruitment and production of PGs and cytokines *(28,30,31,41)*.

Inflammatory Cell Recruitment/Elicitation Models

Eicosanoids, in particular LTB_4 and other 5-LO products, have been demonstrated to be important inflammatory cell chemotactic factors. Their involvement in various pathophysiologic models can be studied in eicosanoid-deficient mice.

Peritonitis Models

Peritonitis can be induced in mice by numerous methods, such as bacterial challenge or formation of immune complexes. A challenge of sterile glycogen injected intraperitoneally elicits predominantly neutrophils. 5-LO, or leukocyte-type 12-LO, deficiency did not affect the recruitment of neutrophils in response to glycogen *(17,33)*. However, 5-LO deficiency did result in a dramatic reduction of infiltrating cells in immune-complex–induced peritonitis *(17)*. This finding has potentially important implications for the role of 5-LO products in immune complex disorders. It should be emphasized that

---

tous response is significantly blunted in the 5-LO–deficient mouse ear whereas the wild-type ear shows increased dermal thickness, and numerous congested blood vessels. E, epidermis; D, dermis; C, cartilage, M, muscle. Size bar equals 100 μm. Ear thickness (μm) averaged over 30 points on two separate ear sections was 185 ± 9.2 and 302 ± 15 for wild-type vehicle and arachidonic acid-treated; 188 ± 6.6 and 201 ± 5.5 for 5-LO–deficient vehicle and arachidonic acid-treated, respectively.

the absence of 5-LO products in mice did not result in a uniformly reduced infiltration of inflammatory cells at other sites. Thus, when immune complex formation was induced in dorsal skin, there was no significant difference in neutrophil elicitation between wild-type and knockout mice *(23)*.

A noninduced suppurative peritonitis was observed in some, but not all, COX-2–deficient mice at 8 wk of age *(30)*. Submucosal edema of the bowel wall, inflammatory cell infiltrates consisting primarily of neutrophils, and focal accumulation of bacteria were observed. The mice with peritonitis had a splenic myeloid hyperplasia. At present, there are no explanations for these findings.

Polyacrylamide Gel and Air Pouch Models

Similar to the carrageenan-induced paw edema model, injection of polyacrylamide, or air, under the dorsal skin leads to robust inflammatory responses, which include inflammatory cell invasion and release of eicosanoids such as LTB_4 and PGE_2. Experiments with 5-LO–deficient mice of the C57BL/6 × 129 Sv hybrid background did not yield evidence for an involvement of 5-LO products in the recruitment of neutrophils in the polyacrylamide model because influx was similar to wild-type mice *(42)*. This result is in direct contrast to the effects of the putative specific 5-LO inhibitor ABT-761, which did dramatically reduce neutrophil influx *(42)*.

In a 6-d air pouch model, after stimulation with carrageenan, absence of COX-2 expression yielded defective macrophage recruitment *(41)*, but similar numbers of total white blood cells were recovered in lavages from wild-type and COX-1– and COX-2–deficient mice.

Collagen-Induced Arthritis Model

An experimental model of human rheumatoid arthritis in the mouse consists of immunizing mice with heterologous type II collagen in the tail, followed by administration of interleukin(IL)-1, which potentiates the development of the disease *(43)*. The model, usually performed in mice of the DBA/1 genetic strain, is dependent on both cellular and humoral immunity to the immunizing antigen.

To investigate the role of LTs in this model, Griffiths et al. *(24)* generated FLAP-deficient mice on the DBA/1 genetic background. They found that the severity of collagen-induced arthritis (analyzed as swelling and redness in paws) was reduced at all time points compared to wild-type animals, even though serum anticollagen antibody levels were nearly equivalent in both groups. In the knee joint cavity, wild-type mice had extensive disease consisting of considerable leukocyte infiltration of the synovial connective tissue, plasma protein extravasation into the synovial cavity, and variable amounts of articular cartilage destruction. By contrast, FLAP-deficient mice, in general, showed no signs of inflammatory cells in the joint cavity or surrounding synovial tissue. The articular cartilage was intact, although there were regions of extensive depletion of proteoglycans. These studies correlated nicely with a previous one in which a specific LTB_4 receptor antagonist blocked collagen-induced arthritis *(44)*.

Allergic Airway Inflammation

Asthma is a chronic inflammatory disease of complex etiology *(45)*. Characteristic symptoms include an exaggerated response of the airways to nonspecific stimuli, inflammation associated with eosinophilic infiltrates, and intermittent airway obstruction. LTs have well-documented roles in the pathophysiology of asthma based on past studies with LO inhibitors and receptor antagonists *(15,16)*. Their mechanism of action and precise involvement in the development of the disease are not completely understood. Mouse "asthma-like" models have been developed that recapitulate the hallmark symptoms of the disease *(46)*. In most cases, the allergic airway inflammation is induced by an initial ip challenge of an antigen like ovalbumin, followed by a series of aerosol antigen exposures over a 2–4 wk regimen.

5-LO–deficient mice and wild-type controls were sensitized and serially exposed to aerosols of ovalbumin *(47)*. Airway resistance was measured in response to intravenous methacholine. Wild-type mice developed a significant increase in cholinergic responsiveness whereas the knockout mice displayed responses that were similar to nonsensitized mice *(47)*. The enhanced responsiveness in the wild-type mice was of a similar magnitude to the response observed in challenge tests with human asthmatics. Pronounced eosinophilia was observed in the airways and bronchoalveolar lavage of wild-type mice *(47,48)*. Of the total bronchoalveolar lavage cells in these mice, 70–80% consisted of eosinophils. Knockout mice had approximately one-half the total lavage cells, and only a fraction of the eosinophils, compared with the wild-type mice following antigen sensitization and aerosolized challenges. These results were observed in both 129 Sv strain mice and the hybrid C57BL/6 × 129 Sv strain mice *(48)*. It should be mentioned, however, that in terms of the immune response, total IgE and ovalbumin-specific IgG levels were elevated significantly in the wild-type mice, but to a substantially lesser degree in the 5-LO–deficient mice. These results indicate that 5-LO products may directly influence the immune response in this model. In fact, LTB_4 has been shown by in vitro studies to enhance IgE secretion from IL-4–stimulated human lymphocytes *(49,50)*. Thus, alterations in the immune response in this particular model could account for the diminished airway hyperresponsiveness and eosinophilia observed in the knockout mice. Studies are under way to examine this possibility.

Since late 1996 or early 1997, the anti-LT agents, Accolate™ (also known as zafirlukast, an LTD_4 receptor antagonist) and Zyflo™ (zileuton, a 5-LO inhibitor) have been used in the clinic for treatment of asthma *(51)*. By inhibiting the action of LTs at airway smooth muscle, sensory C fibers that innervate the epithelium, mucus secreting cells, and inflammatory cells *(16)*, these agents can reduce the inflammation of this disease, which is showing signs of increased prevalence in urban industrialized nations. Henderson et al. *(52)* demonstrated that zileuton abolished eosinophilia in ovalbumin-treated wild-type mice but that it did not affect the airway hyperresponsiveness, in contrast to studies with 5-LO–deficient mice. The reason for these apparent discrepancies has not been determined yet. Nevertheless, 5-LO or FLAP knockout mice may prove useful for teasing out the mechanisms of action of these drugs, or basic mechanisms of asthma pathogenesis, although mice can display different responses to LTs than humans *(53)*. The reduction of airway hyperresponsiveness and eosinophilic inflammation in 5-LO–deficient mice could possibly be owing to shunting of arachidonic acid metabolism to other prostanoids, such as PGE_2, which is known to affect the immune response. It will be important to determine the roles, if any, of PGs in this model, by either using COX-deficient mice, or selective COX inhibitors administered to 5-LO–deficient mice. Additionally, rescue of the phenotype found in 5-LO–deficient mice with enzyme expressed in the appropriate inflammatory cells (possibly by adenovirus gene transfer, or bone marrow reconstitution) at different time points during development of airway inflammation in the mice will be a critical experiment to understand acquisition of the airway hyperresponsiveness and inflammation.

Bacterial/Parasite Infections and Inflammation/Host Defense
Schistosomiasis

Schistosoma mansoni eggs, laid by adult female worms, are transported via the portal circulation where they become lodged in the presinusoidal capillaries. An eosinophil-rich, T-cell–dependent granuloma ensues *(54)*. Previous studies with LO inhibitors, but not COX inhibitors, have indicated a significant reduction in the size of synchronous primary lung granulomas, which form around schistosome eggs injected into mice *(55)*. Since 5- and 12/15-LO products are synthesized abundantly by eosinophils and macrophages, they represent candidate mediators of inflammation in schistosomiasis. To test this, 5-LO and 12/15-LO knockout mice were infected with *S. mansoni (56)*. Eight weeks after infection, 5-LO–deficient mice developed smaller granulomas around liver-deposited schistosome eggs compared to wild-type or 12/15-LO–deficient mice *(56)*. However, there were no obvious differences in cellular composition of the granulomas among the three different groups. All three groups of mice were infected to a similar degree as measured by schistosome antigen, suggesting comparable worm burdens. Likewise, there were no alterations in eosinophils in peritoneal exudates or peripheral blood. Could altered cytokine levels explain the diminished granuloma size in 5-LO–deficient mice? Preliminary evidence suggested that IL-10, but not IL-4 or interferon-γ, gene expression was altered (diminished) in the knockout mice. These results would suggest that the difference in granuloma size is not the result of a relative shift in Th1/Th2 cytokine profiles. IL-10 plays a regulatory role in chronic granulomatous inflammation *(57)*, and the interplay of 5-LO products and this cytokine will have to be explored further.

Inflammation in response to schistosome egg antigen was also tested in the ear swelling assay. Both immediate and delayed-type hypersensitivity responses were significantly lower in 5-LO–deficient mice when compared to wild-type controls or 12/15-LO–deficient mice *(56)*. 5-LO, therefore, appears to be an important contributor to granulomatous inflammation and antigen-mediated hypersensitivity responses in murine *S. mansoni* infections, but is clearly not the sole mediator of inflammation.

Nippostrongylus brasiliensis Infection

Gastrointestinal nematodes cause host immune and inflammatory responses that lead to their expulsion *(58)*. Mice infected with these parasites make a Th2-type cytokine response, and expulsion of some is IL-4–dependent. Mast cells and eosinophils are key cells involved in the response, and given that these cells are capable of synthesis of large quantities of bioactive LTs, it was important to investigate 5-LO product involvement in gastrointestinal parasite expulsion. The data so far with 5-LO knockout mice and expulsion of *N. brasiliensis* have been equivocal (i.e., 5-LO products probably contribute to some extent to worm expulsion, but that extent is relatively small and variable among experiments) (unpublished observations).

IL-4 enhances cholinergic neural control of mouse small intestinal smooth muscle through an LTD_4-dependent mechanism in studies using 5-LO knockout mice *(59)*. During parasitic infection, mast cells come into close proximity with cholinergic nerves, and mast cell release of LTD_4 may increase sensitivity of these nerves to stimulation, leading to altered motility. Although a direct role for LTD_4 in parasite expulsion is not likely a major factor, other yet-undefined roles of LTs in the inflammatory response, perhaps related to mucus secretion, may become apparent with further studies.

Klebsiella pneumoniae *Infection*

The importance of 5-LO products in an experimental model of bacterial pneumonia was tested *(60)*. After an intratracheal instillation of the Gram-negative organism *K. pneumoniae*, wild-type mice developed a severe bacteremia, which was present to a significantly lesser degree in knockout mice *(60)*. This resulted in more deaths in the wild-type group. However, recruitment of neutrophils was not impaired in the 5-LO knockout mice, even though LTB_4 synthesis could not be detected. On the other hand, the ability of alveolar macrophages to phagocytose and kill the bacteria was diminished significantly, which may have contributed to the difference in mortality. These findings, therefore, indicate that 5-LO products can be important in bacterial host defense, at least in this particular murine model.

Vascular Permeability Changes in Inflammation

Vascular permeability changes are one of the key events in acute inflammation, and some studies have looked at this function in mice defective for lipid mediator signaling. Murata et al. *(36)* reported that the vascular permeability change (measured as extractable Pontamine sky blue dye) of intradermally injected bradykinin was potentiated by both PGE_2 and prostacyclin in wild-type mice, but the response to prostacyclin was abolished in prostacyclin-receptor–deficient mice.

In platelet-activating factor (PAF)-injected mice, there were no significant differences in vascular permeability between 5-LO–deficient and wild-type mice, measured as changes in hematocrit and leakage of Evan's blue dye in airway tissues *(61)*. Alterations in vascular permeability, therefore, could not explain the drastic differences in survival between the two groups of mice in PAF-induced shock *(17,61)*.

Inflammatory Pain Responses

Since prostacyclin receptor mRNA had been shown to colocalize with substance P mRNA in neurons of the dorsal root ganglion *(62)*, prostacyclin-receptor–deficient mice were examined for various pain responses *(36)*. Prostacyclin was not involved in nociceptive signals at the spinal and supraspinal levels. However, in the acetic-acid–induced writhing test to examine the extent of prostacyclin receptors in inflammatory pain, there was a strong reduction in the number of writhes in the deficient mice *(36)*. The reduction was similar to that seen in indomethacin-pretreated wild-type mice. Intraperitoneal injection of prostacyclin, but not PGE_2, could mimic the writhing response induced by acetic acid, and this response was absent in the knockout mice. Thus, the prostacyclin receptor is capable of transducing pain responses in some inflammatory models.

"Physiological" Inflammation

Natural reproductive processes such as ovulation, luteolysis, cyclical uterine events, and implantation resemble, in many ways, classical inflammatory reactions *(63)*. For instance, in the mouse, the invasiveness of trophoblasts is so influential that the blastocyst penetrates the endothelium *(64)*. The stroma then responds under the influence of progesterone to undergo an implantation/decidual reaction, with changes in vascular permeability, blood flow, and edema being important events. Prostanoids have been implicated in several aspects of these reproductive functions. Thus, in embryo transfer experiments, it was found that COX-2–deficient mice undergo reduced implantation, with fewer responding mice and smaller implantation sites, indicating that maternal PG production is necessary to establish a successful pregnancy *(65)*. Mahler et al. *(66)* noted that ovulation was defective in COX-2–deficient mice but did not elaborate on the mechanism. It appears that ovarian granulosa cells in these mice may not properly contact the oocyte.

In FP-receptor–deficient mice, implantation was normal *(35)*. Both ovulation and fertilization were also unaffected by disruption of the FP-receptor gene. These results indicate that a PG other than $PGF_{2\alpha}$ is involved in these processes. However, in elegant studies by Sugimoto et al. *(35)* with FP-receptor–deficient mice, evidence indicated that $PGF_{2\alpha}$ induces luteolysis, leading to decreased progesterone levels, induction of oxytocin receptor mRNA, and parturition. $PGF_{2\alpha}$'s myometrial contractile activity was not essential for this process, but it may induce luteolysis via apoptosis of luteal cells.

Conclusions and Future Directions

The use of eicosanoid-mediator–deficient mice and those defective in eicosanoid receptor signaling is still at an early stage. Remarkable achievements have been accomplished already with the nine gene-disrupted lines of mice (*see* Table 1) since the first description of 5-LO–deficient mice was reported in late 1994 *(17)*. With the increased availability of these mice to other investigators in their respective fields of research, it is anticipated that further developments into the biology and pathophysiology of inflammatory disorders will be made. Atherosclerosis, asthma, inflammatory bowel disease, to mention a few, are disorders with significant inflammatory components, that can be studied in LO, COX, or eicosanoid-receptor–deficient mice. Several different LOs are expressed in skin *(38,39,67,68)*. Their contribution to the vast array of skin inflammatory lesions and defects in different strains of mice can be an important area of future study. Interesting studies on tumorigenesis are beginning to emerge that implicate the role of COX-2 derived prostanoids in tumor growth and function *(69)*.

The involvement of prostacyclin, rather than PGE_2, in pain and certain inflammatory responses is intriguing. Having uncovered new roles for prostacyclin, in addition to its antiplatelet and vasodilatory actions, it will be interesting to see the results from other eicosanoid-receptor–deficient mice. The precise elucidation of reproductive functions of the various prostanoids is coming to fruition, after decades, dating back to the initial discovery of the compounds in semen in the early 1930s, and the discovery of their actions on uterine smooth muscle *(70)*.

Studies, especially with COX-deficient mice, have yielded conundrums. Many of the experiments with NSAIDs known to be effective against either COX-1 or COX-2, or both, and that reduce inflammation, are not borne out with experiments performed in COX-1– or COX-2–deficient mice. Why are there fewer NSAID-induced gastric lesions in COX-1–deficient mice when one would expect the opposite? Why do COX-2–deficient mice show normal inflammatory responses in some models? Are there compensatory mechanisms, or do some uncharacterized developmental abnormalities mask the usual phenotype observed with COX inhibitors? Most studies with LT-deficient mice have not yielded surprising or strange results. Data obtained with these mice have cor-

Table 1
Targeted Disruption of Genes Involved in Lipid Mediator Pathways

Disrupted gene (gene locus name)	Phenotype/major findings
5-LO (*Alox5*)	• Diminution of inflammation in some models (arachidonic acid-induced ear edema, immune complex- and zymosan-induced peritonitis, allergic airway "asthma") • Reduced severity of PAF-induced shock
Leukocyte-type 12/15-LO (*Alox12l*)	• No obvious abnormalities • In vitro alterations in zymosan-induced LDL oxidation
Platelet-type 12-LO (*Alox12p*)	• hyperresponsive ADP-induced platelet aggregation
Cyclooxygenase-1 (*Ptgs1*)	• Decreased inflammatory response in arachidonic acid-induced ear edema model • No gastric pathology and less susceptibility to NSAID-induced gastric lesions • Delayed onset of parturition
Cyclooxygenase-2 (*Ptgs2*)	• Renal developmental abnormalities • Normal inflammatory responses in arachidonic acid and TPA ear and carrageenan paw edema models • Mitigation of endotoxin-induced hepatocellular cytotoxicity • Infertility and reduced litter size • Diminished papilloma formation in carcinogenesis model
5-LO-activating protein	• Reduced severity of collagen-induced arthritis • Blunted inflammatory responses similar to those seen in 5-LO–deficient mice
FP receptor (*Ptgfr*)	• Parturition failure
Prostacyclin receptor (*Ptgir*)	• Increased susceptibility to thrombosis • Reduced inflammatory and pain responses
Cytosolic phospholipase A$_2$	• Abnormal parturition • Reduced allergic airway inflammation responses • Less edema and smaller infarct size in cerebral artery ischemia model

roborated many of the past findings with specific anti-LT compounds. 12-LO–deficient mice have not yet provided definitive clues to these enzymes' function. The combined input of members throughout the scientific community with interests in eicosanoid function should help to answer the many unsolved questions and yet-to-be discovered roles of this fascinating group of lipid autocoids.

Acknowledgments

The author wishes to express his gratitude to collaborators past and present, and laboratory members for their scientific contributions relating to this chapter. The author's contributions have been supported in part by NIH grants HL53558 and HL58464.

References

1. Needleman, P., Turk, J., Jakschik, B. A., Morrison, A. R., and Lefkowith, J. B. (1986) Arachidonic acid metabolism. *Ann. Rev. Biochem.* **55**, 69–102.

2. Samuelsson, B. (1983) Leukotrienes: mediators of immediate hypersensitivity reactions and inflammation. *Science* **220**, 568–575.

3. Bergström, S., Danielsson, H., and Samuelsson, B. (1964) *Biochim. Biophys. Acta* **90**, 207–210.

4. van Dorp, D. A., Beerthuis, R. K., Nugteren, D. H., and Vonkeman, H. (1964) *Biochim. Biophys. Acta* **90**, 204–207.

5. Borgeat, P. and Samuelsson, B. (1979) Transformation of arachidonic acid by rabbit polymorphonuclear leukocytes: Formation of a novel dihydroxyeicosatetraenoic acid. *J. Biol. Chem.* **254**, 2643–2646.

6. Murphy, R. C., Hammarström, S., and Samuelsson, B. (1979) Leukotriene C: A slow-reacting substance from murine mastocytoma cells. *Proc. Natl. Acad. Sci. USA* **76**, 4275–4279.

7. Ferreira, S. H., Moncada, S., and Vane, J. R. (1971) Indomethacin and aspirin abolish prostaglandin release from the spleen. *Nature—New Biology* **231**, 237–239.

8. Flower, R., Gryglewski, R., Herbaczynska-Cedro, K., and Vane, J. R. (1972) Effects of anti-inflammatory drugs on prostaglandin biosynthesis. *Nature—New Biology* **238**, 104–106.

9. Xie, W., Chipman, J. G., Robertson, D. L., Erickson, R. L., and Simmons, D. L. (1991) Expression of a mitogen-responsive gene encoding prostaglandin synthase is regulated by mRNA splicing. *Proc. Natl. Acad. Sci. USA* **88**, 2692–2696.

10. Kujubu, D. A., Fletcher, B. S., Varnum, B. C., Lim, R. W., and Herschman, H. R. (1991) TIS10, a phorbol ester tumor promoter-inducible mRNA from Swiss 3T3 cells, encodes a novel prostaglandin synthase/cyclooxygenase homologue. *J. Biol. Chem.* **266**, 12,866–12,872.

11. Herschman, H. R. (1996) Prostaglandin synthase 2. *Biochim. Biophys. Acta* **1299**, 125–140.

12. Smith, W. L., Garavito, R. M., and DeWitt, D. L. (1996) Prostaglandin endoperoxide H synthases (cyclooxygenases)-1 and -2. *J. Biol. Chem.* **271**, 33,157–33,160.

13. Ford-Hutchinson, A. W., Bray, M. A., Doig, M. V., Shipley, M. E., and Smith, M. J. (1980) Leukotriene B, a potent chemokinetic and aggregating substance released from polymorphonuclear leukocytes. *Nature* **286**, 264,265.

14. Samuelsson, B., Dahlén, S.-E., Lindgren, J.-Å, Rouzer, C. A., and Serhan, C. N. (1987) Leukotrienes and lipoxins: Structures, biosynthesis and biological effects. *Science* **237**, 1171–1175.

15. Henderson, W. R. (1994) The role of leukotrienes in inflammation. *Ann. Intern. Med.* **121**, 684–697.

16. Hay, D. W. P., Torphy, T. J., and Undem, B. J. (1995) Cysteinyl leukotrienes in asthma: old mediators up to new tricks. *Trends Pharm. Sci.* **16**, 304–309.

17. Chen, X.-S., Sheller, J. R., Johnson, E. N., and Funk, C. D. (1994) Role of leukotrienes revealed by targeted disruption of the 5-lipoxygenase gene. *Nature* **372**, 179–182.

18. Goulet, J. L., Snouwaert, J. N., Latour, A. M., Coffman, T. M., and Koller, B. H. (1994) Altered inflammatory responses in leukotriene-deficient mice. *Proc. Natl. Acad. Sci. USA* **91**, 12,852–12,856.

19. Carlson, R. P., O'Neill-Davis, L., Chang, J., and Lewis, A. J. (1985) Modulation of mouse ear edema by cyclooxygenase and lipoxygenase inhibitors and other pharmacologic agents. *Agents and Actions* **17**, 197–204.

20. Young, J. M., Wagner, B. M., and Spires, D. A. (1983) Tachyphylaxis in 12-O-tetradecanoylphorbol acetate- and arachidonic acid-induced ear edema. *J. Invest. Dermatol.* **80**, 48–52.

21. Chen, X.-S., Naumann, T. A., Kurre, U., Jenkins, N. A., Copeland, N. G., and Funk, C. D. (1995) cDNA cloning, expression, mutagenesis, intracellular localization and gene chromosomal assignment of mouse 5-lipoxygenase. *J. Biol. Chem.* **270**, 17,993–17,999.

22. Funk, C. D., Hoshiko, S., Matsumoto, T., Rådmark, O., and Samuelsson, B. (1989) Characterization of the human 5-lipoxygenase gene. *Proc. Natl. Acad. Sci. USA* **86**, 2587–2591.

23. Funk, C. D. (1996) The molecular biology of mammalian lipoxygenases and the quest for eicosanoid functions using lipoxygenase deficient mice. *Biochim. Biophys. Acta* **1304**, 65–84.

24. Griffiths, R. J., Smith, M. A., Roach, M. L., Stock, J. L., Stam, E. J., Milici, A. J., Scampoli, D. N., Eskra, J. D., Byrum, R. S., Koller, B. H. (1997) Collagen-induced arthritis is reduced in 5-lipoxygenase-activating protein deficient mice. *J. Exp. Med.* **185**, 1123–1129.

25. Byrum, R. S., Goulet, J. L., Griffiths, R. J., and Koller, B. H. (1997) Role of the 5-lipoxygenase-activating protein (FLAP) in murine acute inflammatory responses. *J. Exp. Med.* **185,** 1065–1075.

26. Kraemer, S. A., Meade, E. A., and DeWitt, D. L. (1992) Prostaglandin endoperoxide synthase gene structure: Identification of the transcriptional start site and 5' flanking regulatory sequences. *Arch. Biochem. Biophys.* **293,** 391–400.

27. Wen, P. Z., Warden, C., Fletcher, B. S., Kujubu, D. A., Herschman, H. R., and Lusis, A. J. (1993) Chromosomal organization of the inducible and constitutive prostaglandin synthase/ cyclooxygenase genes in mouse. *Genomics* **15,** 458–460.

28. Langenbach, R., Morham, S. G., Tiano, H. F., Loftin, C. D., Ghanayem, B. I., Chulada, P. C., Mahler, J. F., Lee, C. A., Goulding, E. H., Kluckman, K. D., Kim, H. S., and Smithies, O. (1995) Prostaglandin synthase 1 gene disruption in mice reduces arachidonic acid-induced inflammation and indomethacin-induced gastric ulceration. *Cell* **83,** 483–492.

29. Fletcher, B. S., Kujubu, D. A., Perrin, D. M., and Herschman, H. R. (1992) Structure of the mitogen-inducible TIS10 gene and demonstration that the TIS10-encoded protein is a functional prostaglandin G/H synthase. *J. Biol. Chem.* **267,** 4338–4344.

30. Morham, S. G., Langenbach, R., Loftin, C. D., Tiano, H. F., Vouloumanos, N., Jennette, J. C., Mahler, J. F., Kluckman, K. D., Ledford, A., Lee, C. A., and Smithies, O. (1995) Prostaglandin synthase 2 gene disruption causes severe renal pathology in the mouse. *Cell* **83,** 473–482.

31. Dinchuk, J. E., Car, B. D., Focht, R. J., Johnston, J. J., Jaffee, B. D., Covington, M. B., Contel, N. R., Eng, V. M., Collins, R. J., and Czerniak, P. M. (1996) Renal abnormalities and an altered inflammatory response in mice lacking cyclooxygenase II. *Nature* **378,** 406–409.

32. Chen, X.-S., Kurre, U., Jenkins, N. A., Copeland, N. G., and Funk, C. D. (1994) cDNA cloning, expression, mutagenesis of C-terminal isoleucine, genomic structure and chromosomal localizations of murine 12-lipoxygenases. *J. Biol. Chem.* **269,** 13,979–13,987.

33. Sun, D. and Funk, C. D. (1996) Disruption of 12/15-lipoxygenase expression in peritoneal macrophages. Enhanced utilization of the 5-lipoxygenase pathway and diminished oxidation of LDL. *J. Biol. Chem.* **271,** 24,055–24,062.

34. Johnson, E. N., Brass, L. F., and Funk, C. D., Increased platelet sensitivity to ADP in mice lacking platelet-type 12-lipoxygenase, *Proc. Natl. Acad. Sci. USA* **95,** 3100–3105.

35. Sugimoto, Y., Yamasaki, A., Segi, E., Tsuboi, K., Aze, Y., Nishimura, T., Oida, H., Yoshida, N., Tanaka, T., Katsuyama, M., Hasumoto, K., Murata, T., Hirata, M., Ushikubi, F., Negishi, M., Ichikawa, A., and Narumiya, S. (1997) Failure of parturition in mice lacking the prostaglandin F receptor. *Science* **277,** 681–683.

36. Murata, T., Ushikubi, F., Matsuoka, T., Hirata, M., Yamasaki, A., Sugimoto, Y., Ichikawa, A., Aze, Y., Tanaka, T., Yoshida, N., Ueno, A., Oh-ishi, S., and Narumiya, S. (1997) Altered pain perception and inflammatory response in mice lacking prostacyclin receptor. *Nature* **388,** 678–682.

37. Inoue, H., Mori, T., and Koshihara, Y. (1988) Sulfidopeptide-leukotrienes are major mediators of arachidonic acid-induced mouse ear edema. *Prostaglandins* **36,** 731–739.

38. Hussain, H., Shornick, L. P., Shannon, V. R., Wilson, J. D., Funk, C. D., Pentland, A. P., and Holtzman, M. J. (1994) Human skin contains a microsomal-type arachidonate 12-lipoxygenase that appears identical to the platelet isoform and is selectively induced in germinal layer keratinocytes in psoriasis. *Am. J. Physiol.* **266,** C243–C253.

39. Takahashi, Y., Reddy, G. R., Ueda, N., Yamamoto, S., and Arase, S. (1993) Arachidonate 12-lipoxygenase of platelet-type in human epidermal cells. *J. Biol. Chem.* **268,** 16,443–16,448.

40. Levy, L. (1969) Carrageenan paw edema in the mouse. *Life Sci.* **8,** 601–606.

41. Chulada, P. C., Lee, C. A., Morham, S. G., Tiano, H. F., and Langenbach, R. (1996) Inflammatory responses in cyclooxygenase-deficient mice. Abstract presented at the Keystone symposia, Lipid mediators: Recent advances in molecular biology, understanding of regulation and pharmacology, Keystone, CO, no. 103, p. 9.

42. Harris, R. R., Wilcox, D., Funk, C. D., Bell, R. L., Brooks, C. D. W., and Carter, G. W. (1995) Polyacrylamide gel induced inflammation in mice: Effect of disruption of 5-lipoxygenase (5LO) gene. *Inflamm.* **44(Suppl. 3),** 221–222, abstract 01/02.

43. Wooley, P. H., Luthra, H. S., Stuart, J. M., and David, C. S. (1981) Type II collagen-induced arthritis. 1. MHC (I-region) linkage and antibody correlates. *J. Exp. Med.* **154,** 688–700.

44. Griffiths, R. J., Pettipher, E. R., Koch, K., Farrell, C. A., Breslow, R., Conklyn, M. J., Smith, M. A., Hackman, B. C., Wimberly, D. J., Milici, A. J. et al. (1995) Leukotriene B_4 plays a critical role in the progression of collagen-induced arthritis. *Proc. Natl. Acad. USA* **92,** 517–521.

45. McFadden, E. R. and Gilbert, I. A. (1992) Asthma. *N. Engl. J. Med.* **327,** 1928–1937.

46. Po, Y.-T., Larsen, G. L., and Irvin, C. G. (1995) Utility of mice in investigating asthma pathogenesis. *Eur. Resp. Rev.* **5,** 224–230.

47. Irvin, C. G., Tu, Y.-P., Sheller, J. R., and Funk, C. D. (1997) 5-Lipoxygenase products are necessary for ovalbumin-induced responsiveness in mice. *Am. J. Physiol.* **272,** L1053–L1058.

48. Funk C. D, Chen, X. S., Sheller, J. R., Tu, Y.-P., and Irvin, C. G. (1997) The role of 5-lipoxygenase products in a mouse model of allergic airway inflammation, "Eicosanoids, Aspirin and Asthma," in *Lung Biology in Health and Disease, vol.114: Eicosanoids, Aspirin, and Asthma* (Szczeklik, A., Grzlewski, R., and Vane, J. R., eds.), pp. 187–200.

49. Yamaoka, K. A., Claesson, H.-E., and Rosén, A. (1989) Leukotriene B_4 enhances activation, proliferation, and differentiation of human B lymphocytes. *J. Immunol.* **143,** 1996–2000.

50. Yamaoka, K. A., Dugas, B., Paul-Eugene, N., Mencia-Huerta, J. M., Braquet, P., and Kolb, J. P. (1994) Leukotriene B_4 enhances IL-4-induced IgE production from normal human lymphocytes. *Cell Immunol.* **156,** 124–134.

51. Smith, L. J. (1996) Leukotrienes in asthma: the potential therapeutic role of antileukotriene agents. *Arch. Intern. Med.* **156,** 2181–2189.

52. Henderson, W. R., Lewis, D. B., Albert, R. K., Zhang, Y., Lamm, W. J. E., Chiang, G. K. S., Jones, F., Eriksen, P., Tien, Y., Jonas, M., and Chi, E. Y. (1996) The importance of leukotrienes in airway inflammation in a mouse model of asthma. *J. Exp. Med.* **184,** 1483–1494.

53. Martin, T. R., Gerard, N. P., Galli, S., and Drazen, J. M. (1988) Pulmonary responses to bronchoconstrictor agonists in the mouse. *J. Appl. Physiol.* **64,** 2318–2323.

54. Wynn, T. A., Eltoum, I., Cheever, A. W., Lewis, F. A., Gause, W. C., and Sher, A. (1993) Analysis of cytokine mRNA expression during primary granuloma formation induced by eggs of *Schistosoma mansoni. J. Immunol.* **151,** 1430–1440.

55. Kunkel, S. L., Chensue, S. W., Mouton, C., and Higashi, G. I. (1984) Role of lipoxygensae products in murine pulmonary granuloma formation. *J. Clin. Invest.* **74,** 514–524.

56. Secor, W. E., Powell, M. R., Morgan, J., Wynn, T. A., and Funk, C. D. (1998) Mice deficient for 5-lipoxygenase, but not 12-lipoxygenase, display altered immune responses during infection with *Schistosoma mansoni, Prostaglandens and Other Lipid Methods,* in press.

57. Stadecker, M. J. (1994) The shrinking schistosomal egg granuloma: how accessory cells control T cell-mediated pathology. *Exp. Parasitol.* **79,** 198–201.

58. Else, K. J., Finkelman, F. D., Maliszewski, C. R., and Grencis, R. K. (1994) Cytokine-mediated regulation of chronic intestinal helminth infection. *J. Exp. Med.* **179,** 347–351.

59. Goldhill, J., Morris, S. C., Maliszewski, C., Urban, J. F., Funk, C. D., Finkelman, F. D., and Shea-Donahue, T. (1997) Interleukin-4 modulates cholinergic neural control of mouse small intestinal longitudinal muscle. *Am. J. Physiol.* **272,** G1135–G1140.

60. Bailie, M. B., Standiford, T. J., Laichalk, L. L., Coffey, M. J., Strieter, R., and Peters-Golden, M. (1996) Leukotriene-deficient mice manifest enhanced lethality from *Klebsiella* pneumonia in association with decreased alveolar macrophage phagocytic and bactericidal activities. *J. Immunol.* **157,** 5221–5224.

61. Johnson, E. N., Sun, D., Chen, X.-S., and Funk, C. D. (1998) Lipoxygenase gene disruption studies—status and applications, in *Lipoxygenases and Their Products: Biological Functions,* in press.

62. Oida, H., Namba, T., Sugimoto, Y., Ushikubi, F., Ohishi, H., Ichikawa, A., and Narumiya, S. (1995) *In situ* hybridization studies of prostacyclin receptor mRNA expression in various mouse organs. *Br. J. Pharmacol.* **116,** 2828–2837.

63. Epsey, L. L. (1994) Current status of the hypothesis that mammalian ovulation is comparable to an inflammatory reaction. *Biol. Reprod.* **50,** 233–238.

64. Finn, C. A. (1996) Why do women menstruate? Historical and evolutionary review. *Eur. J. Obstet., Gynecol. & Reprod. Biol.* **70,** 3–8.

65. Trzaskos, J. M., Lim, H., Das, S. K., BazDresch, M., Focht, R., Dinchuk, J., and Dey, S. K. (1996) Impaired decidualization and embryo implantation contribute to reduced fertility in COX2 null mice. Abstract presented at the Keystone symposia, Lipid mediators: Recent advances in molecular biology, understanding of regulation and pharmacology, Keystone, CO, no. 110, p. 11.

66. Mahler, J. F., Davis, B. J., Morham, S. G., and Langenbach, R. (1996) Disruption of cyclooxygenase genes in mice. *Toxicol. Path.* **24,** 717–719.
67. Funk, C. D., Keeney, D. S., Oliw, E. H., Boeglin, W. E., and Brash, A. R. (1996) Functional expression and cellular localization of a mouse epidermal lipoxygenase. *J. Biol. Chem.* **271,** 23,338–23,344.
68. Jisaka, M., Boeglin, W. E., Kim, R. B., Nanney, L. B., and Brash, A. R. (1997) Molecular cloning and functional expression of a phorbol ester-inducible 8*S*-lipoxygenase from mouse skin. *J. Biol. Chem.* **272,** 24,410–24,416.
69. Oshima, M., Dinchuk, J. E., Kargman, S. L., Oshima, H., Hancock, B., Kwong, E., Trzaskos, J. M., Evans, J. F., and Taketo, M. M. (1996) Suppression of intestinal polyposis in Apc$^{\Delta716}$ knock-out mice by inhibition of cyclooxygenase 2 (Cox-2) *Cell* **87,** 803–809.
70. Kurzrok, R., and Lieb, C. C. (1930) Biochemical studies of human semen. II. The action of semen on the human uterus. *Proc. Soc. Exp. Biol. Med.* **28,** 268–272.

6

Isoprostanes in the Assessment of Oxidant Stress In Vivo

Muredach P. Reilly, Domenico Pratico, Paul Lanken, Norman Delanty, Joshua Rockach, John Lawson, and Garret A. FitzGerald

Introduction

Oxidative stress is believed to play an important pathophysiological role in a variety of cardiovascular disorders, including atherosclerosis *(1)* and ischemia-reperfusion injury *(2)*. Epidemiological studies have related the incidence of certain diseases inversely to the estimated intake of dietary antioxidants *(3,4)*. Furthermore, data from certain animal models of oxidative stress lend indirect support for this hypothesis *(5,6)*. However, difficulty in assessing oxygen radical generation in vivo has proven to be the major limitation to the understanding of this mechanism of human disease. Traditional in vitro assays of malondialdehyde and lipid hydroperoxides are thought to be fallible when applied to clinical investigation because of such factors as ex vivo generation of products, inaccuracy of assay methodology, and the instability and nonspecificity of the analytes *(7,8)*. Alternative approaches rely on the measurement of indices of free radical generation explicitly induced ex vivo, such as copper-induced low-density lipoprotein (LDL) oxidation and the generation of spin traps *(9,10)*. However, it is unclear how indices of LDL oxidizability relate to oxidant stress in vivo. Consequently, the relationship of oxidant stress to human disease remains unclear. Furthermore, there is little information on the actual in vivo antioxidant effects of vitamin C or E in humans. Thus, there is little biochemical basis for choice of disease and dose selection when such compounds are studied in phase III clinical trials *(11,12)*.

From: *Molecular and Cellular Basis of Inflammation*
Edited by: C. N. Serhan and P. A. Ward © Humana Press Inc., Totowa, NJ

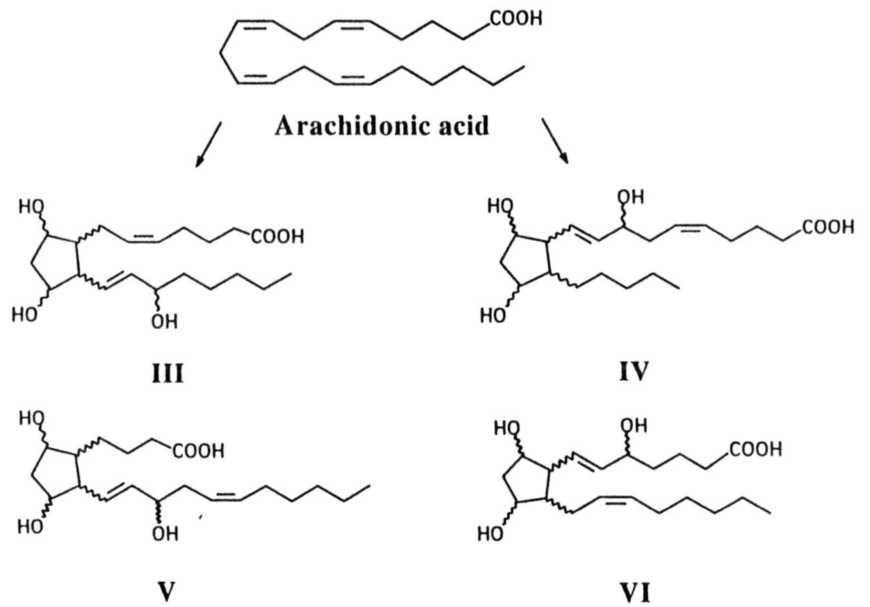

Fig. 1. F_2 isoprostane structures. Bold type denotes proposed nomenclature. Names in parentheses represent previously used terminology.

Isoeicosanoids

Isoeicosanoids, isomers of enzymatically derived eicosanoids, are free radical catalyzed products of arachidonic acid *(13)*. They include members of the F, D, and E isoprostanes (iPs), isothromboxanes, and isoleukotrienes *(14–17)*. The formation of prostaglandin (PG)-like autooxidation products of arachidonate has been known for some time *(18)*. However, it was the observation of Morrow et al. *(19)* that F_2 isoprostanes (iPFs) were present in biological fluids that prompted investigation of these compounds as potential indices of oxidant stress in vivo *(19)*. The utility of these compounds as indices of oxidant stress has been supported by a number of investigations *(20–24)*. Attention has been focused primarily on the originally described iPFs. Recently, their nomenclature (Fig. 1) has been revised *(25)*. Theoretically, up to 64 iPFs may be formed. However, few have been characterized in any detail. Attention was focused initially on iPF$_{2\alpha}$-III (formerly known as 8-iso PGF$_{2\alpha}$) because of its biological activity in vitro *(26,27)*.

Biological Activity of iPF$_{2\alpha}$-III

iPF$_{2\alpha}$-III is a potent vasoconstrictor of renal, pulmonary, coronary, and cerebral arterial circulations and may function as a mitogen *(26–29)*. These actions are blocked by thromboxane receptor (TP) antagonists. By contrast to thromboxane (TX) analogs, iPF$_{2\alpha}$-III induces shape change without irreversible aggregation *(27,30,31)*. However, it fails to activate either of the cloned splice variants of the human TX receptor or the cloned PGF$_{2\alpha}$ receptor at concentrations that are likely to circulate in vivo *(30)*. Thus, any biological role is likely to be in the immediate microenvironment of its formation, and its autacoidal importance is presently unclear. However, its generation by platelets, monocytes, and in LDL exposed to oxidants in vitro *(32,33)* suggest a potential role for this iP in contributing to the effects of oxidant stress in the vasculature in vivo. The biological role of other isoeicosanoids remains largely unexplored. Unlike iPF$_{2\alpha}$-III, 8,12-iso iPF$_{2\alpha}$-III activates PGF$_{2\alpha}$ receptors (FPs) in preference to TPs, stimulating mitogenesis in NIH 3T3 cells *(34)*. Again, this occurs in a saturable and receptor specific manner; however, the biological importance of this iP in vivo is also unclear. Although iPs may act as incidental ligands at membrane PG receptors, it has been suggested that they may also activate specific iP receptors *(35)*. However, definitive pharmacologic evidence for iP receptors has yet to be produced, and none have been cloned.

Analysis of iPs

Several approaches to the measurement of iPFs have been employed. These include the estimation of "total" iPFs, the use of immunoassays for iPF$_{2\alpha}$-III, and the measurement of specific iPFs using gas chromatography-mass spectrometry (GC-MS). Morrow et al. estimate iPFs using a GC-MS-based, selected ion monitoring assay, employing an isotope-labeled PGF$_{2\alpha}$ internal standard *(20)*. They have applied this technique to estimate levels of iPs bound to lipid in tissues, freely circulating in plasma, and excreted in urine *(20)*. Despite its attractions, this method has some intrinsic limitations. The specificity and precision of the assay is limited by the absence of an iP internal standard, given that PGF$_{2\alpha}$ elutes at a distance from the iPFs. It makes assumptions about quantitative recovery of iPs through purification and extraction procedures that cannot be validated. Indeed, this method failed to identify the small cyclooxygenase (COX)-dependent contribution to iPF$_{2\alpha}$-III generation in vitro *(32)*. Both this approach and the use of GC-MS in specific iP analysis may be confounded by imperfect resolution of iP peaks on the GC. Application of liquid chromatography MS-MS to iP analysis is likely to address this issue. The presence of abundant circulating phospholipids in plasma renders measurements in this matrix susceptible to iPF formation ex vivo. Similarly, COX-dependent formation of iPF$_{2\alpha}$-III by platelets activated ex vivo, analogous to ex vivo formation of TXB$_2$ *(36)*, may confound plasma-based measurement of primary iPFs. A major metabolite of iPF$_{2\alpha}$-III has recently been identified and may permit refinement of the current approach to estimate formation of this compound in plasma *(37)*. Immunoassays for iPF$_{2\alpha}$-III have been developed and applied to in vitro and in vivo studies *(38)*. However, although the assays were validated quantitatively by GC-MS analysis of iPF$_{2\alpha}$-III, they have not been tested for crossreactivity with the other iPFs or their metabolites that may be formed in settings in which they are applied in vivo. For the present, they also must be viewed as semiquantitative.

Given that up to 64 iPF isomers in four structural classes may exist *(39)*, we considered it judicious to develop assays for specific isomers. We also favored urine as a target matrix over plasma; it may be obtained noninvasively and, given the relative absence of phospholipid in urine compared to plasma, it is likely to be less susceptible to iP formation ex vivo. Our prior experience, using both plasma and urine to estimate eicosanoid biosynthesis, suggests that qualitatively distinct information is unlikely to be provided by a plasma-based assay *(40)*. Given its biological activity, we initially developed an assay for the iPF$_{2\alpha}$-III isomer using a GC-MS, employing isotope-labeled iPF$_{2\alpha}$-III as an internal standard *(32)* and have applied it to the estimation of urinary levels. More recently, we have developed assays for other isomers using similar techniques.

COX-Dependent Formation of iPF$_{2\alpha}$-III

Our initial studies examining the formation of iPF$_{2\alpha}$-III by human platelets and monocytes in vitro yielded surprising results. We found that iPF$_{2\alpha}$-III, but not other iPFs, could be formed by an aspirin-sensitive mechanism in platelets *(32)*. Semipurified platelet COX-1 was confirmed as the source of iPF$_{2\alpha}$-III in these studies. Whereas platelets contain only the constitutive form of COX, COX-1, human monocytes contain both COX-1 and the more readily inducible form of the enzyme, COX-2. Monocytes, treated with bacterial lipopolysaccharide to induce COX-2, were also found to generate iPF$_{2\alpha}$-III, as well as conventional PGs, by a mechanism suppressed by selective COX-2 inhibitor *(33)*. Interestingly, these cells, when activated with zymosan in the presence of LDL, formed iPF$_{2\alpha}$-III in a free radical-dependent manner. This was inhibited by antioxidants, but not COX-2 inhibitors.

The formation of iPF$_{2\alpha}$-III in a COX-dependent manner raised concerns as to its utility as an index of oxidant stress in vivo, particularly as activation of platelets or monocytes may be a feature of many syndromes putatively associated with oxidant stress. For example, this is true of cigarette smoking and coronary reperfusion with thrombolytics or angioplasty *(41,42)*. To address this issue, we examined the effects of aspirin administration on iPF$_{2\alpha}$-III and TXB$_2$ formation in normal volunteers and in chronic cigarette smokers *(22)*. Low-dose aspirin completely suppressed platelet COX-1 activity, as reflected by serum TXB$_2$ levels (>98% suppression) and resulted in marked inhibition of in vivo TX generation, as reflected by an approx 75% reduction in urinary excretion of the 11-dehydro metabolite of TXB$_2$. By contrast, although aspirin resulted in a partial inhibition of serum iPF$_{2\alpha}$-III, there was no reduction in urinary excretion of this iP. This suggested that the enzymatic pathway contributed trivially, if at all, to overall iPF$_{2\alpha}$-III excretion in urine, even in a syndrome of COX-1 activation.

Given the need to exclude the involvement of this pathway in multiple clinical settings which COX activation and free radical generation might coincide *(43)*, we developed an assay for a distinct iPF that is not formed by the COX pathway. We have synthesized an internal standard for this class VI isomer, iPF$_{2\alpha}$-VI (formerly known as IPF$_{2\alpha}$-I), and developed a GC-MS–based assay for its determination *(44,45)*. iPF$_{2\alpha}$-VI is more abundant in human urine than iPF$_{2\alpha}$-III, it is not formed by platelets or monocytes in a COX-dependent manner, and urinary levels are not suppressed by high-dose indomethacin or chronic aspirin administration in healthy volunteers *(45)*. We have recently examined the coordinate formation of both iPFs in human syndromes of oxidant stress *(46,47)*.

iPFs in Human Disease

The striking increase in iPs in animal models of oxidant stress *(48,49)* suggested that their measurement could be an important development in assessing the role of oxidant stress in specific vascular disorders. They are remarkably stable compounds and are not subject to formation ex vivo when stored appropriately *(19,45)*. Initially, the authors concentrated on the measurement of iPF$_{2\alpha}$-III in urine. Excretion proved to be remarkably constant in healthy individuals. There was no circadian variation or differences between genders. Similarly, moderate exercise did not alter excretion, but levels tended to increase with age.

Cigarette Smoking

Cigarette smoke is a source of many free radicals *(50)* and may result in platelet *(41)* and neutrophil activation *(51)* in vivo with further amplification of free radical generation. Furthermore, cigarette smoking is associated with endothelial dysfunction in vivo *(52)*, as well as increased rates of acute thrombosis *(53)*. Increased urinary excretion of 8-oxoDg, an index of free radical catalyzed DNA adduct formation, has been described in apparently healthy chronic cigarette smokers *(54)*. Morrow et al. *(20)* reported increased plasma and urinary total iPFs in individuals who smoke. Similarly, the we have shown that smoking resulted in a dose-dependent increase in urinary $iPF_{2\alpha}$-III levels in human volunteers *(22)*. Furthermore, levels dropped significantly when these individuals quit smoking or were supplemented high-dose vitamin C, which is deficient in smokers *(55)*.

Ischemic-Reperfusion Syndromes

Oxidant stress has been implicated in vascular reperfusion following a period of ischemia. Examples include the regional myocardial stunning seen in animal models of coronary occlusion/reperfusion *(6)* and in some patients following thrombolytic therapy *(56)*, as well as the global myocardial dysfunction seen after coronary artery bypass surgery *(57)*. We previously shown increased urinary $iPF_{2\alpha}$-III in a number of syndromes of myocardial reperfusion *(24)*. Levels were significantly elevated, coincident with Doppler documented reperfusion, in a canine model of coronary thrombolysis. Similarly, excretion was enhanced coincident with cross clamp release, compared to preoperative and 24-h postoperative values in subjects undergoing elective coronary artery bypass surgery. Recently, we have extended these observations to include patients undergoing reperfusion for myocardial infarction *(46)*. Urinary excretion of both $iPF_{2\alpha}$-III and $iPF_{2\alpha}$-VI was markedly increased coincident with angiographically documented reperfusion in patients treated with thrombolytic agents and percutaneous transluminal coronary angioplasty (PTCA) for myocardial infarction (Fig. 2). There was a minor increment in iPF excretion after diagnostic coronary arteriography and elective PTCA. Notably, there was a striking correlation between the urinary levels of both iPFs, suggesting that lipid peroxidation, rather than COX activation, was the common mechanism of iP formation in this setting. Urinary $iPF_{2\alpha}$-III levels, measured by immunoassay, were found to be not significantly elevated in a recent study of patients with acute ischemic stroke *(58)*. However, a formal study of iP generation during documented ischemia-reperfusion in the cerebral circulation of humans has not been reported.

Hypercholesterolemia and Atherosclerosis

Oxidative modification of LDL is thought to play a critical role in atherogenesis. The evidence is largely configured on "proatherogenic" properties conferred on LDL by its oxidation in vitro *(1,59)*, the identification of receptors for oxidatively modified LDL in human monocyte/macrophages and other cells *(60)*, its presence in human atherosclerotic plaque *(61)*, and the apparent efficacy of antioxidants in some *(5)*, but not all *(62)*, animal models of atherogenesis *(5)*. However, direct evidence of increased oxidant stress in vivo remains to be established.

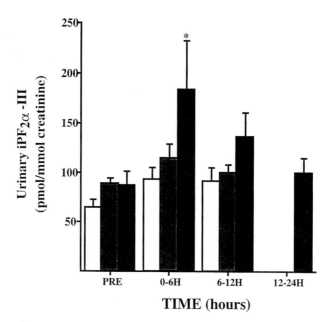

Fig. 2. Urinary iPF$_{2\alpha}$-III levels (mean SEM; pmol/mmol creatinine) increase markedly in the first 6 h following angiographically documented reperfusion for acute myocardial infarction (black bars; $n = 10$). There is a minor increase in iPF$_{2\alpha}$-III levels following diagnostic coronary angiography (white bars; $n = 11$) and elective angioplasty (shaded bars, $n = 15$).

We and others have demonstrated that iPFs are formed in LDL, coincident with lipid peroxides, when it is oxidized in vitro *(24,63,64)*. This is true for LDL exposed to copper or to more physiologically relevant oxidant signals, such as peroxynitrite or coincubation with activated endothelial cells. Recently, we have demonstrated increased levels of both iPF$_{2\alpha}$-III and iPF$_{2\alpha}$-VI in atherosclerotic vessels compared to normal arterial segments *(65)*. Furthermore, iPF$_{2\alpha}$-III immunolocalized to mono-cyte/macrophages and vascular smooth muscle cells in human atherosclerotic plaque. Recently, "total" iPFs have also been found in atherosclerotic plaque *(66)*. Therefore, we designed specific studies to assess the generation of both iPF$_{2\alpha}$-III and iPF$_{2\alpha}$-VI in patients with homozygous familial hypercholesterolemia (HFH) and also in more moderate hypercholesterolemia *(47)*. Urinary excretion of these iPs was increased in both groups of hypercholesterolemic patients compared to their respective controls (Fig. 3A). Furthermore, the concentration of iPF$_{2\alpha}$-III esterified in LDL was elevated in HFH patients and correlated with urinary excretion of this compound. LDL and urinary iP levels remained elevated in hypercholesterolemic subjects compared to controls when corrected for arachidonic acid. There was a striking correlation between urinary levels of both iPs (Fig. 3B), as in patients undergoing PTCA for myocardial infarction, supporting lipid peroxidation as the common mechanism of iP formation. Given the potentially distinct mechanisms that might result in free radical generation in smokers, one might anticipate an even greater increment in dyslipidemic individuals who smoke cigarettes. Elevated levels of immunoreactive iPF$_{2\alpha}$-III have recently been reported in hyper-cholesterolemic patients *(67)*.

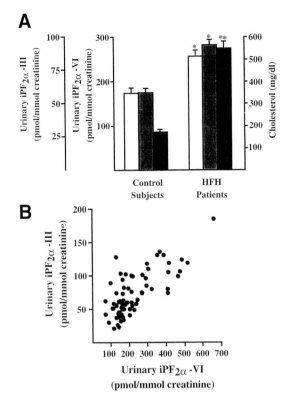

Fig. 3. (A) Urinary iPF$_{2\alpha}$-III (white bar; $p < 0.0005$) and iPF$_{2\alpha}$-VI (shaded bar; $p < 0.0005$) excretion is increased in 12-h urine samples from HFH patients ($n = 38$) compared to age- and gender-matched control subjects ($n = 38$). There is marked elevation in serum cholesterol (black bar; $p < 0.0001$) in these patients compared to controls. (B) Correlation ($r = 0.67$; $p < 0.0001$, $n = 74$) of urinary iPF$_{2\alpha}$-III and iPF$_{2\alpha}$-VI levels in HFH patients and control subjects.

Adult Respiratory Distress Syndrome (ARDS)

ARDS is an end stage of diverse forms of lung disease *(68)*. Several studies suggest that reactive oxygen species generated by polymorphonuclear leukocytes may damage pulmonary epithelium in this syndrome *(69,70)*. Furthermore, oxidatively modified proteins and increased lipid peroxidation have been reported in patients with ARDS *(71,72)*. The authors performed a number of studies to assess iPF generation in ARDS. Urine was collected from patients at high risk for ARDS who were admitted to the medical intensive care unit (MICU) on ventilators, and from age- and gender-matched nonventilated patients admitted to a general medical ward. Retrospectively, 8 of 13 patients admitted to the MICU fulfilled clinical criteria for ARDS. Urinary levels of iPF$_{2\alpha}$-III (Fig. 4) were heterogeneously distributed in the ARDS patients, but were markedly elevated (median [range] 250 [80–1607]; $n = 8$) compared to nonARDS, ventilated MICU patients (100 [30–152]; $n = 5$, $p < 0.01$) and non-MICU controls (85 [28–146]; $n = 16$, $p < 0.005$). To explore the relationship between the clinical course of ARDS and iPF excretion, serial 8 h urine samples were collected from a subgroup of MICU patients ($n = 8$) over a 3 d period. There was a significant correlation between

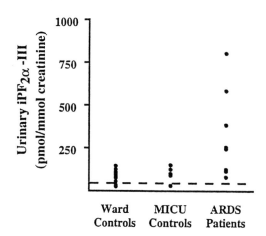

Fig. 4. Urinary iPF$_{2\alpha}$-III excretion (pmol/mol creatinine; median [range]) is elevated in ARDS patients (250 [80–1607]; $n = 8$) compared to non-ARDS mechanically ventilated control patients (100 [30–152]; $n = 5$, $p < 0.01$) and nonventilated general ward control patients (85 [28–146]; $n = 16$, $p < 0.005$).

oxygen requirements, as reflected by inhaled F$_{IO_2}$, and urinary iPF$_{2\alpha}$-III excretion over time ($r = 0.8$; $n = 3$, $p < 0.0005$) in acute phase ARDS patients (Fig. 5), but not in patients in the late phase of ARDS ($r = 0.4$; $n = 3$, $p = 0.2$) or in ventilated patients without ARDS ($r = 0.3$; $n = 2$, $p = 0.33$). These preliminary data suggest that there is a marked increase in oxidant stress, as determined by urinary iPF excretion, in ARDS patients and that the highest levels are seen in those patients in the acute stage of the illness.

Conclusion

Measurement of urinary iPFs offers a quantitatively accurate, yet noninvasive approach to determine free radical generation in vivo. Such assays have already been used to confirm increased oxidant stress in certain clinical settings. It is likely that they will afford a biochemical rationale for the dose selection of antioxidant drugs and the choice of appropriate disease targets for intervention with such agents. Given the number of iPF isomers, the potential for their enzymatic formation, and their likely differential metabolism, the use of specific iPF assays seems desirable at present. The development of simpler and less cumbersome assays will facilitate the application of these techniques to a wider clinical field. Indeed, methods for the simultaneous estimation of multiple isomers and their metabolites are presently being developed. Elucidation of the importance of iPFs as incidental PG receptor ligands, the characterization of putative specific iPF receptors, and a more extensive understanding of their biological activities will clarify the possible autacoidal role of these compounds in vivo.

Acknowledgment

This work was supported by grants from the Wellcome Trust and the National Institutes of Health (DHL 54500).

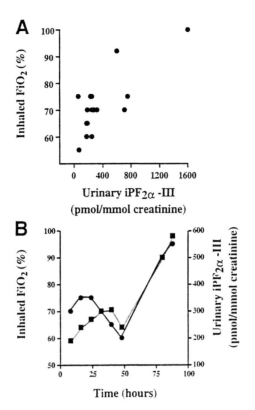

Fig. 5. **(A)** Correlation ($r = 0.8; p < 0.0005$) of urinary $iPF_{2\alpha}$-III and inhaled oxygen levels in patients with acute ARDS ($n = 3$). **(B)** An example of the time course of urinary excretion of $iPF_{2\alpha}$-III (squares) and oxygen requirements (circles) in a patient with acute ARDS.

References

1. Steinberg, D., Parthasarathy, S., Carew, T. E., Khoo, J. C., and Witztum, J. L. (1989) Beyond cholesterol: Modification of low-density lipoprotein that increases its atherogenicity. *N. Engl. J. Med.* **320,** 915–924.
2. Bolli, R. (1992) Myocardial 'stunning' in man. *Circulation* **86,** 1671–1691.
3. Rimm, E. B., Stampfer, M. J., Ascherio, A., Giovannucci, E., Colditz, G. A., and Willett, W. C. (1993) Vitamin E consumption and the risk of coronary heart disease in men. *N. Engl. J. Med.* **328,** 1450–1456.
4. Hertog, M. J. L., Feskens, E. J. M., Hollman, P. C. H., Katan, M. B., and Kromhout, D. (1993) Dietary antioxidant flavinoids and risk of coronary heart disease: The Zutphen elderly study. *Lancet* **324,** 1007–1011.
5. Carew, T. E., Schwencke, D., and Steinberg, D. (1987) Antiatherogenic effect of probucol unrelated to its hypocholesterolemic effect: Evidence that antioxidants *in vivo* can selectively inhibit low density lipoprotein degradation in macrophage-rich fatty streaks and slow the progression of atherosclerosis in the Watanabe Heritable Hyperlipidemic rabbit. *Proc. Natl. Acad. Sci. USA* **84,** 7725–7729.
6. Li, X.-Y., McCay, P. B., Zughaib, M., Jeroudi, M. O., Triana, F., and Bolli, R. (1993) Demonstration of free radical generation in the "stunned" myocardium in the conscious dog and identification of major differences between conscious and open-chest dogs. *J. Clin. Invest.* **92,** 1025–1041.
7. Halliwell, B. and Chirico, S. (1993) Lipid peroxidation: its mechanism, measurement and significance. *Am. J. Clin Nutr.* **57(Suppl.),** 715S–725S.

8. Holley, A. E. and Cheeseman, K. H. (1992) Measuring free radical reactions in vivo. *Br. Med. Bulletin* **49,** 494–505.

9. Esterbauer, H., Striegl, G., Puhl, H., and Rotheneder, M. (1989) Continuous monitoring of *in vitro* oxidation of human low density lipoprotein. *Free Rad. Res. Commun.* **6,** 67–75.

10. Coghlan, J. G., Flitter, W. D., Holley, A. E., Norell, M., Mitchell, A. G., Isley, C. D., and Slater, T. F. (1991) Detection of free radicals and cholesterol hydroperoxides in blood taken from the coronary sinus of man during percutaneous transluminal coronary angioplasty. *Free Rad. Res. Commun.* **14,** 409–417.

11. Hennekens, C. H., Buring, J. E., Manson, J., Stampfer, M., Rosner, B., Cook, N. R., Belanger, C., LaMotte, F., Gaziano, J. M., Ridker, P. M., Willet, W., and Peto, R. (1996) Lack of effect of long-term supplementation with beta carotene on the incidence of malignant neoplasms and cardiovascular disease. *N. Engl. J. Med.* **334,** 1145–1149.

12. Stephens, N. G., Parsons, P. M., Kelly, F., Cheeseman, K., Mitchinson, M. J., and Brown, M. J. (1996) Randomized controlled trial of vitamin E in patients with coronary disease: Cambridge Heart Antioxidant Study. *Lancet* **347,** 781–786.

13. Patrono, C. and FitzGerald, G. A. (1997) Isoprostanes: Potential markers of oxidant stress in atherothrombotic disease. *Arterioscl. Thromb. Vasc. Biol.* **17,** 2309–2315 (brief review).

14. Morrow, J. D. and Roberts, L. J. II (1996) The isoprostanes: Current knowledge and directions for future research. *Biochem. Pharmacol.* **51,** 1–9.

15. Morrow, J. D., Minton, T. A., Mukundan, C. R., Campbell, M. D., Zackert, W. E., Daniel, V. C., Badr, K. F., and Roberts, L. J. II (1994) Free radical-induced generation of isoprostanes *in vivo*: Evidence for the formation of D-ring and E-ring isoprostanes. *J. Biol. Chem.* **269,** 4317–4326.

16. Morrow, J. D., Awad, J. A., Wu, A., Zackert, W. E., Daniel, V. C., and Roberts, L. J. II (1996) Nonenzymatic free radical-catalyzed generation of thromboxane-like compounds (isothromboxanes) in vivo. *J. Biol. Chem.* **271,** 23,185–23,190.

17. Harrison, K. A. and Murphy, R. C. (1995) Isoleukotrienes: Biologically active free radical products of lipid peroxidation. *J. Biol. Chem.* **270,** 17,273–17,278.

18. O'Connor, D. E., Mihelich, E. D., and Coleman, M. C. (1984) Stereochemical course of the autooxidative cyclization of lipid hydroperoxides to prostaglandin-like bicyclo endoperoxides. *J. Am. Chem. Soc.* **106,** 3577–3584.

19. Morrow, J. D., Hill, K. E., Burk, R. F., Nammour, T. M., Badr, K. F., and Roberts, L. J. II (1990) A series of prostaglandin F_2-like compounds are produced *in vivo* in humans by a noncyclooxygenase, free radical-catalyzed mechanism. *Proc. Natl. Acad. Sci. USA* **87,** 9383–9387.

20. Morrow, J. D., Frei, B., Longmire, A. W., Gaziano, J. M., Lynch, S. M., Shyr, Y., Strauss, W. E., Oates, J. A., and Roberts, L. J. II (1995) Increase in circulating products of lipid peroxidation (F_2-isoprostanes) in smokers. *N. Engl. J. Med.* **332,** 1198–1203.

21. Gopaul, N. K., Nourooz-Zadeh, J., Mallet, A. I., and Anggard, E. E. (1994) Formation of F_2-isoprostanes during aortic endothelial cell-mediated oxidation of low density lipoprotein. *FEBS Lett.* **348,** 297–300.

22. Reilly, M. P., Delanty, N., Lawson, J. A., and FitzGerald, G. A. (1996) Modulation of oxidant stress *in vivo* in chronic cigarette smokers. *Circulation* **94,** 19–25.

23. Delanty, N., Reilly, M., Pratico, D., Fitzgerald, D. J., FitzGerald, G. A. (1996) 8-Epi $PGF_{2\alpha}$: specific analysis of an isoeicosanoid as an index of oxidant stress *in vivo. Br. J. Clin. Pharmacol.* **42,** 15–19.

24. Delanty, N., Reilly, M. P., Pratico, D., Lawson, J. A., McCarthy, J., Wood, A. E., Ohnishi, S. T., Fitzgerald, D. J., and FitzGerald, G. A. (1997) 8-Iso $PGF_{2\alpha}$ generation during coronary reperfusion: a potential quantitative marker of oxidant stress *in vivo. Circulation* **95,** 2492–2499.

25. Rokach, J., Khanapure, S. P., Hwang, S.-W., Adiyaman, M., Lawson, J. A., and FitzGerald, G. A. (1998) Nomenclature of isoprostanes: A proposal. *Prostaglandins*, in press.

26. Takahashi, K., Nammour, T. M., Fukunaga, M., Ebert, J., Morrow, J. D., Roberts, L. J. II, Hoover, R. L., and Badr, K. F. (1992) Glomerular actions of a free radical generated novel prostaglandin, 8-epi-prostaglandin $F_{2\alpha}$ in the rat: Evidence for interaction with thromboxane A_2 receptors. *J. Clin. Invest.* **90,** 136–141.

27. Yin, K., Halushka, P. V., Yan, Y. T., and Wong, P. Y. (1994) Antiaggregatory activity of 8-epi-prostaglandin F_2 alpha and other F-series prostanoids and their binding to thromboxane A_2/ prostaglandin H_2 receptors in human platelets. *J. Pharmacol. Exp. Ther.* **270,** 1192–1196.

28. Mobert, J., Becker, B. F., Zahler, S., and Gerlach, E. (1997) Hemodynamic effects of isoprostanes (8-iso prostaglandin $F_{2\alpha}$ and $E_{2\alpha}$) in isolated guinea pig heart. *J. Cardiovasc. Pharmacol.* **29,** 789–794.

29. Hoffman, S. W., Moore, S., and Ellis, E. F. (1997) Isoprostanes: Free radical-generated prostaglandins with constrictor effects on cerebral arterioles. *Stroke* **28,** 844–849.

30. Pratico, D., Smyth, E. M., Violi, F., and FitzGerald, G. A. (1996) Local amplification of platelet function by 8-epi $PGF_{2\alpha}$ is not mediated by thromboxane receptor isoforms. *J. Biol. Chem.* **271,** 14,916–14,924.

31. Kinsella, B. T., O'Mahony, D. J., and FitzGerald, G. A. (1997) The human thromboxane A_2 receptor α isoform (TPα) functionally couples to the G proteins Gq and G11 *in vivo* and is activated by the isoprostane 8-epi $PGF_{2\alpha}$. *J. Pharmacol. Exp. Ther.* **281,** 957–964.

32. Pratico, D., Lawson, J. A., and FitzGerald, G. A. (1995) Cyclooxygenase-dependent formation of the isoprostane, 8-epi prostaglandin $PGF_{2\alpha}$. *J. Biol. Chem.* **270,** 9800–9808.

33. Pratico, D. and FitzGerald, G. A. (1996) Generation of 8-epi prostaglandin $PGF_{2\alpha}$ by human monocytes. *J. Biol. Chem.* **271,** 8919–8924.

34. Kunapuli, P., Lawson, J. A., Rokach, J. A., and FitzGerald, G. A. (1997) Functional characterization of the ocular $PGF_{2\alpha}$: activation by the isoprostane 12-epi $PGF_{2\alpha}$. *J. Biol. Chem.* **272,** 27,147–27,154.

35. Fukunaga, M., Makita, N., Roberts, L. J. II, Morrow, J. D., Takahashi, K., and Badr, K. F. (1993) Evidence for the existence of F_2-isoprostanes receptors on rat vascular smooth muscle cells. *Am. J. Physiol.* **264,** 1619–1624.

36. Catella, F., Healy, D., Lawson, J., and FitzGerald, G. A. (1986) 11–dehydro-thromboxane B_2: an index of thromboxane formation in the human circulation. *Proc. Natl. Acad. Sci. USA* **83,** 5861–5865.

37. Roberts, L. J. II, Moore, K. P., Zackert, W. E., Oates, J. A., and Morrow, J. D. (1996) Identification of the major urinary metabolite of the F_2-isoprostanes, 8-iso-$PGF_{2\alpha}$ in humans. *J. Biol. Chem.* **271,** 20,617–20,620.

38. Wang, Z., Ciabattoni, G., Creminon, C., Lawson, J. A., FitzGerald, G. A., Patrono, C., and Maclouf, J. (1995) Immunoassay of urinary 8-epi $PGF_{2\alpha}$. *J. Pharmacol. Exp. Ther.* **275,** 94–100.

39. Waugh, R. J. and Murphy, R. C. (1996) Mass spectrometric analysis of four regioisomers of F_2-isoprostanes formed by free radical oxidation of arachadonic acid. *J. Am. Soc. Mass Spectrom.* **7,** 490–499.

40. FitzGerald, G. A., Pedersen, A. K., and Patrono, C. (1983) Analysis of prostacyclin and thromboxane A_2 biosynthesis in cardiovascular disease. *Circulation* **67,** 1174–1177.

41. Nowak, J., Murray, J. J., Oates, J. A., and FitzGerald, G. A. (1987) Biochemical evidence of a chronic abnormality in platelet and vascular function in healthy individuals who smoke cigarettes. *Circulation* **76,** 6–14.

42. Fitzgerald, D. J., Catella, F., Roy, L., and FitzGerald, G. A. (1988) Platelet activation *in vivo* after intravenous streptokinase in patients with acute myocardial infarction. *Circulation* **77,** 142–150.

43. Klein, T., Reutter, F., Schweer, H., Seyberth, H. W., and Nusing, R. M. (1997) Generation of the isoprostane 8-epi-prostaglandin $F_{2\alpha}$ *in vitro* and *in vivo* via cyclooxygenases. *J. Pharmacol. Exp. Ther.* **282,** 1658–1665.

44. Adiyaman, M., Lawson, J. A., Hwang, S.-W., Khanapure, S. P., FitzGerald, G. A., and Rokach, J. (1996) Total synthesis of a novel isoprostane $IPF_{2\alpha}$-I and its identification in biological fluids. *Tetrahedron Lett.* **37,** 4849–4852.

45. Pratico, D., Barry, O. P., Lawson, J. A., Adiyaman, M., Huang, S.-W., Khanapure, H., Rokach, J., and FitzGerald, G. A. (1998) $IPF_{2\alpha}$-I: a novel index of lipid peroxidation in humans. *Proc. Natl. Acad. Sci. USA,* **95,** 3449–3454.

46. Reilly, M. P., Delanty, N., Roy, L., O'Callaghan, P., Crean, P., Rokach, J., and FitzGerald, G. A. (1997) Increased formation of the isoprostanes, isoprostane $F_{2\alpha}$-I and 8-epi prostaglandin $PGF_{2\alpha}$, in acute coronary angioplasty: evidence for oxidant stress during coronary reperfusion in humans. *Circulation* **96,** 3314–3320.

47. Reilly, M. P., Delanty, N., Tremoli, E., Rader, D., and FitzGerald, G. A. (1996) Elevated levels of 8-epi prostaglandin $PGF_{2\alpha}$ in familial hypercholesterolemia: evidence of oxidative stress in vivo. *Circulation* **94,** I-683 (abstract).

48. Morrow, J. D., Awad, J. A., Kato, T., Takahashi, K., Badr, K. F., Roberts, L. J. II, and Burk, R. F. (1992) Formation of novel noncyclooxygenase-derived prostanoids (F_2-isoprostanes) in car-

bon tetrachloride hepatotoxicity: An animal model of lipid peroxidation. *J. Clin. Invest.* **90,** 2502–2507.

49. Awad, J. A., Morrow, J. D., Hill, K. E., Roberts, L. J. II, and Burk, R. F. (1994) Detection and localization of lipid peroxidation in selenium and vitamin E-deficient rats using F_2-isoprostanes. *J. Clin. Invest.* **95,** 2611–2619.

50. Pryor, W. A. and Stone, K. (1993) Oxidants in cigarette smoke: radicals, hydrogen peroxide, peroxynitrate and peroxynitrite. *Ann. NY Acad. Sci.* **686,** 12–27.

51. Freedman, D. S., Flanders, W. D., Barboriak, J. J., Malarcher, A. M., and Gates, L. (1996) Cigarette smoking and leukocyte subpopulations in men. *Ann. Epidemiol.* **6,** 299–306.

52. Zeiher, A. M., Schachinger, V., and Minners, J. (1995) Long-term cigarette smoking impairs endothelial-dependent coronary arterial vasodilator function. *Circulation* **92,** 1094–1100.

53. Burke, A. P., Farb, A., Malcom, G. T., Liang, Y. H., Smialek, J., and Virmani, R. (1997) Coronary risk factors and plaque morphology in men with coronary disease who died suddenly. *N. Engl. J. Med.* **336,** 1276–1282.

54. Loft, S., Astrup, A., Buemann, B., and Poulsen, H. E. (1994) Oxidative DNA damage correlates with oxygen consumption in humans. *FASEB J.* **8,** 534–537.

55. Schectman, G., Byrd, J. C., and Gruchow, H. W. (1989) The influence of smoking on vitamin C status in adults. *Am. J. Public Health* **79,** 158–162.

56. Galli, M., Marcassa, C., Bolli, R., Gianuzzi, P., Temporelli, P. L., Imparato, A., Silva Oreggo, P. L., Giubbini, R., Giordano, A., and Tavazzi, L. (1994) Spontaneous delayed recovery of reperfusion and contraction after the first 5 weeks after anterior infarction. *Circulation* **90,** 1386–1397.

57. Tortolani, A. J., Powell, S. R., Misik, V., Weglicki, W. B., Pogo, G. J., and Kramer, J. H. (1993) Detection of alkoxyl and carbon-centered free radicals in coronary sinus blood from patients undergoing elective cardioplegia. *Free Rad. Biol. Med.* **14,** 421–426.

58. van Kooten, F., Ciabattoni, G., Patrono, C., Dippel, D. W., and Koudstaal, P. J. (1997) Platelet activation and lipid peroxidation in patients with acute ischemic stroke. *Stroke* **28,** 1557–1563.

59. Esterbauer, H., Dieber-Rothenender, M., Waeg, G., Striegl, G., and Jurgens, G. (1990) Biochemical, structural, and functional properties of oxidized low-density lipoprotein. *Chem. Res. Toxicol.* **3,** 77–92.

60. Mazzone, T. and Chait, A. (1982) Autoregulation of the modified low density lipoprotein receptor in human monocyte-derived macrophages. *Arteriosclerosis* 487–492.

61. Rosenfeld, M. E., Khoo, J. C., Miller, E., Parthasarathy, S., Palinski, W., and Witztum, L. J. (1991) Macrophage-derived foam cells freshly isolated from rabbit atherosclerotic lesions degrade modified lipoproteins, promote oxidation of low-density lipoproteins and contain oxidation-specific lipid-protein adducts. *J. Clin. Invest.* **87,** 90–100.

62. Munday, J., Thompson, K. G., James, K. A. G., and Manktelow, B. W. (1998) Dietary antioxidants do not reduce fatty streak formation in the C57BL/6 mouse atherosclerosis model. *Arterioscl. Thromb. Vasc. Biol.* **18,** 114–119.

63. Lynch, S. M., Morrow, J. D., Roberts, L. J. II, and Frei, B. (1994) Formation of noncyclooxygenase-derived prostanoids (F_2-isoprostanes) in plasma and low density lipoprotein exposed to oxidative stress *in vitro*. *J. Clin. Invest.* **93,** 998–1004.

64. Gopaul, N. K., Nourooz-Zadeh, J., Mallet, A. I., and Anggard, E. E. (1994) Formation of F_2-isoprostanes during aortic endothelial cell-mediated oxidation of low density lipoprotein *FEBS Lett.* **348,** 297–300.

65. Pratico, D., Iuliano, L., Mauriello, A., Spagnoli, S., Lawson, J. A., Rokach, J., Maclouf, J., Violi, F., and FitzGerald, G. A. (1997) Localization of distinct F_2 isoprostanes in human atherosclerotic lesions. *J. Clin. Invest.* **100,** 2028–2034.

66. Gniwotta, C., Morrow, J. D., Roberts, L. J. II, and Kühn, H. (1997) Prostaglandin F_2-like compounds, F_2-isoprostanes, are present in increased amounts in human atherosclerotic lesions. *Arter. Thromb. Vasc. Biol.* **17,** 3236–3241.

67. Davi, G., Alessandrini, P., Mezzetti, A., Minotti, G., Bucciarelli, T., and Costantini, F. (1997) *In vivo* formation of 8-epi-prostaglandin F_2 is increased in hypercholesterolemia. *Arter. Thromb. Vasc. Biol.* **17,** 3230–3235.

68. Demling, R. H. (1995) The modern version of the adult respiratory distress syndrome. *Ann. Rev. Med.* **46,** 193–202.

69. Helfin, A. C. and Brigham, K. L. (1981) Prevention by granulocyte depletion of increased lung vascular permeability of sheep lung following endotoxemia. *J. Clin. Invest.* **68,** 1253–1260.

70. Zimmerman, G. A., Renzetti, A. D., and Hill, H. R. (1983) Functional and metabolic activity of granulocytes from patients with adult respiratory distress syndrome: evidence for activated neutrophils in the pulmonary circulation. *Am. Rev. Respir. Dis.* **127,** 290–300.

71. Krsek-Staples, J. A., Kew, R. R., and Webster, R. O. (1992) Ceruloplasmin and transferrin levels are altered in serum and bronchoalveolar lavage fluid of patients with respiratory distress syndrome. *Am. Rev. Respir. Dis.* **145,** 1009–1015.

72. Quinlan, G. J., Evans, T. W., and Gutteridge, J. M. C. (1994) Linoleic acid and protein thiol changes suggestive of oxidative damage in the plasma of patients with adult respiratory distress syndrome. *Free Rad. Res.* **20,** 299–304.

7

Isoprostanes as Markers
of Lipid Peroxidation in Atherosclerosis

L. Jackson Roberts II and Jason D. Morrow

Introduction

Cardiovascular disease is one of the leading causes of morbidity and mortality in the United States. Central to the process of atherogenesis is the uptake of LDL by macrophages resulting in formation of foam cells in the vascular wall. Thus, insights into the mechanism that leads to the uptake of LDL by macrophages are key to understanding the pathogenesis of atherosclerosis. Native LDL is not internalized by macrophages. However, chemical modification of LDL apolipoprotein B-100 converts the LDL into a ligand for scavenger receptors on macrophages, which leads to rapid uptake of the modified LDL *(1–3)*. Because the scavenger pathway of LDL uptake lacks feedback inhibition by intracellular cholesterol content, massive accumulation of modified LDL can occur, resulting in foam cell formation.

Considerable evidence suggests that oxidation of LDL is the mechanism responsible for the conversion of LDL to an atherogenic form in vivo. Human epidemiologic studies have found an inverse association between the intake of antioxidants and risk of cardiovascular disease (*see* ref. *4*). Several studies have also demonstrated that antioxidants attenuate the development of atherosclerosis in experimental animals (*see* ref. *5*). LDL extracted from atherosclerotic lesions has been shown to resemble oxidized LDL *(6)*, and antibodies against oxidized LDL react with atherosclerotic lesions but not normal vascular walls *(7)*. In addition, specific products of lipid peroxidation have also been localized in atherosclerotic lesions *(8)*. Multiple potential mechanisms for LDL oxidation have been proposed (*see* ref. *5*). LDL that has been sufficiently modified by oxidation to be recognized by scavenger receptors is more electronegative than native

From: *Molecular and Cellular Basis of Inflammation*
Edited by: C. N. Serhan and P. A. Ward © Humana Press Inc., Totowa, NJ

LDL, which has been attributed to the loss of lysine residues on the LDL ApoB-100 protein resulting from the generation of reactive aldehyde decomposition products of lipid peroxidation, which form Schiff base adducts with lysine ε-amino groups *(8–11)*.

In addition to foam cell formation, oxidation of LDL may also contribute in other ways to atherosclerotic cardiovascular disease. Oxidized LDL is toxic to vascular cells *(12)* and promotes recruitment of monocytes/macrophages into the vascular wall (*see* ref. *5*). Oxidized LDL can impair vascular endothelial function by inactivating and inhibiting the release of nitric oxide (NO') *(13,14)*. Oxidized LDL also promotes thrombosis via its effects on platelet function and the coagulation/fibrinolytic systems *(15–17)*. In addition, oxidized LDL can inhibit lecithin:cholesterol acyltransferase, which would impair the antiatherogenic reverse cholesterol transport pathway *(18)*.

There has been considerable interest in the development of reliable noninvasive approaches that might provide an index of oxidation susceptibility and thus atherosclerotic risk. Such an indicator could identify individuals at high risk who might benefit from antioxidant therapy and could also be used to monitor the efficacy of antioxidant therapy to suppress lipid peroxidation. However, methods that have been developed to assess lipid peroxidation in vivo notably lack either specificity or sensitivity or are too invasive for human investigation *(19)*. In 1990, the authors reported the discovery of a novel series of prostaglandin (PG)-like compounds that are formed nonenzymatically independent of the cox (cox) enzyme by free radical–induced peroxidation of arachidonic acid *(20)*. Because these compounds are isomeric to cox-derived PGs, they have been termed "Isoprostanes" (IsoPs). The F-ring IsoPs (F_2-IsoPs), which are $PGF_{2\alpha}$-like compounds, are stable molecules and are present in all normal biological fluids and tissues at levels that can be easily detected. Following the initial discovery of IsoPs, a body of evidence has emerged suggesting that measurement of IsoPs represents one of the most reliable approaches to assess oxidative stress status and lipid peroxidation in vivo (*see* refs. *21–23*). In this report, the authors summarize data that have been obtained that support the value of utilizing measurements of IsoPs as a marker of lipid peroxidation and its potential application as an index of atherosclerotic risk.

Biochemistry of Formation of Isoprostanes

Figure 1 outlines the mechanism of formation of F_2-IsoPs. Abstraction of an allylic hydrogen from arachidonic acid by a free radical at the sites indicated results in the formation of three arachidonoyl radical species. Addition of molecular oxygen to these arachidonoyl radicals leads to the formation of four peroxyl radicals. The peroxyl radicals then undergo endocyclization with further addition of molecular oxygen to yield four PGG_2-like bicycylic endoperoxide intermediates. The endoperoxides are then reduced by naturally occurring reducing substances to yield four F_2-IsoP regioisomers. Recently the authors published a nomenclature system for the IsoPs based on the carbon number on which the side chain hydroxyl group is located with the carboxyl carbon being designated carbon number one *(24)*. Accordingly, the regioisomers depicted in Fig. 1 are designated 15-, 8-, 12-, and 5-series F_2-IsoPs. Each of these regioisomers is theoretically comprised of 8 racemic diastereomers for a total of 64 different compounds. Evidence has recently been obtained both in vitro and in vivo for the generation of all four of the F_2-IsoP regioisomers that are predicted by the proposed mechanism of

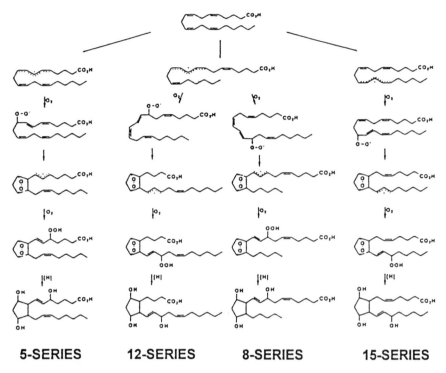

5-SERIES   12-SERIES   8-SERIES   15-SERIES

Fig. 1. Biochemical pathway for the formation of F_2-IsoPs by nonenzymatic free-radical–induced peroxidation of arachidonic acid. Four regioisomers are formed, each of which is theoretically comprised of eight racemic diastereomers. According to the nomenclature system established for IsoPs *(24)*, the four regioisomers are designated as 5-, 12-, 8-, and 15-series based on the carbon number on which the side-chain hydroxyl is located; the carboxyl carbon is carbon number one.

formation *(25,26)*. Of these the 15- and 5- series regioisomer compounds are formed in greater abundance compared with the 8- and 12-series regioisomer compounds. This finding is understandable because the addition of molecular oxygen at two different sites of a single arachidonoyl radical leads to the formation of both 8- and 12-series regioisomer compounds, whereas the 15- and 5-series regioisomer compounds each derive from a single arachidonoyl radical.

In the scheme shown in Fig. 1, the IsoP endoperoxide intermediates are reduced to form F_2-IsoPs IsoPs. It has been shown that the cox-derived PGH_2 is unstable in aqueous solvents and undergoes rearrangement to form PGE_2 and PGD_2 *(27)*. In addition, a mechanism has been described by which the endoperoxides might also undergo non-enzymatic rearrangement to form thromboxane (TX) *(28)*. Thus, if the IsoP endoperoxides are not efficiently reduced to F_2-IsoPs, they would also be expected to undergo rearrangement. In this regard, the authors have shown that the IsoP endoperoxides do undergo rearrangement in vivo, resulting in the formation of abundant quantities of E_2-IsoPs, D_2-IsoPs, and isothromboxanes *(29,30)*.

A unique aspect of the formation of IsoPs is that they are formed *in situ* esterified to tissue lipids and then released preformed *(31)*. By contrast, arachidonic acid must be released in free form prior to metabolism by the cox enzyme to form PGs. Of considerable interest is that molecular modeling of phosphatidylcholine with an F_2-IsoP esterified at the *sn*-2 position reveals it to be a profoundly distorted molecule that would be expected to greatly alter the fluidity and integrity of cellular membranes, a well-known deleterious effect of lipid peroxidation *(31)*.

IsoPs as Markers of Lipid Peroxidation In Vivo

As mentioned, the lack of reliable noninvasive methods to accurately assess oxidative stress status in vivo has been a major impediment in attempts to explore the role of free radicals in the pathogenesis of human disease. In this regard, quantification of F_2-IsoPs has emerged as a significant advance in this area *(21–23)*. Stable isotope dilution gas chromatography mass spectrometric methods of assay have been developed for measurement of F_2-IsoPs *(32–34)*. More recently, immunoassays have been developed for specific measurement of one of the F_2-IsoPs, 15-F_{2t}-IsoP (8-iso-$PGF_{2\alpha}$) *(34)* and are available commercially (Oxford Biomedical Research, Oxford, MI, and Cayman Chemical, Ann Arbor, MI). Immunoassays for this F_2-IsoP were developed because it possesses potent biological activity *(vide infra)* and has been shown to be formed in abundance in vivo *(35)*. A method utilizing immunoaffinity purification of 15-F_{2t}-IsoP coupled with quantification by mass spectrometry has also been described *(36)*. One of the 5-series F_2-IsoPs, namely, 5-F_{2t}-IsoP, has also been detected in human urine by mass spectrometry, but immunoassays for this compound have not yet been developed *(37)*.

F_2-IsoPs are present at readily detectable levels in every biological fluid and tissue thus far examined and, interestingly, exceed those of cox-derived PGs by more than one order of magnitude. This allows the definition of a normal range such that modest increases in the formation of F_2-IsoPs can be reliably established. In established animal models of free radical injury, levels of F_2-IsoPs have been shown to increase dramatically *(20,38–40)*. Studies have also been undertaken directly comparing the efficacy of measuring F_2-IsoPs with two of the most commonly used methods that have been utilized to assess lipid peroxidation, namely, measurement of malondialdehyde (MDA) and lipid hydroperoxides, in an animal model of lipid peroxidation, that being administration of CCl_4 to rats *(41,42)*. The fold increase in the formation of F_2-IsoPs induced by CCl_4 far exceeded that for either MDA or lipid hydroperoxides. This discrepancy was particularly striking in the case of MDA in which levels of F_2-IsoPs detected in the liver of CCl_4-treated rats, exceeded levels of MDA by as much as ~30-fold. Further, plasma concentrations of F_2-IsoPs increased a mean of ~25-fold in CCl_4-treated rats whereas lipid hydroperoxides could not be detected in the circulation even in this setting of severe oxidant injury using a highly sensitive mass spectrometric method of assay. The reason(s) that the measurement of F_2-IsoPs proved to be a much more sensitive indicator of lipid peroxidation in these studies is unclear but may involve differences in the rate of metabolic clearance.

As mentioned, one of the unique aspects of the formation of IsoPs is that they are initially formed in situ esterified in tissue lipids and subsequently released preformed by phospholipases. This can be a very dynamic process in that the timing of sampling for measurement of free compounds in biological fluids can be critical. On the other hand, measurement of levels of IsoPs esterified in tissue lipids can provide a valuable approach to directly localize oxidant injury in key tissues of interest. This is accomplished by measuring free compounds following hydrolysis of a lipid extract of tissue *(32,33)*. Although measurement of levels of F_2-IsoPs esterified in tissue lipids is

Table 1
Levels of F_2-IsoPs Esterified in 3 mL of Unfractionated Plasma
and Lipoprotein Subfractions Isolated from Another 3 mL of the Same Plasma in Two Subjects

Lipoprotein fractions	Subject 1: F_2-IsoPs (pgs)	Subject 2: F_2-IsoPs (pgs)
Unfractioned total	435	585
VLDL	67	42
LDL	102	112
HDL	199	232
Bottom[a]	65	89
Sum	433	475

[a]Presumably contains a small quantity of HDL + F_2-IsoPs not associated with lipoproteins.

primarily utilized in experimental animals because it is invasive, the high degree of sensitivity of the mass spectrometric method of analysis can allow the measurement of levels of esterified F_2-IsoPs in small biopsy samples of human tissue (unpublished observation).

Use of Measurements of IsoPs
to Assess Oxidative Modification of Plasma Lipoproteins

Measurement of F_2-IsoPs esterified in plasma lipids can provide a unique approach to directly explore the LDL oxidation hypothesis of atherosclerosis. Previously, it has been generally agreed that there is no conclusive evidence that native lipoproteins contain products of fatty acid oxidation *(43)*. However, the authors have found that F_2-IsoPs esterified in plasma lipids can be detected at a level of 119 ± 22 pg/mL plasma from normal volunteers. However, this level of F_2-IsoPs does not reflect an oxidative modification of LDL sufficient to be recognized by scavenger receptors on macrophages because native LDL isolated from normal volunteers is not taken up by macrophages. Nonetheless, measurements of F_2-IsoPs esterified in plasma lipoproteins can be utilized to explore whether pathological states are associated with alterations in the extent of oxidation of plasma lipoproteins. An important question that remains unanswered, however, is whether enhanced levels of F_2IsoPs esterified in lipoproteins in the plasma compartment have predictive value for the development of atherosclerosis in the vascular wall. Although far from conclusive, some data has been obtained that at least suggest that there may be a positive association between these two parameters (*vide infra*).

Most of the data the authors have obtained for measuring levels of F_2-IsoPs esterified in lipoproteins was derived from measurements of F_2-IsoPs esterified in total plasma lipids, rather than isolated lipoproteins. This can provide a general index of the extent of oxidation of lipoproteins because the vast majority of esterified lipids in plasma are contained in the lipoproteins. This approach has primarily been used to avoid the potential for artifactual formation of IsoPs by autoxidation during the process of isolation and separation of the individual lipoprotein subclasses. However, the authors have obtained data regarding the distribution of F_2-IsoPs esterified in the different lipoprotein fractions using a rapid method for their isolation and separation (OptiPrep Accurate Chemical and Scientific, Westbury, NY). The results of these measurements in lipoproteins isolated from 3 mL of plasma from two normal volunteers are shown in Table 1. Interestingly, the HDL fraction was found to contain the highest amount of F_2-IsoPs. This is consistent with previous data that have suggested that HDL is more readily oxidized than LDL *(44)*. VLDL was found to contain the lowest amount of F_2-IsoPs and

LDL was intermediate. The fraction eluting at the bottom of the gradient presumably contains a small quantity of HDL plus F_2-IsoPs not associated with lipoproteins. Notably, the sum of all fractions was nearly identical with the level measured in the same amount of unfractionated plasma. This result suggests that F_2-IsoPs were not generated by autoxidation to any appreciable extent during the isolation of lipoprotein fractions using this method. These preliminary results suggest that it may be possible to utilize this approach to assess specifically the extent of oxidation of plasma LDL.

IsoPs and Atherosclerosis in Experimental Animals

A Role for Superoxide in Atherogenesis

Vascular endothelial cells and smooth muscle cells have been shown to oxidatively modify LDL and evidence suggests a role for superoxide in this process *(45,46)*. Oxidized LDL and superoxide also inactivate and inhibit the release of the endothelium-derived vasodilator nitric oxide (NO$^{\bullet}$) *(13,14,47,48)*. Thus, endothelial Cu/Zn superoxide dismutase activity may be important in maintaining endothelial vasodilator function mediated by NO$^{\bullet}$. Superoxide inactivates NO$^{\bullet}$ by combining with NO$^{\bullet}$ to produce the oxidant peroxynitrite, which potently induces the formation of IsoPs in LDL *(49,50)*. To explore these relationships, the authors recently determined the effect of suppression of Cu/Zn superoxide dismutase activity through the production of dietary copper deficiency in rats on endothelial vasodilator function and levels of F_2-IsoPs esterified in plasma lipids *(51)*. In control Cu-replete animals, levels of F_2-IsoPs esterified in plasma lipids were 263 ± 40 pg/mL whereas levels in the Cu-deficient animals were 2.5-fold higher (665 ± 156 pg/mL) ($p < 0.05$ vs control) (Fig. 2). Interestingly, plasma-esterified F_2-IsoP levels were strongly correlated inversely to the arterial relaxation in response to the endothelial-dependent vasodilator acetylcholine ($r = -0.83, p = 0.0009$) (Fig. 2), but not to the endothelial-independent vasodilators Ca^{2+} ionophore A23187 ($r = -0.34, p = 0.29$) and NO$^{\bullet}$ ($r = -0.13, p = 0.71$). These findings suggest important roles both for Cu/Zn superoxide dismutase in maintaining endothelial vasodilator function mediated by NO$^{\bullet}$ and for superoxide in the oxidation of lipoproteins in vivo.

IsoPs in a Rabbit Model of Atherosclerosis

Several studies in rabbit models of atherosclerosis have found a preventive effect of antioxidant administration on atherogenesis (*see* ref. *5*). Thus, it was of interest to explore whether levels of F_2-IsoPs may be increased in a rabbit model of atherosclerosis and to determine the effect of administration of the antioxidant butylated hydroxytoluene (BHT) on IsoP formation. The authors measured levels of F_2-IsoPs esterified in plasma lipids from four rabbits fed a high-fat/high-cholesterol diet (0.5% cholesterol, 10% corn oil) and four rabbits fed a normal diet (Fig. 3). Levels of F_2-IsoPs esterified in plasma lipids in the high-fat/high-cholesterol fed group were markedly increased compared to control animals fed a normal diet—by 15.6-fold ($p < 0.03$). It had previously been shown that administration of BHT at a dose of 3 g/d significantly reduced the development of atherosclerosis in high-fat/high-cholesterol fed rabbits by ~70% *(52,53)*. Interestingly, administration of 3 g/d BHT to four rabbits fed a high-fat/high-cholesterol diet reduced levels of F_2-IsoPs by a similar extent, ~70% ($p < 0.03$), without significantly altering plasma cholesterol levels. These findings are of considerable interest as it relates to the potential value of measuring levels of F_2-IsoPs esterified in plasma lipids as a predictive index of atherogenesis in the vascular wall. In this regard,

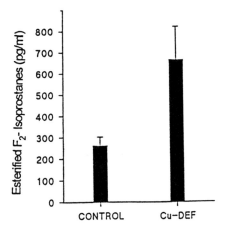

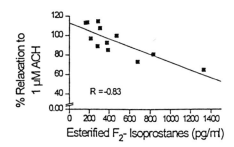

Fig. 2. **(Top)** Levels of F_2-IsoPs esterified in plasma lipids of control Cu-replete and Cu-deficient rats. **(Bottom)** Correlation between plasma esterified F_2-IsoPs levels from Cu-replete and Cu-deficient rats and the vascular relaxation response in aortas harvested from the same animals to the endothelial-dependent vasodilator acetylcholine (1 μ*M*) ($r = -0.083$, $p = 0.0009$). The percent reduction in tension (relaxation) was compared to the contraction produced by 1 μ*M* of phenylephrine.

levels of F_2-IsoPs esterified in plasma lipids were dramatically elevated in the animals that developed severe atherosclerosis, and administration of BHT, which significantly inhibited atherogenesis in these animals, also markedly suppressed levels of F_2-IsoPs.

IsoPs in a Canine Model of Cardiac Ischemia/Reperfusion Injury

A role for free radicals in ischemia/reperfusion injury is well established *(54,55)*. As discussed subsequently (*vide infra*), IsoPs can potently contract coronary arteries *(56)*. Thus, if the formation of IsoPs is enhanced during cardiac ischemia/reperfusion, this could have a deleterious effect by compromising coronary blood flow. Thus, the authors explored whether the formation of F_2-IsoPs is enhanced in a canine model of cardiac ischemia/reperfusion injury. In these experiments, the left anterior descending artery was occluded in three dogs for a period of 85 min, followed by reperfusion for 4 h. Blood samples were obtained from the coronary sinus for measurement of F_2-IsoPs at baseline prior to ischemia and at various times during the reperfusion period. Plasma concentrations of F_2-IsoPs increased, reaching a maximum at 180 min during the

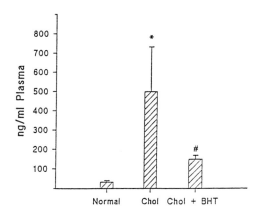

Fig. 3. Levels of F_2-IsoPs esterified in plasma lipids in rabbits fed a control diet (normal), rabbits fed a high-fat/high-cholesterol diet (Chol), and rabbits fed a high-fat/high-cholesterol diet that were treated with the antioxidant BHT (3 g/d) (Chol + BHT). $^*p$ <0.03 vs normal; $^\#p$ <0.03 vs Chol.

reperfusion period in all three animals. The mean increase in the plasma concentrations of F_2-IsoP above baseline was 3.9 ± 1.3-fold (Fig. 4).

These findings are consistent with data recently published demonstrating that the urinary excretion of F_2-IsoPs increased significantly in a canine model of coronary thrombolysis and, more importantly, also in humans during thrombolytic therapy for acute myocardial infarction *(57)*.

Collectively, these data indicate that the formation of IsoPs can be enhanced during cardiac ischemia/reperfusion injury, which suggests a potential role for these compounds to compromise myocardial blood flow in this setting because of their ability to potently induce coronary vasoconstriction.

Human Studies Utilizing Measurements of IsoPs to Explore the Oxidation Hypothesis of Atherosclerosis

IsoPs in Smokers

A link between cigarette smoking and risk of cardiovascular disease is well established *(58)*. However, the underlying mechanism(s) for this effect is not fully understood. The gaseous phase of cigarette smoke has been shown to contain numerous potent oxidants and exposure of LDL to the gaseous phase of cigarette smoke in vitro induces oxidation of the LDL lipids *(59,60)*. Thus, the authors explored the hypothesis that smoking induces an oxidative stress and specifically determined whether lipoproteins in individuals who smoke contain higher levels of F_2-IsoPs, indicative of a greater degree of oxidative modification. The authors studied ten individuals who smoked heavily (>30 cigarettes/d) and 10 age- and sex-matched nonsmoking normal volunteers *(61)*. Figure 5 (top) shows the results of these studies. Figure 5 (left) shows free F_2-IsoPs concentrations in plasma. The connecting lines link the age- and sex-matched subjects. Plasma concentrations of F_2-IsoPs were significantly elevated in the smokers compared to the nonsmokers ($p = 0.02$), although there was considerable interindividual variation. Figure 5 (right) shows the levels of F_2-IsoPs esterified in plasma lipids. Again,

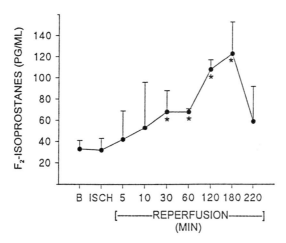

Fig. 4. Plasma concentrations (pg/mL) of F_2-IsoPs in coronary sinus blood from dogs obtained at baseline and various times following induction of cardiac ischemia produced by occlusion of the anterior descending coronary artery and reperfusion. B = baseline level prior to occlusion of the anterior descending coronary artery. ISCH = level at the end of 85 min of ischemia. 5–120 = levels at indicated times from 5 to 120 min during the reperfusion period. *$p \leq 0.02$ vs baseline.

levels were significantly higher in the smokers compared to nonsmokers ($p = 0.03$). Confirmation that these differences in levels of F_2-IsoPs between smokers and non-smokers were owing to cigarette smoking was obtained by measuring levels of F_2-IsoPs following 2 wk of abstinence from smoking in 8 of the 10 smokers who successfully abstained from smoking (Fig. 5, bottom). The lines connect the data obtained before and after smoking cessation in the same subject. In all subjects, levels of F_2-IsoPs both free in the circulation and esterified to plasma lipoproteins were significantly lower 2 wk following abstinence from smoking ($p = 0.03$ and $p = 0.02$, respectively). The occurrence of enhanced formation of IsoPs in smokers has also subsequently been confirmed in studies by others *(36,62)*. Collectively, these findings suggest strongly that smoking causes an oxidative stress and the finding that smokers have elevated levels of F_2-IsoPs esterified in plasma lipids also supports the hypothesis that the link between smoking and risk of cardiovascular disease may be attributed to enhanced oxidation of LDL.

IsoPs in Patients with Polygenic Hyercholesterolemia

It has been well established that patients with hypercholesterolemia have an increased risk for the development of atherosclerosis. Thus, it was of interest to determine whether levels of F_2-IsoPs were increased in patients with hypercholesterolemia.

Levels of F_2-IsoPs esterified in plasma lipids were determined in seven patients with polygenic hypercholesterolemia (Fig. 6). Levels in patients with hypercholesterolemia were found to be significantly increased a mean of 3.4-fold (range 1.7–7.5-fold) above levels measured in normal controls ($p < 0.001$). In these patients, cholesterol levels ranged from 211 to 310 mg/dL, triglycerides ranged from 68 to 822 mg/dL, HDL cholesterol ranged from 36–62 mg/dL, and LDL cholesterol ranged from 119 to 227 mg/dL. Interestingly, there was no correlation between levels of F_2-IsoPs and lipid levels in

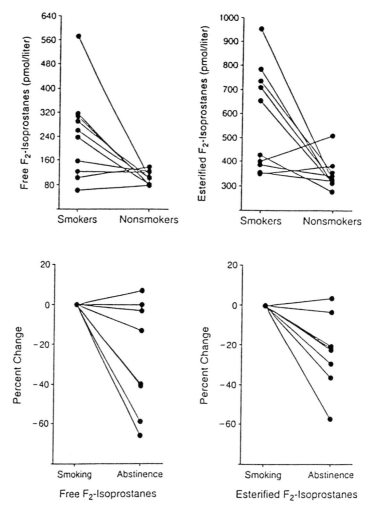

Fig. 5. Levels of free **(top left)** and esterified F_2-IsoPs **(top right)** in plasma from smokers and nonsmokers. The dots representing subjects who smoked are each connected to a dot representing a nonsmoker matched to the subject for age and sex. Percent change in the levels of free **(bottom left)** and esterified F_2-IsoPs **(bottom right)** in plasma from smokers after 2 wk of abstinence from smoking. Each dot on the right represents the change for an individual subject.

these patients ($r = -0.36$, $p = 0.41$ for triglycerides; $r = -0.33$, $p = 0.46$ for total cholesterol; $r = 0.48$, $p = 0.27$ for HDL; $r = -0.16$, $p = 0.76$ for LDL). The ratio of levels of F_2-IsoPs to total cholesterol and triglycerides actually varied by as much 57- and 20-fold, respectively. In addition, the authors measured plasma arachidonic acid content in three of these patients and in six normal controls. In the normal individuals, the ratio of F_2-IsoPs levels to arachidonic acid content varied a maximum of 1.8-fold. However, in the patients with hypercholesterolemia, the ratio varied as much as 4.8-fold. For example, in one patient, the levels of F_2-IsoPs and arachidonic acid were 403 pg/mL and 11.3 mg/mL, respectively. By contrast, in another patient, the level of F_2-IsoPs was much lower (280 pg/mL), but the level of arachidonic acid was much higher (37.0 mg/mL). These data suggest that the finding of high levels of F_2-IsoPs in patients

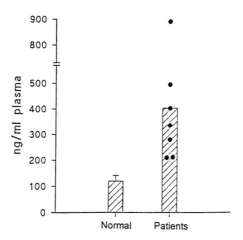

Fig. 6. Levels of esterified F_2-IsoPs in normal healthy subjects and patients with polygenic hypercholesterolemia defined as total serum cholesterol level >200 mg/dL. Dots denotes data from the individual subjects. p <0.001 for mean level in patients vs normal controls.

with hypercholesterolemia is not owing simply to the presence of more lipid, i.e., arachidonic acid substrate. Rather, these data suggest that hypercholesterolemia is associated with enhanced oxidative stress. The underlying basis for this intriguing observation, however, remains obscure. Interestingly, a recent preliminary report also found that the urinary excretion of F_2-IsoPs was also increased in patients with type II hypercholesterolemia by a mean of 2.5-fold, which was suppressed by approx 60% with vitamin E treatment (600 mg/d) *(63)*.

IsoPs in Patients with Diabetes

Patients with diabetes are well known to have an increased incidence of atherosclerotic vascular disease. Interestingly, the formation of F_2-IsoPs was recently found to be induced in vascular smooth muscle cells in vitro by elevated glucose concentrations *(64)*. Thus, the authors explored whether there was evidence for enhanced oxidative stress in vivo in patients with diabetes. In this study, the authors compared levels of F_2-IsoPs esterified in plasma lipids in 61 patients who underwent coronary angiography. In this group were 15 patients with diabetes. The extent of coronary atherosclerosis in the diabetic patients was similar to that in the 46 nondiabetic individuals. Plasma esterified levels of F_2-IsoPs measured in the diabetic patients (33.4 ± 4.8 pg/mL, mean ± SEM) were found to be modestly but significantly increased compared to levels measured in the nondiabetic patients (22.2 ± 1.9 pg/mL, p <0.02). Gopaul et. al. have also reported similar findings, in which they found a mean 3.3-fold increase in free F_2-IsoP concentrations in plasma of diabetic patients compared to nondiabetic healthy control subjects *(65)*.

Correlation Between Plasma Concentrations of Homocysteine and IsoPs

High plasma levels of homocysteine have been found to be an independent risk factor for cardiovascular disease *(66)*. The mechanism by which hyperhomocysteinemia

Table 2.
Lipid and F_2-IsoP Levels in Human Vessel Walls

Parameter	Arterial lesions	Umbilical veins	Significance
Free cholesterol (μg/mg dry wt)	5.39 ± 4.20 (n = 9)	1.52 ± 0.74 (n = 10)	p = 0.011
Cholesterol esters[a] (μg/mg dry wt)	1.88 ± 1.50 (n = 9)	0.08 ± 0.07 (n = 10)	p = 0.001
F_2-IsoPs (pg/mg wet wt)	27.1 ± 21.4 (n = 10)	1.37 ± 0.37 (n = 10)	p = 0.001
F_2-IsoPs (pg/mg dry wt)	75.9 ± 59.3 (n = 10)	11.7 ± 6.2 (n = 10)	p = 0.003
Ratio: F_2-IsoPs/ arachidonic acid (mg/g)	15.0 ± 12.0 (n = 10)	3.8 ± 1.8 (n = 10)	p = 0.009

[a]Sum of cholesterol linoeate and cholesterol arachidonate.

induces atherosclerosis is not fully understood, but promotion of LDL oxidation has been suggested *(67–69)*. The authors recently explored the relationship between total plasma concentrations of homocysteine and F_2-IsoPs in 100 Finnish male participants in the Antioxidant Supplementation in Atherosclerosis Prevention (ASAP) study (Voutillainen, S., Morrow, J. D., Roberts, L. J. II, Alfthan, G., Alhe, H., Nyyerssonen, K., and Lalenen, J. T., manuscript submitted). The mean plasma total homocysteine and F_2-IsoP concentrations were 11.1 μmol/L and 29.6 ng/L, respectively. The simple correlation coefficient for association between plasma concentrations of homocysteine and F_2-IsoPs was 0.40 ($p < 0.0001$). Plasma concentrations of F_2-IsoPs increased linearly across quintiles of homocysteine levels. The mean (95% confidence interval) plasma concentration of F_2-IsoPs was 47.5% greater in 20% of individuals with the highest homocysteine levels compared to the 20% of individuals with the lowest homocysteine plasma concentrations. The finding of a positive correlation between plasma concentrations of F_2-IsoPs and homocysteine supports the suggestion, but does not prove cause and effect, that the mechanism underlying the link between high homocysteine levels and risk for cardiovascular disease may be attributed to enhanced lipid peroxidation.

IsoPs in Human Athersclerotic Plaques

In accordance with the LDL oxidation hypothesis of atherosclerosis, levels of F_2-IsoPs should be higher in atherosclerotic plaques than in normal vascular tissue. To address this issue, the authors measured levels of F_2-IsoPs in fresh advanced atherosclerotic plaque tissue removed during carotid artery thrombarterectomy ($n = 10$), and compared these with levels measured in normal human umbilical veins removed from the placenta immediately after delivery ($n = 10$) *(69)*. Levels of F_2-IsoPs esterified in vascular tissue normalized to both wet wt and dry wt were significantly higher in atherosclerotic plaques compared to normal vascular tissue (Table 2). A better measure of the actual extent of oxidation, however, would be obtained by normalizing the data to the amount of arachidonic acid content of the tissue since this is the substrate for IsoP formation. When the data were normalized to arachidonic acid content, the F_2-IsoP/arachidonic acid ratio was approximately fourfold higher than the ratio in normal vascular tissue ($p = 0.009$). This finding indicates that unsaturated fatty acids in atherosclerotic plaques are more extensively oxidized than lipids in normal vascular tissue. These findings are also in accord with data from others that have also found increased amounts of other lipid peroxidation products in human atherosclerotic plaques *(70–72)*, including the localization of F_2-IsoPs in atherosclerotic plaque tissue to foam cells and vascular smooth muscle cells *(73)*.

Suppression of IsoP Formation by Antioxidants

Consistent with epidemiology studies that have established an inverse association between antioxidant intake and risk for cardiovascular disease, several studies have shown that administration of antioxidants suppresses atherogenesis in experimental animal models of atherosclerosis *(5)*. However, only limited data have been obtained, to date, evaluating the efficacy of antioxidants to prevent cardiovascular disease in humans. The results of human trials on the relationship between antioxidants and coronary artery disease have been recently summarized *(4)*. In addition to the studies in which the primary end point evaluated is cardiac events, a recent study reported data from the Cholesterol Lowering Atherosclerosis Study that suggested that high vitamin E supplementation (≥ 100 IU/d) was associated with significantly less progression of early preintrusive carotid artery atherosclerosis compared to low vitamin E users in patients not treated with lipid-lowering drugs ($p = 0.03$) *(74)*. However, no effect was seen in individuals who had a high intake of vitamin C (≥ 250 mg/d).

Critical to such studies in humans is information regarding which doses and combinations of antioxidants are most efficacious in suppressing oxidation of LDL. The conclusion at an NIH workshop convened to address this issue was that "we simply do not have enough information to determine which antioxidant (or combination of antioxidants) offers the best hope or how much of each should be administered" *(75)*. One major reason that this information is lacking is that the clinical pharmacology of antioxidants has not been carefully defined, which can be attributed to the lack of a reliable method to quantitatively determine the effect of antioxidants to suppress oxidative stress in vivo in humans. Most of the data that has been obtained in an attempt to assess the efficacy of administration of various antioxidants to inhibit LDL oxidation was derived from studies in which the susceptibility of LDL to oxidation is determined ex vivo *(76)*. However, whether such data can be accurately extrapolated to predict what occurs in vivo is highly questionable *(4)*.

Thus, the authors sought to obtain data that would support the notion that quantification of F_2-IsoPs could provide a valuable approach to define the clinical pharmacology of antioxidants. Toward this goal, they have obtained considerable data that clearly demonstrate that modulation of antioxidant status greatly influences the formation of F_2-IsoPs. For example, significantly enhanced formation of F_2-IsoPs was found to occur in rats rendered deficient in vitamin E, even in the absence of the administration of an oxidant to induce their formation *(39)*. Interestingly, two of the most prominent pathologic manifestations of vitamin E deficiency in rats are cardiac and skeletal muscle myopathy, and levels F_2-IsoPs in tissues of vitamin E–deficient rats were highest in cardiac and skeletal muscle. Se deficiency in rats also augments the overproduction of F_2-IsoPs in vitamin E–deficient rats *(77)*. Furthermore, Se deficiency and depletion of glutathione levels profoundly augments the production of F_2-IsoPs in rats treated with the oxidant diquat *(40)*.

Conversely, the administration of antioxidants has been shown to suppress the formation of F_2-IsoPs both in vitro and in experimental animals and humans in vivo. For example, H_2O_2-induced-formation of IsoPs in renal tubular epithelial cells in vitro was

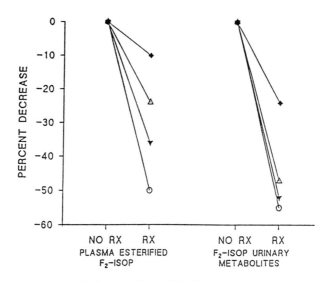

Fig. 7. Percent change in the levels of esterified F_2-IsoPs in plasma **(left)** and the urinary excretion of F_2-isoprostane metabolites **(right)** in normal volunteers before treatment (No Rx) and after 2 wk treatment (Rx) with a combination of vitamin E, vitamin C, and β-carotene. The same symbol before and after treatment denotes data from the same subject.

found to be inhibited by the 21-aminosteroid antioxidant U-74389G *(78)*. Cisplatin was also found to induce IsoP formation in these cells, which could be inhibited by *N*-acetylcysteine *(79)*. The authors also found that levels of F_2-IsoPs esterified in the kidneys of rats increase with advancing age, which can be prevented by long-term administration of vitamin E *(80)*. Administration of antioxidant 21-amino-steroids or the reducing agent methylene blue also was shown to significantly inhibit the marked increase in the formation of IsoPs in rats in which an oxidant injury was induced by administration of CCl_4 *(20,42)*. As discussed previously, the authors also demonstrated that administration of BHT significantly suppressed levels of F_2-IsoPs esterified in plasma lipids in rabbits fed a high-fat/high-cholesterol diet. More recently, they carried out a pilot study to determine whether administration of anti-oxidants would also suppress IsoP formation in humans. They were particularly interested in determining the effect of antioxidant administration on levels of F_2-IsoPs esterified in plasma lipids because of its potential relevance as an index of atherosclerotic risk. They administered a combination of vitamin C (4 g/d), vitamin E (3200 IU/d), and β-carotene (300 mg/d) for a period of 2 wk to five normal volunteers. High doses were used in this pilot study because of the short duration of treatment, which was insufficient to achieve a steady-state effect of the lipophilic antioxidants, vitamin E, and β-carotene *(81,82)*. Figure 7 shows the results expressed as percent decrease from baseline levels measured prior to administration of antioxidants. The authors found a significant maximum reduction approaching 60% both in levels of F_2-IsoPs esterified in plasma lipids ($p < 0.05$) and in the excretion of urinary F_2-IsoP metabolites that they had identified *(83)* ($p = 0.02$). Furthermore there was roughly a similar rank order of suppression for levels esterified in plasma lipids and urinary excretion of metabolites. The results of this pilot study provide proof of concept that the clinical pharmacology of antioxidants can be defined using measurements of F_2-IsoPs as a quantitative index of the effect of these agents to suppress lipid peroxidation in vivo in humans.

More recently, the authors assessed the effect of administration of 200 mg of d-α-tocopherol (natural vitamin E) alone, 500 mg of slow release vitamin C alone, and the two antioxidants in combination in a cohort of 100 Finnish males enrolled in the ASAP trial. After 1 yr of treatment, plasma concentrations of F_2-IsoPs were measured to determine the effect of the treatment regimens on endogenous lipid peroxidation. Vitamin E administration was found to significantly reduce plasma concentrations of F_2-IsoPs by 20.9% (95% confidence interval, 7.5–34.3%, $p = 0.003$). Vitamin C supplementation alone did not have a significant effect on plasma concentrations of F_2-IsoPs ($p = 0.536$). Vitamin C has been shown to reduce tocopherol radicals, thus regenerating vitamin E *(84,85)*. Based on this effect, it was anticipated that vitamin C might have an interactive effect with vitamin E to further suppress lipid peroxidation, even though the authors found that vitamin C alone had no significant effect on suppressing plasma F_2-IsoP concentrations. Surprisingly, however, levels of F_2-IsoPs were not suppressed further with the addition of vitamin C to vitamin E, and actually tended to be higher in the group treated with both vitamin E and C compared to levels in the group with vitamin E alone, although this did not reach statistical significance ($p = 0.322$).

These data obtained in the ASAP study contrast with what has been observed to occur in one study with supplementation of smokers with vitamin E and C *(62)*. Although this was a small study involving only four to seven volunteers, administration of vitamin C (2 g/d) alone significantly suppressed the increase in the urinary excretion of F_2-IsoPs that occurred in the smokers. By contrast, vitamin E alone (800 IU/d) had no effect. Supplementation with vitamin E in addition to vitamin C had no additional effect on suppressing the urinary excretion of F_2-IsoPs compared to vitamin C alone. These findings are difficult to reconcile with the findings in the ASAP study. However, the ability of these antioxidants to suppress overproduction of IsoPs associated with smoking may be different from the situation in which these agents are used in chemoprevention in normal individuals, who are not under an oxidative stress. One might also speculate that these differences might be related to differences in plasma levels of vitamin C. The authors and others have found that smokers exhibit a selective reduction in plasma levels of vitamin C *(61)*. By contrast, subjects in the ASAP Finnish study had normal plasma concentrations of vitamin C. This possibility is supported by the finding that vitamin C supplementation (2 g/d) in nonsmokers and smokers, who were documented to have low plasma concentrations of vitamin C, prevented the increased monocyte adhesiveness to endothelium seen in smokers but did not affect monocyte adhesiveness in vitamin C–replete nonsmokers *(86)*. Supplementation of smokers who had been placed on a low vitamin C diet ($\leq$30 mg/d) with 1 g/d vitamin C significantly enhanced the resistance of LDL to oxidation ex vivo *(87)* whereas this effect has not been found to occur with vitamin C supplementation in normal volunteers *(88,89)*. Nonetheless, these findings highlight the importance of defining the clinical pharmacology of antioxidants in the situation in which they are targeted for use.

Biological Actions of IsoPs Relevant to Atherosclerosis and Cardiovascular Disease

Two of the IsoPs tested thus far have been found to exert potent biological actions that may have relevance to atherogenesis and cardiovascular disease. The side chains of the IsoPs are predominantly oriented *cis* in relation to the cyclopentane ring *(90)*. Thus, two IsoPs that would be expected to form are $15\text{-}F_{2t}$-IsoP ($8\text{-iso-PGF}_{2\alpha}$) and $15\text{-}E_{2t}$-IsoP (8-iso-PGE_2). $15\text{-}F_{2t}$-IsoP has been shown to be produced in abundance in vivo *(35)*. Both of these IsoPs have been found to be potent vasoconstrictors of renal and pulmonary vasculature *(20,29,91–94)*. Initially, it was found that the vasoconstricting actions of $15\text{-}F_{2t}$-IsoP could be abrogated by the TX receptor antagonsist SQ29548 *(91)*. This suggested that vasoconstricting activity of $15\text{-}F_{2t}$-IsoP was mediated by TX receptors. However, subsequent studies have provided evidence suggesting that the mechanism by which $15\text{-}F_{2t}$-IsoP and $15\text{-}E_{2t}$-IsoP cause vasoconstriction may be via interaction with a unique receptor *(94–100)*. In this context, the ability of TX receptors to antagonize the vasoconstriction of these IsoPs suggests that the receptor that mediates the vascular effects of these IsoPs may be structurally similar to the TX receptor. $15\text{-}F_{2t}$-IsoP has also been shown to induce the release of endothelin-1, a potent vasoconstrictor, from vascular endothelium *(101)*. Of potential relevance to coronary artery and cerebrovascular disease is that $15\text{-}F_{2t}$-IsoP potently contracts cerebral arteries and that both $15\text{-}F_{2t}$-IsoP and $15\text{-}E_{2t}$-IsoP have been found to potently contract coronary arteries *(56,102)*. As shown previously, the production of F_2-IsoPs increases strikingly in a canine model of cardiac ischemia/reperfusion injury (Fig. 3). Further, the formation of F_2-IsoPs increases acutely during thrombolytic therapy in patients with mycocardial infarction *(57)*. Thus, the formation of $15\text{-}F_{2t}$-IsoP and $15\text{-}E_{2t}$-IsoP under these circumstances in the heart may have adverse effects by reducing coronary blood flow. It is of considerable interest that TX receptor antagonists have been found to significantly reduce myocardial damage in an animal model of cardiac ischemia/reperfusion injury, whereas aspirin was ineffective despite complete inhibition of platelet TX production *(103)*. Although the explanation for this intriguing observation is not known, it was speculated that it might be attributed to inhibition of the coronary vasoconstricting actions of IsoPs. Further, $15\text{-}F_{2t}$-IsoP induces proliferation in vascular smooth muscle cells, an effect that may also have relevance to intimal thickening of vascular walls that occurs in atherosclerotic vascular disease *(97)*. $15\text{-}F_{2t}$-IsoP can also augment the action of agonists of platelet aggregation *(98,104)*. This effect could contribute to promote thrombosis, which is the precipitating event in acute myocardial infarction and stroke, and promote platelet aggregation in patients with carotid artery artherosclerosis, which plays a causative role in transient cerebral ischemic episodes.

Novel Reactive Products of the IsoP Pathway Capable of Converting LDL to an Atherogenic Form

In the mid-1980s, Salomon et al. reported the discovery that PGH_2 undergoes rearrangement to form ketoaldehdye acyclic derivatives, which have been termed levuglandins owing to their structural similarity to levulinic acid *(105)*. Recently, in collaboration with Salomon et al., the authors explored whether the IsoP endoperoxide intermediates might also undergo rearrangement to form isolevuglandins (Fig. 8). The authors' interest in this possibility stems from the fact that these compounds have the potential to be highly cytotoxic and mutagenic because they are extraordinarily reactive molecules that readily form covalent adducts with proteins and DNA *(106)*. Their reactivity exceeds that of other reactive aldehydes that have been identified as products of lipid peroxidation, e.g. MDA and 4-hydroxynonenal, by several orders of

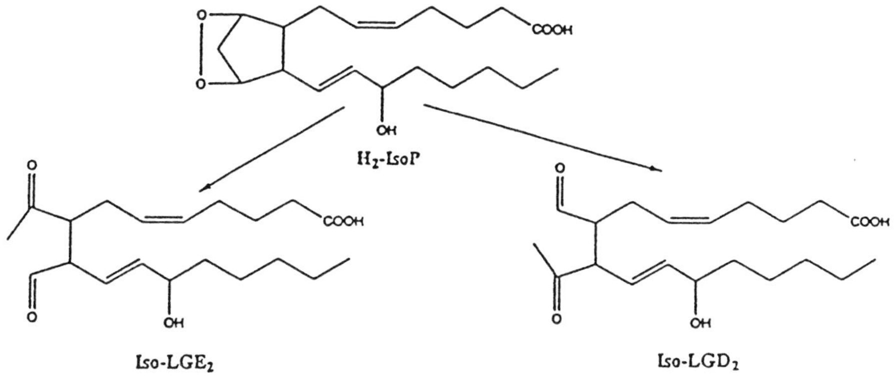

Fig. 8. Biochemical pathway for the formation of isolevuglandin E_2 and isolevuglandin D_2 by rearrangement of isoprostane endoperoxides. Four isolevuglandin regioisomers would be formed from the four isoprostane endoperoxide regioisomers (Fig. 1), each of which would be theoretically comprised of eight racemic diastereomers. For simplicity, only the representative structure of the 15-series compounds without stereochemical designations is depicted.

magnitude. The possibility that isolevuglandins may be formed during oxidation of LDL may have considerable relevance to the oxidation hypothesis of atherosclerosis because of their potential to form adducts with ApoB-100. As mentioned previously, adduction of reactive decomposition products of lipid peroxidation with ε-amino groups on ApoB-100 is believed to be the key process responsible for the conversion of LDL to an atherogenic form *(11)*. This notion would be supported by the authors' demonstration that oxidation of LDL in vitro induces the formation of prodigious quantities of IsoPs *(50,107)*, and the recent demonstration by Salomon et al. that levuglandin E_2 converts LDL to an atherogenic form with an efficiency that far exceeds that for 4-hydroxynonenal and MDA *(108)*.

Recently the authors explored whether isolevuglandins are formed during oxidation of arachidonic acid in vitro and found that, under these conditions, the amounts of isolevuglandins formed actually exceeded the amounts of F_2-IsoPs formed by several-fold (Brand, C. J., Solomon, R. G., Morrow, J. D., and Roberts, L. J. II, manuscript in preparation). The remarkable proclivity of these compounds to adduct to proteins (within a time frame of minutes) precludes their detection in protein containing biological fluids and tissues. Thus, the authors have recently undertaken studies utilizing electrospray tandem mass spectrometry to identify the nature of isolevuglandin protein adducts and to develop methodology for their detection and quantification in vivo. They have found that isolevuglandins initially form pyrrole adducts with lysine residues that then readily oxidize to lactam and hydroxylactam adducts. Further, they have been able to detect the presence of isolevuglandin lactam and hydroxylactam adducts on LDL ApoB-100 following oxidation of LDL in vitro. This latter provocative finding provides a strong rationale to pursue studies assessing the relative contribution of isolevuglandins with that of other reactive decomposition products of lipid peroxidation in the conversion of LDL to an atherogenic form. The discovery that these highly reactive levuglandin-like molecules are produced as products of the IsoP pathway also opens numerous other avenues for future investigation. To facilitate such studies, the authors have recently accomplished the total synthesis of an isolevuglandin derived from the 12-series IsoP endoperoxide regioisomer *(109)*.

Summary

A considerable body of evidence has been obtained that strongly supports the hypothesis that oxidative modification of LDL is a key process by which LDL is converted to an atherogenic form that is taken up by macrophages to form foam cells. The discovery of IsoPs has proven to be an important advance in the ability to assess oxidative stress status in vivo. The authors' finding that IsoPs can be detected esterified in lipoproteins, even in normal healthy individuals, may provide a unique and valuable approach to directly assess the extent of lipoprotein, and specifically LDL, oxidation in humans to identify individuals who may be at risk for atherosclerotic disease and who would potentially benefit from antioxidant therapy. In this regard, increased levels of IsoPs esterified in plasma lipids have been detected in humans with disorders known to be associated with an increased risk for cardiovascular disease. However, whether enhanced levels of IsoPs esterified in lipoproteins in the plasma compartment accurately predicts enhanced ahterogenesis in the vascular wall remains to be established. Nonetheless, the use of IsoP measurements should provide a valuable approach to define the clinical pharmacology of antioxidants. Such information would greatly inform clinical trials aimed at assessing the efficacy of antioxidants to prevent atherosclerosis and provide a basis for rational interpretation of results of trials that have been completed or will be forthcoming from trials that are currently under way. Furthermore, a more complete understanding of the biological actions of IsoPs and related compounds generated via the IsoP pathway, e.g., isolevuglandins, may provide valuable insights into how these compounds might participate as mediators of oxidant injury in general and specifically in the pathogenesis and pathophysiology of atherosclerotic vascular disease.

Acknowledgments

This work was supported by grants GM42056, GM15431, and DK48837 from the National Institutes of Health. The authors extend their special appreciation to their many collaborators listed as coauthors on referenced manuscripts. They also greatly appreciate the contributions of Drs. Eliott Sigal and Jan Mahoney in the studies with the rabbit model of atherosclerosis, and Drs. Chuck Chasten and Catherine Venturini in the studies with the canine model of cardiac ischemia/reperfusion.

References

1. Goldstein, J. L., Ho, Y. K., Basu, S. K., and Brown, M. S. (1979) Binding site on macrophages that mediates uptake and degradation of acetylated low density lipoprotein, producing massive cholesterol deposition. *Proc. Natl. Acad. Sci. USA* **76,** 333–337.
2. Henriksen, T., Mahoney, E. M., and Steinberg, D. (1981) Enhanced macrophage degradation of low density lipoprotein previously incubated with cultured endothelial cells: recognition by receptor for acetylated low density lipoproteins. *Proc. Natl. Acad. Sci. USA* **78,** 6499–6503.
3. Sparrow, C. P., Parthasarathy, S., and Steinberg, D. (1989) A macrophage receptor that recognizes oxidized low density lipoprotein but not acetylated low density lipoprotein. *J. Biol. Chem.* **264,** 2599–2604.
4. Diaz, M. N., Frei, B., Vita, J. A., and Keaney, J. F., Jr. (1997) Antioxidants and atherosclerotic heart disease. *N. Engl. J. Med.* **337,** 408–416.

5. Berliner, J. A. and Heinecke, J. W. (1996) The role of oxidized lipoproteins in atherogenesis. *Free Rad. Biol. Med.* **20,** 707–727.

6. Yla-Herttuala, S., Palinski, W., and Rosenfeld, M. E. (1989) Evidence for the presence of oxidatively modified low density lipoprotein in atherosclerotic lesions of rabbit and man. *J. Clin. Invest.* **84,** 1086–1095.

7. Palinski, W., Rosenfeld, M. E., Yla-Herttuala, S., Gurtner, G. C., Socher, S. S., Butler, S. W., Parthasarathy, S., and Carew, T. E. (1989) Low density lipoprotein undergoes oxidative modification in vivo. *Proc. Natl. Acad. Sci. USA* **86,** 1372–1376.

8. Esterbauer, H., Gebicki, J., Puhl, H., and Jurgens, G. (1992) The role of lipid peroxidation and antioxidants in oxidative modification of LDL. *Free Rad. Biol. Med.* **13,** 341–390.

9. Steinbrecher, U. P. (1987) Oxidation of human low density lipoprotein results in derivatization of lysine residues of apolipoprotein B by lipid decomposition products. *J. Biol. Chem.* **262,** 3603–3608.

10. Esterbauer, H., Jurgens, G., Quehenberger, O., and Koller, E. (1987) Autoxidation of human low density lipoprotein: loss of polyunsaturated fatty acids, vitamin E, and generation of aldehydes. *J. Lipid Res.* **28,** 495–509.

11. Zhang, H. F., Yang, Y. H., and Steinbrecher, U. P. (1993) Structural requirements for the binding of modified proteins to the scavenger receptor of macrophages. *J. Biol. Chem.* **268,** 5535–5542.

12. Morel, D. W., Hessler, J. R., and Chisolm, G. M. (1983) Low density lipoprotein cytotoxicity induced by free radical peroxidation of lipid. *J. Lipid Res.* **24,** 1070–1076.

13. Chin, J. H., Azhar, S., and Hoffman, B. B. (1992) Inactivation of enothelial derived relaxing factor by oxidized lipoproteins. *J. Clin. Invest.* **89,** 10–18.

14. Kugiyama, K., Kerns, S. A., Morrisett, J. D., Roberts, R., and Henry, P. D. (1990) Impairment of endothelium-dependent relaxation by lysolecithin in modified low-density lipoproteins. *Nature* **344,** 160–162.

15. Drake, T. A., Hannani, K., Fei, H., Lavi, S., and Berliner, J. A. (1991) MM-LDL induces tissue factor expression in cultured human endothelial cells. *Am. J. Path.* **138,** 601–607.

16. Aviram, M. (1989) Modified forms of low density lipoprotein affect platelet aggregation in vitro. *Thromb. Res.* **53,** 561–567.

17. Tippin, P. G., Davenport, P., Gallicchio, M., Filonzi, E. L., Apostolopoulos, J., and Wojita, J. (1993) Atheromatous plaque macrophages produce PAI-1 and simulate its production by endothelial cells and smooth muscle cells. *Am. J. Pathol.* **143,** 875–885.

18. Bielicki, J. K., Forte, T. M., and McCall, M. R. (1996) Minimally oxidized LDL is a potent inhibitor of lecithin:cholesterol acytransferase activity. *J. Lipid Res.* **37,** 1012–1021.

19. Halliwell, B. and Grootveld, M. (1987) The measurement of free radical reactions in humans. *FEBS Lett.* **213,** 9–14.

20. Morrow, J. D., Hill, K. E., Burk, R. F., Nammour, T. M., Badr, K. F., and Roberts, L. J. II (1990) A series of prostaglandin F_2-like compounds are produced in vivo in humans by a non-cox, free radical catalyzed mechanism. *Proc. Natl. Acad. Sci. USA* **87,** 9383–9387.

21. Morrow, J. D., and Roberts, L. J. II (1996) The isoprostanes: current knowledge and directions for future research. *Biochem. Pharmacol.* **51,** 1–9.

22. Roberts, L. J. II and Morrow, J. D. (1997) The generation and actions of isoprostanes. *Biochem. Biophys. Acta* **1345,** 121–135.

23. Morrow, J. D. and Roberts, L. J., II. (1997) The isoprostanes: unique bioactive products of lipid peroxidation. *Prog. Lip. Res.* **36,** 1–21.

24. Taber, D. F., Morrow, J. D., and Roberts, L. J. II (1997) A nomenclature system for the isoprostanes. *PGs* **53,** 63–67.

25. Waugh, R. J., and Murphy, R.C. (1996) Mass spectrometric analysis of four regioisomers of F_2-isoprostanes formed by free radical oxidation of arachidonic acid. *J. Am. Soc. Mass. Spectrom.* **1,** 490–499.

26. Waugh, R. J., Morrow, J. D., Roberts, L. J. II, and Murphy, R. C. (1997) Identification and relative quantitation of F_2-isoprostane regioisomers formed in vivo in the rat. *Free Rad. Biol. Med.* **23,** 943–954.

27. Hamberg, M. and Samuelsson, B. (1973) Detection and isolation of an endoperoxide intermediate in prostaglandin biosynthesis. *Proc. Natl. Acad. Sci. USA* **70,** 899–903.

28. Hecker, M. and Ullrich, V. (1989) On the mechanism of prostacyclin and thromboxane A2 biosynthesis. *J. Biol. Chem.* **264,** 141–150.

29. Morrow, J. D., Minton, T. A., Mukundan, C. R., Campbell, M. D., Zackert, W. E., Daniel, V. C., Badr, K. F., Blair, I. A., and Roberts, L. J. II (1994) Free radical induced generation of isoprostanes in vivo: evidence for the formation of D-ring and E-ring isoprostanes. *J. Biol. Chem.* **269**, 4317–4326.

30. Morrow, J. D., Awad, J. A., Zackert, W. E., Daniel, V. C., and Roberts, L. J. II (1996) Free radical-induced generation of thromboxane-like compounds (isothromboxanes) in vivo. *J. Biol. Chem.* **38**, 23,185–23,190.

31. Morrow, J. D., Awad, J. A., Boss, H. J., Blair, I. A., and Roberts, L. J. II (1992) Non-cox-derived prostanoids (F_2-isoprostanes) are formed in situ on phospholipids. *Proc. Natl. Acad. Sci. USA* **89**, 10,721–10,725.

32. Morrow, J. D. and Roberts, L. J. II (1994) Mass spectrometry of prostanoids: F_2-isoprostanes produced by non-cox free radical-catalyzed mechanism. *Methods Enzymol.* **233**, 163–174.

33. Morrow, J. D. and Roberts, L. J. II (1998) Mass spectrometric quantification of F_2-isoprostanes in biological fluids and tissues as a measure of oxidant stress. *Methods Enzymol.*, **300**, 3–12.

34. Wang, A., Ciabationi, G., Creminon, C., Lawson, J., FitzGerald, G. A., Patrono, C., and Maclouf, J. (1995) Immunological characterization of urinary 8-epi-prostaglandin $F_{2\alpha}$ excretion in man. *J. Pharmacol. Exp. Ther.* **275**, 94–100.

35. Morrow, J. D., Minton, T. A., Badr, K. F., and Roberts, L. J. II. (1994) Evidence that the F_2-isoprostane, 8-epi-prostaglandin $F_{2\alpha}$, is formed in vivo. *Biochim. Biophys. Acta* **1210**, 244–248.

36. Bachi, A., Zuccato, E., Baraldi, M., Fanelli, R., and Chiabrando, C. (1996) Measurement of urinary 8-epi-prostaglandin $F_{2\alpha}$, a novel index of lipid peroxidation in vivo, by immunoaffinity extraction/gas chromatography-mass spectrometry. Basal levels in smokers and nonsmokers. *Free Rad. Biol. Med.* **20**, 619–624.

37. Adiyaman, M., Lawson, J. A., Hwang, S. W., Khanapure, S. P., FitzGerald, G. A., and Rokach, J. (1996) Total synthesis of a novel isoprostane $IPF_{2\alpha}$-I and its identification in biological fluids. *Tetrahedron Lett.* **37**, 4849–4852.

38. Morrow, J. D., Awad, J. A., Kato, T., Takahashi, K., Badr, K. F., Roberts, L. J. II, and Burk, R. F. (1992) Formation of non-cox derived prostanoids (F_2-isoprostanes) in carbon tetrachloride heptotoxicity, an animal model of lipid peroxidation. *J. Clin. Invest.* **90**, 2502–2507.

39. Awad, J. A., Morrow, J. D., Hill, K. E., Roberts, L. J. II, and Burk, R. F. (1994) Detection and localization of lipid peroxidation in vitamin E and selenium deficient rats using F_2-isoprostanes. *J. Nutr.* **124**, 810–816.

40. Awad, J. A., Burk, R. F., and Roberts, L. J. II (1994) Effect of selenium deficiency and glutathione modulating agents on diquat toxicity and lipid peroxidation. *J. Pharmacol. Exp. Thera.* **270**, 858–864.

41. Longmire, A. W., Swift, L. L., Roberts, L. J. II, Awad, J. A., Burk, R. F., and Morrow, J. D. (1994) Effect of oxygen tension on the generation of F_2-isoprostanes and malondialdehyde in peroxidizing rat liver microsomes. *Biochem. Pharmacol.* **47**, 1173–1177.

42. Matthews, W. R., Mckenna, R., Guido, D. M., Petre, T. W., Jolly, R. A., Morrow, J. D., and Roberts, L. J. II (1993) A comparison of gas chromatography-mass spectrometry assays for in vivo lipid peroxidation. *Proceedings of the 41st ASMS Conference on Mass Spectrometry and Allied Topics*, 865A–865B.

43. Halovet, P. and Collen, D. (1994) Oxidized lipoproteins in atherosclerosis and thrombosis. *FASEB J.* **8**, 1279–1284.

44. Suzukawa, M., Ishikawa, T., Yoshida, H., and Nakamura, H. (1995) Effect of in vivo supplementation with low-dose vitamin E on susceptibility of low density lipoprotein and high density lipoprotein to oxidative modification. *Am. J. Nutr.* **14**, 46–52.

45. Heinecke, J. W., Baker, L., Rosen, H., and Chait, A. (1986) Superoxide-mediated modification of low density lipoprotein by arterial smooth muscle cells. *J. Clin. Invest.* **77**, 757–761.

46. Steinbrecher, U. P. (1988) Role of superoxide in endothelial cell modification of LDL. *Biochim. Biophys. Acta* **959**, 20–30.

47. Gryglewski, R. J., Palmer, R. M., and Moncada, S. (1986) Superoxide anion is involved in the breakdown of endothelium-derived relaxing factor. *Nature* **320**, 453–456.

48. Huie, R. E. and Padmaja, S. (1993) The reaction of NO with superoxide. *Free Rad. Res. Commun.* **18**, 195–199.

49. Beckman, J. S., Beckman, T. W., Chen, J., Marshall, P. A., and Freeman, B. A. (1990) Apparent hydroxyl radical production by peroxynitrate: implications for endothelial injury from nitric oxide and superoxide. *Proc. Natl. Acad. Sci. USA* **87**, 1620–1624.

50. Moore, K. P., Darley-Usmar, V., Morrow, J. D., and Roberts, L. J. II. (1995) Formation of F_2-isoprostanes during oxidation of human low density lipoprotein and plasma by peroxynitrite. *Circ. Res.* **77,** 335–341.

51. Lynch, S. M., Frei, B., Morrow, J. D., Roberts, L. J. II, Xu, A., Jackson, T., Reyna, R., Klevay, L. M., Vita, J. A., and Keaney, J. F. (1997) Vascular superoxide dismutase deficiency impairs endothelial vasodilator function through direct inactivation of nitric oxide and increased lipid peroxidation. *Arterioscl. Thromb. Vasc. Biol.,* **17,** 2975–2981.

52. Xiu, R. J., Ying, F. X., Berglund, L., Henriksson, P., and Bjorkhem, I. (1994) The antioxidant butylated hydroxytoluene prevents early cholesterol-induced microcirculatory changes in rabbits. *J. Clin. Invest.* **93,** 2732–2737.

53. Bjorkhem, I., Henriksson-Freyschuss, A., Breuer, O., Diczfalusyt, U., Berglund, L., and Henriksson, P. (1991) The antioxidant butylated hydroxytoluene protects against atherosclerosis. *Arterioscl. Thromb.* **11,** 15–22.

54. McCord, J. M. (1987) Oxygen-derived radicals: a link between reperfusion injury and inflammation. *Fed. Proc.* **46,** 2402–2406.

55. Werns, S. W. and Lucchesi, B. R. (1990) Free radical and ischemic tissue injury. *TIPS* **11,** 161–166.

56. Mobert, J., Becker, B. F., Zahler, S., and Gerlach, E. (1997) Hemodynamic effects of isoprostanes (8-iso-prostaglandin $F_{2\alpha}$ and E_2) in isolated guinea pig hearts. *J. Cardiovasc. Pharmacol.* **29,** 789–794.

57. Delanty, N., Reilly, M. B., Pratico, M. D., Lawson, J. A., McCarthy, M. B., Wood, A. E., Ohnishi, S. T., FitzGerald, D. J., and FitzGerald, G. A. (1997) 8-epi-$PGF_{2\alpha}$ generation during coronary reperfusion. *Circulation* **95,** 2492–2499.

58. Kannel, W. B. (1981) Update on the role of cigarette smoking in coronary disease. *Am. Heart J.* **101,** 319–328.

59. Church, D. F. and Pryor, W. A. (1985) Free-radical chemistry of cigarette smoke and its toxicological implications. *Environ. Health Perspect.* **64,** 111–126.

60. Frei, B., Forte, T. M., Ames, B. N., and Cross, C. E. (1991) Gas phase oxidants of cigarette smoke induce lipid peroxidation and changes in lipoprotein properties in human blood plasma: protective effect of ascorbic acid. *Biochem. J.* **277,** 133–138.

61. Morrow, J. D., Frei, B., Atkinson, A. W., Gaziano, M., Lynch, S. M., Shyr, Y., Strauss, W. E., Oates, J. A., and Roberts, L. J. II (1995) Increase in circulating products of lipid peroxidation (F_2-isoprostanes) in smokers. Smoking as cause of oxidant damage. *N. Engl. J. Med.* **332,** 1198–1203.

62. Reilly, M., Delanty, N., Lawson, J. A., and FitzGerald, G. A. (1996) Modulation of oxidant stress in vivo in chronic cigarette smokers. *Circulation* **94,** 19–25.

63. Davi, G., Alessandrini, P., Mezzetti, A., Minotti, G., Bucciarelli, A., Costatini, F., Cipollone, F., Bon, G., Ciabattoni, G., and Patrono, C. (1997) In vivo formation of 8-epi-prostaglandin $F_{2\alpha}$ in hypercholesterolemia. *Arterioscl. Thromb. Vasc. Biol.* **17,** 3230–3235.

64. Natarajan, R., Lanting, L., Gonzales, N., and Nadler, J. (1996) Formation of and F_2-isoprostane in vascular smooth muscle cells by elevated glucose and growth factors. *Am. J. Physiol.* **271** (*Heart Circ. Physiol.* **40**), H159–H165.

65. Gopaul, N. K., Anggard, E. E., Mallet, A. I., Beteridge, D. J., Wolff, S. P., and Nourooz-Zadey, J. (1995) Plasma 8-epi-$PGF_{2\alpha}$ are elevated in individuals with non-insulin dependent diabetes mellitus. *FEBS Lett.* **368,** 225–229.

66. Boushey, C. J., Beresford, S. A., Omenn, G. S., and Motulsky, A. G. (1995) A quantitative assessment of plasma homocysteine as a risk factor for vascular disease: probable benefits of increasing folic acid intakes. *J. Am. Med. Assoc.* **274,** 1049–1057.

67. Berwanger, C. S., Jeremy, J. Y., and Stansby, G. (1995) Homocysteine and vascular disease. *Br. J. Surg.* **82,** 726–731.

68. Mayer, E. L., Jacobsen, D. W., and Robinson, K. (1996) Homocysteine and coronary atherosclerosis. *J. Am. Coll. Cardiol.* **27,** 517–527.

69. Gniwotta, C., Morrow, J. D., Roberts, L. J. II, and Kuhn, H. (1997) Prostaglandin F_2-like compounds, F_2-isoprostanes, are present in increased amounts in human atherosclerotic lesions. *Arterioscl. Thromb. Vasc. Biol.,* **17,** 3236–3241.

70. Harland, W. A., Gilbert, J. D., Steel, G., and Brooks, J. W. (1971) Lipids in human atheroma. *Atheroscl.* **13,** 239–243.

71. Kuhn, H., Belkner, J., Wiesner, R., Schewe, T., Lankin, V. A., and Tikhaze, A. K. Structure elucidation of oxygenated lipids in human atherosclerotic lesions. *Eicosanoids* **5**, 17–22.
72. Folck, V. A., Nivar-Aristy, R. A., Krajewski, L. P., and Cathcardt, M. K. (1995) LOX contributes to the oxidation of lipids in human atherosclerotic plaques. *J. Clin. Invest.* **96**, 504–510.
73. Pratico, D., Lulianl, L., Mauriello, A., Spagnoli, L., Lawson, J. A., Maclouf, J., Violi, F., and Fitzgerald, G. A. (1997) Localization of distinct F_2-isoprostanes in human atherosclerotic lesions. *J. Clin. Invest.* **100**, 2028–2034.
74. Azen, S. P., Qian, D., Mack, W. J., Sevanian, A., Selzer, R. H., Liu, C. R., and Hodis, H. N. (1996) Effect of supplementary antioxidant vitamin intake on carotid arterial wall intima-media thickness in a controlled clinical trial of cholesterol lowering. *Circulation* **94**, 2369–2372.
75. Steinberg, D. and Workshop Participants. (1992) Antioxidants in the prevention of human atherosclerosis. *Circulation* **85**, 2338–2344.
76. Keaney, J. F., Jr. and Frei, B. (1994) Antioxidant protection of low-density lipoprotein and its role in the prevention of atherosclerotic vascular disease, in *Natural Antioxidants in Human Health and Disease* (Frei, B., ed.), Academic, San Diego, CA, pp. 303–352.
77. Awad, J. A., Morrow, J. D., Hill, K. E., Roberts, L. J. II, and Burk, R. F. (1994) Detection and localization of lipid peroxidation in selenium- and vitamin E-deficient rats using F_2-isoprostanes. *J. Nutr.* **124**, 810–816.
78. Salahudeen, A., Bach, K., Morrow, J. D., and Roberts, L. J. II (1995) Hydrogen peroxide induces 21-aminosteroid-inhibitable F_2-isoprostane production and cytolysis in renal tubular epithelial cells. *J. Am. Soc. Nephrol.* **6**, 1300–1303.
79. Salahudeen, A., Wilson, P., Pande, R., Poovala, V., Kanji, V., Ansari, N., Morrow, J. D., and Roberts, L. J. II (1998) Cisplatin induces N-acetylcysteine suppressible F_2-isoprostane production and injury in renal tubular epithelial cells. *J. Am. Soc. Nephrol.*, in press.
80. Reckelhoff, J. F., Kanji, V., Racusen, L., Schmidt, A. M., Yan, S. D., Morrow, J. D., and Roberts, L. J. II (1998) Vitamin E ameliorates enhanced renal lipid peroxidation and accumulation of F2-isoprostane in aging kidneys. *Am. J. Physiol.*, **274**, R767–R774.
81. Poor, D. L., Bierer, T. L., Merchen, N. R., Fahey, G. C., Murphy, M. R., and Erdman, J. W. (1992) Evaluation of the preruminant calf as a model for the study of human carotenoid metabolism. *J. Nutr.* **122**, 262–268.
82. Karpinski, K. and Hidiroglou, M. (1990) Monitoring vitamin E pools in sheep tissue and plasma after intravenous dosing of radiotocopherol. *Br. J. Nutr.* **63**, 375–386.
83. Awad, J. A., Morrow, J. D., and Roberts, L. J. II (1993) Identification of metabolites of noncox-derived prostaglandin-like compounds (F_2-isoprostanes) in human urine and plasma. *J. Biol. Chem.* **268**, 4161–4169.
84. Kagan, V. E., Sebinova, E. A., Forte, T., Scita, G., and Packer, L. (1992) Recycling of vitamin E in human low density lipoproteins. *J. Lipid Res.* **33**, 385–397.
85. Constantinescu, A., Han D., and Packer, L. (1993) Vitamin E recycling in human erythrocyte membranes. *J. Biol. Chem.* **268**, 10,906–10,903.
86. Weber, C., Erl, W., Weber, K., and Weber, P. C. (1996) Increased adhesiveness of isolated monocytes to endothelium is prevented by vitamin C intake in smokers. *Circulation* **93**, 1488–1492.
87. Fuller, C. J., Grundy, S. M., Norkus, E. P., and Jialal, I. (1996) Effect of ascorbate supplementation on low density lipoprotein oxidation in smokers. *Atherosclerosis* **119**, 139–150.
88. Reaven, P. D., Khouw, A., Beltz, W. F., Parthasarathy, S., and Witztum, J. L. (1993) Effect of dietary antioxidant combinations in humans: protection of LDL by vitamin E but not beta-carotene. *Arterioscl. Thromb.* **13**, 590–600.
89. Belcher, J. D., Balla, J., Balla, G., Jacobs, D. R., Jr., Gross, M., Jacob, H. S., and Vercellotti, G. M. (1993) Vitamin E, LDL and endothelium: Brief oral vitamin supplementation prevents oxidized LDL-mediated vascular injury in vitro. *Arterioscl. Thromb.* **13**, 1779–1789.
90. O'Conner, D. E., Mihelich, E. D., and Coleman, M. C. (1981) Isolation and characterization of bicycloendoperoxides derived from methyl linolenate. *J. Am. Chem. Soc.* **103**, 222–224.
91. Takahashi, K., Nammour, T. M., Fukunaga, M., Ebert, J., Morrow, J. D., Roberts, L. J. II, Hoover, R. L., and Badr, K. F. (1992) Glomerular actions of a free radical-generated novel prostaglandin, 8-epi-prostaglandin $F_{2\alpha}$, in the rat. *J. Clin. Invest.* **90**, 136–141.
92. Kang, H. K., Morrow, J. D., Roberts, L. J. II, Newman, J. H., and Banerjee, M. (1993) Airway and vascular effects of 8-epi-prostaglandin $F_{2\alpha}$ in isolated perfused rat lung. *J. Appl. Physiol.* **74**, 460–465.

93. Banerjee, M., Ho Kang, K., Morrow, J. D., Roberts, L. J. II, and Newman, J. H. (1992) Effects of a novel prostaglandin, 8-epi-PGF$_{2\alpha}$, in rabbit lung in situ. *Am. J. Physiol.* **263**, H660–H663.

94. Fukunaga, M., Takahashi, K., and Badr, K. (1993) Vascular smooth muscle action and receptor interactions of 8-iso-PGE$_2$, an E$_2$-isoprostane. *Biochem. Biophys. Res. Commun.* **195**, 507–515.

95. Morrow, J. D., Minton, T. A., and Roberts, L. J., II. (1992) The F$_2$-isoprostane, 8-epi-prostaglandin F$_{2\alpha}$, a potent agonist of the vascular thromboxane/endoperoxide receptor, is a platelet thromboxane/endoperoxide receptor antagonist. *PGs* **44**, 155–163.

96. Longmire, A. W., Roberts, L. J. II, and Morrow, J. D. (1994) Actions of the E$_2$-isoprostane, 8-iso-PGE$_2$, on the platelet thromboxane/endoperoxide receptor in humans and rats: additional evidence for the existence of a unique isoprostane receptor. *PGs* **48**, 247–256.

97. Fukunaga, M., Makita, N., Roberts, L. J., II, Morrow, J. D., Takahashi, K., and Badr. K. F. (1993) Evidence for the existence of F$_2$-isoprostane receptors on rat vascular smooth muscle cells. *Am. J. Physiol.* **264**, C1619–C1624.

98. Pratico, D., Smyth, E. M., Violi, F., and FitzGerald, G. A. (1996) Local amplification of platelet function by 8-epi-prostaglandin F$_{2\alpha}$ is not mediated by thromboxane receptor isoforms. *J. Biol. Chem.* **271**, 14,916–14,924.

99. Yura, T., Fukunaga, M., Grygorczyk, T., Makita, N., Takahashi, K., and Badr, K. F. (1995) Molecular and functional evidence for the distinct nature of F$_2$-isoprostane receptors on rat vascular smooth muscle cells. *Adv. Prostaglandin Thromboxane Leukotriene Res.* **23**, 237–239.

100. Fukunaga, M., Yura, T., Grygorczyk, R., and Badr, K. F. (1997) Evidence for the distinct nature of F$_2$-isoprostane receptors from those of thromboxane A$_2$. *Am. J. Physiol.* **272**, F477–F483.

101. Fukunaga, M., Yura, T., and Badr, K. F. (1995) Stimulatory effect of 8-epi-PGF$_{2\alpha}$, an F$_2$-isoprostane, on endothelin-1 release. *J. Cardiovasc. Pharmacol.* **26(Suppl. 3)**, S51–S52.

102. Hoffman, S. W., Moore, S., and Ellis, E. F. (1997) Isoprostanes: free radical-generated PGs with constrictor effects on cerebral arterioles. *Stroke* **28**, 844–849.

103. Gomoll, A. W. and Ogletree, M. L. (1994) Failure of aspirin to interfere with the cardioprotective effects of ifetroban. *Eur. J. Pharmacol.* **271**, 471–479.

104. Yin, K., Halushka, P. V., Yu-ting, Y., and Wong, P. Y-K. (1994) Antiaggregatory activity of 8-epi-prostaglandin F$_{2\alpha}$ and other F-series prostanoids and their binding to thromboxane A$_2$/prostaglandin H$_2$ receptors in human platelets. *J. Pharmacol. Exp. Ther.* **270**, 1192–1196.

105. Salomon, R. G., Miller, D. B., Zagorski, M. G., and Coughlin, D. J. (1984) Solvent-induced fragmentation of prostaglandin endoperoxides: new aldehyde products from PGH$_2$ and a novel intramolecular 1,2-hydride shift during endoperoxide fragmentation in aqueous solution. *J. Am. Chem. Soc.* **106**, 6049–6060.

106. Salomon, R. G., Jirousek, M. B., Ghosh, S., and Sharma, R. B. (1987) Prostaglandin endoperoxides 21: covalent binding of levuglandin E$_2$ with proteins. *PGs* **34**, 643–656.

107. Lynch, S. M., Morrow, J. D., Roberts, L. J. II, and Frei, B. (1994) Formation of non-cycooxygenase derived prostanoids (F$_2$-isoprostanes) in human plasma and isolated low density lipoproteins exposed to metal ion-dependent and -independent oxidative stress. *J. Clin. Invest.* **93**, 998–1004.

108. Hoppe, G., Subbanagounder, G., O'Neil, J., Salomon, R. G., and Hoff, H. F. (1997) Macrophage recognition of LDL modified by levuglandin E$_2$, an oxidation product of arachidonic acid. *Biochim. Biophys. Acta* **1344**, 1–5.

109. Subbanagounder, G., Salomon, R. G., Murthi, K. K., Brame, C., and Roberts, L. J. II (1997) Total synthesis of iso[4]-levuglandin E$_2$. *J. Org. Chem.* **62**, 7658–7666.

8

Structure and Regulation of NADPH Oxidase of Phagocytic Leukocytes

Insights from Chronic Granulomatous Disease

Paul G. Heyworth, John T. Curnutte, and John A. Badwey

Production of Reactive Oxygen Species by Phagocytic Leukocytes: A Brief Overview

When phagocytic cells of the immune system (neutrophils, monocytes, macrophages, and eosinophils) come into contact with opsonized microorganisms or a wide range of soluble stimuli, their consumption of oxygen increases dramatically (reviewed in refs. *1–3*). A multicomponent NADPH oxidase system drives this respiratory burst by catalyzing the one electron reduction of oxygen to superoxide (O_2^-):

$$NADPH + 2O_2 \rightarrow NADP^+ + H^+ + 2O_2^- \qquad (1)$$

The phagocyte NADPH oxidase is composed of at least five unique protein components (Fig. 1). Two components, gp91-*phox* and p22-*phox* (phagocyte oxidase [*phox*]) are integral to the plasma and specific granule membranes. These proteins are subunits of flavocytochrome-b_{558} *(4–6)* that contains both the flavin and heme centers involved in the transport of electrons from NADPH to oxygen *(7,8)*. Three other well-characterized components, p40-*phox*, p47-*phox*, and p67-*phox* *(9–12)*, are found in the cytosol of resting neutrophils in which they exist in a high molecular weight complex *(13,14)*, probably associated with the submembranous cytoskeleton. On stimulation of the respiratory burst, p40-*phox*, p47-*phox*, and p67-*phox* translocate to the membrane and become associated with the membrane-bound components to form a fully active catalytic complex *(12,15–17)* (Fig. 1, right). In addition to these five *phox* components, the small GTP-binding proteins Rac and Rap1A are involved in the NADPH oxidase sys-

From: *Molecular and Cellular Basis of Inflammation*
Edited by: C. N. Serhan and P. A. Ward © Humana Press Inc., Totowa, NJ

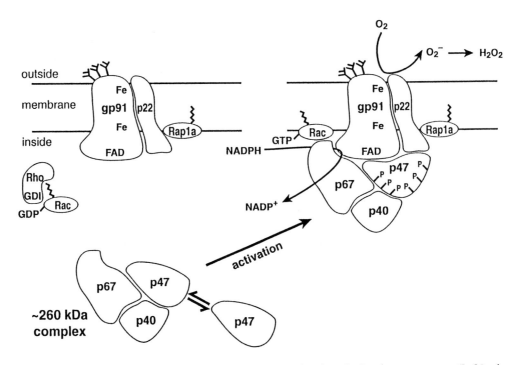

Fig. 1. Model of phagocyte NADPH oxidase activation. In its dormant state **(left)**, the oxidase is composed of membrane-bound and cytosolic (or cytoskeleton-associated) protein components. The former include gp91-*phox* and p22-*phox*, which together form flavocytochrome-b_{558}. Rap1, a small GTP-binding protein, is also present in the membrane, physically and perhaps functionally associated with the cytochrome. The cytosolic components include p40-*phox*, p47-*phox*, and p67-*phox*, which exist in a complex with a molecular mass of ~260 kDa. A pool of free, monomeric p47-*phox* is also present in cytosol prepared from resting neutrophils. In its inactive, GDP-bound state, the small GTP-binding protein Rac (Rac2 in human neutrophils) is also cytosolic and is bound to RhoGDP-dissociation inhibitor (GDI). On stimulation **(right)**, p47-*phox*, p67-*phox*, and p40-*phox* become associated with the plasma membrane primarily through interactions between p47-*phox* and the subunits of the cytochrome. This translocation process is accompanied by, and perhaps requires (1) the release of Rac from RhoGDI, its conversion to an active (GTP-bound) state, and its association with the plasma membrane; and (2) the multisite phosphorylation of p47-*phox*. In a manner that is not yet fully understood, binding of the cytosolic components activates the flavocytochrome to catalyze the transfer of electrons from NADPH to oxygen, via the flavin and heme redox centers. The compartment labeled "inside" is the cytoplasmic space; "outside" refers to either the extracellular or the phagosomal space.

tem. Rac1 or Rac2 is required for NADPH oxidase activity *(18,19)*, and Rap1A is physically and perhaps functionally associated with flavocytochrome-b_{558} *(20)*.

NADPH oxidase plays a critical role in nonspecific host defense. Superoxide is converted to hydrogen peroxide, hydroxyl radicals, and hypohalous acids (e.g., HOCl), all of which are powerful antimicrobial agents and, as such, are essential in the killing and digestion of bacteria, fungi, and parasites *(21)*. Phagocytes contain many other microbicidal agents, such as defensins and proteases *(22)*, which together with O_2^- and its derivatives form a fearsome antimicrobial system.

Unfortunately, in contrast to its beneficial role in host defense, activation of NADPH oxidase can also lead to severe tissue damage by O_2^- and its derivatives, contributing to the pathogenesis of inflammatory disease *(1,23)*. For example, in patients with adult respiratory distress syndrome in which large numbers of neutrophils accumulate in the lungs, there is extensive indirect evidence that O_2^- generated by neutrophil NADPH oxidase can directly cause the acute capillary-alveoli wall injury that results in alveolar flooding and respiratory failure *(24)*. Similarly, NADPH oxidase–derived oxygen metabolites are likely to cause the microvascular damage of lung and tissue associated with ischemia-reperfusion in patients with trauma and myocardial infarction *(23,25)*. The prolonged generation of oxygen radicals by phagocytes in situations of chronic inflammation (e.g., in ulcerative colitis and in the lungs of smokers) also contributes to dysplasia and eventual malignant transformation *(26,27)*.

Given the potentially destructive nature of O_2^-, it is not surprising that NADPH oxidase is highly regulated at multiple levels *(1)*. At one level, there are plasma membrane receptors specific for several ligands that, in many cases, are both chemoattractants and (at higher concentrations) stimulators of NADPH oxidase. These stimuli are released at sites of inflammation and include *N*-formyl peptides secreted by bacteria, the complement fragment C5a, interleukin-8, and platelet activating factor *(28)*. At a second level, receptor-linked GTP-binding proteins mediate the activation of phosphatidylinositol metabolism by activating phospholipase C, resulting in rapid increases in inositol phosphate, diacylglycerol, and calcium. These second messengers in turn lead to the activation of an array of enzymes including protein kinase C (PKC) and phospholipase D, both of which have been implicated in NADPH oxidase activation *(29,30)*. A final level of control is provided by the apparent physical separation of the oxidase into membrane-bound and soluble components.

The importance of the phagocyte NADPH oxidase in host defense is made apparent by the consequences of gene mutations affecting any one of four of the *phox* components (gp91-*phox*, p22-*phox*, p47-*phox*, or p67-*phox*), resulting either in the absence of any gene product or in the synthesis of defective proteins *(21,31,32)*. Chronic granulomatous disease (CGD), a rare syndrome caused by these mutations, is characterized by a total absence (or in a few instances, very low levels) of O_2^- production by phagocytes of effected individuals. Consequently, these patients are highly susceptible to life-threatening bacterial and fungal infections from the time of birth. This chapter will focus on insights into the NADPH oxidase system provided by the study of patients with CGD.

Components of the NADPH Oxidase System and the Molecular Basis of CGD

Flavocytochrome-b$_{558}$

The low-potential (–245 mV) flavocytochrome-b_{558} is the membrane-bound redox center of the NADPH oxidase system and consists of two subunits, gp91-*phox* and p22-*phox*, in a 1:1 stoichiometry *(33,34)*. Each cytochrome molecule contains two heme moieties and one FAD group *(7,8,35)*. The gp91-*phox* subunit of the cytochrome is a heavily glycosylated integral membrane protein *(36)*. Figure 2 shows one possible membrane-spanning model of the protein based on hydropathy plots and interactions of specific domains with cytosolic subunits *(37,38)*. Other models of gp91-*phox* topology

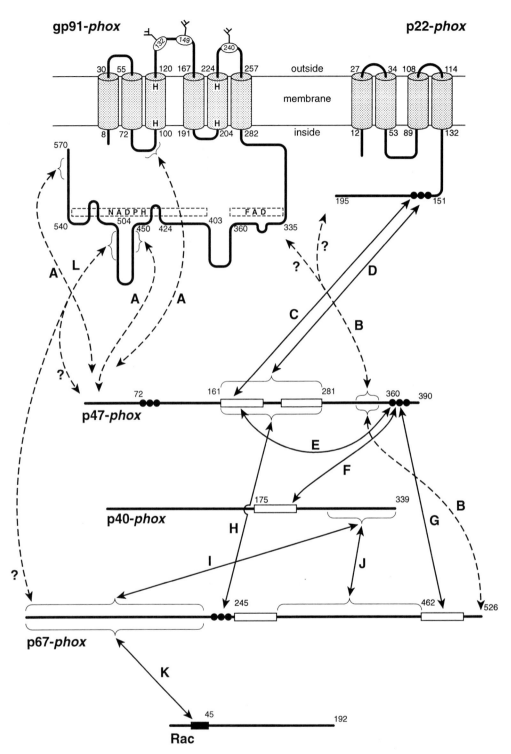

Fig. 2. Interactions among components of the NADPH oxidase system. The six known protein components of the phagocyte NADPH oxidase are shown in schematic form. Rap1A is not shown as no specific sites of interaction have been identified between it and the flavocytochrome subunits. Arrows indicate interactions for which there is some experimen-

have been proposed (e.g., *see* ref. *31*) in which the N-terminus of the protein is extracellular rather than cytosolic. The presence of a highly hydrophobic region between amino acids 100 and 120 that contains two histidines possibly involved in heme ligation, and the suggestion by De Leo et al. *(38)* that amino acids 86–93 form a site of interaction with p47-*phox*, led the authors to formulate the model depicted in Fig. 2.

At present it is unclear whether both heme groups of flavocytochrome-b_{558} are contained within gp91-*phox* or if one is shared between gp91-*phox* and p22-*phox* *(39)*. The most likely candidates for serving as heme ligands are the four histidines located within the predicted membrane-spanning regions of gp91-*phox* (residues 101, 115, 209, 222) and the only invariant histidine in p22-*phox* (residue 94), which is also predicted to be within the membrane *(40)*. The only other histidine in p22-*phox* (amino acid 72) is known to be polymorphic *(41)* and is replaced by tyrosine in the porcine protein *(42)*. Careful examination of sequence homologies and supporting biochemical data led several authors to propose that both the FAD- and NADPH-binding domains of the NADPH oxidase are contained within the gp91-*phox* subunit *(7,8,43)*. The evidence is fully described in the appropriate references and discussed again (*see* Structure–Function Information) in the context of CGD mutations. A three-dimensional model of the C-terminal half of gp91-*phox* has been proposed based on the crystal structure of spinach ferridoxin reductase *(44)*.

A membrane-spanning model of p22-*phox* is also shown in Fig. 2. For clarity in this figure, p22-*phox* and gp91-*phox* are shown as isolated proteins, but in reality they are tightly physically associated with each other, although exact points of contact are as yet unknown. Beyond serving as a possible heme binding site (*see* above), the precise role of p22-*phox* is unclear. It is apparently involved in stablizing the gp91-*phox* subunit during processing *(45)*, and formation of the gp91-*phox*/p22-*phox* heterodimer is important for the stability of the two subunits *(46)*. Moreover, p22-*phox* clearly acts as a docking site for p47-*phox*, thus enabling membrane association of all the cytosolic components. The cytoplasmic C-terminal domain of p22-*phox* contains two proline-rich Src homology 3 (SH3)-binding domains, and there is good evidence that at least one of them (amino acids 151–160) interacts directly with p47-*phox* *(47–50)*.

The Soluble phox Components

The original identification of p47-*phox* as a phosphoprotein *(51)*, and subsequent cloning and sequencing of p47-*phox* *(52,53)*, p40-*phox* *(12)*, and p67-*phox* *(54)*, have been discussed at length in the original papers and subsequent reviews *(1,13,31,55)*. For the purpose of this chapter, the authors will focus on some important structural

---

tal evidence, but the interactions do not all necessarily occur within the cell (*see text*). Solid arrows are used where the specific domains or regions of the protein (bracketed) that interact have been identified on both components. Broken arrows are used where an interacting domain has been identified on one component but the site of interaction on the second component is unknown. If the identity of the second component is in doubt the broken arrow bifurcates and is marked with a question mark. ☐, SH3 domains; •••, proline-rich domains; and ■, the "effector" region of Rac. Numbering of amino acids is from the N-terminus of each protein. gp91-*phox* and p22-*phox* are shown in more detail in Figs. 4 and 5, respectively. Selected references are as follows: **(A)** *(37,38)*; **(B)** *(126,127)*; **(C)** *(47,128)*; **(D)** *(48–50,93)*; **(E)** *(49,50)*; **(F)** *(129,130)*; **(G)** *(49,129,131)*; **(H)** *(93,128)*; **(I)** *(132)*; **(J)** *(129,133,134)*; **(K)** *(105,107,109)*; **(L)** *(85,114)*.

features of these molecules that allow them to interact with one another and with the subunits of flavocytochrome b_{558}.

p47-*phox* contains two SH3 domains that occur in tandem in the center of the linearized molecule (Fig. 2). SH3 domains are found in a large number of proteins involved in signal transduction *(56)* and consist of approx 50 amino acids forming an exposed hydrophobic ligand-binding site that can interact with proline-rich sequences *(57,58)*. Two such proline-rich sequences are also contained within the sequence of p47-*phox* (amino acids 72–80 and 360–370). In the unstimulated cell, there is good evidence that the C-terminal proline-rich domain of p47-*phox* interacts with the N-terminal SH3 domain of the same molecule *(49,50)*. Another important structural feature of p47-*phox* is the large number of positively charged basic residues in the C-terminal region of the protein. This part of the protein is also rich in serines, which, in close proximity to basic residues, form favorable sites for phosphorylation by PKC and other protein kinases *(52,53)*. Between seven and nine serines within this region are phosphorylated concomitant with activation of the oxidase *(59,60)*.

p67-*phox* has a highly acidic C-terminal region and like p47-*phox* contains two SH3 domains and a proline-rich sequence (amino acids 227–234) (Fig. 2). Low-level phosphorylation of p67-*phox* has been reported but estimates of the stoichiometry of phosphorylation (mol phosphate/mol protein) suggest that it is probably not of physiological significance *(61–63)*. In addition to a single, central SH3 domain in p40-*phox*, the N-terminal half of the protein has some homology with p47-*phox* *(12)*.

The precise roles of p40-*phox*, p47-*phox*, and p67-*phox* in the NADPH oxidase are unclear. Cross and Curnutte have provided evidence that p47-*phox* and p67-*phox* have individual roles in regulating the redox activity of the oxidase *(64,65)*. Their data suggest that p67-*phox* facilitates electron flow from NADPH to the flavin center and that p47-*phox* controls the subsequent step from FAD to heme. Others have proposed that p67-*phox* actually contains a binding site for NADPH *(66)*, but that is hard to reconcile with the current dogma that the FAD- and NADPH-binding sites coexist (as one would expect) on gp91-*phox*. One function of p47-*phox* is certainly that of a docking protein, for it is principally through p47-*phox* that the other cytosolic proteins can associate with the flavocytochrome (*see below*). In cell-free NADPH oxidase systems, p40-*phox*, unlike the other *phox* components and Rac, is not required for O_2^--generating activity *(7,67)*. In fact, it can inhibit such systems and downregulate the oxidase in a transfected cell model *(68)*.

GTP-Binding Proteins

Rac1 and Rac2, two very closely related members of the Rho family of GTP-binding proteins *(69)*, were purified from phagocytes and shown to mediate the known GTP requirement of the NADPH oxidase *(18,19,70–72)*. Rac1 and Rac2 are 90% identical, but whereas Rac1 is expressed in a wide variety of cell types, Rac2 is apparently restricted to cells of myeloid and lymphoid origin *(69)*. A third member of this family, Rac3, has recently been cloned and sequenced. Rac3 has 92 and 89% identity to Rac1 and Rac2, respectively, but it is unknown whether it can substitute for Rac1 and Rac2 in the phagocyte NADPH oxidase *(73)*. Rap1A is physically associated with flavocytochrome-b_{558} *(20)* and functionally involved in oxidase activity *(74,75)*. These properties have been reviewed recently *(76)* and will not be discussed further in this chapter.

Molecular Basis of CGD

The hallmark of CGD is the total absence or severely diminished levels of O_2^- production by the NADPH oxidase of phagocytic leukocytes. The disease is uncommon, occurring in approx 1 in 250,000 individuals, and is genetically and biochemically heterogeneous (for reviews *see* refs. *21,31,* and *55*). As shown in Table 1, the genetic heterogeneity of CGD arises because any one of four genes encoding *phox* components can be affected, resulting in either X-chromosome–linked or autosomal recessive modes of inheritance. Mutations in the gene for gp91-*phox* (CYBB, Xp21.1) cause the X-linked form of the disease, which accounts for nearly two-thirds of all cases. As would be expected from the genetics, the vast majority of these patients are males. The autosomal recessive forms of the disease, accounting for the remaining 36% of cases, are equally divided among males and females. The affected genes in these patients encode p22-*phox* (CYBA, 16q24), p47-*phox* (NCF1, 7q11.23), or p67-*phox* (NCF2, 1q25). There are no reports of CGD resulting from mutations in the gene for p40-*phox* (NCF, 22q13.1), but the level of this protein is severely diminished in the phagocytes of patients lacking p67-*phox* (A67°CGD) (Table 1) *(12,77)*.

The biochemical heterogeneity of CGD arises from the diverse (and poorly understood) functions of the affected proteins, and from the many different mutations within the genes for gp91-*phox* and p22-*phox*. These mutations can result in (1) undetectable levels of the affected component, (2) decreased levels with normal or subnormal activity, or (3) normal levels of inactive protein *(78)*. Table 1 shows the current classification scheme for these different forms of CGD, together with some relevant biochemical data. The subtype nomenclature given in Table 1 will be used throughout the remainder of this chapter.

Animal Models of CGD

In the absence of naturally occurring animal models of CGD, two groups have successfully generated murine models of the disease. Dinauer et al. *(79)* generated a model of X-linked CGD by gene targeting of CYBB, the gene encoding gp91-*phox*. As would be predicted, phagocytes of affected hemizygous males lacked detectable flavocytochrome-b_{558} subunits by immunoblot and generated no O_2^-. Using a similar targeted disruption technique, a p47-*phox* knockout mouse has also been created *(80)*. The mouse models mimic human CGD in that they have increased susceptibility to both bacterial *(79,81)* and fungal infections *(82)*. Both models have recently been used to demonstrate the effectiveness of gene transfer using retroviral vectors and murine bone marrow cells *(83,84)*.

These and similar models will be valuable for testing the safety and efficiency of different models of gene transfer, and in elucidating the role of phagocyte-generated reactive oxygen species in inflammation.

Interactions Among Components
of the NADPH Oxidase System

Interactions among the protein components of the phagocyte NADPH oxidase are the subject of a rapidly growing and rather confusing literature. The confusion arises because many of the interactions observed, with a variety of techniques, appear to be mutually exclusive unless one constructs overly complicated models of the activation process. Some of the techniques (e.g., yeast two-hybrid system, dot-blot assays), in the

Table 1
Classification of CGD

Component affected	Gene locus	Subtype[a]	Frequency (% of all CGD cases)	Cytochrome b spectrum (% of normal)	Cytosolic components[b] (% of normal)			O$_2^-$ production (% of normal)
					p40	p47	p67	
gp91-*phox*	Xp21.1	X91°	56	0	100	100	100	0
		X91⁻	5	3–30	100	100	100	3–30
		X91⁺	3	100	100	100	100	0
p22-*phox*	16q24	A22°	6	0	100	100	100	0
		A22⁺	1	100	100	100	100	0
p47-*phox*	7q11.23	A47°	23	100	<100[c]	0	<100[c]	0–1
p67-*phox*	1q25	A67°	6	100	10–20	<100[c]	0	0–1

[a]The letter represents the mode of inheritance (X-linked [X] or autosomal recessive [A]); the number indicates the *phox* component that is genetically affected. The superscript symbols indicate whether the level of the affected protein component is undetectable (°), decreased (−), or normal (+) as measured by immunoblot analysis.

[b]By immunoblot analysis.

[c]Anecdotal evidence suggests that these components are present at levels less than normal in some patients.

absence of supporting data, reveal interactions that *can* occur between proteins or isolated domains of proteins, but are not selective for those that *do* occur within the normal phagocyte. This complexity and confusion is evident in Fig. 2, which depicts many of the reported interactions with selected references. As DeLeo et al. *(2)* and Leusen et al. *(85)* have recently reviewed this subject in detail, this section will focus on aspects of the oxidase in which these interactions play a critical role.

The High Molecular Mass Complex of Soluble Oxidase Components

When resting neutrophils are fractionated following breakage by nitrogen cavitation or sonication, all the p40-*phox* and p67-*phox* together with one-third to one-half the cellular content of p47-*phox* are found in a high molecular mass (~260 kDa) complex in the soluble cytosolic fraction *(14,86)*. The remaining p47-*phox* exists as a monomer in these preparations. Although p40-*phox* and p67-*phox* appear to be present in equimolar amounts, the exact stoichiometry of the three *phox* components within the complex is unclear *(12)*, and the possibility that it contains additional proteins (e.g., cytoskeletal elements) cannot be excluded.

By contrast to these physical methods of cell breakage, when resting or stimulated neutrophils are solubilized with the detergent Triton X-100, p67-*phox* and most of the p40-*phox* are sedimented with the cytoskeleton-enriched insoluble fraction (Heyworth et al., unpublished observations; refs. *87* and *88*). p47-*phox* is present in the Triton X-100–soluble fraction of resting cells and becomes associated with the cytoskeleton only on cell activation. This is good evidence that p67-*phox* (or p40-*phox*) interacts directly with cytoskeletal proteins, but no direct physical association has been demonstrated.

These results initially seem contradictory to the concept of a cytosolic complex containing p40-*phox*, p47-*phox*, and p67-*phox*, but this can be resolved if one imagines that the intact complex is linked to the submembranous cytoskeleton, rather than being dispersed throughout the cytosol. In this model, for which there is some recent experimental evidence *(89)*, disruption of neutrophils by nitrogen cavitation would release the intact complex from the cytoskeleton whereas disruption in Triton X-100 would preferentially break the bonds between p47-*phox* and the other constituents of the complex. Such a model would place the soluble NADPH oxidase components in close proximity to the flavocytochrome-b_{558} subunits, with which they must interact to form a catalytic system. On activation, increases in affinity between the soluble and membrane-bound components would then lead to the phenomenon of translocation, as discussed below.

Irrespective of the exact composition and subcellular localization of the 260-kDa complex, there is abundant evidence that the complex is stabilized by multiple protein-protein interactions, in both the resting and activated phagocyte (for references *see* Fig. 2). These are likely to include interactions between SH3 and proline-rich domains within the proteins (e.g., Fig. 2F–H), as well as interactions between p67-*phox* and p40-*phox* outside these domains (Fig. 2I,J). The stability of the complex appears to be dependent on the presence of p67-*phox* because in its absence (in A67° CGD) p47-*phox* and the small amount of p40-*phox* remaining exist only in their monomeric forms *(13,90)*. In the absence of p47-*phox*, p40-*phox* and p67-*phox* remain associated with each other in an ~210-kDa complex, suggesting that the primary association of p40-*phox* is with p67-*phox*, rather than p47-*phox*. This is consistent with the original identification of p40-*phox* in immunoprecipitates of p67-*phox* *(12)*.

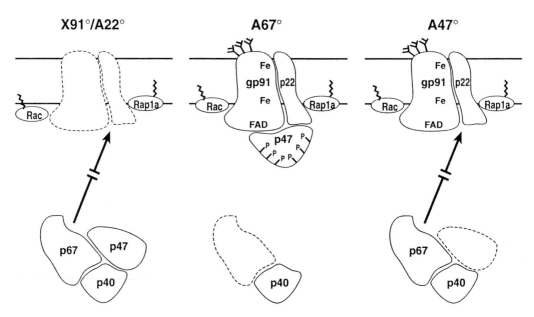

Fig. 3. Defective translocation of the cytosolic NADPH oxidase components in the different forms of CGD. In X91° and A22° CGD, the absence of either gp91-*phox* or p22-*phox*
leads to the secondary loss of the other cytochrome component. In these forms of the disease,
none of the cytosolic *phox* components become associated with the plasma membrane on
neutrophil activation. Rac translocation occurs but to a lesser extent than in normal neutrophils. In A67° CGD, normal translocation of p47-*phox* is observed, but p40-*phox* (present at
only 10–20% of normal levels) does not associate with the membrane. In A47° CGD, neither
p67-*phox* nor p40-*phox* translocate on neutrophil stimulation, indicating that these components associate with the membrane (and cytochrome-b_{558}) primarily by virtue of their interaction with p47-*phox*. In A47° and A67° CGD, Rac2 associates with the membrane in a
normal manner. Broken lines indicate missing components in the different forms of CGD.

Translocation of Soluble Oxidase Components

When phagocytic leukocytes are stimulated to generate O_2^-, the soluble oxidase components, p40-*phox*, p47-*phox*, p67-*phox*, and Rac, translocate from the cytosol to the
plasma membrane. Up to 10% of the cellular content of these proteins is found in membrane fractions isolated from activated neutrophils *(16,17,91)*. Similar experiments with
CGD neutrophils have shown an interesting and informative pattern of translocation, as
summarized in Fig. 3.

In flavocytochrome-deficient forms of the disease (X91° and A22° CGD), there was
no translocation of p40-*phox*, p47-*phox*, or p67-*phox* from the cytosol to the membrane
on stimulation of neutrophils, suggesting that one or both components of the
flavocytochrome act as a membrane docking site for the soluble components (Fig. 3,
left) *(12,17)*. Rac translocation was greatly decreased in the absence of the flavocytochrome (*see* next section). In A67° CGD, there was apparently normal translocation of p47-*phox*, but no detectable translocation of p40-*phox* (Fig. 3, middle) *(17,92)*,
whereas in the absence of p47-*phox* (A47° CGD), neither p40-*phox* nor p67-*phox* translocated (Fig. 3, right) *(17,92)*. Similar results for p47-*phox* and p67-*phox* have been

obtained with a transfected cell model capable of O_2^- generation *(93)*. Translocation of the cytosolic *phox* components therefore depends not only on the flavocytochrome but also on p47-*phox*, suggesting that this protein plays a central role in NADPH oxidase assembly.

This conclusion is supported by studies that have explored the interactions between the soluble and membrane-bound oxidase components. From Fig. 2 it is clear that the majority of interactions likely to account for activation-dependent translocation occur between the subunits of flavocytochrome-b_{558} and p47-*phox*. To date no direct association of either p67-*phox* or p40-*phox* with the flavocytochrome subunits has been reported, consistent with their apparent dependence on p47-*phox* for translocation. The principal interactions that mediate p47-*phox* association with the flavocytochrome are those between (1) the SH3 domains of p47-*phox* and proline-rich region(s) in the C-terminal tail of p22-*phox* (Fig. 2C,D); (2) multiple sites on gp91-*phox* and unknown regions of p47-*phox* (Fig. 2A); and (3) a region encompassing amino acids 323–342 of p47-*phox* and an unknown domain in the flavocytochrome (Fig. 2B).

Although p47-*phox* appears to have a predominant role in the assembly of the soluble oxidase components at the plasma or phagosomal membrane, there is good evidence that p67-*phox* must also be able to interact with the flavocytochrome. First, A47° (but not X91° or A22°) CGD neutrophils are capable of producing low levels of intracellular oxidants (e.g., hydrogen peroxide) *(94,95)*, a fact that may contribute to the less severe clinical picture in this form of the disease *(21)*. Second, in cell-free NADPH oxidase activation systems, high concentrations of p67-*phox* (together with GTP-bound Rac) can facilitate electron flow, in the absence of p47-*phox* *(64,65,96,97)*. Any interaction between p67-*phox* and the flavocytochrome (without p47-*phox* to stabilize it) may be of too low an affinity or be too transient for detection by crude biochemical techniques. The site(s) of interaction is unknown, but it has been argued that p67-*phox* is a better candidate than p47-*phox* for binding to and moving the putative coil structure of gp91-*phox* that lies over the NADPH-binding cleft in the inactive state (Fig. 2L) *(44,85)*. This model would certainly be consistent with the view that p67-*phox* regulates electron flow from NADPH to the flavin *(64,65)*.

Interactions Between Rac and Phagocyte Oxidase Components

On activation of NADPH oxidase by phorbol myristate acetate (PMA) or FMLP and possibly under the influence of lipid mediators, Rac separates from its GDI and becomes stably associated with the plasma membrane *(91,98–101)*. Based on experiments with X91° CGD neutrophils, in which the authors saw greatly reduced (by approx 75%) levels of Rac in the plasma membrane, they proposed that flavocytochrome-b_{558} is required for maximum stability of the GTP-binding protein in the membrane of activated neutrophils *(99)*. The remaining low level of Rac translocation in the absence of flavocytochrome, in addition to results from cell-free translocation experiments, suggested that Rac is able to associate with a site in the membrane distinct from the gp91-*phox*/p22-*phox* heterodimer. The authors and Dusi et al. *(92,99,102)* have reported that the translocation of Rac2 in A47° and A67° CGD is normal or near normal, indicating that its association with the membrane is independent of the soluble *phox* proteins (Fig. 3). Others have suggested that Rac2 fails to translocate in the absence of p47-*phox* *(101)*. With Rac1, Dusi et al. *(92,102)* saw a different pattern, suggesting that its translocation was dependent not only on the presence but also the translocation of p67-*phox*, consistent with the binding studies described below. It is important to note, however, that Philips et al. *(103)* have demonstrated that the association of Rac with the membrane is not required for O_2^- generation, and in at least two reports no stable association of Rac with the membrane was observed *(85,103,104)*. It is possible that the membrane association of Rac is an epiphenomenon, occurring solely by virtue of its exposed C-terminal geranylgeranyl group.

Rac is essential for phagocyte NADPH oxidase activity, but its precise role remains unknown. Clearly an important step in determining its role is to identify the target proteins within the oxidase complex with which it interacts. To date most of the evidence points not to the membrane-bound flavocytochrome, but to the cytosolic/cytoskeletal-associated protein p67-*phox*. GTP-bound, but not GDP-bound, Rac bound to a glutathione-*S*-transferase (GST)-p67-*phox* fusion protein but not to GST-p47-*phox*. Rho, a closely related GTP-binding protein, interacted with neither *phox* subunit. Rac1 bound to the N-terminal 199 amino acids of p67-*phox* (i.e., neither SH3 domain was required) and mutated forms of Rac that failed to interact with p67-*phox* greatly supported lower levels of superoxide generation in a cell-free assay system *(105)*.

Several additional studies have provided support for the view that p67-*phox* is a target for Rac in NADPH oxidase activation. Prigmore et al. *(106)*, using a nitrocellulose binding assay, detected an interaction between rp67-*phox* and both Rac1 and CDC42Hs, a closely related protein with approx 70% identity that has no or very weak NADPH oxidase–stimulating activity. Using the yeast two-hybrid system in a semiquantitative assay, Dorseuil et al. *(107)* showed that the binding of p67-*phox* to Rac2 is approximately six-fold greater than its binding to Rac1. They found no evidence for a direct interaction between Rac and p40-*phox*, p47-*phox*, or the cytochrome subunits.

The use of Rac1-CDC42Hs chimeras has localized the domain specifying oxidase activity to the N-terminal 40 amino acids of Rac. Point mutations within this domain diminished cell-free oxidase activation and abolished the interaction with p67-*phox (108)*. These findings are supported by a recent study of Rac interactions with p67-*phox*, which has the virtue of combining functional steady-state kinetic measurements of O_2^- generation with direct physical measurements of Rac and p67-*phox* interaction *(109)*. Rac1 and Rac2 bound to p67-*phox* with a 1:1 stoichiometry and with K_d values of 120 and 60 nM, respectively. Point mutations within the Rac1 "effector" region (amino acid 26–45) greatly increased the K_d for binding to p67-*phox* and the concentration of Rac required in a cell-free O_2^--generating system. Point mutations within the so-called "insert" region (amino acids 124–135) of Rac1 did not change the affinity of the protein for p67-*phox*, but did decrease its ability to activate the NADPH oxidase. Based on these data, the authors proposed a model in which the Rac "effector" region binds to p67-*phox* (Fig. 2), the "insert" region interacts with a different component, possibly flavocytochrome-b_{558}, and the isoprenylated C-terminus binds to the membrane *(109,110)*.

Structure–Function Information Derived from Mutations That Occur in CGD

Mutations in the Subunits of Flavocytochrome-b$_{558}$

Mutations in gp91-phox

Over 220 mutations causing X-linked CGD have been identified in the gene for gp91-*phox*. A comprehensive review of all these mutations is beyond the scope of this chapter, but further details are available in recent reviews *(21,31)* and in databases accessible on the Internet.*

Deletions (ranging from several million to a single nucleotide) and insertions account for approx 35% of the characterized mutations in X-CGD. The remaining 65% consist of nucleotide substitutions, which can be subdivided into (1) splice site mutations leading to misprocessing of mRNA (16%); (2) nonsense mutations causing premature termination of protein synthesis (26%); and (3) missense mutations causing substitution of a single amino acid (23%). The final category of mutations provides the most information about the different domains of gp91-*phox*. Although most mutations lead to the total absence or greatly diminished levels of protein (X91°or X91$^-$ CGD) and are relatively uninformative, 11 of the 43 characterized missense mutations, plus one in-frame deletion, a splice site mutation, and an in-frame deletion/insertion cause X91$^+$ CGD. The phagocytes of these patients contain normal levels of nonfunctional protein. These mutations are shown on a membrane-spanning model of gp91-*phox* in Fig. 4 and are discussed in more detail below.

Two mutations at amino acid 54 have been described, 54Arg→Gly and 54Arg→Ser, and both result in normal levels of stable gp91-*phox* and inactive cytochrome-b_{558}. The effect of the 54Arg→Gly mutation has not been well characterized *(111)*, but cytochrome with the 54Arg→Ser mutation has a slightly shifted absorbance spectrum. The mutant cytochrome permitted normal translocation of p47-*phox* and p67-*phox*, and the NADPH-binding and flavin regions of the protein appeared to function normally. However, the heme centers did not become reduced and no O_2^- was generated *(95)*. Potentiometric measurements revealed two nonidentical heme centers with midpoint potentials of −220 and −300 mV, compared to −225 and −265 mV in normal cytochrome b_{558}. In the mutant cytochrome, the decrease in midpoint potential of one heme center by 35 mV appears to prevent the transfer of electrons from FAD via the heme groups to oxygen. The authors proposed that 54Arg, close to the extracellular surface of a membrane-spanning domain, could interact with the propionyl side chain of a heme group forming a ligand with one of the histidines in the adjoining membrane segment (amino acids 100–120) (Fig. 4) *(35)*.

A recent report described a patient with X91$^+$ CGD in which an in-frame triplet nucleotide deletion caused the loss of phenylalanine at position 215 or 216 *(113)*. Based on analysis of the heme spectrum, the patient's neutrophils contained <2% of normal levels of flavocytochrome-b_{558}, and p22-*phox* was undetectable by flow cytometry. Surprisingly, immunoblot analysis revealed normal levels of gp91-*phox* in neutrophil membrane preparations. These findings suggest that deletion of 215Phe or 216Phe, predicted to be in a membrane-spanning domain between two histidines that potentially serve as heme ligands (Fig. 4), not only interferes with the ability of the gp91-*phox* to bind heme but also impairs its interaction with p22-*phox*, leading to instability of this subunit.

A single missense mutation (341Thr→Lys) causing X91$^+$ CGD has been found in the proposed FAD-binding region of gp91-*phox* *(111)*. The resulting flavocytochrome

---

*An X-CGD database with patients listed by accession number is available at http://www.helsinki.fi/science/signal/databases/x-cgdbase.html *(111)*, and a table of X-CGD mutations in order of affected nucleotide(s) is available at http://seconde.scripps.edu/is199724.html#A1 *(112)*.

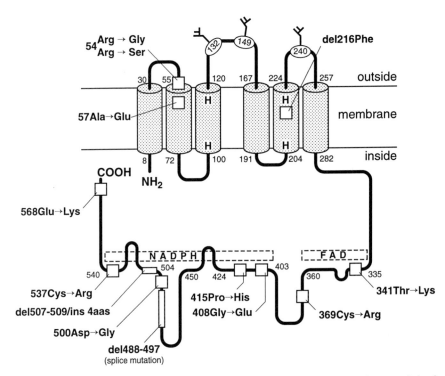

Fig. 4. Mutations causing X91⁺ CGD shown on a membrane-spanning model of gp91-*phox*. The four histidines (residues 101, 115, 209, and 222) likely to bind the two heme groups of the flavocytochrome are shown by single-letter code (H) in two of the membrane-spanning domains. Asparagines identified as being glycosylated *(36)* are identified by their residue numbers (132, 149, and 240). The proposed FAD and NADPH-binding domains are based on data and sequence comparisons in refs. *7, 8,* and *43*. Open boxes indicate 13 mutations known to cause X91⁺ CGD *(see text* for more details). Stippled cylinders indicate likely membrane spanning domains, and numbering of amino acids is from the N-terminus.

has not been biochemically characterized. One might expect the heme signal to be normal, but binding of FAD and electron transport through the flavin center to be adversely affected.

As shown in Fig. 4, several X91⁺ mutations have been identified within the proposed NADPH-binding domains of gp91-*phox* or in loops exposed to the cytosol near this region. The 408Gly→Glu mutation leads to normal levels of inactive flavocytochrome-b_{558} and greatly decreased translocation of p47-*phox* and p67*phox* (*31*). As Leusen et al. *(85)* have noted, 408Gly is likely to be buried in the protein and unavailable for direct binding to cytosolic proteins. This suggests that the mutation must disturb neighboring domains or loops that interact with the soluble components. Decreased translocation of cytosolic components was also seen in neutrophils from one patient with a 369Cys→Arg substitution in a loop between the putative FAD- and NADPH-binding domains *(85)*, and another patient with a 500Asp→Gly mutation in the 20-amino acid coil, believed to cover the NADPH binding cleft in the noncatalytic state *(44,114)*. This coil has been identified by peptide inhibition studies as a binding region for either p47-*phox* or p67-*phox* (Fig. 2).

Translocation of p47-*phox* and p67-*phox* was not disrupted in neutrophils from a patient with a 415Pro→His mutation *(17,115)*. However, gp91-*phox* in neutrophil membranes from this patient showed no binding of 2-azido-NADP, a photoaffinity label that bound nonmutant gp91-*phox* *(8)*. This finding lends weight to the argument that gp91-*phox* contains the NADPH-binding site and that the flavocytochrome alone performs the catalytic activities of the oxidase *(116)*.

Two rather unusual mutations occur in or adjacent to the NADPH-binding region. The first is a splice-site mutation (ag→gg at the 3' end of intron 11) that activates a cryptic splice site and leads to the expression of gp91-*phox* with 10 amino acids deleted (deletion of 488–497) *(117)*. The flavocytochrome-b_{558} was spectrally and quantitatively normal, but the neutrophils generated O_2^- at only 6% of the normal rate. As the deletion is located within the 20-amino acid coil mentioned above, it is likely that it disrupts the interaction with the cytosolic components and/or prevents proper access of NADPH to its binding site. The second unusual mutation involves the deletion of five and insertion of eight nucleotides in exon 12 of the gp91-*phox* gene. In the resulting protein, the amino acids 507Gln508Lys509Thr are deleted, and HisIleTrpAla are inserted *(118)*. Formation of the complete NADPH oxidase complex occurred in the affected neutrophils (i.e., p47-*phox* and p67-*phox* translocated normally) but no O_2^- was generated, consistent with the location of the mutation in an NADPH-binding domain.

The cysteine at position 537, recently found to be mutated to arginine in an X91$^+$ CGD patient *(111)* is in a CysGly motif that is highly conserved in other NAD(P)H-dependent flavoproteins *(7)*. It is therefore likely that 537Cys plays an important role in the catalysis of electron flow from NADPH to FAD, and that the mutation disrupts this process. Finally, the 568Glu→Lys mutation (the third amino acid from the C-terminus) is in a region of the protein tentatively identified by Rotrosen et al. *(7)* as acting as a flavin-shielding domain in the absence of substrate NADPH. This region also provides a site of interaction with p47-*phox* (*see* Fig. 2 and references therein).

It is noteworthy that although only 4 of 22 missense mutations (or in-frame deletions) in the N-terminal half of gp91-*phox* lead to normal levels of flavocytochrome, over half (10 out of 19) of these types of mutations occurring in the C-terminal cytosolic domain result in X91$^+$ CGD. It seems that minor changes within the membrane-spanning half of the protein are more likely to lead to an unstable product, perhaps by interfering with heme binding or association with the p22-*phox* subunit during processing *(45,46)*. The cytosolic portion of the protein is less susceptible to single amino acid changes or small deletions, but when mutations occur they cause protein dysfunction by altering the NADPH- or FAD-binding domains, or by disrupting important interactions with the cytosolic components.

p22-phox

Although the number of individuals affected is far fewer, the molecular basis of A22 CGD appears to be as heterogeneous as that of X91 CGD. Ten different mutations have been identified in the gene for p22-*phox* from nine affected families. Of five known missense mutations causing changes in single amino acids (Table 2), four presumably result in unstable product as no protein has been detected by immunoblot. Only a single mutation (467 C→A) has been identified that results in A22$^+$ CGD. Interestingly, the resulting protein has a substitution of 156Pro→Gln, within a proline-rich region of the intracellular C-terminal tail of p22-*phox* (Fig. 5) *(119)*. This region serves as a

Table 2
Mutations in the Gene for p22-*phox*

cDNA nucleotide change[a]	Mutation	Amino acid change	CGD type	Reference
>10 kb	Deletion	Not applicable	A22°	*41*
158 A→T	Missense	53Glu→Val	A22°	*135*
G between 166 C and 172 A	Insertion	Frameshift	A22°	*135*
244 C	Deletion	Frameshift	A22°	*41*
269 G→A	Missense	90Arg→Gln	A22°	*41,136*
281 A→G	Missense	94His→Arg	A22°	*136*
5' intron 4 gt→at	Splice site	Deletion of exon 4	A22°	*136*
354 C→A	Missense	118Ser→Arg	A22°	*41*
5' intron 5 gt→ct	Splice site	Deletion of exon 5	A22°	*31*
467 C→A	Missense	156Pro→Gln	A22+	*119*

[a]The cDNA numbering system used here follows the convention that +1 is the A of the ATG initiator codon. This differs from the numbering of the GenBank sequence; for p22-*phox* (GenBank accession nos. M21186 and J03774), subtract 28 from the GenBank sequence number to arrive at the number used here.

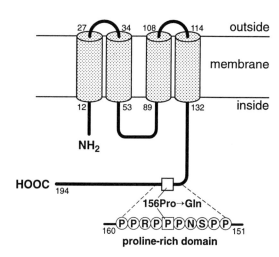

Fig. 5. Model of p22-*phox* showing a single known mutation causing A22+ CGD. Stippled cylinders indicate likely membrane-spanning domains. The position of the 156Pro→Gln mutation is shown by an open square within the SH3-binding proline-rich domain of the cytosolic C-terminal portion of the protein.

binding site for an SH3 domain of p47-*phox* (Fig. 2). In PMA-activated neutrophils from the affected patient, the translocation of p47-*phox* and p67-*phox* to the plasma membrane was greatly diminished. Similarly, in a cell-free translocation assay, neutrophil membranes from the patient failed to bind detectable levels of the cytosolic oxidase components *(48)*. Thus, it appears that the proline-rich region (amino acids 151–160) does indeed play an important functional role, perhaps a dominant role, in promoting membrane association of p47-*phox* and p67-*phox*. The substitution of proline at position 156 with glutamine appears to disrupt the interaction between p47-*phox* and the flavocytochrome. To the authors' knowledge, this is the first mutation identified that

Table 3
Mutations in the Gene for p67-*phox*

cDNA nucleotide change[a]	Mutation	Amino acid change	CGD type	Reference
55–63 AAGAAGGAC	Deletion	19–21 LysLysAsp	A67°	*137*
170–172 AGA or 171–173 GAA or 172–174 AAG	Deletion	Deletion of 58Lys	A67[-b]	*120,138*
233 G→A	Missense	78Gly→Glu	A67°	*139*
5' intron 3 gt→gc	Splice site	Deletion of exon 3	A67°	*140*
304 C→T	Nonsense	102 Arg→stop	A67°	*137*
5' intron 4 gt→at	Splice site	Deletion of exon 3 and 4, or exon 4, or last nucleotides of exon 4	A67°	*137*
AG after 397 A (or 399 G)	Insertion	Frameshift	A67°	*141*
479 A→T and 481 A→G	Double missense	160–161AspLys→ValGlu	A67°	*142*
5' intron 9 gt→at	Splice site	Deletion of exon 8 and 9	A67°	*143*
1169–1173 CTAAG	Deletion	Frameshift	A67°	*137*
1183 C→T	Missense	395Arg→Trp	A67°	*137*

[a]Subtract 67 from Genbank numbering (accession no. M32011).
[b]Patient is heterozygous for this mutation and an undefined deletion of 11–13 kb in the other allele.

disrupts the binding between an SH3 domain and a proline-rich region and causes a genetic disease.

Mutations in Cytosolic Components

Mutations in p67-phox

To date 11 mutations in the gene for p67-*phox* have been characterized (*see* Table 3). These mutations are distributed among 12 A67 patients (for a total of 24 affected alleles) and are discussed in more detail in the papers cited in Table 3. In all but one of these patients, the p67-*phox* protein is undetectable (A67°CGD), and the mutations are therefore relatively uninformative about the structure and function of the protein. The single exception is a female CGD patient who is a compound heterozygote for a large deletion of 11–13 kb in one allele of the p67-*phox* gene and a triplet nucleotide deletion that predicts the in-frame deletion of 58Lys in the other *(120)*. The mutant p67-*phox*Δ58Lys is apparently expressed and stable because neutrophils from the patient contained approximately one-half the normal amount of p67-*phox* as measured by quantitative immunoblot. Some interesting biochemical findings have been reported on the phagocytes of this patient. First, no translocation of either p47-*phox* or p67-*phox*Δ58Lys occurred on stimulation of affected neutrophils with PMA or zymosan. Second, GTP-loaded Rac1 bound to a GST-p67-*phox* fusion protein in a dot-blot assay but failed to bind to a GST-p67-*phox*Δ58Lys fusion protein, indicating that the deletion of 58Lys in p67-*phox* disrupts the interaction with the GTP-binding protein. The authors concluded that interaction between p67-*phox* and Rac1 is essential for translocation of p47-*phox* and p67-*phox* and the assembly of an active oxidase at the membrane. There are, however, two important caveats. First, it is somewhat surprising that translocation of p47-*phox* did not occur in these affected neutrophils as several studies have shown that in the absence of p67-*phox* (e.g., in A67°CGD), the association of p47-*phox* with the plasma membrane is normal or near normal (*see* Translation of Soluble Oxidase Components). These previous studies indicate, therefore, that the binding of Rac to p67-*phox* is *not* essential for the interaction of p47-*phox* with the flavocytochrome. It is possible that te deletion of 58Lys produces a dominant negative form of p67-*phox* that prevents the complex of cytosolic oxidase components from associating with the membrane. The second caveat arises because the authors were unable to detect any binding of Rac2 to wild-type p67-*phox* in their dot-blot assay, although at least two studies have indicated that Rac2 has a higher affinity for p67-*phox* than Rac1 *(107,109)*. It remains uncertain how the Δ58Lys mutation prevents activation of O_2^- generation, but it is likely that this and similar mutants will be informative in understanding the role of Rac-p67-*phox* interactions.

Mutations in p47-phox and the Identification of a Pseudogene

By contrast to other forms of the disease, in which the majority of mutations are family specific, a single common mutation has been reported in over 60 patients worldwide with A47°CGD *(31,121–124)*. All but four of these individuals appeared to be homozygous for the mutation, a dinucleotide deletion (ΔGT) at a GTGT repeat at the beginning of exon 2 that predicts a frameshift and a premature stop codon at amino acid 51. In one of the four patients who are apparently heterozygous for ΔGT, a single nucleotide deletion (502 G) has also been observed *(123)*.

An examination of normal genomic DNA revealed, surprisingly, that in 34 healthy individuals, not only the normal GTGT sequence was present in the PCR product, but also a superimposed sequence with the ΔGT (Fig. 6). This suggested that a very similar gene (e.g., a pseudogene) was coamplified and cosequenced with the normal p47-*phox* gene in these experiments. The generation of p47-*phox* clones from three different types of human genomic libraries, containing either the GTGT sequence or the GT deletion, confirmed the existence in the normal population of a gene with ΔGT *(125)*. In addition to the GT deletion, the isolated pseudogene clones contained nine single bp substitutions within exonic regions as well as a number of differences within introns that differentiated them from the p47-*phox* wild-type gene. Genomic DNA from normal controls and A47°CGD patients was analyzed for the presence of two of these additional pseudogene markers *(124)*. Seventeen of 20 patients homozygous for the ΔGT mutation were also homozygous for a pseudogene-specific CG→TG transversion in intron 1. Seven of these 17 patients were also homozygous for a 20-bp duplication in intron 2, and therefore possessed only pseudogene-specific alleles at all three positions. Genomic DNA from all healthy donors possessed both p47-*phox* gene and pseudogene alleles based on the analysis of these markers. It is evident from these studies that recombination events (e.g., crossovers with deletions, gene conversions) between the p47-*phox* gene and a highly homologous pseudogene are the main cause of A47°CGD.

Future Studies

The elucidation of the phagocyte NADPH oxidase and our understanding of CGD have progressed in unison. The discovery of many of the oxidase components has resulted from the study of different forms of CGD. Similarly, the molecular and biochemical dissection of the oxidase system has led to our understanding of the molecular mechanisms causing the disease. It is likely that all components specific to the oxidase are now known and although CGD mutational analysis may provide further clues, other approaches will also be necessary to wrestle the final secrets from the NADPH oxidase

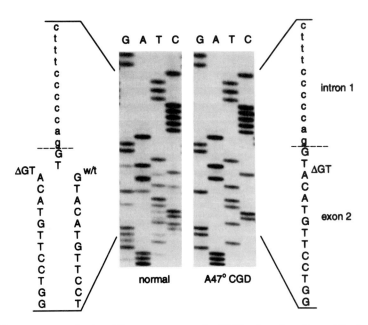

Fig. 6. Sequence analysis of human genomic DNA showing the p47-*phox* gene and pseudogene. Genomic DNA derived from a normal individual and a patient with A47° CGD was amplified by PCR and sequenced. In all normal individuals analyzed, two superimposed sequences were observed starting after the first GT at the beginning of exon 2. They correspond to the wild-type p47-*phox* gene sequence and to the sequence of a highly homologous pseudogene in which one GT of the GTGT tandem repeat is deleted (ΔGT), causing a frameshift and a premature stop at codon 51 (not shown) *(125)*. The A47° CGD patient shows only the pseudogene sequence. Recombination events between the wild-type gene and the pseudogene probably cause the majority of cases of A47° CGD. Dashed lines show the intron/exon boundaries, with the intronic and exonic sequence shown in lower case and upper case letters, respectively.

system. Sophisticated biochemical, cytochemical, and genetic studies will be required to answer some of the questions still facing investigators in this field. These include (1) What are the specific roles of the cytosolic *phox* components in the assembly and activation of the system? (2) What are the roles of the GTP-binding proteins, Rac and Rap1A? (3) How is electron transport regulated through the FAD and heme centers of the flavocytochrome? (4) Which kinases and phosphatases regulate the cycle of phosphorylation and dephosphorylation of p47-*phox* that appears to regulate its association and possibly dissociation from the flavocytochrome? (5) What are the specific cytoskeletal elements with which the oxidase components interact? It is likely to be the coordinated regulation of the cytoskeleton and NADPH oxidase activation that allows O_2^- to be generated at specific sites (e.g., regions of the plasma membrane attached to the substratum or forming phagosomes) rather than globally, throughout the periphery of the cell *(3)*. This additional control mechanism would help prevent the promiscuous release of reactive oxygen species and limit their damage to cells and tissues that occurs during the inflammatory process.

Acknowledgments

This work was supported by grants AI24838 and CA68276 (P.G.H.), and AI23323, and DK50015 (J.A.B.) from the National Institutes of Health. The authors are grateful to Valerie Moreau for her help in preparing the manuscript, Deborah Noack for running the sequencing gel in Fig. 6, and the staff of TSRI Biomedical Graphics for their assistance with the artwork.

References

1. Morel, F., Doussiere, J., and Vignais, P. V. (1991) The superoxide-generating oxidase of phagocytic cells: Physiological, molecular and pathological aspects. *Eur. J. Biochem.* **201,** 523–546.
2. DeLeo, F. R. and Quinn, M. T. (1996) Assembly of the phagocyte NADPH oxidase: Molecular interaction of oxidase proteins. *J. Leukocyte Biol.* **60,** 677–691.
3. Robinson, J. M. and Badwey, J. A. (1995) The NADPH oxidase complex of phagocytic leukocytes: A biochemical and cytochemical view. *Histochemistry* **103,** 163–180.
4. Dinauer, M. C., Orkin, S. H., Brown, R., Jesaitis, A. J., and Parkos, C. A. (1987) The glycoprotein encoded by the X-linked chronic granulomatous disease locus is a component of the neutrophil cytochrome b complex. *Nature* **327,** 717–720.
5. Parkos, C. A., Allen, R. A., Cochrane, C. G., and Jesaitis, A. J. (1987) Purified cytochrome *b* from human granulocyte plasma membrane is comprised of two polypeptides with relative molecular weights of 91,000 and 22,000. *J. Clin. Invest.* **80,** 732–742.
6. Segal, A. W. (1987) Absence of both cytochrome b_{-245} subunits from neutrophils in X-linked chronic granulomatous disease. *Nature* **326,** 88–91.
7. Rotrosen, D., Yeung, C. L., Leto, T. L., Malech, H. L., and Kwong, C. H. (1992) Cytochrome b_{558}: the flavin-binding component of the phagocyte NADPH oxidase. *Science* **256,** 1459–1462.
8. Segal, A. W., West, I., Wientjes, F., Nugent, J. H. A., Chavan, A. J., Haley, B., Garcia, R. C., Rosen, H., and Scrace, G. (1992) Cytochrome b_{-245} is a flavocytochrome containing FAD and the NADPH-binding site of the microbicidal oxidase of phagocytes. *Biochem. J.* **284,** 781–788.
9. Curnutte, J. T., Scott, P. J., and Mayo, L. A. (1989) Cytosolic components of the respiratory burst oxidase: Resolution of four components, two of which are missing in complementing types of chronic granulomatous disease. *Proc. Natl. Acad. Sci. USA* **86,** 825–829.
10. Volpp, B. D., Nauseef, W. M., and Clark, R. A. (1988) Two cytosolic neutrophil oxidase components absent in autosomal chronic granulomatous disease. *Science* **242,** 1295–1297.
11. Nunoi, H., Rotrosen, D., Gallin, J. I., and Malech, H. L. (1988) Two forms of autosomal chronic granulomatous disease lack distinct neutrophil cytosol factors. *Science* **242,** 1298–1301.
12. Wientjes, F. B., Hsuan, J. J., Totty, N. F., and Segal, A. W. (1993) p40–*phox*, a third cytosolic component of the activation complex of the NADPH oxidase to contain *src* homology 3 domains. *Biochem. J.* **296,** 557–561.
13. Heyworth, P. G., Peveri, P., and Curnutte, J. T. (1992) Cytosolic components of NADPH oxidase: Identity, function, and role in regulation of oxidase activity, in *Cellular and Molecular Mechanisms of Inflammation, vol. 4, Biological Oxidants: Generation and Injurious Consequences* (Cochrane, C. G. and Gimbrone, M. A., Jr., eds.), Academic, San Diego, CA, pp. 43–81.
14. Park, J.-W., Ma, M., Ruedi, J. M., Smith, R. M., and Babior, B. M. (1992) The cytosolic components of the respiratory burst oxidase exist as a M_r (approx.) 240,000 complex that acquires a membrane-binding site during activation of the oxidase in a cell-free system. *J. Biol. Chem.* **267,** 17,327–17,332.
15. Heyworth, P. G., Shrimpton, C. F., and Segal, A. W. (1989) Localization of the 47 kDa phosphoprotein involved in the respiratory-burst NADPH oxidase of phagocytic cells. *Biochem. J.* **260,** 243–248.
16. Clark, R. A., Volpp, B. D., Leidal, K. G., and Nauseef, W. M. (1990) Two cytosolic components of the human neutrophil respiratory burst oxidase translocate to the plasma membrane during cell activation. *J. Clin. Invest.* **85,** 714–721.
17. Heyworth, P. G., Curnutte, J. T., Nauseef, W. M., Volpp, B. D., Pearson, D. W., Rosen, H., and Clark, R. A. (1991) Neutrophil NADPH oxidase assembly: Translocation of p47-*phox* and p67-*phox* requires interaction between p47-*phox* and cytochrome b_{558}. *J. Clin. Invest.* **87,** 352–356.

18. Abo, A., Pick, E., Hall, A., Totty, N., Teahan, C. G., and Segal, A. W. (1991) Activation of the NADPH oxidase involves the small GTP-binding protein p21^{rac1}. *Nature* **353,** 668–670.

19. Knaus, U. G., Heyworth, P. G., Evans, T., Curnutte, J. T., and Bokoch, G. M. (1991) Regulation of phagocyte oxygen radical production by the GTP-binding protein Rac 2. *Science* **254,** 1512–1515.

20. Quinn, M. T., Parkos, C. A., Walker, L., Orkin, S. H., Dinauer, M. C., and Jesaitis, A. J. (1989) Association of a Ras-related protein with cytochrome b of human neutrophils. *Nature* **342,** 198–200.

21. Curnutte, J. T. (1995) Disorders of phagocyte function, in *Hematology: Basic Principles and Practice* (Hoffman, R., Benz, E. J., Jr., Shattil, S. J., Furie, B., Cohen, H. J., and Silberstein, L. E., eds.), Churchill Livingstone, New York, pp. 792–818.

22. Lehrer, R. I. and Ganz, T. (1990) Antimicrobial polypeptides of human neutrophils. *Blood* **76,** 2169–2181.

23. Weiss, S. J. (1989) Tissue destruction by neutrophils. *N. Engl. J. Med.* **320,** 365–376.

24. Simon, R. H. and Ward, P. A. (1992) Adult respiratory distress syndrome, in *Inflammation: Basic Principles and Clinical Correlates* (Gallin, J. I., Goldstein, I. M., and Snyderman, R., eds.), Raven, New York, pp. 999–1016.

25. Seekamp, A., Mulligan, M. S., Till, G. O., and Ward, P. A. (1993) Requirements for neutrophil products and L-arginine in ischemia-reperfusion injury. *Am. J. Pathol.* **142,** 1217–1226.

26. Weitzman, S. A. and Gordon, L. I. (1990) Inflammation and cancer: Role of phagocyte-generated oxidants in carcinogenesis. *Blood* **76,** 655–663.

27. Schraufstatter, I. U. and Jackson, J. H. (1992) Early injury of cells by external oxidants and the consequences of DNA damage, in *Cellular and Molecular Mechanisms of Inflammation, vol. 4, Biological Oxidants: Generation and Injurious Consequences* (Cochrane, C. G. and Gimbrone, M. A., Jr., eds.), Academic, San Diego, CA, pp. 21–41.

28. Snyderman, R. and Uhing, R. J. (1992) Chemoattractant stimulus-response coupling, in *Inflammation: Basic Principles and Clinical Correlates* (Gallin, J. I., Goldstein, I. M., and Snyderman, R., eds.), Raven, New York, pp. 421–439.

29. Heyworth, P. G. and Badwey, J. A. (1990) Protein phosphorylation associated with the stimulation of neutrophils: modulation of superoxide production by protein kinase C and calcium. *J. Bioenerg. Biomemb.* **22,** 1–26.

30. Rossi, F., Grzeskowiak, M., Della Bianca, V., Calzetti, F., and Gandini, G. (1990) Phosphatidic acid and not diacylglycerol generated by phospholipase D is functionally linked to the activation of the NADPH oxidase by fMLP in human neutrophils. *Biochem. Biophys. Res. Commun.* **168,** 320–327.

31. Roos, D., De Boer, M., Kuribayashi, F., Meischl, C., Weening, R. S., Segal, A. W., Åhlin, A., Nemet, K., Hossle, J. P., Bernatowska-Matuszkiewicz, E., and Middleton-Price, H. (1996) Mutations in the X-linked and autosomal recessive forms of chronic granulomatous disease. *Blood* **87,** 1663–1681.

32. Segal, A. W. (1996) The NADPH oxidase and chronic granulomatous disease. *Mol. Med. Today* **2,** 129–135.

33. Wallach, T. M. and Segal, A. W. (1996) Stoichiometry of the subunits of flavocytochrome b_{558} of the NADPH oxidase of phagocytes. *Biochem. J.* **320,** 33–38.

34. Huang, J., Hitt, N. D., and Kleinberg, M. E. (1995) Stoichiometry of p22-*phox* and gp91-*phox* in phagocyte cytochrome b_{558}. *Biochemistry* **34,** 16,753–16,757.

35. Cross, A. R., Rae, J., and Curnutte, J. T. (1995) Cytochrome b_{-245} of the neutrophil superoxide-generating system contains two nonidentical hemes: Potentiometric studies of a mutant form of gp91-*phox*. *J. Biol. Chem.* **270,** 17,075–17,077.

36. Wallach, T. M. and Segal, A. W. (1997) Analysis of glycosylation sites on gp91-*phox*, the flavocytochrome of the NADPH oxidase, by site-directed mutagenesis and translation in vitro. *Biochem. J.* **321,** 583–585.

37. Rotrosen, D., Kleinberg, M. E., Nunoi, H., Leto, T. L., Gallin, J. I., and Malech, H. L. (1990) Evidence for a functional cytoplasmic domain of phagocyte oxidase cytochrome b_{558}. *J. Biol. Chem.* **265,** 8745–8750.

38. DeLeo, F. R., Yu, L., Burritt, J. B., Loetterle, L. R., Bond, C. W., Jesaitis, A. J., and Quinn, M. T. (1995) Mapping sites of interaction of p47-*phox* and flavocytochrome b with random-sequence peptide phage display libraries. *Proc. Natl. Acad. Sci. USA* **92,** 7110–7114.

39. Quinn, M. T., Mullen, M. L., and Jesaitis, A. J. (1992) Human neutrophil cytochrome *b* contains multiple hemes: evidence for heme associated with both subunits. *J. Biol. Chem.* **267,** 7303–7309.

40. Parkos, C. A., Dinauer, M. C., Walker, L. E., Allen, R. A., Jesaitis, A. J., and Orkin, S. H. (1988) Primary structure and unique expression of the 22-kilodalton light chain of human neutrophil cytochrome b. *Proc. Natl. Acad. Sci. USA* **85,** 3319–3323.

41. Dinauer, M. C., Pierce, E. A., Bruns, G. A. P., Curnutte, J. T., and Orkin, S. H. (1990) Human neutrophil cytochrome *b* light chain (p22-*phox*): gene structure, chromosomal location, and mutations in cytochrome-negative autosomal recessive chronic granulomatous disease. *J. Clin. Invest.* **86,** 1729–1737.

42. Zhou, Y. and Murtaugh, M. P. (1994) Cloning and expression of the gene encoding the porcine NADPH oxidase light-chain subunit (p22-*phox*). *Gene* **148,** 363–367.

43. Sumimoto, H., Sakamoto, N., Nozaki, M., Sakaki, Y., Takeshige, K., and Minakami, S. (1992) Cytochrome b_{558}, a component of the phagocyte NADPH oxidase, is a flavoprotein. *Biochem. Biophys. Res. Commun.* **186,** 1368–1375.

44. Taylor, W. R., Jones, D. T., and Segal, A. W. (1993) A structural model for the nucleotide binding domains of the flavocytochrome b$_{-245}$ b-chain. *Protein Sci.* **2,** 1675–1685.

45. Porter, C. D., Parkar, M. H., Verhoeven, A. J., Levinsky, R. J., Collins, M. K. L., and Kinnon, C. (1994) p22-*phox*-deficient chronic granulomatous disease: Reconstitution by retrovirus-mediated expression and identification of a biosynthetic intermediate of gp91-*phox. Blood* **84,** 2767–2775.

46. Yu, L., Zhen, L., and Dinauer, M. C. (1997) Biosynthesis of the phagocyte NADPH oxidase cytochrome b_{558}: role of heme incorporation and heterodimer formation in maturation and stability of gp91-*phox* and p22-*phox* subunits. *J. Biol. Chem.* **272,** 27,288–27,294.

47. Sumimoto, H., Hata, K., Mizuki, K., Ito, T., Kage, Y., Sakaki, Y., Fukumaki, Y., Nakamura, M., and Takeshige, K. (1996) Assembly and activation of the phagocyte NADPH oxidase: specific interaction of the N-terminal Src homology 3 domain of p47-*phox* with p22-*phox* is required for activation of the NADPH oxidase. *J. Biol. Chem.* **271,** 22,152–22,158.

48. Leusen, J. H. W., Bolscher, B. G. J. M., Hilarius, P. M., Weening, R. S., Kaulfersch, W., Seger, R. A., Roos, D., and Verhoeven, A. J. (1994) [156]Pro → Gln substitution in the light chain of cytochrome b_{558} of the human NADPH oxidase (p22-*phox*) leads to defective translocation of the cytosolic proteins p47-*phox* and p67-*phox. J. Exp. Med.* **180,** 2329–2334.

49. Leto, T. L., Adams, A. G., and De Mendez, I. (1994) Assembly of the phagocyte NADPH oxidase: binding of Src homology 3 domains to proline-rich targets. *Proc. Natl. Acad. Sci. USA* **91,** 10,650–10,654.

50. Sumimoto, H., Kage, Y., Nunoi, H., Sasaki, H., Nose, T., Fukumaki, Y., Ohno, M., Minakami, S., and Takeshige, K. (1994) Role of Src homology 3 domains in assembly and activation of the phagocyte NADPH oxidase. *Proc. Natl. Acad. Sci. USA* **91,** 5345–5349.

51. Segal, A. W., Heyworth, P. G., Cockcroft, S., and Barrowman, M. M. (1985) Stimulated neutrophils from patients with autosomal recessive chronic granulomatous disease fail to phosphorylate a M_r-44000 protein. *Nature* **316,** 547–549.

52. Volpp, B. D., Nauseef, W. M., Donelson, J. E., Moser, D. R., and Clark, R. A. (1989) Cloning of the cDNA and functional expression of the 47-kilodalton cytosolic component of human neutrophil respiratory burst oxidase. *Proc. Natl. Acad. Sci. USA* **86,** 7195–7199.

53. Lomax, K. J., Leto, T. L., Nunoi, H., Gallin, J. I., and Malech, H. L. (1989) Recombinant 47-kilodalton cytosol factor restores NADPH oxidase in chronic granulomatous disease. *Science* **245,** 409–412.

54. Leto, T. L., Lomax, K. J., Volpp, B. D., Nunoi, H., Sechler, J. M. G., Nauseef, W. M., Clark, R. A., Gallin, J. I., and Malech, H. L. (1990) Cloning of a 67-kD neutrophil oxidase factor with similarity to a noncatalytic region of p60[c-src]. *Science* **248,** 727–730.

55. Thrasher, A. J., Keep, N. H., Wientjes, F., and Segal, A. W. (1994) Chronic granulomatous disease. *Biochim. Biophys. Acta Mol. Basis Dis.* **1227,** 1–24.

56. Pawson, T. (1995) Protein modules and signalling networks. *Nature* **373,** 573–580.

57. Musacchio, A., Noble, M., Pauptit, R., Wierenga, R., and Saraste, M. (1992) Crystal structure of a Src-homology 3 (SH3) domain. *Nature* **359,** 851–855.

58. Ren, R., Mayer, B. J., Cicchetti, P., and Baltimore, D. (1993) Identification of a ten-amino acid proline-rich SH3 binding site. *Science* **259,** 1157–1161.

59. Rotrosen, D. and Leto, T. L. (1990) Phosphorylation of neutrophil 47-kDa cytosolic oxidase factor: translocation to membrane is associated with distinct phosphorylation events. *J. Biol. Chem.* **265,** 19,910–19,915.

60. El Benna, J., Faust, L. P., and Babior, B. M. (1994) The phosphorylation of the respiratory burst oxidase component p47-*phox* during neutrophil activation: phosphorylation of sites recognized by protein kinase C and by proline-directed kinases. *J. Biol. Chem.* **269,** 23,431–23,436.

61. Dusi, S. and Rossi, F. (1993) Activation of NADPH oxidase of human neutrophils involves the phosphorylation and the translocation of cytosolic p67-*phox*. *Biochem. J.* **296,** 367–371.

62. Heyworth, P. G., Ding, J., Erickson, R. W., Lu, D. J., Curnutte, J. T., and Badwey, J. A. (1996) Protein phosphorylation in neutrophils from patients with p67-*phox*-deficient chronic granulomatous disease. *Blood* **87,** 4404–4410.

63. El Benna, J., Dang, P. M. C., Gaudry, M., Fay, M., Morel, F., Hakim, J., and Gougerot-Pocidalo, M. A. (1997) Phosphorylation of the respiratory burst oxidase subunit p67-*phox* during human neutrophil activation: regulation by protein kinase C-dependent and independent pathways. *J. Biol. Chem.* **272,** 17,204–17,208.

64. Cross, A. R., Yarchover, J. L., and Curnutte, J. T. (1994) The superoxide-generating system of human neutrophils possesses a novel diaphorase activity: evidence for distinct regulation of electron flow within NADPH oxidase by p67-*phox* and p47-*phox*. *J. Biol. Chem.* **269,** 21,448–21,454.

65. Cross, A. R. and Curnutte, J. T. (1995) The cytosolic activating factors p47-*phox* and p67-*phox* have distinct roles in the regulation of electron flow in NADPH oxidase. *J. Biol. Chem.* **270,** 6543–6548.

66. Smith, R. M., Connor, J. A., Chen, L. M., and Babior, B. M. (1996) The cytosolic subunit p67-*phox* contains an NADPH-binding site that participates in catalysis by the leukocyte NADPH oxidase. *J. Clin. Invest.* **98,** 977–983.

67. Abo, A., Boyhan, A., West, I., Thrasher, A. J., and Segal, A. W. (1992) Reconstitution of neutrophil NADPH oxidase activity in the cell-free system by four components: p67-*phox*, p47-*phox*, p21*rac*1, and cytochrome b_{-245}. *J. Biol. Chem.* **267,** 16,767–16,770.

68. Sathyamoorthy, M., De Mendez, I., Adams, A. G., and Leto, T. L. (1997) p40-*phox* down-regulates NADPH oxidase activity through interactions with its SH3 domain. *J. Biol. Chem.* **272,** 9141–9146.

69. Didsbury, J., Weber, R. F., Bokoch, G. M., Evans, T., and Snyderman, R. (1989) *Rac*, a novel *ras*-related family of proteins that are botulinum toxin substrates. *J. Biol. Chem.* **264,** 16,378–16,382.

70. Knaus, U. G., Heyworth, P. G., Kinsella, B. T., Curnutte, J. T., and Bokoch, G. M. (1992) Purification and characterization of rac 2: A cytosolic GTP-binding protein that regulates human neutrophil NADPH oxidase. *J. Biol. Chem.* **267,** 23,575–23,582.

71. Mizuno, T., Kaibuchi, K., Ando, S., Musha, T., Hiraoka, K., Takaishi, K., Asada, M., Nunoi, H., Matsuda, I., and Takai, Y. (1992) Regulation of the superoxide-generating NADPH oxidase by a small GTP-binding protein and its stimulatory and inhibitory GDP/GTP exchange proteins. *J. Biol. Chem.* **267,** 10,215–10,218.

72. Kwong, C. H., Malech, H. L., Rotrosen, D., and Leto, T. L. (1993) Regulation of the human neutrophil NADPH oxidase by *rho*-related G-proteins. *Biochemistry* **32,** 5711–5717.

73. Haataja, L., Groffen, J., and Heisterkamp, N. (1997) Characterization of *RAC3*, a novel member of the Rho family. *J. Biol. Chem.* **272,** 20,384–20,388.

74. Maly, F.-E., Quilliam, L. A., Dorseuil, O., Der, C. J., and Bokoch, G. M. (1994) Activated or dominant inhibitory mutants of Rap1A decrease the oxidative burst of Epstein-Barr virus-transformed human B lymphocytes. *J. Biol. Chem.* **269,** 18,743–18,746.

75. Gabig, T. G., Crean, C. D., Mantel, P. L., and Rosli, R. (1995) Function of wild-type or mutant Rac2 and Rap1a GTPases in differentiated HL60 cell NADPH oxidase activation. *Blood* **85,** 804–811.

76. Quinn, M. T. (1996) Role of small GTP-binding proteins in leukocyte signal transduction, in *Signal Transduction in Leukocytes: G Protein-Related and Other Pathways* (Lad, P. M., Kaptein, J. S., and Lin, C.-K. E., eds.), CRC, Boca Raton, FL, pp. 75–142.

77. Zhan, S. X., Vazquez, N., Zhan, S. L., Wientjes, F. B., Budarf, M. L., Schrock, E., Ried, T., Green, E. D., and Chanock, S. J. (1996) Genomic structure, chromosomal localization, start of transcription, and tissue expression of the human p40-*phox*, a new component of the nicotinamide adenine dinucleotide phosphate-oxidase complex. *Blood* **88,** 2714–2721.

78. Curnutte, J. T., Orkin, S. H., and Dinauer, M. C. (1994) Genetic disorders of phagocyte function, in *The Molecular Basis of Blood Diseases* (Stamatoyannopoulos, G., Nienhuis, A. W., Majerus, P. W., and Varmus, H., eds.), W. B. Saunders, Philadelphia, pp. 493–540.

79. Pollock, J. D., Williams, D. A., Gifford, M. A. C., Li, L. L., Du, X., Fisherman, J., Orkin, S. H., Doerschuk, C. M., and Dinauer, M. C. (1995) Mouse model of X-linked chronic granulomatous disease, an inherited defect in phagocyte superoxide production. *Nature Genet.* **9**, 202–209.

80. Jackson, S. H., Gallin, J. I., and Holland, S. M. (1995) The p47-*phox* mouse knock-out model of chronic granulomatous disease. *J. Exp. Med.* **182**, 751–758.

81. Dinauer, M. C., Deck, M. B., and Unanue, E. R. (1997) Mice lacking reduced nicotinamide adenine dinucleotide phosphate oxidase activity show increased susceptibility to early infection with *Listeria monocytogenes*. *J. Immunol.* **158**, 5581–5583.

82. Morgenstern, D. E., Gifford, M. A. C., Li, L. L., Doerschuk, C. M., and Dinauer, M. C. (1997) Absence of respiratory burst in X-linked chronic granulomatous disease mice leads to abnormalities in both host defense and inflammatory response to *Aspergillus fumigatus*. *J. Exp. Med.* **185**, 207–218.

83. Björgvinsdóttir, H., Ding, C. J., Pech, N., Gifford, M. A., Li, L. L., and Dinauer, M. C. (1997) Retroviral-mediated gene transfer of gp91-*phox* into bone marrow cells rescues defect in host defense against *Aspergillus fumigatus* in murine X-linked chronic granulomatous disease. *Blood* **89**, 41–48.

84. Mardiney, M. III, Jackson, S. H., Spratt, S. K., Li, F., Holland, S. M., and Malech, H. L. (1997) Enhanced host defense after gene transfer in the murine p47-*phox*-deficient model of chronic granulomatous disease. *Blood* **89**, 2268–2275.

85. Leusen, J. H. W., Verhoeven, A. J., and Roos, D. (1996) Interactions between the components of the human NADPH oxidase: Intrigues in the *phox* family. *J. Lab. Clin. Med.* **128**, 461–476.

86. Someya, A., Nagaoka, I., and Yamashita, T. (1993) Purification of the 260 kDa cytosolic complex involved in the superoxide production of guinea pig neutrophils. *FEBS Lett.* **330**, 215–218.

87. Nauseef, W. M., Volpp, B. D., McCormick, S., Leidal, K. G., and Clark, R. A. (1991) Assembly of the neutrophil respiratory burst oxidase: protein kinase C promotes cytoskeletal and membrane association of cytosolic oxidase components. *J. Biol. Chem.* **266**, 5911–5917.

88. Curnutte, J. T., Erickson, R. W., Ding, J., and Badwey, J. A. (1994) Reciprocal interactions between protein kinase C and components of the NADPH oxidase complex may regulate superoxide production by neutrophils stimulated with a phorbol ester. *J. Biol. Chem.* **269**, 10,813–10,819.

89. Wientjes, F. B., Segal, A. W., and Hartwig, J. H. (1997) Immunoelectron microscopy shows a clustered distribution of NADPH oxidase components in the human neutrophil plasma membrane. *J. Leukocyte Biol.* **61**, 303–312.

90. Heyworth, P. G., Ellis, B. A., and Curnutte, J. T. (1997) Stoichiometry of the cytosolic NADPH oxidase components in their multiprotein complex in normal and chronic granulomatous disease (CGD) neutrophils. *Blood* **90**, 19a(abstract).

91. Quinn, M. T., Evans, T., Loetterle, L. R., Jesaitis, A. J., and Bokoch, G. M. (1993) Translocation of Rac correlates with NADPH oxidase activation: evidence for equimolar translocation of oxidase components. *J. Biol. Chem.* **268**, 20,983–20,987.

92. Dusi, S., Donini, M., and Rossi, F. (1996) Mechanisms of NADPH oxidase activation: translocation of p40-*phox*, Rac1 and Rac2 from the cytosol to the membranes in human neutrophils lacking p47-*phox* or p67-*phox*. *Biochem. J.* **314**, 409–412.

93. De Mendez, I., Adams, A. G., Sokolic, R. A., Malech, H. L., and Leto, T. L. (1996) Multiple SH3 domain interactions regulate NADPH oxidase assembly in whole cells. *EMBO J.* **15**, 1211–1220.

94. Vowells, S. J., Fleisher, T. A., Sekhsaria, S., Alling, D. W., Maguire, T. E., and Malech, H. L. (1996) Genotype-dependent variability in flow cytometric evaluation of reduced nicotinamide adenine dinucleotide phosphate oxidase function in patients with chronic granulomatous disease. *J. Pediatr.* **128**, 104–107.

95. Cross, A. R., Heyworth, P. G., Rae, J., and Curnutte, J. T. (1995) A variant X-linked chronic granulomatous disease patient (X91$^+$) with partially functional cytochrome *b*. *J. Biol. Chem.* **270**, 8194–8200.

96. Freeman, J. L. and Lambeth, J. D. (1996) NADPH oxidase activity is independent of p47-*phox* in vitro. *J. Biol. Chem.* **271**, 22,578–22,582.

97. Koshkin, V., Lotan, O., and Pick, E. (1996) The cytosolic component p47-*phox* is not a *sine qua non* participant in the activation of NADPH oxidase but is required for optimal superoxide production. *J. Biol. Chem.* **271,** 30,326–30,329.
98. Abo, A., Webb, M. R., Grogan, A., and Segal, A. W. (1994) Activation of NADPH oxidase involves the dissociation of p21^{rac} from its inhibitory GDP/GTP exchange protein (rhoGDI) followed by its translocation to the plasma membrane. *Biochem. J.* **298,** 585–591.
99. Heyworth, P. G., Bohl, B. P., Bokoch, G. M., and Curnutte, J. T. (1994) Rac translocates independently of the neutrophil NADPH oxidase components p47-*phox* and p67-*phox*: evidence for its interaction with flavocytochrome b_{558}. *J. Biol. Chem.* **269,** 30,749–30,752.
100. Chuang, T.-H., Bohl, B. P., and Bokoch, G. M. (1993) Biologically active lipids are regulators of Rac-GDI complexation. *J. Biol. Chem.* **268,** 26,206–26,211.
101. El Benna, J., Ruedi, J. M., and Babior, B. M. (1994) Cytosolic guanine nucleotide-binding protein Rac2 operates *in vivo* as a component of the neutrophil respiratory burst oxidase: transfer of Rac2 and the cytosolic oxidase components p47-*phox* and p67-*phox* to the submembranous actin cytoskeleton during oxidase activation. *J. Biol. Chem.* **269,** 6729–6734.
102. Dusi, S., Donini, M., and Rossi, F. (1995) Mechanisms of NADPH oxidase activation in human neutrophils: p67-*phox* is required for the translocation of rac 1 but not of rac 2 from cytosol to the membranes. *Biochem. J.* **308,** 991–994.
103. Philips, M. R., Feoktistov, A., Pillinger, M. H., and Abramson, S. B. (1995) Translocation of p21^{rac2} from cytosol to plasma membrane is neither necessary nor sufficient for neutrophil NADPH oxidase activity. *J. Biol. Chem.* **270,** 11,514–11,521.
104. Le Cabec, V., Möhn, H., Gacon, G., and Maridonneau-Parini, I. (1994) The small GTP-binding protein rac is not recruited to the plasma membrane upon NADPH oxidase activation in human neutrophils. *Biochem. Biophys. Res. Commun.* **198,** 1216–1224.
105. Diekmann, D., Abo, A., Johnston, C., Segal, A. W., and Hall, A. (1994) Interaction of Rac with p67-*phox* and regulation of phagocytic NADPH oxidase activity. *Science* **265,** 531–533.
106. Prigmore, E., Ahmed, S., Best, A., Kozma, R., Manser, E., Segal, A. W., and Lim, L. (1995) A 68-kDa kinase and NADPH oxidase component p67-*phox* are targets for Cdc42Hs and Rac1 in neutrophils. *J. Biol. Chem.* **270,** 10,717–10,722.
107. Dorseuil, O., Reibel, L., Bokoch, G. M., Camonis, J., and Gacon, G. (1996) The Rac target NADPH oxidase p67-*phox* interacts preferentially with Rac2 rather than Rac1. *J. Biol. Chem.* **271,** 83–88.
108. Kwong, C. H., Adams, A. G., and Leto, T. L. (1995) Characterization of the effector-specifying domain of Rac involved in NADPH oxidase activation. *J. Biol. Chem.* **270,** 19,868–19,872.
109. Nisimoto, Y., Freeman, J. L. R., Motalebi, S. A., Hirshberg, M., and Lambeth, J. D. (1997) Rac binding to p67-*phox*: Structural basis for interactions of the Rac1 effector region and insert region with components of the respiratory burst oxidase. *J. Biol. Chem.* **272,** 18,834–18,841.
110. Kreck, M. L., Freeman, J. L., Abo, A., and Lambeth, J. D. (1996) Membrane association of Rac is required for high activity of the respiratory burst oxidase. *Biochemistry* **35,** 15,683–15,692.
111. Roos, D., Curnutte, J. T., Hossle, J. P., Lau, Y. L., Ariga, T., Nunoi, H., Dinauer, M. C., Gahr, M., Segal, A. W., Newburger, P. E., Giacca, M., Keep, N. H., and van Zwieten, R. (1996) X-CGDbase: A database of X-CGD-causing mutations. *Immunol. Today* **17,** 517–521.
112. Heyworth, P. G., Curnutte, J. T., Rae, J., Noack, D., and Cross, A. R. (1996) Hematologically important mutations: X-linked chronic granulomatous disease—an update. *Blood Cells Mol. Dis.* **23,** 443–450.
113. Jendrossek, V., Ritzel, A., Neubauer, B., Heyden, S., and Gahr, M. (1997) An in-frame triplet deletion within the gp91-*phox* gene in an adult X-linked chronic granulomatous disease patient with residual NADPH-oxidase activity. *Eur. J. Haematol.* **58,** 78–85.
114. Leusen, J. H. W., De Boer, M., Bolscher, B. G. J. M., Hilarius, P. M., Weening, R. S., Ochs, H. D., Roos, D., and Verhoeven, A. J. (1994) A point mutation in gp91-*phox* of cytochrome b_{558} of the human NADPH oxidase leading to defective translocation of the cytosolic proteins p47-*phox* and p67-*phox*. *J. Clin. Invest.* **93,** 2120–2126.
115. Dinauer, M. C., Curnutte, J. T., Rosen, H., and Orkin, S. H. (1989) A missense mutation in the neutrophil cytochrome b heavy chain in cytochrome-positive X-linked chronic granulomatous disease. *J. Clin. Invest.* **84,** 2012–2016.
116. Koshkin, V. and Pick, E. (1993) Generation of superoxide by purified and relipidated cytochrome b_{559} in the absence of cytosolic activators. *FEBS Lett.* **327,** 57–62.

117. Schapiro, B. L., Newburger, P. E., Klempner, M. S., and Dinauer, M. C. (1991) Chronic granulomatous disease presenting in a 69-year-old man. *N. Engl. J. Med.* **325,** 1786–1790.

118. Azuma, H., Oomi, H., Sasaki, K., Kawabata, I., Sakaino, T., Koyano, S., Suzutani, T., Nunoi, H., and Okuno, A. (1995) A new mutation in exon 12 of the gp91-*phox* gene leading to cytochrome b-positive X-linked chronic granulomatous disease. *Blood* **85,** 3274–3277.

119. Dinauer, M. C., Pierce, E. A., Erickson, R. W., Muhlebach, T. J., Messner, H., Orkin, S. H., Seger, R. A., and Curnutte, J. T. (1991) Point mutation in the cytoplasmic domain of the neutrophil p22-*phox* cytochrome b subunit is associated with a nonfunctional NADPH oxidase and chronic granulomatous disease. *Proc. Natl. Acad. Sci. USA* **88,** 11,231–11,235.

120. Leusen, J. H. W., De Klein, A., Hilarius, P. M., Åhlin, A., Palmblad, J., Smith, C. I. E., Diekmann, D., Hall, A., Verhoeven, A. J., and Roos, D. (1996) Disturbed interaction of p21-*rac* with mutated p67-*phox* causes chronic granulomatous disease. *J. Exp. Med.* **184,** 1243–1249.

121. Casimir, C. M., Bu-Ghanim, H. N., Rodaway, A. R. F., Bentley, D. L., Rowe, P., and Segal, A. W. (1991) Autosomal recessive chronic granulomatous disease caused by deletion at a dinucleotide repeat. *Proc. Natl. Acad. Sci. USA* **88,** 2753–2757.

122. Iwata, M., Nunoi, H., Yamazaki, H., Nakano, T., Niwa, H., Tsuruta, S., Ohga, S., Ohmi, S., Kanegasaki, S., and Matsuda, I. (1994) Homologous dinucleotide GT or TG deletion in Japanese patients with chronic granulomatous disease with p47-*phox* deficiency. *Biochem. Biophys. Res. Commun.* **199,** 1372–1377.

123. Volpp, B. D. and Lin, Y. (1993) In vitro molecular reconstitution of the respiratory burst in B lymphoblasts from p47-*phox*-deficient chronic granulomatous disease. *J. Clin. Invest.* **91,** 201–207.

124. Roesler, J., Görlach, A., Rae, J., Hopkins, P. J., Patino, P., Lee, P., Curnutte, J. T., and Chanock, S. J. (1995) Recombination events between the normal p47-*phox* gene and a highly homologous pseudogene are the main cause of autosomal recessive chronic granulomatous disease (CGD). *Blood* **86,** 260a (abstract).

125. Görlach, A., Lee, P., Roesler, J., Hopkins, P. J., Christensen, B., Green, E. D., Chanock, S. J., and Curnutte, J. T. (1997) A p47-*phox* pseudogene carries the most common mutation causing p47-*phox*-deficient chronic granulomatous disease. *J. Clin. Invest.* **100,** 1907–1918.

126. DeLeo, F. R., Nauseef, W. M., Jesaitis, A. J., Burritt, J. B., Clark, R. A., and Quinn, M. T. (1995) A domain of p47-*phox* that interacts with human neutrophil flavocytochrome b_{558}. *J. Biol. Chem.* **270,** 26,246–26,251.

127. DeLeo, F. R., Ulman, K. V., Davis, A. R., Jutila, K. L., and Quinn, M. T. (1996) Assembly of the human neutrophil NADPH oxidase involves binding of p67-*phox* and flavocytochrome b to a common functional domain in p47-*phox*. *J. Biol. Chem.* **271,** 17,013–17,020.

128. De Mendez, I., Homayounpour, N., and Leto, T. L. (1997) Specificity of p47-*phox* SH3 domain interactions in NADPH oxidase assembly and activation. *Mol. Cell. Biol.* **17,** 2177–2185.

129. Fuchs, A., Dagher, M. C., Fauré, J., and Vignais, P. V. (1996) Topological organization of the cytosolic activating complex of the superoxide-generating NADPH-oxidase: pinpointing the sites of interaction between p47-*phox*, p67-*phox* and p40-*phox* using the two-hybrid system. *Biochim. Biophys. Acta Mol. Cell Res.* **1312,** 39–47.

130. Ito, T., Nakamura, R., Sumimoto, H., Takeshige, K., and Sakaki, Y. (1996) An SH3 domain-mediated interaction between the phagocyte NADPH oxidase factors p40-*phox* and p47-*phox*. *FEBS Lett.* **385,** 229–232.

131. Finan, P., Shimizu, Y., Gout, I., Hsuan, J., Truong, O., Butcher, C., Bennett, P., Waterfield, M. D., and Kellie, S. (1994) An SH3 domain and proline-rich sequence mediate an interaction between two components of the phagocyte NADPH oxidase complex. *J. Biol. Chem.* **269,** 13,752–13,755.

132. Wientjes, F. B., Panayotou, G., Reeves, E., and Segal, A. W. (1996) Interactions between cytosolic components of the NADPH oxidase: p40-*phox* interacts with both p67-*phox* and p47-*phox*. *Biochem. J.* **317,** 919–924.

133. Fuchs, A., Dagher, M.-C., and Vignais, P. V. (1995) Mapping the domains of interaction of p40-*phox* with both p47-*phox* and p67-*phox* of the neutrophil oxidase complex using the two-hybrid system. *J. Biol. Chem.* **270,** 5695–5697.

134. Tsunawaki, S., Kagara, S., Yoshikawa, K., Yoshida, L. S., Kuratsuji, T., and Namiki, H. (1996) Involvement of p40-*phox* in activation of phagocyte NADPH oxidase through association of its carboxyl-terminal, but not its amino-terminal, with p67-*phox*. *J. Exp. Med.* **184,** 893–902.

135. Hossle, J. P., De Boer, M., Seger, R. A., and Roos, D. (1994) Identification of allele-specific p22-*phox* mutations in a compound heterozygous patient with chronic granulomatous disease by mismatch PCR and restriction enzyme analysis. *Hum. Genet.* **93,** 437–442.

136. De Boer, M., De Klein, A., Hossle, J.-P., Seger, R., Corbeel, L., Weening, R. S., and Roos, D. (1992) Cytochrome b_{558}-negative, autosomal recessive chronic granulomatous disease: Two new mutations in the cytochrome b_{558} light chain of the NADPH oxidase (p22-*phox*). *Am. J. Hum. Genet.* **51,** 1127–1135.

137. Patiño, P. J., Rae, J., Erickson, R. W., Ding, J., Garcia de Olarte, D., and Curnutte, J. T. (1996) Molecular characterization of autosomal recessive chronic granulomatous disease caused by a deficiency of the NADPH oxidase component p67-*phox*. *Blood* **88,** 622a (abstract).

138. Åhlin, A., De Boer, M., Roos, D., Leusen, J., Smith, C. I. E., Sundin, U., Rabbani, H., Palmblad, J., and Elinder, G. (1995) Prevalence, genetics and clinical presentation of chronic granulomatous disease in Sweden. *Acta Paediatr.* **84,** 1386–1394.

139. De Boer, M., Hilarius-Stokman, P. M., Hossle, J.-P., Verhoeven, A. J., Graf, N., Kenney, R. T., Seger, R., and Roos, D. (1994) Autosomal recessive chronic granulomatous disease with absence of the 67-kD cytosolic NADPH oxidase component: Identification of mutation and detection of carriers. *Blood* **83,** 531–536.

140. Tanugi-Cholley, L. C., Issartel, J.-P., Lunardi, J., Freycon, F., Morel, F., and Vignais, P. V. (1995) A mutation located at the 5' splice junction sequence of intron 3 in the p67-*phox* gene causes the lack of p67-*phox* mRNA in a patient with chronic granulomatous disease. *Blood* **85,** 242–249.

141. Nunoi, H., Iwata, M., Tatsuzawa, S., Onoe, Y., Shimizu, S., Kanegasaki, S., and Matsuda, I. (1995) AG dinucleotide insertion in a patient with chronic granulomatous disease lacking cytosolic 67-kD protein. *Blood* **86,** 329–333.

142. Bonizzato, A., Russo, M. P., Donini, M., and Dusi, S. (1997) Identification of a double mutation (D160V-K161E) in the p67-*phox* gene of a chronic granulomatous disease patient. *Biochem. Biophys. Res. Commun.* **231,** 861–863.

143. Aoshima, M., Nunoi, H., Shimazu, M., Shimizu, S., Tatsuzawa, O., Kenney, R. T., and Kanegasaki, S. (1996) Two-exon skipping due to a point mutation in p67-*phox*-deficient chronic granulomatous disease. *Blood* **88,** 1841–1845.

9

Recruitment of γ/δ T-Cells and Other T-Cell Subsets to Sites of Inflammation

Mark A. Jutila

Introduction

Effective immune responses against pathogens require the migration of diverse sets of lymphoid cells into tissues that occurs both under homeostatic conditions and during inflammation associated with infection. Most mature naive α/β T-cells recirculate from the blood into secondary lymphoid organs, such as lymph nodes and Peyer's patches on a continual basis. They reenter the blood via the lymphatics. This process of recirculation provides the naive T-cell access to the organs of the body that collect antigen from epithelial surfaces, somatic tissues, and blood. Once T-cells respond to antigen, become activated, proliferate, and eventually develop into memory cells, they exhibit different trafficking behaviors, preferentially homing to extra-lymphoid sites of inflammation, such as inflamed skin or arthritic joints. In some instances, inflammation leads to the tissue-specific accumulation of distinct memory α/β T-cell subsets. Other specialized T-cells, such as γ/δ T-cells, exhibit trafficking patterns similar to memory α/β T-cells (preference for extralymphoid sites of inflammation). γ/δ T-cells can also exhibit constitutive homing to noninflamed, epithelial cell–associated tissues (reviewed in refs. *1–12*).

It is hypothesized that the directed migration of T-cells into tissues contributes to the efficiency of the immune response. The constitutive migration or homing of naive α/β T-cells to the various secondary lymph organs provides a mechanism for the immune system to continuously "probe" for specific antigen that has entered the body. The selective migration of memory effector cells to extralymphoid sites of inflammation/infection provides a mechanism to ensure that the cell type most effective in eliminating a pathogen is delivered to the actual site of infection. The migration of γ/δ T-cells

From: *Molecular and Cellular Basis of Inflammation*
Edited by: C. N. Serhan and P. A. Ward © Humana Press Inc., Totowa, NJ

into inflammatory sites as well as their selective trafficking to virtually all portals of entry into the body (epithelial-associated tissues), places these cells in the "first line of defense" against invading pathogens.

The process of lymphocyte trafficking is controlled, in part, by specific adhesive interactions between the circulating cell and the vascular endothelium lining vessels in a given tissue. Lymphocytes follow a multistep process involving rolling along and eventual tight adhesion to the vascular wall, followed by transendothelial migration. Specific adhesion receptor/ligand pairs control each of these steps. This chapter will provide a brief overview of the trafficking of naive and memory α/β T-cells and γ/δ T-cells, with an emphasis on the adhesion proteins regulating the very initial interaction of the lymphocyte with the vascular endothelium (rolling). Myeloid cells, such as neutrophils and monocytes, also accumulate in inflammatory tissues, many times using the same molecular mechanisms as lymphocytes, but a discussion of these cells is beyond the scope of this chapter. In most instances, reviews will be cited for much of the background information. Papers will be cited that deal with issues directly relevant to this chapter (e.g., adhesion proteins on memory T-cell subsets, background on γ/δ T-cells).

Overview of T-Cell Subsets

As mentioned, the trafficking of T-cells exhibits tissue-, inflammation-, and T-cell–subset specificity. The T-cell phenotypes that exhibit different migration potentials are quite distinct. Brief overviews of the T-cell subsets shown to follow different trafficking pathways are presented next.

Naive and Memory α/β T-Cells

α/β T-cells, defined by their T-cell receptor for antigen (Tcr), comprise the majority of the T-cell pool and are the predominant cell that has been studied in the context of immune responses. These cells express CD3 and, generally, either CD4 or CD8. The latter surface antigens correlate with restriction to MHC class II or class I antigens, respectively. Naive α/β T-cells are simply defined as cells that have not yet encountered antigen (reviewed in refs. *1, 2*, and *5*). This population is composed of a large repertoire of T-cells with different Tcrs for antigen. Once a naive α/β T-cell encounters its specific antigen, it may or may not undergo expansion and effector cell development *(5)*. Expansion involves enlargement of the T-cell and the turning on of a number of genes, which control their proliferation and production of immune mediators. As this effector cell response subsides, the α/β T-cell enters the memory T-lymphocyte stage *(1–3,5)*. Memory α/β T-cells have the capacity for a more rapid and vigorous response to recall antigen, which then leads to the development of a second effector stage. These secondary effector cells produce large quantities of cytokines and are extremely potent immune cells. These latter characteristics enhance the host secondary immune responses against reinfection (reviewed in ref. *5*).

Naive and memory α/β T-cells are phenotypically distinct. They can be identified by expression of different surface antigens as well as by the pattern of cytokines they produce. The most common surface markers used to distinguish naive and memory T-cells are the different CD45 isoforms (reviewed in refs. *1* and *5*). In general, naive α/β T-cells preferentially express high molecular mass forms of CD45 called CD45RB in mice and CD45RA in humans *(1,5)*. Memory α/β T-cells, on the other hand, preferentially express low molecular mass isoforms called CD45RO. Though the CD45 isoforms are used extensively in the analyses of naive and memory T-cells, their selective expression is not absolute, and cells at different stages of development or proliferation can express both isoforms *(1,13)*.

Of particular relevance, expression of different adhesion proteins can also be used to distinguish naive and memory α/β T-cells. Resting naive α/β T-cells express low levels of different integrins, such as CD11a/CD18 (LFA-1) and members of the β1 integrin family (such as VLA4), and α4/β7. They also express low levels of CD44, a receptor for hyaluronate. Naive T-cells homogeneously express high levels of L-selectin (reviewed in refs. *1*, *3*, and *6*). After conversion to an effector/memory T lymphocyte, expression of many of the integrins and CD44 increases, whereas L-selectin is selectively downregulated on some cells *(1,5)*. Some memory α/β T-cells, which are found in cutaneous sites of inflammation, express an adhesion molecule called cutaneous lymphocyte antigen (CLA) *(4,14–17)*. Memory T-cells from the gut express high levels of α4/β7 integrin *(4,18–20)*. The altered expression of adhesion proteins is important in regulating the change in the trafficking behavior of memory T-cells, which will be addressed in the discussion of migration pathways.

As mentioned, naive and memory α/β T-cells can also be distinguished by the cytokines they produce as well as expression of cytokine receptors. As expected, naive α/β T-cells, when artificially activated in vitro, produce few cytokines (predominantly IL-2) and express low levels of IL-2 receptors *(5)*. The cytokine production profiles of memory α/β T-cells are dramatically different from that of naive T-cells, both qualitatively and quantitatively *(5)*. Indeed, in some animals, effector/ memory T-cells can be further subdivided into subsets, called Th1 and Th2, based simply on the type of cytokine they produce. Th1 cells produce cytokines that drive inflammatory and cell-mediated immune (CMI) responses, whereas Th2 cells predominantly drive antibody responses. Impressively, effective host immune responses against different pathogens can be enhanced by selectively driving either a Th1 or Th2 T-cell response *(21)*.

γ/δ *T-Cells*

γ/δ T-cells are *bona fide* T-cells. They express CD3 and recognize antigen via receptors (γ/δ Tcrs) molecularly similar to those on conventional T-cells (α/β). The Tcrs they express are antigenically unique and identified by specific antibodies *(22,23)*. In spite of their potential for considerable diversity, γ/δ Tcr specificities are quite limited. And, although γ/δ T-cells that react with classical MHC I and II have been isolated, many appear to react with other nonclassical MHC gene products as well, possibly providing a faster and more encompassing immunological response *(24–27)*. Several reports suggest that γ/δ T-cells may recognize "unconventional antigens," such as heat shock proteins and nonpeptide (carbohydrate) antigens *(28–32)*. Unlike α/β T-cells, most γ/δ T-cells lack significant expression of CD4 and CD8 (some do express low levels of either antigen). Lineage-specific markers distinct from Tcr, such as the WC1 antigen in ruminants, have been characterized for these cells as well *(33–35)*. γ/δ T-cells have the potential to produce Th1 and Th2 cytokines *(36)*. Some reports suggest that these cells contribute to the initial host response to various infectious agents, which include parasitic, bacterial, and viral pathogens, and tumors, contributing to what is referred to as "the first line of defense" *(12)*. This hypothesis is consistent with their anatomical location at the portals of entry in nonlymphatic tissues, such as the skin and gut, and sites of inflammation *(12,23,37,38–44)*.

In addition to functions that are beneficial to the host, γ/δ T-cells appear to be associated with and may indirectly contribute to overt pathological processes. Accumulation of γ/δ T-cells occurs in chronic inflammatory tissues, such as inflamed synovia *(41,42)*, and in lesions associated with human autoimmune diseases, such as lupus erythematosius *(43)* and scleroderma *(44)*. Since many γ/δ T-cells respond to heat shock proteins, including those released by stressed mammalian cells, as well as a variety of other unusual antigens, their presence in inflamed tissues may lead to deleterious "autoimmune-like" reactions *(29)*. As such, understanding how and why γ/δ T-cells go to inflammatory sites is an important goal.

Most analyses of γ/δ T-cells have been done in mice and humans. However, there have been a limited number of excellent studies of these cells in sheep and cattle. The most striking observation to come from these studies is that γ/δ T-cells represent the predominant T-cell population found in the circulation of newborn sheep and cattle *(23,37)* (It has been found that their percentages exceed 70% of the T-cell pool in some calves.) Large numbers of γ/δ T-cells can also be found in the gut and spleen. Based on their sheer number, it is likely that they perform critically important functions in ruminants (vs those in other animals in which their numbers are much smaller).

Migration Pathways of T-Cell Subsets

To fully appreciate the complexity of T-cell migration into inflammatory sites (inducible trafficking), one must understand the migration pathways that are used under homeostatic conditions (constitutive migration). For simplicity, the author will discuss these as separate and distinct events. However, it is acknowledged that even constitutive lymphocyte homing could be defined as an inducible process regulated by immune stimulation and/or other events associated with development. Thus, in this latter view, all trafficking pathways are inducible (inflammation driven) and differ only in the degree of induction. Another aspect of T-cell trafficking in both constitutive and inducible migration is that tissue-specific pathways are followed by some specific T-cell subsets *(1,4)*. Table 1 lists these pathways and the phenotypes of T-cells that follow them. The list is not intended to imply that these pathways and phenotypes are absolute; it simply serves as a framework for discussion. In reality, there is considerable crossover among the pathways.

Constitutive Migration (Lymphocyte Homing)

It has been known since the early 1960s that lymphocytes continuously migrate from the blood into various lymphoid tissues, such as peripheral lymph nodes and Peyer's patches of the gut, during a process originally called "lymphocyte homing" *(8,45)*. The homing process gives lymphocytes the opportunity to continuously probe virtually all sites of the body for specific antigen. Naive α/β T-lymphocytes have the functional capacity to enter virtually all lymphoid tissues *(1–6,8,45)*. If antigen is not found, the lymphocyte enters the lymphatic system and eventually reenters the circulation via the thoracic duct to begin the process again, which takes approx 1–2 d. If antigen is found, the lymphocyte responds, proliferates, and performs its specific function—antibody production, T-helper activity, or T-cytolytic activity.

Activated and memory α/β T-lymphocytes exhibit different patterns of constitutive recirculation through secondary lymphoid tissue *(1,4,5)*. Considerable debate has sur-

Table 1
Migration Pathways Followed by T-Cell Subsets

Tissue-selective pathway	T-cell subset[a]	Degree of involvement
Peripheral lymph nodes	Naive T cells	++++
	Memory T-cells	
	Lselhi/α4/β1^{hi}	++
	γ/δ T-cells	+
Peyer's patches	Naive T-cells	++++
	Memory T-cells	
	α4/β7^{hi}	++
	γ/δ T-cells	?
Lamina propria	Naive T-cells	+/–
	Memory T-cells	
	α4/β7 hi	+++
	γ/δ T-cells	?
Skin	Naive T-cells	+/–
	Memory T-cells	
	Th1	++++
	CLA^{hi}	++++
	γ/δ T-cells	++++

[a]L-sel., L-selectin; CLA, cutaneous lymphocyte-associated antigen.

rounded the ability of activated or memory T-cells to recirculate through these tissues *(46–49)*. In vivo trafficking studies in sheep showed that these cells preferentially migrate to extralymphoid sites of inflammation. Indeed, memory α/β T-cells are the predominant lymphocyte isolated from the lymphatics draining extralymphoid sites of inflammation, such as in the skin *(1,50)*. This was taken as support for the hypothesis that memory lymphocytes do not extravasate via the vascular system into secondary lymphoid organs and that they only accumulate in these tissues by collection through the draining lymphatics. This led investigators to study potential mechanisms that could explain why memory T-cells are not delivered to secondary lymphoid organs via the vascular system. Some groups have suggested that memory cells lack certain adhesion molecules, such as L-selectin, which prevent their entry *(5,51,52)*, whereas others have suggested that the function of certain adhesion molecules on memory cells is altered. For example, it has been suggested that L-selectin acts as a signaling molecule on naive, but not memory T-cells, and that this signaling function is important for the entry of the T-cell into the lymph node *(53)*.

More importantly, the authors of the early in vivo trafficking studies never concluded that memory α/β T-cells could not traffic to lymph nodes or Peyer's patches, only that their potential to do so was greatly reduced *(1,2,7,50)*. Recent studies, which have been done to directly address this issue, have shown that memory or activated lymphocytes clearly have the capacity to enter secondary lymphoid organs via the vascular system *(46–48)*. An interesting difference in the homing of naive or memory α/β T-cells into lymph nodes detected in a recent study was the finding that memory cells traverse into and move through and out of the tissues much faster than naive T-cells *(48)*. Thus, some of the reduced trafficking of memory cells can be explained by the time point at which measurements were made.

Interestingly, trafficking of memory or activated T-cells through secondary lymphoid organs is tissue selective, either via the vascular bed in the specific tissue or via the draining lymphatics (Table 1). Memory or activated T-cells from mucosal sites preferentially migrate back to mucosal sites when reinfused into the animal *(1,4,9, 18,54–58)*. Likewise, memory cells isolated from peripheral sites preferentially migrate back to those sites *(50,57)*. The tissue-specific migration of memory T-cells likely contributes to the efficiency of the immune response, by ensuring that cells that have previously contacted antigen in a tissue preferentially migrate back to the same tissue *(1)*. The precise mechanisms accounting for tissue-selective accumulation of these T-cells are not completely understood, but likely involve selective trafficking mechanisms. However, a recent study suggests that tissue-selective apoptosis may also be involved *(47)*.

Inflammation-Associated Migration (Inducible Trafficking)

Inducible trafficking occurs during the host response to tissue inflammation triggered by trauma or infection. Prior to these insults, trafficking into nonlymphoid tissues is minimal, with the resulting inflammatory event upregulating migration of different leukocyte types into the inflamed tissue. If inflammation progresses (chronic), lymphocytes comprise the majority of the inflammatory cells that enter the affected site. Inducible lymphocyte trafficking leads to the accumulation of a sufficient number of cells in order to mount an effective peripheral host response. In most instances, inducible trafficking is beneficial; however, if inflammation continues unabated, overt tissue damage can occur and chronic inflammatory disease such as arthritis ensues *(59)*.

Under most circumstances, memory/effector α/β T-cells are a major lymphocyte population that migrate into extralymphoid sites of inflammation *(1,4)*, such as skin *(50)*, arthritic joint *(60)*, lung *(16)*, and lamina propria *(19)*. Naive α/β T-cells are rarely found in these sites, although clear examples of low numbers of naive T-cells in certain inflammatory reactions have been documented *(1)*. The accumulation of effector/memory cells in extralymphoid sites of inflammation is beneficial in most instances. As discussed above, these cells provide a more rapid and vigorous immune response. However, these same characteristics may contribute to overt pathological processes, such as in arthritis and, perhaps, the development of autoimmune reactions.

Extensive analysis of the migration pathways of Th1 and Th2 cell has not been done. Recently, Th1 cell lines have been shown to selectively migrate into inflamed skin when reinfused into the animal *(61,62)*. Th1 cells, through production of IFN-γ and other cytokines, likely contribute to the inflammatory reaction. The selective accumulation of these cells in extralymphoid sites of inflammation may be important for the CMI responses they induce. CMI responses require direct cell contact with the infectious agent or the infected host cell, which is likely located outside the lymphoid system in many instances.

As mentioned in the introduction, γ/δ T-cells also accumulate in inflammatory lesions and follow inducible migration pathways. Indeed, the migration of γ/δ T-cells is quite similar to the pathways followed by effector/memory α/β T-cells *(7)*. However, γ/δ T-cells in newborn calves exhibit this homing phenotype prior to significant antigen exposure. In young calves, few γ/δ T-cells are found in secondary lymphoid tissues, such as peripheral lymph nodes, whereas large numbers are found in extralymphoid, epithelial-associated sites in the skin, gut mucosa, lung, female reproductive tract, mammary gland, and regions of inflammation, as well as being blood borne *(23,37,38–44)*. Injection of cytokines or mitogens into the skin dramatically increases the migration of γ/δ T-cells into the tissue *(10,37,63–65)*.

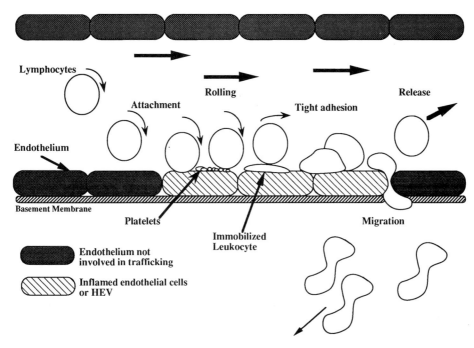

Fig. 1. Multistep process of lymphocyte migration into tissues.

The migration of T-cells into tissues following inflammation is not the same in all organs. Indeed, considerable tissue specificity is seen in the type of T-cell that migrates into a given inflamed tissue (Table 1). Skin and gut mucosa provide the best examples of inducible, tissue-specific T-cell migration. For example, inflammation in the skin leads to the accumulation of CLA bright T-cells in humans, which also fall within the Th1 subset in mice *(14–17,61,62,66–69)*. By contrast, inflammation in the gut mucosa leads to accumulation of α4/β7 bright/CLA negative T-cells *(18–20)*. Inflammation in lung tissue also leads to the selective accumulation of defined T-cell subsets *(16)*. The selective accumulation of these different subsets is probably important in the type of immune response that occurs in the specific tissue.

Lymphocyte/Endothelial Cell Interactions Involved in T-Cell Trafficking

An area of intense investigation has been the characterization of molecular mechanisms that control constitutive and inducible as well as tissue– and lymphocyte–subset-specific trafficking. The process of lymphocyte trafficking involves a complex series of events that leads to the recruitment of cells from the rapid flow of blood into specific tissues. This process involves initial recognition of the vessel wall during blood flow (represented by attachment and rolling of the lymphocyte along the endothelium), subsequent tight adhesion (sometimes aggregation) to endothelial cells, and, finally, transendothelial migration and accumulation in the underlying tissue (Fig. 1). In some instances, lymphocytes may roll on platelets or other leukocytes immobilized on the endothelium. Not all lymphocytes enter a given tissue, even after initiating rolling;

these cells release and reenter the circulation. Some cells that are "preactivated" and have a high propensity for adhesion may not require the rolling step and may stop almost immediately on interacting with the vessel wall.

Each step of extravasation is controlled by distinct receptor/ligand interactions, which mediate adhesion between the lymphocyte and endothelium and extracellular matrix, and activation and migration of the leukocyte. In secondary lymphoid tissues, rolling interactions are controlled by lymphocyte adhesion molecules, which are constitutively active and recognize constitutively expressed ligands on endothelial cells (high endothelial venules [HEV] in mice and humans). In inflamed tissues, rolling interactions are controlled by induced ligands on endothelial cells or immobilized cells, such as platelets. Tight adhesion and transendothelial migration are controlled by different lymphocyte adhesion molecules, which require a signal for function and recognize both constitutive and inducible endothelial cell ligands. Soluble factors (chemotactic factors) released by tissues are believed to be one signal that induces the transition from rolling to a permanently bound cell and causes directed migration of the leukocyte into the underlying tissue. Different combinations of receptor/ligand pairs and production of different chemotactic factors are thought to regulate constitutive, inflammation-induced, as well as tissue-selective trafficking of different lymphocyte subsets. The reader is directed to many different reviews that outline various presentations of this model *(70–74)*. Direct support for this model has come from in vitro adhesion assays done under physiological flow and intravital microscopy experiments in which the interaction of lymphocytes with the vascular wall is directly examined in vivo *(75–82)*.

Adhesion Molecules Involved in Trafficking of T-Cell Subsets

As predicted from the model described in the previous section, specific adhesion molecule/ligand pairs contribute to the specificity of lymphocyte trafficking. A large number of adhesion proteins, expressed by both lymphocytes and endothelial cells, that mediate rolling and/or tight adhesion have been defined. Table 2 lists lymphocyte/endothelial-cell adhesion molecules involved in the initial step of trafficking (rolling). Some of these molecules also mediate tight adhesion. The adhesion molecules that direct lymphocyte trafficking into secondary lymphoid organs or into extralymphoid sites of inflammation in many cases are the same, although clear differences exist. Those molecules that have been shown to be involved in constitutive or inflammation-induced trafficking are outlined next. Molecules involved in lymphocyte rolling will be emphasized.

Adhesion Molecules Involved in Constitutive Lymphocyte Homing

Here I will focus on naive α/β T-lymphocyte homing to peripheral vs mucosal lymphoid organs. Lymphocyte homing to these sites occurs continuously; thus the adhesion molecules that initiate the interaction of the T-cell with the vascular wall must be constitutively and functionally expressed on the lymphocyte as well as endothelium. Analysis of the expression of different adhesion molecules on naive cells gives clues about which are important in the trafficking of these cells. As outlined above, naive α/β T-cells express high levels of L-selectin and moderate to very low levels of different

Table 2
Defined Leukocyte and Endothelial Cell Adhesion Molecules Regulating
the Initial Event (Rolling) in Lymphocyte Homing to Secondary Lymphoid Organs
and Sites of Inflammation

Lymphocyte adhesion molecule	Ligand	Function
L-selectin	PNAd (CD34, others) on endothelium	Naive lymphocyte homing to peripheral lymph nodes
	MAdCAM-1 modified with specific CHO	Naive lymphocyte homing to Peyer's patches endothelium
	PSGL-1 modified with specific CHO on leukocytes	Leukocyte on leukocyte rolling
α4/β7	MAdCAM-1 on endothelium	Naive and memory T-cell homing to Peyer's patches
	VCAM-1 on endothelium	Memory T-cell homing to extralymphoid sites of inflammation
α4/β 1		
PSGL-1 modified with specific CHO	P-selectin/E-selectin on endothelium and platelets (P-selectin)	Th1 T-cell homing to inflamed skin
CLA	E-selectin on endothelium	Memory T-cell homing to inflamed skin

[a]CLA, cutaneous lymphocyte-associated antigen; PSGL-1, P-selectin glycoprotein ligand-1; PNAd, peripheral lymph node addressin; MAdCAM-1, mucosal addressin cell adhesion molecule-1; VCAM-1, vascular cell adhesion molecule-1; CHO, carbohydrate.

integrins, such as LFA-1 or α4/β1. From these studies, one could predict that L-selectin has a predominant role in the trafficking of naive T-cells through secondary lymphoid organs of the body.

Homing to Peripheral Lymph Nodes

L-selectin is perhaps the best characterized lymphocyte adhesion molecule involved in homing (8,83–85). It was originally described as the peripheral lymph node homing receptor because antibodies against it almost completely blocked lymphocyte adhesion to HEV (venules used by lymphocytes to enter lymphoid tissues in mice and humans) in peripheral and mesenteric lymph nodes, but only partially blocked adhesion to HEV in Peyer's patches (83). L-selectin belongs to the selectin family of adhesion molecules, which also includes E- and P-selectin expressed by endothelial cells. All selectins have an N-terminal mammalian C type lectin domain, which mediates the adhesive activity of the receptor by recognition of defined carbohydrate moieties on target cells (84–86). L-selectin specifically binds large molecular mass glycoproteins expressed by HEV that are recognized by the MECA 79 monoclonal antibody (MAb) (87,88). The MECA79 antigens have been collectively called the peripheral lymph node addressin (PNAd), and two of the predominant MECA 79 reactive species have been molecularly characterized: GlyCAM-1 (89), which is an L-selectin ligand of 60 kDa, and CD34 (90,91), a 90-kDa conventional transmembrane protein. Although L-selectin binds each of these molecules, it is not essential to trafficking since GlyCAM-1 is secreted and lymphocyte homing in mice deficient in CD34 is not reduced *(92)*. Another large molecular mass glycoprotein of 200 kDa has been shown to bind L-selectin, which could be the essential ligand, but it has not been molecularly characterized *(93)*. Another 90-kDa antigen may also be important *(92)*. A common feature of the PNAd species is that they require fucose and sulfate to bind L-selectin *(84–86,94)*. Also, mice deficient in fucosyl transferase type VII, an enzyme required to produce selectin carbohydrate binding structures, lack L-selectin ligands on their HEV and exhibit almost a total lack of lymphocyte homing to peripheral lymph nodes *(95)*.

The L-selectin/PNAd interaction initiates the tethering or rolling of naive α/β T-lymphocytes along HEV. Antibodies directed against L-selectin completely inhibit this interaction *(4,88,96)*. Following G-protein–dependent signaling events triggered by L-selectin binding or by factors such as chemokines immobilized along the vessel wall, the adhesive activity of the lymphocyte is upregulated *(4,81)*. This upregulation involves adhesion proteins belonging to the integrin family on the lymphocyte, such as LFA-1, and the Ig superfamily on the endothelium, such as intercellular adhesion molecule-1 (ICAM-1) *(81)*.

Homing to Peyer's Patches

Homing of naive α/β T-cells into mucosal lymphoid tissues has also been well defined. Mucosal lymphoid tissue HEV express a molecule called mucosal addressin cell adhesion molecule-1 (MAdCAM-1), which serves as a ligand for lymphocyte rolling as well as tight adhesion *(98,99)*. MAdCAM-1 has regions similar to the domains in Ig superfamily adhesion molecules, such as ICAM-1 and vascular adhesion molecule-1 (VCAM-1), as well as a region that can express MECA 79 reactive epitopes (PNAd) *(98,99)*. These features of MAdCAM-1 allow it to interact with multiple adhesion molecules on the T-cell. For example, naive α/β T-cells expressing L-selectin can roll on mucosal HEV expressing MAdCAM-1 decorated by PNAd *(81,99)*. Once rolling is initiated, integrins are activated, which mediate tight adhesion *(81)*. As in lymph nodes, LFA-1 is important in the tight adhesion of T-cells to mucosal HEV through binding ICAM-1.

The integrin $\alpha4/\beta7$ serves a unique function as another specific counterreceptor for MAdCAM-1. $\alpha4/\beta7$ was originally defined as a mucosal homing receptor and given the name lymphocyte Peyer's patch adhesion molecule *(100)*. $\alpha4/\beta7$ specifically binds MAdCAM-1, leading to both rolling and tight adhesion *(101,102)*. Therefore, two different molecules on naive T-cells can initiate tethering interactions on MAdCAM-1: $\alpha4/\beta7$ and L-selectin *(4,81,101,102)*. $\alpha4/\beta7$ serves a second role in contributing to permanent adhesion; it can also bind VCAM-1, but this interaction is not important in mucosal homing *(103)*.

Adhesion Molecules Involved in Inflammation-Induced Lymphocyte Trafficking

Infection or other insults to extralymphoid tissue can lead to T-cell migration via inducible adhesion pathways, distinguishing them from the pathways used in lymphocyte homing. In general, naive α/β T-cells do not migrate in appreciable numbers into extralymphoid tissues, whereas memory cell subsets and γ/δ T-cells do. As with naive T-cells, analysis of the expression of adhesion molecules on memory α/β T-cells and γ/δ T-cells provides clues to the function of specific receptor/ligand pairs in different inflammatory settings. In humans and large animals, such as sheep or cows, memory α/β T-cells are heterogeneous with respect to L-selectin expression—positive as well as negative subsets are clearly present in the peripheral blood and in different tissues *(104–107)*. By contrast, most murine memory T-cells are thought to be L-selectin negative *(5,53)*. Human memory T-cells heterogeneously express α4/β7 as well as another adhesion molecule called CLA, which is a receptor for E-selectin *(see* discussion on E-selectin) *(14–20)*. Other adhesion molecules, such as CD44, LFA-1, and α4/β1 are homogeneously expressed at high levels on memory α/β T-cells *(5)*. These expression patterns suggest that the adhesion proteins selectively expressed by memory T-cells could be involved in the migration of different subsets into specific tissues, whereas the ones that may be expressed by all cells are involved in a common step used in all sites.

Analysis of adhesion molecule expression by Th1 or Th2 cells has been difficult because of the lack of defined antigenic markers for these cells to use in flow cytometric analyses. Analysis of in vitro expanded mouse Th1 and Th2 clones has shown that the former expresses ligands for both E- and P-selectin. This was shown through the use of recombinant selectin Ig chimeras *(61,62)*. The Th1 cells express a form of P-selectin glycoprotein ligand-1 (PSGL-1) that supports the binding of P-selectin *(62)*.

Few expression analyses of adhesion molecules have been done on γ/δ T-cells. In humans, γ/δ T-cells express L-selectin, CLA, and different leukocyte integrins *(14,80,108)*. Our laboratory has done extensive work on γ/δ T-cells in cattle in which they represent the predominant T-cell at birth. It has been found that bovine γ/δ T-cells homogeneously express three to five times the level of L-selectin as other T-cells *(107)*. By contrast, they express equivalent levels of CD18, CD44, and α4/β7 *([107]*, Jutila, M. A., unpublished). Bovine γ/δ T-cells do not express CLA, but they have receptors for E-selectin, P-selectin, and a potentially new selectin-like adhesion molecule that has recently been identified *(37,76,109)*—all ligands found in sites of inflammation.

From expression studies, we can predict that bovine γ/δ T-cells have an unusual capacity to bind to multiple adhesion molecules, in both uninflamed and inflamed tissues. However, even though they express high levels of L-selectin and bind to HEV, this adhesive phenotype does not correlate with migration of the bovine γ/δ T-cell into the peripheral lymph node *(107)*. γ/δ T-cells avidly bind to PNAd-positive venules in peripheral lymph nodes, but they do not proceed with migration into the underlying tissue *(107)*. Thus, it must be kept in mind that simply expressing a specific adhesive phenotype does not always predict whether a migration pathway will be followed.

The expression analyses point to roles for a variety of different adhesion molecules in regulating the inducible trafficking of T-cells. Next, the author will focus on E-, P-, and L-selectin, because they regulate rolling, their expression profiles or the profiles of their respective ligands suggest that they are involved in tissue-selective inducible T-cell migration, and their function has been analyzed extensively. VCAM-1-mediated interactions will also be briefly discussed.

E-Selectin Mediated Lymphocyte Migration

E-selectin is a selectin family member restricted to endothelium whose binding specificity is for carbohydrates expressed by leukocytes similar to those bound by L-selectin *(86)*. Most uninflamed endothelium does not express E-selectin. However, E-selectin is upregulated on endothelial cells by inflammatory mediators, such as TNF-α or IL-1 (reviewed in refs. *84–86*). In vivo, E-selectin has been shown to be expressed in different sites of inflammation, including dermal inflammatory lesions and arthritis—sites associated with memory and/or γ/δ T-cell accumulation *(14,15,37,41,60)*. In 1990 two different groups showed that subsets of human memory T-cells bind E-selectin *(15,110)*. In 1993 Walcheck et al. *(39)* showed that bovine γ/δ T-cells also avidly bind E-selectin. In subsequent experiments using in vitro flow assays, E-selectin has been shown to support rolling interactions of human memory T-cells and bovine γ/δ T-cells *(75–78)*. Recently, Th1 cells have been shown to bind E-selectin *(61)*.

Prior to showing that a subset of human memory α/β T-cells bound E-selectin, Picker et al. *(15)* showed that an antigen they termed CLA antigen is preferentially expressed by T-cells that accumulate in diverse inflammatory reactions in the skin. It was later shown that CLA, which comprises a group of lymphocyte surface glycoproteins decorated by selectin-binding carbohydrates, serves as the counterreceptor for E-selectin as PNAd does for L-selectin *(111)*. In peripheral blood and appendix, CLA is found on only a small subset of memory cells. By contrast, CLA is found on >50% of the memory cells from peripheral lymph nodes, particularly those draining cutaneous sites. Interestingly, all CLA positive T-cells are also L-selectin positive *(16,17)*. Picker et al. *(14)* proposed that the CLA/E-selectin interaction preferentially directs specific subsets of human memory cells to the inflamed dermis. Supporting this hypothesis, immunohistological analyses showed that E-selectin is consistently and preferentially found in inflamed skin *(15)*. Furthermore, CLA is not found on memory T-cells from tissues such as the gut.

The binding of bovine γ/δ T-cells to E-selectin also correlates with an ability of these cells to migrate to inflamed dermis *(37,63)*. In support of the Picker et al. *(14)* hypothesis that E-selectin serves as a skin-specific adhesion molecule, Walcheck et al. *(37)* have shown that E-selectin is consistently detected in dermal lesions as well as in inflamed peripheral lymph nodes, whereas they have been unable to find E-selectin in inflamed Peyer's patches, lamina propria, or stomach (Jutila, M. A., unpublished). Unlike human T-cells, bovine γ/δ T-cells are not stained by antibodies directed against CLA. Two different approaches to define the γ/δ T-cell receptor for E-selectin have been used. In the first, immobilized purified E-selectin on sepharose beads was used in an affinity column to isolate a predominant 250-kDa glycoprotein from the surface of bovine γ/δ T-cells *(37)*. In another approach, an E-selectin/Ig chimera to precipitate biotin surface-labeled membrane protein from γ/δ T-cells was used, and the same 250-kDa ligand described above as well as an additional ligand of 180–200 kDa were isolated. A similar approach on human T-cells uncovered 200–220-kDa and 260-kDa ligands, which are believed to be analogous to the molecules isolated from bovine lymphocytes, as well as a 130-kDa ligand *(112)*. The molecular masses of these ligands identified by the E-selectin chimera are very similar to the molecular species that comprise CLA *(14)*.

In vivo blocking studies have also supported a role for E-selectin in directing the traffic of T-cells into inflamed skin. By targeting E-selectin, selective inhibition of T-cell subset recruitment can be achieved. For example, anti–E-selectin MAbs block the migration of α/β and γ/δ T-cells into delayed type hypersensitivity (DTH) reactions induced by phytohemagglutinin (PHA) in pigs *(10,63,64)*. E-selectin has been shown to be important in directing cells to DTH reactions in primates *(113)*. Lymphocyte migration (Th1 cells) into inflamed mouse skin can also be blocked by anti–E-selectin MAbs *(61)*. An MAb directed against both L- and E-selectin blocks the migration of bovine γ/δ T-cells into acute dermal lesions (Jutila, M. A., unpublished). Gene knockout mice have also supported an important role for E-selectin in directing T-cell migration to chronic inflammation associated with DTH reactions *(114)*.

P-Selectin Mediated Lymphocyte Trafficking

P-selectin is expressed by both inflamed endothelial cells and platelets (reviewed in refs. *84–86*). It is stored in granules of both cell types and can be rapidly translocated to the cell surface where it mediates adhesion, again, by binding specific carbohydrates on target cells. Like E-selectin, subsets of memory T-cells and γ/δ T-cells bind P-selectin *(75–77,115)*. A major difference, however, in the binding to P-selectin is that it does not correlate with CLA expression *(75,76)*. Subsets of human memory T-cells express PSGL-1, a glycoprotein ligand for P-selectin originally defined on neutrophils, which binds P-selectin *(115)*. Bovine γ/δ T-cells also bind P-selectin and although antibodies against human PSGL-1 do not crossreact in cattle, it is likely that a PSGL-1-like molecule serves as the γ/δ T-cell ligand. P-selectin/Ig chimera precipitates a surface protein from γ/δ T-cells with the same molecular mass as PSGL-1, and enzymes, such as *O*-sialoglycoprotease and low-dose chymotrypsin, that inhibit the function of PSGL-1 block γ/δ T-cell binding to P-selectin *(116)*. P-selectin also supports mouse Th1 T-cell binding *(62)*.

P-selectin is found on vessels in a greater number of tissues than E-selectin *(86)*. Unlike E-selectin, P-selectin is also expressed by activated platelets, which can be found along vessel walls in many different inflammatory lesions *(86)*. Thus, P-selectin has the potential of regulating a greater array of inflammatory reactions and resulting accumulation of T-cells. Antibody-blocking studies in mice have shown that the migration of Th1 T-cells into inflamed skin is blocked by anti–P-selectin MAbs *(61)*. Similar findings in the skin have been shown in other studies *(117)*. Gene knockout mice have also supported a role for P-selectin in regulating T-cell migration into DTH reactions in mouse skin *(114)*. Therefore, as with E-selectin, inhibition of P-selectin does impact the trafficking of T-cells. Since P- and E-selectin bind different T-cell subsets, subset-selective inhibition can be acheived by blocking one or the other of these adhesion proteins.

L-Selectin Mediated Lymphocyte Trafficking
During Inflammation

Naive α/β T-cells express high levels of L-selectin, which they use to enter secondary lymphoid organs. However, CLA-positive, as well as other memory α/β T-cells, are also L-selectin bright *(16,84,85,105)*. These cells most likely use L-selectin in migration through lymph nodes, but the question remains whether ligands for L-selectin in extralymphoid sites of inflammation exist. PNAd can be induced on vessels in chronically inflamed human and bovine skin (*[118,119]*, Jutila, M. A., unpublished). The author has done limited MAb blocking experiments in calves and found that anti–L-selectin MAb can block a significant portion of the migration of T-cells into a skin lesion induced by endotoxin (Jutila, M. A., unpublished). Additional evidence that L-selectin is involved in the migration of T-cells into inflamed skin has come from studies of L-selectin–deficient mice. Lymphocyte migration to skin during allograft rejection is reduced *(120)*. Interestingly, there have been no reports of PNAd expression in inflamed mouse skin; thus, the nature of the L-selectin ligands in this setting remains unclear.

Although it is generally assumed that the primary role of L-selectin in mediating leukocyte extravasation is adhesion to endothelial cells, it does mediate another type of adhesive interaction that most likely contributes to the magnitude of the inflammatory response. In 1994 it was shown that once neutrophils become immobilized on the vascular endothelium, they can serve as the adhesive substrate for continual recruitment of newly arriving neutrophils (Fig. 1). This neutrophil/neutrophil interaction is completely blocked by anti–L-selectin MAbs *(121)*. One leukocyte ligand for L-selectin is PSGL-1 *(122)*, but antibodies that completely block PSGL-1 function only partially inhibit leukocyte-on-leukocyte rolling, suggesting that other ligands probably exist *(122)*.

Although leukocyte-on-leukocyte rolling is well accepted for neutrophils, it is not clear to what extent lymphocytes participate in this interaction. It has been shown that adherent monolayers of bovine γ/δ T-cells avidly support rolling interactions of other γ/δ T-cells, which are completely blocked by anti-L–selectin MAb *(116)*. By contrast, studies by other groups have been unable to demonstrate L-selectin ligands on human lymphocytes *(123)*. However, subsets of human memory T-cells express functional PSGL-1 *(115)*; therefore, under certain circumstances, human lymphocytes may have the potential to interact with each other via L-selectin.

VCAM-1/α4/β1–Mediated Lymphocyte Trafficking

A very important inflammation-associated adhesion system of relevance to T-cells is the α4/β1/VCAM-1 interaction *(4,124–131)*. Indeed, a search of literature data bases on VCAM-1 reveals publications numbering in the thousands; however, here characteristics of this adhesive interaction will only be briefly outlined.

VCAM-1/α4/β1 interactions are generally restricted to mononuclear cells, although recent studies suggest that neutrophils may also use this pathway in some animals *(132)*. VCAM-1 is expressed on endothelial cells in a variety of different inflammatory lesions in which it avidly supports T-cell binding via α4/β1 (reviewed in refs. *4* and *128*). A requisite for this interaction is high expression of α4/β1 on the T-cell, which is a common feature of memory cells *(4,128)*. The α4/β1/VCAM-1 interaction can result in selectin-independent lymphocyte rolling as well as tight adhesion *(4,79,123, 128,129)*. Since α4/β1 is expressed at high levels on most, if not all, memory T-cells, selective inhibition of memory T-cell subset migration most likely cannot be accomplished by targeting this interaction. It would be predicted that far more general effects on T-cell migration would be achieved. Indeed, this has been shown in vivo. α4/β1/VCAM-1 interactions are important in psoriasis *(69)* and other cutaneous inflammatory lesions *(131)*. One of the more impressive in vivo effects of blocking this interaction has been shown in the brain. Antibodies against α4/β1 prevent experimental autoimmune encephalomyelitis *(132)*.

Other Adhesion Molecules Mediating Lymphocyte Trafficking

There are other receptor/ligand pairs that are critically important in regulating T-cell migration into sites of inflammation. Some of these pairs are briefly mentioned next, and the reader is directed to recent reviews providing more detailed information on them *(6,8,70,72,74,84–87,133,134)*.

MAdCAM-1 can be expressed outside of mucosal tissues, such as in the pancreas of NOD diabetic mice, where it can contribute to inflammation-induced lymphocyte trafficking. Antibodies against β7 integrins block the progression of the disease *(135)*. The interactions of LFA-1 with ICAM-1, ICAM-2, and/or ICAM-3 are critical in both constitutive and inflammation-induced trafficking of T-cells *(134)*. These interactions control both lymphocyte/endothelial cell binding, as well as lymphocyte/antigen-presenting cell interactions within the tissue. Vascular adhesion protein-1 (VAP-1) is another adhesion molecule thought to be important in regulating T-cell traffic into some inflammatory lesions *(136)*. However, VAP-1 has only been defined in humans; thus, animal studies of its role in vivo have not been done.

Finally, functional analyses and other studies of adhesion molecule expression on memory T-cells suggests that other undefined adhesion molecules exits. For example, memory T-cells from inflamed lung lack L-selectin and CLA, suggesting that they use other adhesion systems to enter this tissue *(16)*. Jones et al. *(137)* has shown that T-cell rolling on 24 h in vitro-stimulated endothelial cells is independent of the known adhesion proteins. Jutila et al. *(109)* have recently shown that γ/δ T-cell rolling on 24-h cytokine-activated endothelial cells is not blocked by antiE-selectin or L-selectin MAbs. They have generated MAbs against these endothelial cells that completely block the rolling interaction. Preliminary characterization of the endothelial cell antigen suggests that it is unlike other previously described adhesion proteins.

Summary

Lymphocyte migration into tissues is essential for effective immune responses against disease-causing pathogens. Lymphocyte trafficking exhibits tissue, inflammation, and subset specificity which is probably important in increasing the efficiency of the host immune response. The selective accumulation of certain T-cell subsets into given uninflamed and inflamed tissues is a fascinating aspect of the mammalian immune system that is conserved in animals as diverse as mice, sheep, cows, and humans. Adhesion proteins expressed by endothelial cells lining venules in tissues and the lymphocyte contribute to the specificity of the lymphocyte trafficking response. Some of the key adhesion molecules that regulate the first step in the process—lymphocyte rolling have been outlined. Selective inhibition of these molecules has the potential to selectively alter the trafficking of defined T-cell subsets. It is likely that most of the adhesion proteins involved in the interactions described have been identified. However, there is still room for the discovery of other molecules.

Ackowledgments

The helpful and critical comments of Dana Hoover, Kemal Aydintug, Eric Wilson, and Jeff Leid are greatly appreciated. This work was supported in part by grants from USDA NRI 96-35204-3580, NIH 1RO1 AI41671-01, and the Montana Agricultural Experiment Station.

References

1. Mackay, C. R. (1993) Homing of naive, memory and effector lymphocytes. *Curr. Opinion Immunol.* **5,** 423–427.
2. Mackay, C. R. (1991) T-cell memory: The connection between function, phenotype and migration pathways. *Immunol. Today* **12,** 189–192.
3. Bradley, L. M. and Watson, S. R. (1996) Lymphocyte migration into tissue: The paradigm derived from CD4 subsets. *Curr. Opinion Immunol.* **8,** 312–320.
4. Butcher, E. C. and Picker, L. J. (1996) Lymphocyte homing and homeostasis. *Science* **272,** 60–66.
5. Swain, S. L., Croft, M., Dubey, C., Haynes, L., Rogers, P., Zhang, X., and Bradley, L. M. (1996) From naive to memory T cells. *Immunol. Rev.* **150,** 143–167.

6. Mackay, C. R. and Imhof, B. A. (1993) Cell adhesion molecules in the immune system. *Immunol. Today* **14,** 99–102.

7. Mackay, C. R. (1991) Skin-seeking memory T cells. *Nature* **349,** 737,738.

8. Picker, L. J. and Butcher, E. C. (1992) Physiological and molecular mechanisms of lymphocyte homing. *Ann. Rev. Immunol.* **10,** 561–591.

9. Springer, T. A. (1994) Traffic signals for lymphocyte recirculation and leukocyte emigration: the multistep paradigm. *Cell* **76,** 301–314.

10. Binns, R. M., Whyte, A., and License, S. T. (1996) Constitutive and inflammatory lymphocyte trafficking. *Vet. Immunol. Immunopathol.* **54,** 97–104.

11. Bluestone, J. A., Khattri, R., Sciammas, R., and Sperling, A. I. (1995) TCR gamma delta T cells: a specialized T-cell subset in the immune system. *Ann. Rev. Cell. Dev. Biol.* **11,** 307–353.

12. Libero, G. (1997) Sentinal function of broadly reactive human γδ T cells. *Immunol. Today* **18,** 22–26.

13. LaSalle, J. M., and Hafler, D. A. (1991) The coexpression of CD45RA and CD45RO isoforms on T cells during the S/G2/M stages of cell cycle. *Cell. Immunol.* **138,** 197–206.

14. Picker, L. J., Michie, S. A., Rott, L. S., and Butcher, E. C. (1990) A unique phenotype of skin-associated lymphocytes in humans: preferential expression of the HECA-452 epitope by benign and malignant T cells at cutaneous sites. *Am. J. Pathol.* **136,** 1053–1068.

15. Picker, L. J., Kishimoto, T. K., Smith, C. W., Warnock, R. A., and Butcher, E. C. (1991) ELAM–1 is an adhesion molecule for skin-homing T cells. *Nature* **349,** 796–799.

16. Picker, L. J., Martin, R. J., Trumble, A., Newman, L. S., Collins, P. A., Bergstresser, P. R., and Leung, D. Y. M. (1994) Differential expression of lymphocyte homing receptors by human memory/effector T cells in pulmonary versus cutaneous immune effector sites. *Eur. J. Immunol.* **24,** 1269–1277.

17. Picker, L. J., Treer, J. R., Ferguson-Darnell, B., Collins, P. A., Bergstresser, P. R., and Terstappen, L. W. M. M. (1993) Control of lymphocyte recirculation in man. II. Differential regulation of the cutaneous lymphocyte-associated antigen, a tissue-selective homing receptor for skin homing T cells. *J. Immunol.* **150,** 1122–1136.

18. Abitorabi, M. A., Mackay, C. R., Jerome, E. H., Osorio, O., Butcher, E. C., and Erle, D. J. (1996) Differential expression of homing molecules on recirculating lymphocytes from sheep gut, peripheral, and lung lymph. *J. Immunol.* **156,** 3111–3117.

19. Farstad, I. N., Halstensen, T. S. Kvale, D., Fausa, O., and Brandtzaeg, P. (1997) Topographic distribution of homing receptors on B and T cells in human gut-associated lymphoid tissue: relation of L-selectin and integrin alpha 4 beta 7 to naive and memory phenotypes. *Am. J. Pathol.* **150,** 187–199.

20. Rott, L. S., Briskin, M. J., Andrew, D. P., Berg, E. L., and Butcher, E. C. (1996) A fundamental subdivision of circulating lymphocytes defined by adhesion to mucosal addressin cell adhesion molecule-1: comparison with vascular cell adhesion molecule-1 and correlation with beta 7 integrins and memory differentiation. *J. Immunol.* **156,** 3727–3736.

21. Mosmann, T. R. and Sad, S. (1996) The expanding universe of T cell subsets: Th1, Th2 and more. *Immunol. Today* **17,** 138–146.

22. Raulet, D. H. (1989) The structure, function, and molecular genetics of the gamma delta T cell receptor. *Ann. Rev. Immunol.* **7,** 175–201.

23. Hein, W. R. and Mackay, C. R. (1991) Prominence of gamma/delta T cells in the ruminant immune system. *Immunol. Today* **12,** 30–34.

24. Rivas, A., Koide, J., Cleary, M. L., and Engleman, E. G. (1989) Evidence for involvement of the γ,δ T cell antigen receptor in cytotoxicity mediated by human alloantigen-specific T cell clones. *J. Immunol.* **142,** 1840–1846.

25. Matis, L. A., Fry, A. M., Cron, R. Q., Cotterman, M. M., Dick, R. F., and Bluestone, J. A. (1989) Structure and specificity of a class II MHC alloreactive γδ T cell receptor heterodimer. *Science* **245,** 746–749.

26. Ciccone, E., Viale, O., Bottino, C., Pende, D., Migone, N., Casorati, G.,Tambussi, G., Moretta, A., and Moretta. L. (1988) Antigen recognition by human T cell receptor γ-positive lymphocytes: specific lysis of allogeneic cells after activation in mixed lymphocyte culture. *J. Exp. Med.* **167,** 1517–1522.

27. Weintraub, B. C., Jackson, M. R., and Hedrick, S. M. (1994) γδ T cells can recognize nonclassical MHC in the absence of conventional antigenic peptides. *J. Immunol.* **153,** 3051–3058.

28. O'Brien, R. L., Happ, M. P., Dallas, A., Cranfill, R., Hall, L., Lang, J., Fu, Y. X., Kubo, R., and Born, W. (1991) Recognition of a single HSP-60 epitope by an entire subset of gamma delta T lymphocytes. *Immunol. Rev.* **121,** 155–170.

29. Haregewoin, A., Singh, B., Gupta, R. S., and Finberg, R. W. (1991) A mycobacterial heat shock protein responsive gamma delta T cell clone also responds to the homologous human heat shock protein: A possible link between infection and autoimmunity. *J. Infect. Dis.* **163,** 156–160.

30. Haregewoin, A., Singh, B., Gupta, R. S., and Finberg, R. W. (1989) Human gamma delta T cells respond to mycobacterial heat-shock protein. *Nature (Lond.)* **340,** 309–312.

31. Born, W., Happ, M. P., Dallas, A., Reardon, C., Kubo, R., Shinnick, T., Brennan, P., and O'Brien, R. (1990) Recognition of heat shock proteins and gamma delta cell function. *Immunol. Today* **11,** 40–43.

32. Pfeffer, K., Schoel, B., Plesnila, N., Lipford, G. B., Kromer, S., Deusch, K., and Wagner, H (1992) A lectin-binding, protease-resistant mycobacterial ligand specifically activates Vγ9+ human γδ T cells. *J. Immunol.* **148,** 575–583.

33. MacHugh, N. D., Wijngaard, P. L. J., Clevers, H. C., and Davis, W. C. (1993) Clustering of monoclonal antibodies recognizing different members of the WC1 gene family. *Vet. Immunol. Immunopathol.* **39,** 155–160.

34. Crocker, G., Sopp, P., Parsons, K., Davis, W. C., and Howard, C. J. (1993) Analysis of the γ/δ T cell restricted antigen WC1. *Vet. Immunol. Immunopathol.* **39,** 137–144.

35. Wijngaard, P. L. J., MacHugh, N. D., Metzelaar, M. J., Romberg, S., Bensaid, A., Pepin, L., Davis, W. C., and Clevers, H. C. (1994) Members of the novel WC1 gene family are differentially expressed on subsets of bovine CD4-CD8-γδ T lymphocytes. *J. Immunol.* **152,** 3476–3482.

36. Ferrick, D. A., Schrenzel, M. D., Mulvania, T., Hsieh. B., Ferlin, W. G., and Lepper, H (1995) Differential production of interferon-gamma and interleukin-4 in response to Th1- and Th2-stimulating pathogens by γ/δ T cells in vivo. *Nature* **373,** 255–257.

37. Walcheck, B., Watts, G., and Jutila, M. A. (1993) Bovine gamma/delta T cells bind E-selectin via a novel glycoprotein receptor: First characterization of a lymphocyte/E-selectin interaction in an animal model. *J. Exp. Med.* **178,** 853–863.

38. Augustin, A., Kubo, R. T., and Sim, G. K. (1989) Resident pulmonary lymphocytes expressing the gamma/delta T-cell receptor. *Nature (Lond.)* **340,** 239–241.

39. Reardon, C., Lefrancois, L., Farr, A., Kubo, R., O'Brien, R., and Born, W. (1990) Expression of gamma/delta T cell receptors on lymphocytes from the lactating mammary gland. *J. Exp. Med.* **172,** 1263–1266.

40. Vietor, H. and Koning, F. (1990) Gamma/delta T-cell receptor repertoire in human peripheral blood and thymus. *Immunogenetics* **31,** 340–346.

41. Brennan, F. M., Londei, M., Jackson, A. M., Hercend, T., Brenner, M. B., Maini, R. N., and Feldmann, M. (1988) T cells expressing gamma delta chain receptors in rheumatoid arthritis. *J. Autoimmun.* **1,** 319–326.

42. Al-Janadi, M., Al-Balla, S., Al-Dalaan, A., and Raziuddin, S. (1993) Cytokine production by helper T cell populations from the synovial fluid and blood in patients with rheumatoid arthritis. *J. Rheumatol.* **20,** 1647–1653.

43. Rajagopalan, S., Zordan, T., Tsokos, G. C., and Datta, S. K. (1990) Pathogenic anti-DNA autoantibody-inducing T helper cell lines from patients with active lupus nephritis: isolation of CD4-8-T helper cell lines that express the gamma delta T-cell antigen receptor. *Proc. Natl. Acad. Sci. USA* **87,** 7020–7024.

44. Kratz, L. E., Boughman, J. A., Pincus, T., Cohen, D. I., and Needleman, B. W. (1990) Association of scleroderma with a T cell antigen receptor gamma gene restriction fragment length polymorphism. *Arthritis Rheum.* **33,** 569–578.

45. Girard, J. P. and Springer, T. A. (1995) High endothelial venules (HEVs): Specialized endothelium for lymphocyte migration. *Immunol. Today* **16,** 449–457.

46. Williams, M. B. and Butcher, E. C. (1997) Homing of naive and memory T lymphocyte subsets to Peyer's patches, lymph nodes and spleen. *J. Immunol.* **159,** 1746–1752.

47. Bode, U., Wonigeit, K., Pabst, R., and Westermann, J. (1997) The fate of activated T cells migrating through the body: Rescue from apoptosis in the tissue of origin. *Eur. J. Immunol.* **27,** 2087–2093.

48. Westermann, J., Geismar, U., Spenholz, A., Bode, U., Sparshott, S. M., and Bell, E. B. (1997) CD4+ T cells of both the nawe and memory phenotype enter rat lymph nodes and Peyer's patches via high endothelial venules: within the tissue their migratory behavior differs. *Eur. J. Immunol.* **27,** 2174–3181.

49. Westermann, J. and Pabst, R. (1996) How organ-specific is the migration of "naive" and "memory" T cells? *Immunol. Today* **17,** 278–282.

50. Mackay, C. R., Marston, W., and Dudler, L. (1992) Altered patterns of T cell migration through lymph nodes and skin following antigen challenge. *Eur. J. Immunol.* **22,** 2205–2210.

51. Bradley, L. M., Atrkins, G. G., and Swain, S. L. (1992) Long-term CD4+ memory T cells from the spleen lack MEL-14, the lymph node homing receptor. *J. Immunol.* **148,** 324–331.

52. Bradley, L. M., Watson, S. R., and Swain, S. L. (1994) Entry of naive CD4 T cells into peripheral lymph nodes requires L-selectin. *J. Exp. Med.* **180,** 2401–2406.

53. Hwang, S. T., Singer, M. S., Giblin, P. A., Yednock, T. A., Bacon, K. B., Simon, S. I., and Rosen, S. D. (1996) GlyCAM-1, a physiologic ligand for L-selectin, activates beta 2 integrins on naive peripheral lymphocytes. *J. Exp. Med.* **184,** 1343–1348.

54. Mackay, C. R., Marston,W. L., and Dudler, L. (1990) Naive and memory T cells show distinct pathways of lymphocyte recirculation. *J. Exp. Med.* **171,** 801–817.

55. Cahill, R. N., Poskitt, D. C., Frost, D. C., and Trnka, Z. (1977) Two distinct pools of recirculating T lymphocytes: migratory characteristics of nodal and intestinal T lymphocytes. *J. Exp. Med.* **130,** 1427–1451.

56. Ottaway, C. A., and Husband, A. J. (1994) The influence of neuroendocrine pathways on lymphocyte migration. *Immunol. Today* **15,** 511–517.

57. Hall, J. G., Hopkins, J., and Orlans, E. (1977) Studies of the lymphocytes in sheep. II. Destination of lymph-borne immunoblasts in relation to their tissue of origin. *Eur. J. Immunol.* **7,** 30–37.

58. Chin, W. and Hay, J. B. (1980) A comparison of lymphocyte migration through intestinal lymph nodes, subcutaneous lymph nodes, and chronic inflammatory sites of sheep. *Gastroenterology* **79,** 1231–1242.

59. Johnson, B. A., Haines, G. K., Harlow, L. A., and Koch, A. E. (1993) Adhesion molecule expression in human synovial tissue. *Arthritis Rheum.* **36,** 137–146.

60. Kohem, C. L., Brezinschek, R. I., Wisbey, H., Tortorella, C., Lipsky, P. E., and Oppenheimer-Marks, N. (1996) Enrichment of differentiated CD45RBdim, CD27-memory T cells in the peripheral blood, synovial fluid, and synovial tissue of patients with rheumatoid arthritis. *Arthritis Rheum.* **39,** 844–854.

61. Austrup, F., Vestweber, D., Borges, E., Lohning, M., Brauer, R., Herz, U., Renz, H., Hallmann, R., Scheffold, A., Radbruch, A., and Hamann, A. (1997) P- and E-selectin mediate recruitment of T-helper-1 but not T-helper-2 cells into inflamed tissues. *Nature* **385,** 81–83.

62. Borges, E., Tietz, W., Steegmaier, M., Moll, T., Hallmann, R., Hamann, A., and Vestweber, D. (1997) P-selectin glycoprotein-1 (PSGL-1) on T helper 1 but not on T helper 2 cells binds to P-selectin and supports migration into inflamed skin. *J. Exp. Med.* **185,** 573–578.

63. Whyte, A., License, S. T., Robinson, M. K., and vanderLienden, K. (1996) Lymphocyte subsets and adhesion molecules in cutaneous inflammation induced by inflammatory agonists: correlation between E-selectin and gamma/delta TcR+ lymphocytes. *Lab. Invest.* **75,** 439–449.

64. Binns, R. M., Whyte, A., License, S. T., Harrison, A. A., Tsang, Y. T., Haskard, D. O., and Robinson, M. K. (1996) The role of E-selectin in lymphocyte and polymorphonuclear cell recruitment into cutaneous delayed hypersensitivity reactions in sensitized pigs. *J. Immunol.* **157,** 4094–4099.

65. Binns, R. M., License, S. T., Harrison, A. A., Keelan, E. T., Robinson, M. K., and Haskard, D. O. (1996) In vivo E-selectin upregulation correlates early with infiltration of PMN, later with PBL entry: MAbs block both. *Am. J. Physiol.* **270,** H183–H193.

66. Santamaria-Babi, L. F., Perez-Soler, M. T., Hauser, C., and Blaser, K. (1995) Skin-homing T cells in human cutaneous allergic inflammation. *Immunol. Res.* **14,** 317–324.

67. Pitzalis, C., Cauli, A., Pipttone, N., Smith, C., Barker, J., Marchesoni, A., Yanni, G., and Panayi, G. S. (1996) Cutaneous lymphocyte antigen-positive T lymphocytes preferentially migrate to the skin but not to the joint in psoriatic arthritis. *Arthritis Rheum.* **39,** 137–145.

68. Santamaria-Babi, L. F., Moser, R., Perez-Soler, M. T., Picker, L. J., Blaser, K., and Hauser, C. (1995) Migration of skin-homing T cells across cytokine-activated human endothelial cell layers involves interaction of the cutaneous lymphocyte-associated antigen (CLA), the very late

antigen-4 (VLA-4), and the lymphocyte function-associated antigen-1 (LFA-1) *J. Immunol.* **154**, 1543–1550.

69. Wakita, H. and Takigawa, M. (1994) E-selectin and vascular cell adhesion molecule-1 are critical for initial trafficking of helper-inducer/memory T cells in psoriatic plaques. *Arch. Dermatol.* **130**, 457–463.
70. Butcher, E. C. (1991) Leukocyte-endothelial cell recognition: Three (or more) steps to specificity and diversity. *Cell* **67**, 1033–1036.
71. Zimmerman, G. A., Prescott, S. M., and McIntyre, T. M (1992) Endothelial cell interactions with granulocytes: Tethering and signaling molecules. *Immunol. Today* **13**, 93–100.
72. Springer, T. A. (1994) Traffic signals for lymphocyte recirculation and leukocyte emigration: The multistep paradigm. *Cell* **76**, 301–314.
73. Kishimoto, T. K. (1991) A dynamic model for neutrophil localization to inflammatory sites. *J. NIH Res.* **3**, 75–77.
74. Jutila, M. A. (1997) Leukocyte trafficking, in *Comprehensive Toxicology*, vol. 5. (Lawrence, D. A., ed.), Elsevier, New York, pp. 201–214.
75. Jutila, M. A., Bargatze, R. F., Kurk, S., Warnock, R. A., Ehsani, N., Watson, S., and Walcheck, B. (1994) Cell surface P- and E-selectin support shear-dependent rolling of bovine γ/δ T cells. *J. Immunol.* **153**, 3917–3928.
76. Alon, R., Rossiter, H., Wang, X., Springer, T. A., and Kupper, T. S. (1994) Distinct cell surface ligands mediate T lymphocyte attachment and rolling on P- and E-selectin under physiological flow. *J. Cell. Biol.* **127**, 1485–1495.
77. Lichtman, A. H., Ding, H., Henault, L., Vachino, G., Camphausen, R., Cumming, D., and Luscinskas, F. W. (1997) CD45RA-RO+ (memory) but not CD45RA+RO– (naive) T cells roll efficiently on E- and P-selectin and vascular cell adhesion molecule-1 under flow. *J. Immunol.* **158**, 3640–3650.
78. Jones, D. A., McIntire, L. V., Smith, C. W., and Picker, L. J. (1994) A two-step adhesion cascade for T cell/endothelial cell interactions under flow conditions. *J. Clin. Invest.* **94**, 2443–2450.
79. Luscinskas, F. W., Ding, H., and Lichtman, A. H. (1995) P-selectin and vascular cell adhesion molecule-1 mediate rolling and arrest, respectively, of CD4+ T lymphocytes on tumor necrosis factor alpha-activated vascular endothelium under flow. *J. Exp. Med.* **181**, 1179–1186.
80. Diavcoc-T. G., Roth, S. J., Morita, C. T., Rosat, J. P., Brenner, M. B., and Springer, T. A. (1996) Interactions of human alpha/beta and gamma/delta T lymphocyte subsets in shear flow with E-selectin and P-selectin. *J. Exp. Med.* **183**, 1193–1203.
81. Bargatze, R. F., Jutila, M. A., and Butcher, E. C. (1995) Distinct roles for L-selectin, and integrins α4β7, and LFA-1 in lymphocyte interactions with HEV *in situ*: the multistep model confirmed and refined. *Immunity* **3**, 99–108.
82. Bargatze, R. F. and Butcher, E. C. (1993) Rapid G protein-regulated activation event involved in lymphocyte binding to high endothelial venules. *J. Exp. Med.* **178**, 367–372.
83. Gallatin, W. M., Weissman, I. L., and Butcher, E. C. (1983) A cell surface molecule involved in organ-specific homing of lymphocytes. *Nature* **304**, 30–34.
84. Tedder, T. F., Steeber, D. A., Chen, A., and Engel, P. (1995) The selectins: Vascular adhesion molecules. *FASEB J.* **9**, 866–873.
85. Kansas, G. S. (1996) Selectins and their ligands: Current concepts and controversies. *Blood* **88**, 3259–3287.
86. McEver, R. P. (1994) Selectins. *Curr. Opinion Immunol.* **6**, 75–84.
87. Streeter, P. R., Rouse, B. T. N., and Butcher, E. C. (1988) Immunologic and functional characterization of a vascular addressin involved in lymphocyte homing into peripheral lymph nodes. *J. Cell. Biol.* **107**, 1853–1862.
88. Berg, E. L., Robinson, M. K., Warnock, R. A., and Butcher, E. C. (1991) The human peripheral lymph node vascular addressin is a ligand for LECAM-1, the peripheral lymph node homing receptor. *J. Cell. Biol.* **114**, 343–349.
89. Lasky, L. A., Singer, M. S., Dowbenko, D., Imai, Y., Henzel, W. J., Grimley, C., Fennie, C., Gillett, N., Watson, S. R., and Rosen, S. D. (1992) An endothelial ligand for the lymphocyte homing receptor. *Cell* **69**, 927–938.
90. Baumheuter, S. Singer, M. S., Henzel, W., Renz, M., Rosen, S. D., and Lasky, L. (1993) Binding of L-selectin to the vascular sialomucin, CD34. *Science* **262**, 436–438.

91. Puri, K. D., Finger, E. B., Gaudernack, G., and Springer, T. A. (1995) Sialomucin CD34 is the major L-selectin ligand in human tonsil high endothelial venules. *J. Cell. Biol.* **131,** 261–270.

92. Suzuki, A., Andrew, D. P., Gonzalo, J. A., Fukumoto, M., Spellberg, J., Hashiyama, M., Takimoto, H., Gerwin, N., Webb, I., Molinex, G., Amakawa, R., Tada, Y., Wakeham, A., Brown, J., McNiece, I., Ley, K., Butcher, E. C., Suda, T., Gutierrez-Ramos, J. C., and Mak, T. W. (1996) CD34-deficient mice have reduced eosinophil accumulation after allergen exposure and show a novel crossreactive 90-kD protein. *Blood* **87,** 3550–3562.

93. Hoke, D., Mebius, R. E., Dybdal, N., Dowbenko, D., Gribling, P., Kyle, C., Baumhueter, S., and Watson, S. R. (1995) Selective modulation of the expression of L-selectin ligands by an immune response. *Curr. Biol.* **5,** 670–678.

94. Imai, Y., Lasky, L. A., and Rosen, S. D. (1993) Sulphation requirement for GlyCAM–1, an endothelial ligand for L-selectin. *Nature* **361,** 555–557.

95. Maly, P., Thall, A. D., Petryniak, B., Rogers, C. E., Smith, P. L., Marks, R. M., Kelly, R. J., Gersten, K. M., Cheng, G., Saunders, T. L., Camper, S. A., Camphousen, R. T., Sullivan, F. X., Isogai, Y., Hindsgaul, O., von Andrian, U. H., and Lowe, J. B. (1996) The FucT-VII $\alpha(1,3)$ fucosyltransferase locus controls lymphocyte homing and blood leukocyte emigration through an essential role in L-, E-, and P-selectin ligand biosynthesis. *Cell* **86,** 643–653

96. von Andrian, U. H. (1996) Intravital microscopy of the peripheral lymph node microcirculation in mice. *Microcirculation* **3,** 287–300.

97. Hamann, A., Jablonski-Westrich, D., Duijvestijn, A., Butcher, E. C., Baisch, H., Harder, R., and Thiele, H.-G. (1988) Evidence for an accessory role of LFA-1 in lymphocyte-high endothelium interaction during homing. *J. Immunol.* **140,** 693–699.

98. Briskin, M. J., McEvoy, L. M., and Butcher, E. C. (1993) MAdCAM-1 has homology to immunoglobin and mucin like adhesion receptors and to IgA1. *Nature* **363,** 461–464.

99. Berg, E. L., McEvoy, L. M., Berlin, C., Bargatze, R. F., and Butcher, E. C. (1993) L-selectin-mediated lymphocyte rolling on MAdCAM-1. *Nature* **366,** 695–698.

100. Hu, M. C., Crowe, D. T., Weissman, I. L., and Holzmann, B. (1992) Cloning and expression of mouse integrin βp (β7): A functional role in Peyer's patch-specific lymphocyte homing. *Proc. Natl. Acad. Sci. USA* **89,** 8254–8258.

101. Berlin, C. Berg, E. L., Briskin, M. J., Andrew, D., Kilshaw, P. J., Holzmann, B., Weissman, I. L., Hamann, A., and Butcher, E. C. (1993) α4/β7 integrin mediates lymphocye binding to the mucosal vascular addressin MAdCAM-1. *Cell* **74,** 185–195.

102. Hamann, A., Andrew, D. P., Jablonski-Westrich, D., Holzmann, B., and Butcher, E. C. (1994) Role of alpha 4-integrins in lymphocyte homing to mucosal tissues in vivo. *J. Immunol.* **152,** 3282–3293.

103. Hahne, M., Lenter, M., Jager, U., Isenmann, S., and Vestweber, D. (1993) VCAM-1 is not involved in LPAM-1 (apha 4 beta p/alpha 4 beta 7) mediated binding of lymphoma cells to high endothelial venules of mucosa-associated lymph nodes. *Eur. J. Cell. Biol.* **61,** 290–298.

104. Mackay, C. R., Marston, W. L., Dudler, L., Spertini, O., Tedder, T. F., and Hein, W. R. (1992) Tissue-specific migration pathways by phenotypically distinct subpopulations of memory T cells. *Eur. J. Immunol.* **22,** 887–895.

105. Tedder, T. F., Matsuyama, T., Rothstein, D., Schlossman, S. F., and Morimoto, C. (1990) Human antigen-specific memory T cells express the homing receptor (LAM-1) necessary for lymphocyte recirculation. *Eur. J. Immunol.* **20,** 1351–1355.

106. Picker, L. J., Treer, J. R., Ferguson-Darnell, B., Collins, P. A., Buck, D., and Terstappen, L. W. M. M. (1993) Control of lymphocyte recirculation in man. I. Differential regulation of the peripheral lymph node homing receptor L-selectin on T cells during virgin to memory cell transition. *J. Immunol.* **150,** 1105–1121.

107. Walcheck, B. and Jutila, M. A. (1993) Bovine gamma/delta T cells express high levels of functional peripheral lymph node homing receptor (L-selectin). *Int. Immunol.* **6,** 81–91.

108. Gal'ea, P. Brezinschek, R., Lipsky, P. E., and Oppenheimer-Marks, N. (1994) Phenotypic characterization of CD4–/alpha beta TCR+ and gamma delta TCR+ T cells with a transendothelial migratory capacity. *J. Immunol.* **153,** 529–542.

109. Jutila, M. A., Wilson, E., and Kurk, S. (1997) Identification and characterization of an adhesion molecule that mediates leukocyte rolling on 24-hour cytokine stimulated bovine endothelial cells under flow conditions. *J. Exp. Med.*, **186,** 1701–1711.

110. Shimizu, Y., Shaw, S., Graber, N., Gopal, T. V., Horgan, K. J., van Seventer, G. A., and Newman, W. (1991) Activation-independent binding of human memory T cells to adhesion molecule ELAM-1. *Nature* **349,** 799–803.

111. Berg, E. L., Yoshino, T., Rott, L. S., Robinson, M. K., Warnock, R. A., Kishimoto, T. K., Picker, L. J., and Butcher, E. C. (1991) The cutaneous lymphocyte antigen is a skin lymphocyte homing receptor for the vascular lectin endothelial cell-leukocyte adhesion molecule 1. *J. Exp. Med.* **174,** 1461–1466.

112. Jones, W., Watts, G., Robinson, M., Vestweber, D., and Jutila, M. A. (1997) Comparison of E-selectin binding glycoprotein ligands on human lymphocytes and neutrophils, and bovine gamma/delta T cells. *J. Immunol.*, **159,** 3574–3583.

113. Silber, A., Newman, W., Sasseville, V. G., Pauley, D., Beall, D., Walsh, D. G., and Ringler, D. J. (1994) Recruitment of lymphocytes during cutaneous delayed hypersensitivity in nonhuman primates is dependent on E-selectin and vascular cell adhesion molecule 1. *J. Clin. Invest.* **93,** 1554–1563.

114. Staite, N. D., Justen, J. M., Sly, L. M., Beaudet, A. L., and Bullard, D. C. (1996) Inhibition of delayed-type contact hypersensitivity in mice deficient in both E-selectin and P-selectin. *Blood* **88,** 2973–2979.

115. Moore, K. L. and Thompson, L. F. (1992) P-selectin (CD62) binds to subpopulations of human memory T lymphocytes and natural killer cells. *Biochem. Biophys. Res. Commun.* **186,** 173–181.

116. Jutila, M. A. and Kurk, S. (1996) Analysis of bovine γ/δ T cell interactions with E-, P-, and L-selectin: Characterization of lymphocyte on lymphocyte rolling and the effects of O-glycoprotease. *J. Immunol.* **156,** 289–296.

117. Tipping, P. G., Huang, X. R., Berndt, M. C., and Holdsworth, S. R. (1996) P-selectin directs T lymphocyte-mediated injury in delayed-type hypersensitivity responses: studies in glomerulonephritis and cutaneous delayed-type hypersensitivity. *Eur. J. Immunol.* **26,** 454–460.

118. Michie, S. A., Streeter, P. R., Bolt, P. A., Butcher, E. C., and Picker, L. J. (1993) The human peripheral lymph node vascular addressin: an inducible endothelial antigen involved in lymphocyte homing. *Am. J. Pathol.* **143,** 1688–1698.

119. Faveeuw, C., Gagnerault, M. C., and Lepault, F. (1994) Expression of homing and adhesion molecules in infiltrated islets of Langerhans and salivary glands of nonobese diabetic mice. *J. Immunol.* **152,** 5969–5978.

120. Tang, M. L., Hale, L. P., Steeber, D. A., and Tedder, T. F. (1997) L-selectin is involved in lymphocyte migration to sites of inflammation in the skin: delayed rejection of allografts in L-selectin-deficient mice. *J. Immunol.* **158,** 5191–5199.

121. Bargatze, R. F., Kurk, S., Butcher, E. C., and Jutila, M. A. (1994) Neutrophils roll on adherent neutrophils bound to cytokine-stimulated endothelium via L-selectin on the rolling cells. *J. Exp. Med.* **180,** 1785–1792.

122. Walcheck, B., Moore, K. L., McEver, R. P., and Kishimoto, T. K. (1996) Neutrophil-neutrophil interactions under hydrodynamic shear stress involve L-selectin and PSGL-1: a mechanism that amplifies initial leukocyte accumulation on P-selectin in vitro. *J. Clin. Invest.* **98,** 1081–1087.

123. Alon, R., Fuhlbrigge, R. C., Finger, E. B., and Springer, T. A. (1996) Interactions through L-selectin between leukocytes and adherent leukocytes nucleate rolling adhesions on selectins and VCAM-1 in shear flow. *J. Cell. Biol.* **135,** 849–865.

124. Newhan, P., Craig, S. E., Seddon, G. N., Schofield, N. R., Rees, A., Edwards, R. M., Jones, E. Y., and Humphries, M. J. (1997) Alpha4 integrin binding interfaces on VCAM-1 and MAdCAM-1: integrin binding sites that play a role in integrin specificity. *J. Biol. Chem.* **272,** 19,429–19,440.

125. Groves, R. W., Ross, E. L., Barker, J. N. W. N., and MacDonald, D. M. (1993) Vascular cell adhesion molecule-1, Expression in normal and diseased skin and regulation in vivo by interferon gamma. *J. Am. Acad. Dermatol.* **29,** 67–72.

126. Abe, Y., Sugisaki, K., and Dannenberg, A. M. Jr. (1996) Rabbit vascular endothelial adhesion molecules: ELAM–1 is most elevated in acute inflammation, whereas VCAM–1 and ICAM–1 predominate in chronic inflammation. *J. Leuk. Biol.* **60,** 692–703.

127. Greenwood, J., Wang, Y., and Calder, V. L. (1995) Lymphocyte adhesion and transendothelial migration in the central nervous system: The role of LFA-1, ICAM-1, VLA-4, and VCAM-1. *Immunology* **86,** 408–415.

128. Picker, L. J. (1994) Control of lymphocyte homing. *Curr. Opinion Immunol.* **6,** 394–406.
129. Berlin, C. R., Bargatze, R. F., Campbell, J. J., von Andrian, U. H., Szabo, M. C., Hasslen, S. R., Nelson, R. D., Berg, E. L., Erlandsen, S. L., and Butcher, E. C. (1995) α4 integrins mediate lymphocyte attachment and rolling under physiologic flow. *Cell* **80,** 413–422.
130. Yednock, T. A., Cannon, C., Fritz, L. C., Sanchez-Madrid, F., Steinman, L., and Karin, N. (1992) Prevention of experimental autoimmune encephalomyelitis by antibodies against alpha 4 beta 1 integrin. *Nature* **356,** 63–66.
131. Hakugawa, J., Bae, S. J., Tanaka, Y., and Katayama, I. (1997) The inhibitory effect of anti-adhesion molecule antibodies on eosinophil infiltration in cutaneous late phase response in Balb/c mice sensitized with ovalbumin. *J. Dermatol.* **24,** 73–79.
132. Reinhardt, P. H., Elliot, J. F., and Kubes, P. (1997) Neutrophils can adhere via alpha4beta1–integrin under flow conditions. *Blood* **89,** 3837–3846.
133. Hogg, N., and Berlin, C. (1995) Structure and function of adhesion receptors in leukocyte trafficking. *Immunol. Today* **16,** 327–330.
134. Osborn, L. (1990) Leukocyte adhesion to endothelium in inflammation. *Cell* **62,** 3–6.
135. Hanninen, A., Salmi, M., Simello, O., Andrew, D., and Jalkanen, S. (1996) Recirculation and homing of lymphocyte subsets: Dual homing specificity of beta 7-integrin (high)-lymphocytes in nonobese diabetic mice. *Blood* **88,** 934–944.
136. Arvilommi, A. M., Salmi, M., Kalimo, K., and Jalkanen, S. (1996) Lymphocyte binding to vascular endothelium in inflamed skin revisited: a central role for vascular adhesion protein-1 (VAP-1) Eur. *J. Immunol.* **26,** 825–833.
137. Jones, D. A., Smith, C. W., Picker, L. J., and McIntire, L. V. (1996) Neutrophil adhesion to 24-hour IL-1 stimulated endothelial cells under flow conditions. *J. Immunol.* **157,** 858–863.

10

The *N*-Formyl Peptide Receptor

Structure, Signaling, and Disease

John S. Mills, Heini M. Miettinen, Michael J. Vlases, and Algirdas J. Jesaitis

Introduction

The chemotaxis of phagocytic leukocytes from the blood to tissues identifies the acute (neutrophil) and chronic (macrophages) inflammatory condition *(1)*. This hallmark process is central to host defense against microorganisms, to mediation of the immune response, and to repair of injured tissues. When unregulated, however, it is also the key vehicle of tissue damage and injury. Consequently, leukocyte chemotaxis, its ligands, and its receptors continue to be the focus of intense study. With a comprehensive molecular understanding of the structure-function relationships of chemotactic activation, intervention that mitigates injury but enhances microbial killing may become possible.

In a little more than a decade, a great deal of information has been gathered about the molecular basis of the chemotactic process and the pivotal role G protein-coupled chemoattractant receptors play in inflammation *(2)*. What has become abundantly clear is that there is, in fact, a multitude of chemotactic cytokines with corresponding seven transmembrane domain receptors *(3,4)*. These receptors not only mediate chemotaxis and initiate a variety of host defense and inflammatory functions *(5,6)* but are also exploited by viruses and other pathogens for infection *(3,7)*. The chemokines are a subject of other chapters in this volume, and their structure, classification, and function is covered sufficiently well there. However, in spite of the intense interest in these systems, fundamental questions remain about the molecular basis of chemokine activation that may be best answered in the classical phagocytic chemotactic receptor systems. Such questions include the nature of the ligand binding site and its effect on conformation of the receptor, transmission of the receptor occupancy signal to trans-

From: *Molecular and Cellular Basis of Inflammation*
Edited by: C. N. Serhan and P. A. Ward © Humana Press Inc., Totowa, NJ

ducing proteins, control of receptor activity, expression, and function in a complex signal transduction network; and, ultimately, what makes a cell move to a chemical stimulus.

The classical chemotactic receptors of phagocytes include the formyl peptide receptor (FPR), the C5a receptor (C5aR), the platelet-activating factor receptor (PAF-R), and the interleukin-8 receptor (IL-8R). These receptors, like the eicosanoid and chemokine receptors, are all members of the G protein-coupled receptor (GPCR) superfamily. The best characterized receptor in this family is neutrophil FPR, which binds bacterial *N*-formyl peptides, such as formyl-met-leu-phe (*f*MLF) *(8)*, formylated peptides derived from mitochondria *(9,10)*, and other as yet unidentified ligands that are released from eukaryotic organisms, such as *Candida albicans* (Edens, H. A., et al., unpublished results). Ligand binding to FPR results in induction of other host-defensive cellular processes, such as chemotaxis, adherence, secretion of lysosomal constituents, and production of superoxide and other inflammatory mediators. Recent focus on the structure and regulation of FPR has brought to light both novel and shared features of the chemotactic system of phagocytes. Two extensive reviews of FPR structure and function have recently been published *(11,12)*. This review attempts to provide additional insights into the structure-function relationships of this system.

Function of FPR in Disease

The role for phagocytes in the pathogenesis of infectious and inflammatory disease derives from their individual cell functions. These include cell polarization, directed motility, specific adhesion, secretion (including superoxide generation), and phagocytosis. Occupancy of FPR has been shown to specifically activate all these functions with the exception of phagocytosis *(2)*. Because these cellular responses have been well characterized with respect to activation by *f*MLF, they have served as a measure of normal leukocyte function against which dysfunction of leukocytes from diseased individuals or models could be examined. The complexity of the problem of identification of the key process in pathogenesis is quickly apparent because of the interplay of functions that affect one another and the ligand receptor systems that mediate their activation. For example, the chemoattractant *f*MLF is known to activate the expression of the adhesion CD11b/CD18 at the cell surface *(13)*. CD11b/CD18 is required for chemotaxis, but an overexpression of this protein might fix a leukocyte in place and thus abrogate the chemotactic process contributing to inflammatory pathogenesis *(13)*. Additionally, the occupancy of FPR stimulates the release of eicosanoid mediators, such as the leukotrienes (LTs) and prostaglandins (PGs), which serve as signals to prime leukocytes, to affect the homeostasis, and to regulate other receptor-mediated effector systems. Finally, new functions for the receptor appear to be emerging that include expression in nonleukocytic cells and possibly as receptors for undefined endogenous ligands *(14–16)* (Edens, H. A., et al., unpublished results). Table 1 summarizes recent literature (since about 1990) describing measurement of *f*MLF-stimulated cellular functions linked to the pathogenesis or manifestation of vascular disease, arthritis, colitis, and periodontitis. A brief summary of these results follows. References for this summary can be found in Table 1.

Table 1
FPR and Disease

Disease	System	Functional effect	FPR#/Kd	Reference
Coronary/ vascular disease	Hu	*f*MLF-aortal contractions; affect tissue monos; high-, low-affinity FPR homologs in nonleukocytic tissue	FPR homolog mRNA, Autorad.	*14*
	Hu	*f*MLF ↓ by adenosine		*161*
	Hu	*f*MLF vasoconstriction ↓ by α-MAC-1 but not in α-LFA-1–treated PMNs; α-ICAM-1 treatment of endothelium also inhibits		*162*
	Hu	*f*MLF ROS and chmtx ↑ after exercise for angina patients, not after angioplasty		*163*
	Hu	*f*MLF adherence and retention of PMNs in coronary venules and arteries after ischemia/reperfusion		*164*
	Hu	*f*MLF-ROS ↓ 1 min after balloon-induced ischemia, ↑ 20 min after reperfusion		*165,166*
	Hu	*f*MLF-ROS ↑ 10%, chmtx 45% 1 min after balloon-induced ischemia/reperfusion		*239*
	Hu	*f*MLF induces transient leuk sequestration in coronary microcirculation that is inhibitable with Ca^{2+} antagonist nisoldipine		*167*
	Hu	*f*MLF inhibits recovery of normal cardiac output after ischemia/reperfusion and exposure to H_2O_2+thrombin+exogenous PMNs		*168*
	Hu	*f*MLF induces ↑ vasoconstriction in femoral arteries		*169*
	Hu	Atrial natriuretic primes primes PMNs to enhance *f*MLF responsiveness in ischemia/reperfusion		*170*
	Hu	*f*MLF induces production of vasoconstrictor, cyclooxygenase products that mediate myotropism in coronary artery tissue		*171*
	Pigs	*f*MLF-ROS elevated in atherosclerotic model and and reduced after supplementation of diet with fish oil		*172*
	Rabbit	*f*MLF ↑ PMN-dependent pulmonary vascular resistance independent of cyclooxygenase or liposygenase products		*173*
	Rat heart	SOD has no effect on PMN/*f*MLF-induced transient vasoconstrictionbradycardia in isolated perfused rat heart		*175*
Rheumatoid arthritis	Hu	Pregnancy supresses inflammation in RA *f*MLF ROS ↓	FPR# =	*176*
	Hu	*f*MLF-induced chmtx ↓ in PMNs from synovium of RA patients vs controls and PB cells		*177*
	Hu	*f*MLF-degranul =; aggr-IgG-degranul ↓ in synovial cells vs control		*178*
	Hu	*f*MLF-ROS ↑ from synovial PMNs vs control or autologous PB cells		*179*
	Hu	Lyme arthritis OspA outer membrane proteins prime PMNs for *f*MLF-ROS and degranulation		*180*
	Hu	NSAID potentiates *f*MLF actin polymerization		*181*

(continued)

Table 1 *(cont.)*

Disease	System	Functional effect	FPR#/Kd	Reference
	Hu	*f*MLF-ROS (±cytokines) ↓ in RA patient PMNs under treatment; = with PMA		*182*
	Hu	*f*MLF-chmtx PB PMNs = ; synovial fluid PMNs ↓; same with IL-8		*183*
	Hu	*f*MLF-intracell H_2O_2 release by chondrocytes (cartilage Mφ)		*184*
	Hu	*f*MLF intracell-Ca^{2+} "exacerbated" in synovial fluid PMNs		*185*
	Hu	C5a, PMA, and *f*MLF-ROS ↓ by flosulide anti-inflammatory	FPR# ↓ 36%	*186*
	Hu	*f*MLF-chmtx in synovial fluid monos = PBL monos; ↓ with C5	FPR# = ; C5aR ↓	*187*
	Hu	*f*MLF-degranulation = in RA PMNs		*188*
	Hu, mouse	Behcet's RA has HLA-B51; HLA-B51 PMNs in diseased, nondiseased, and transgenic mice show ↑ *f*MLF-ROS		*189*
	Hu	PMN random migration ↑; chmtx ↓; juvenile RA PMNs *f*MLF-chmtx ↑ during disease episodes		*190*
	Hu	*f*MLF-ROS ↑ in PBL and synovial fluid PMNs; PAF no priming effect in RA cells		*191*
Colitis	Rat gut	*f*MLF causes ↑ LTB2, not PGE2/TXB2 in TNBS-induced colitis		*192*
	Hu	*f*MLF-ROS inactive UC ↑, UC/colectomy ↑, non-UC colectomy ↑ colon milieu supresses "normal response" ∴ UC = colectomy; PMA responses =	FPR express. =	*193*
	Rat	*f*MLF associates with bile acids and inhibits transcytosis of bile phospholipids and cholesterol		*194*
	Rat	*f*MLF instillation (and AGSG) cause PMN accumulation followed colonic inflammation		*195*
	Rat	Lipophilic antioxidant free radical scavenger tirilazad ↓ tissue edema in IBD rats and ↓ *f*MLF-ROS generated in colonic tissue		*47*
	Hu	Shigella-induced colitis: polarized PMN# ↑ in shigellosis; *f*MLF-polarizations ↑ with colitis complication		*196*
	Hu	Active and quiescent IBD patients have sera that prime PMN *f*MLF-ROS		*197*
	Hu	RD from control, inactive vs active UC patients: show graded suppression of *f*MLF-ROS; 44% of active UC RDs potentiated *f*MLF-ROS; control RDs and inactive RDs were 13 and 18% potentiation; inactive RDs, active RDs ↑ basal PMN ROS		*198*
	Rat	2 wk post TNBS-colitis: *f*MLF (and IL-8,LTB4)-chmtx suppressed; ROS ↑		*199*
	Hu	*C. dificile* enterotoxin A–induced colitis; in elderly; toxin A stimulates chmtx more than *f*MLF		*200*
	Hu	*f*MLFases in gut are reduced in Crohn's disease not in UC		*201*

(continued)

Table 1 *(cont.)*

Disease	System	Functional effect	FPR#/Kd	Reference
	Hu	ƒMLF-ROS ↓ in UC and Crohn's disease PB PMNs; monos ƒMLF-ROS ↑		*202*
	Rabbit	ƒMLF induces release of thrombexane from submucosa and mucosa of control colon; greatly amplified during inflammation		*203*
	Hu	Crohn's disease not UC PMNs, show ↑ FPR#, = Kds; ƒMLF-ROS ↑	FPR# ↑, Kd=	*204*
	Rats/Mice	Colonic instillation ƒMLF, ƒNLF, ƒMet causes marked mucosal edema and PMN infiltration in isolated colon; rectal instillation in mice causes acute rectal inflammation		*174*
Juvenile periodontitis	Hu	PB PMNL chmtx ↓	High-affinity FPR ↓, FPR isoforms ↓	*24*
JP	Hu	Chmtx ↑ (leading front method)		*205*
JP	Hu	ƒMLF/C5a-induced Ca^{2+} response ↑		*206*
JP	Hu	↓ ƒMLF binding and displaceable binding @ 23°C ƒMLF secretion normal	FPR# ↓	*207*
JP	Hu	ƒMLF and complement chmtx ↓ caused by serum effects		*208*
JP	Hu	ƒMLF chmtx rate ↓		*209*
LJP	Hu	Prepubertal JP chmtx = from age-matched controls JP chmtx ↓ relative to adults; CD11b = relative to controls		*210*
JP	Hu	ƒMLF-ROS, ƒMLF-elastase secretion unaffected		*211*
JP	Hu	Reduced antibody binding to ƒMLF-binding protein on PMNs from JP patients		*25*
LJP	Hu	Gp110 and FPR ↓ correlated to chmtx ↓ FPR# ↓		*212*
LJP	Hu	ƒMLF-aggregation ↓ in JP; ↑ in AP and post-JP		*213*
LJP	Hu	100% patient's PMNs show ƒMLF chmtx ↓; 30% patient's PMNs show phagocytosis ↓		*214*
LJP	Hu	ƒMLF-DAGK markedly ↓ in 60% LJP patients PMNs; DAGK inhibitor R59022 ↓ chmtx and ↑ ROS		*22*
LJP	Hu	In LJP PMNs, ƒMLF-DAG levels ↑, R59022 has no effect on ƒMLF-DAG		*23*
LJP	Hu	In Fc non-Fc zymosan phagocytosis, ƒMLF-ROS ↑; FcR, CR1, CR3 levels = in LJP PMNs		*215*
LJP	Hu	LJP patient sera ↓ chmtx, ↓ FPR# ; TNF-α, α-IL-2 block inhibition; AP and LJP patient sera w/o chmtx defect had no effect	FPR# ↓	*216*
LJP	Hu	Ca^{2+}-PKC ↓ for LJP PMNs, correlated with ↓ chmtx		*217*
LJP	Hu	2nd phase ƒMLF-Ca^{2+} in control and LJP PMNs		*218*
LJP	Hu	PMN migration ↓ but ƒMLF-chmtx = skin window test)		*219*
LJP	Hu	Bacterial extract factor primes ƒMLF-ROS production; factor heat resistant, proteinaceous, not endotoxin		*220,221*
LJP/JP	Hu	Chmtx and phagocytosis ↓		*222*
RPJP	Hu	Opsonized zymosan and ƒMLF-chmtx and ROS ↓; PMA-ROS normal		*223*

(continued)

Table 1 *(cont.)*

Disease	System	Functional effect	FPR#/Kd	Reference
PJP/RPJP	Hu	Chmtx ↓ (Boyden chamber)		*224*
JP/RPP	Hu	Significantly enhanced random migration in JP @ 1–10 n*M* *f*MLF chmtx ↓, JP @ > 1 µ*M* *f*MLF chmtx ↑; in RPP chmtx ↓ in as many as 85% PMN/monos, RPP random migration ↑ in as many as 63% PMN/monos		*225*
JP/RPP	Hu	Chmtx = in patients and controls		*226*
JP/RPP	Hu	*f*MLF chmtx ↓		*227*
JP/RPP	Hu	*f*MLF chmtx = to control (direct visual observation)		*228*
RPP	Hu	Total cellular β-glucuronidase and *f*MLF-β-glucuronidase release ↑ in gingival PMNs		*229*
RPP	Hu	PBL PMNs from RPP had ↑ amounts of β-glucuronidase and release more after *f*MLF		*230*
RPP	Hu	LPS (*P. gingivalis*) primes RPP PMNs via CD14: *f*MLF-ROS ↑ 2–3-fold; control =		*231*
RPP/AP	Hu	*f*MLF-chmtx, ROS, adherence ↓	FPR# ↓	*232*
RefP	Hu	In refractory periodontitis PB-PMNs, *f*MLF-chmtx		*233*
P/Gingivitis	Hu	Amino-F2 and SnF2 ↑ *f*MLF-ROS in normal PB PMNs		*234*

[a]↑, increased, greater; ↓, decreased, less than; = no change, equal to; a, antibody against; AGSG, Ala-Gly-Ser-Gly; AP, adult periodontitis; chmtx, chemotaxis; DAG, diacylglycerol; DAGK, DAG kinase; *f*MLF, fMet-Leu-Phe; *f*MLF-, *f*MLF induced or stimulated; IBD, inflammatory bowel disease; JP, juvenile periodontitis; leuk, leukocytes; LJP, localized JP; monos, monocytes or macrophages; NSAID, nonsteroidal anti-inflammatory drugs; PB, peripheral blood; PMA, phorbol myristate acetate; PKC, protein kinase C; RA, rheumatoid arthritis; RD, rectal dialysates; ROS, reactive oxygen species; RPP, rapidly progressive JP; SOD, superoxide dismutase; TNBS, trinitrobenzene sulfuric acid; UC, ulcerative colitis.

Vascular Disease

Phagocytes have been implicated in vascular disease because of their participation in atherosclerotic plaque formation *(17)* and in ischemia/reperfusion injury *(18,19)*. Briefly, in vascular disease, as in most inflammatory states, peripheral blood PMNs have been shown to be hyperresponsive to *f*MLF in their production of toxic or reactive oxygen species (ROS). This appears to be true for angina, atherosclerosis, and reperfusion injury after ischemia. Chemotaxis of PMNs is also elevated toward *f*MLF in vascular disease. Because *f*MLF induces leukocyte sequestration in the coronary microcirculation, the connection between infection (source of formylated peptides) and vascular disease would appear to be stronger *(20,21)*. Most recently, a series of interesting studies has suggested a direct role of FPR in vascular function, and perhaps pathology. In rabbits, *f*MLF increases PMN-dependent pulmonary vascular resistance that is independent of cyclooxygenase (COX) and lipoxygenase (LO) products. *f*MLF also induces aortal biphasic contractions and femoral vasoconstriction directly and independent of PMN. The former can be inhibited with adenosine but only partially with nonsteroidal anti-inflammatory drugs. FPR-specific autoradiography and mRNA analysis supports the presence FPR-related receptor in myocardial tissue outside of PMN or vascular tissue macrophages *(14)*.

Rheumatoid Arthritis

In rheumatoid arthritis, PMNs obtained from peripheral blood or synovial fluid also exhibit differences reflected in their responses to ƒMLF. In most cases, ƒMLF-ROS production appears to be elevated, whereas the situation for chemotaxis is mixed. Elevated measures of chemotaxis were found in peripheral blood leukocytes from juvenile arthritis patients. However, in adult arthritis patients the activity of blood leukocytes and synovial leukocytes was depressed. The almost universal increases in ƒMLF-stimulated ROS production were sensitive to mitigation by anti-inflammatory agents and therapy.

Colitis

In colonic tissue, ƒMLF has been shown to induce as well as exacerbate pathogenic inflammation in rats, rabbits, and mice. ƒMLF stimulates the production of LTB_4 (not PGE_2 or TXB_2) in trinitrobenzene sulfuric acid–induced colitis in rat gut but also thromboxane (TX) from mucosa and submucosa of inflamed colons of rabbits. In most cases, the ƒMLF-ROS of peripheral or colonic PMNs is elevated whereas the chemotactic response is reduced. Since the colonic milieu is abundant with bacteria and thus would be expected to be replete with bacterial ƒMLF-like substances, an important question is why inflammation is not normally chronic. Colonic peptidases cleave ƒMet peptides and are reduced in Crohn's disease but not in ulcerative colitis. However, the effects of rectal dialysates are to suppress ƒMLF-ROS production, which is reduced in actively inflamed or inactive ulcerative colitis patients.

Juvenile Periodontitis

Localized juvenile periodontitis (LJP) is an early form of periodontal disease associated with infection with *Actinobacillus actinomycetemcomitans*. The condition is localized to first molars and incisors, results in bone resorption and tooth loss, and is characterized by a high prevalence of compromised neutrophil function. Of 26 reports since 1977 (listed in Table 1) concerned with this disease and the role of ƒMLF, 16 describe impaired neutrophil chemotaxis. ƒMLF-induced cell aggregation, ROS production has also been found to be depressed in specific reports, but either unaffected or enhanced in others. ƒMLF-induced degranulation and production of ROS, in most cases, were elevated in juvenile periodontitis (JP) patients, whereas the Ca^{2+} response observed in other studies was unaffected. Unfortunately, a systematic pooled study from many laboratories has not been attempted to address some of the apparent discrepancies. In fact, there may be a number of defects that affect the ƒMLF-stimulated signal transduction pathway. Most recently, Hurttia et al. *(22,23)* discovered an LJP defect of diacylglycerol kinase (DAGK) in affected PMNs displaying inhibited chemotaxis and elevated levels of ƒMLF-stimulated diacylglycerol-DAG. This finding was supported by the action of R59022, a DAGK inhibitor, which inhibited chemotaxis, increased DAG levels, and increased ROS production in ƒMLF-stimulated normal PMNs, but had no effect on ƒMLF-stimulated DAG levels in PMNs from LJP patients. Additional reports suggest that there may be a defect in FPR in certain LJP patients. Five reports indicated a reduction in FMLF binding sites over matched controls. Perez et al. *(24)* described separation of four differently charged isoforms of FPR that were incompletely represented in JP cells. DeNardin et al. *(25)* identified ƒMLF-binding proteins of atypical M_r by SDS-PAGE that appeared to have reduced immunological reactivity with specific monoclonal antibodies in LJP. Unfortunately, neither of these studies was followed up with an examination of the genetic structure of the FPR locus.

The *N*-Formyl Peptide Receptor Family

Human FPR is a GPCR receptor with seven putative transmembrane spanning domains and three potential N-linked glycosylation sites *(26)*. The effects of amino acid substitutions and modifications of the N- and C-terminals of *f*MLF on FPR binding and activation have been extensively studied *(27–29)*. The N-terminal formyl group, the methionine at position 1, and phenylalanine at position 3 have all been shown to be necessary for the highest affinity binding. Decarboxylation of the phenylalanine markedly reduces activity, but esters or amides of phenylalanine are as active or more active than the free acid. Therefore, the phenylalanine carbonyl oxygen is likely to be involved in hydrogen-bonding interactions with FPR. None of these functional groups is absolutely required for activity, but, rather, each functional group in *f*MLF appears to individually contribute to the overall free energy of ligand binding.

Ten residues that affect *f*MLF binding have been mapped to transmembrane domains II–VII *(30)*, including residues L78 (II-17, helix II, residue 17 of 26 transmembrane spanning residues in the nomenclature used throughout this text), D106 (III-8), L109 (III-11), T157 (IV-18), R201 (V-2), I204 (V-5), R205 (V-6), W254 (VI-16), Y257 (VI-19), and F291 (VII-11). In addition, several residues in the extracellular loop between helices II and III have been shown to affect ligand binding *(31)* indicating that these residues may also be involved in binding, perhaps by folding inward on a binding pocket located between the transmembrane-spanning helices.

Sequences for FPR from numerous species have been determined. Rabbit FPR cDNA encodes a protein that is 78% identical to that of human FPR and binds *f*MLF with high affinity *(32)*. Murine FPR is 76% identical to human FPR, and it exhibits low-affinity binding to *f*MLF *(33)*. Another human gene, FPRL1 (now identified as LXA$_4$R *[34]*), cross-hybridizes with FPR under high-stringency conditions *(35,36)* Lipoxin A$_4$ (LXA$_4$) cDNA encodes a protein whose sequence is 69% identical to that of FPR. FPR and LXA$_4$R transcripts are detected only in differentiated myeloid cells. LXA$_4$R exhibits a much lower binding affinity (K_d > 400 nM) for *f*MLF compared to FPR (K_d = 1 nM), and when expressed in transfected cells, it mediates *f*MLF-stimulated calcium mobilization only at micromolar concentrations of *f*MLF *(37)*. LXA$_4$R binds LXA$_4$ with a high affinity (5 nM) and leukotriene D$_4$ (LTD$_4$)with an intermediate affinity (80 nM) *(34,38)*. A different form of LXA$_4$R has been identified in human umbilical vein endothelial cells that exhibits similar affinities for both LXA$_4$ and LTD$_4$ but its sequence is unknown *(38,39)*. Another receptor related in sequence to LXA$_4$R and FPR is FPRL2 *(37)*. It is 72% identical to LXA$_4$R and 57% identical to FPR, and is present in differentiated myeloid cells but not in neutrophils. The ligand for FPRL2 has not yet been identified, but it exhibits no detectable activation by *f*MLF *(40)*. Thus, human LXA$_4$R is only slightly less homologous to human FPR than are FPRs from two other mammalian species. The close relationships among these receptors provide comparisons that are helpful in determining which amino acid residues are involved in ligand binding. Their high degree of sequence similarity suggests that small changes in sequence, appropriately located in the ligand-binding pocket, can alter ligand specificity.

Rhodopsin as a Template for the Structure of FPR

Several types of evidence provide information about the placement of retinal in rhodopsin. The first is the formation of a retinal Schiff base with K296 (helix VII residue 11) in the seventh transmembrane-spanning helix of opsin *(41)*. Second, analog of retinal have been prepared with photoaffinity labels placed in *(42)* or adjacent to *(43)* the cyclohexene ring of retinal. These photoaffinity labels crosslinked to W265 (VI-19) and several residues in helix III, indicating that the cyclohexene ring lies close to these residues. Third, the counterion to protonated 11-*cis*-retinal has been identified as E113 [III-3] *(44)*, and this counterion is ~3 Å from the C12 of retinal *(45)*. This counterion can be "moved" to residue G90 [II-17] *(46)*, or residue A117 [III-7] *(55)* and still function as a counterion, indicating that E113, G90, and A117 must be close to the Schiff base nitrogen or to the C12 of retinal *(45)*, at least when rhodopsin is in its protonated 11-*cis*-retinal form.

The two-dimensional projection of the structure of rhodopsin has been determined to 6 Å resolution and the three-dimensional (3D) structure has been reconstructed at lower resolution *(48)*. A refinement of this structure has allowed the helical tilt angles of all seven helices to be determined, and density on the extracellular side of the membrane suggested a folded domain *(49)*. In addition, the 3D conformation of 11-*cis*-retinal bound to rhodopsin has been determined by nuclear magnetic resonance (NMR) *(45)*. An approximate structure of rhodopsin was determined by "docking" this NMR structure of 11-*cis*- retinal into the protein *(50)*. Also, a 3D model of the structure of rhodopsin has been constructed by incorporating approximate distance constraints obtained from chemical crosslinking and site-directed mutagenesis *(51)*. Taken together, these data provide a good 3D structure for rhodopsin that can be used for modeling the structures of other GPCR.

Similarities Among Retinal, fMLF, and LXA$_4$

Because the GPCR form a large homologous superfamily, it is reasonable to assume that their respective ligands may act similarly and that the proteins may share certain structural features that mediate their interaction with their respective G proteins. Miettinen et al. *(30)* showed that residues in FPR that affect the binding to *f*MLF analog map in analogous regions to those that affect retinal binding in rhodopsin. Because rhodopsin structure is better understood than other GPCR and because information is available on residues in rhodopsin that are important for retinal binding and G protein activation (*see* Nathans *[52]* for review), it is useful to compare the retinal chromophore of rhodopsin to *f*MLF and ligands of other GPCR. Similarities among the ligands should be reflected in similar residues in their respective receptors. Also, differences among ligands should be reflected in complementary changes in their respective receptors. Figure 1 shows that the structures of all-*trans* retinal, *f*MLF, and LXA$_4$ have very similar dimensions and volumes. The fact that FPR's most closely related receptor, LXA$_4$R binds both the arachidonic acid derivative, LXA$_4$ *(34)*, and *f*MLF *(53)* further emphasizes the similarity between peptide and nonpeptide structures.

A 3D Model of FPR

To determine whether it was indeed possible for *f*MLF to fit between the seven transmembrane helices of FPR, the authors prepared a 3D model of FPR based on the model of rhodopsin reported by Herzyk and Hubbard *(51)*. The sequences of the transmem-

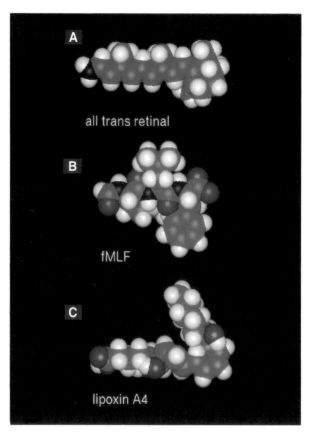

Fig. 1. Similarity of ligand structures. (A) All-*trans*-retinal in its unprotonated Schiff base form. (B) formyl-met-leu-phe-OH in an extended conformation. (C) LXA$_4$ in a conformation in which C17–C20 is bent to be similar to the side chain of Leu in *f*MLF.

brane segments of FPR were selected based on the multiple sequence alignment of GPCRs by Baldwin *(54)* except that helix II was assigned to residues 61–87 rather than 57–83 *(30)*. The basic model was generated using the automated rule-based method described by Herzyk and Hubbard *(51)* with the rhodopsin template on the Swiss-Model 7TM Interface of the Swiss-Prot World Wide Web server.*

A 3D model of FPR that includes a 3D model of *f*MLF placed between the seven transmembrane helices is shown in Fig. 2. The methionine and phenylalanine side chains of *f*MLF are positioned deep within the binding pocket (relative to the extracellular side), whereas the leucine side chain is nearer the extracellular space. The positioning of *f*MLF within the binding pocket was based on data obtained by site-directed mutagenesis *(30)* and photocrosslinking (Mills, J. M., et al., unpublished results). The plane of the *f*MLF phenyl ring was positioned parallel to the helical axes. In this position, the phenyl ring can form close van der Waal's contacts with L109 (III-7) and W254 (VI-18) *(30)*. This places the phenylalanine ring of *f*MLF in a similar position to the cyclohexene ring of retinal, which is close to W265 (VI-18) and helix III in opsin

*World Wide Web address: http://expasy.hcuge.ch/cgi-bin/ProMod-GPCR.pl.

(43). The amine nitrogen of K85 (II-24) is within 2–3 Å of the methionine carbonyl oxygen on *f*MLF—sufficiently close to form a hydrogen bond. This position is based on photocrosslinking data in which FPR residues 84–86 were found to crosslink to a photoactivatable amino acid residue that was used to replace the leucine residue in *f*MLF *(240)*. Figure 1 shows that the methionine carbonyl of *f*MLF is in a similar position to the C-12 of retinal, further justifying the placement of K-85 (II-24) near the methionine carbonyl of *f*MLF. R201 (V-2) and R205 (V-6) are positioned close to the carboxylate oxygen of *f*MLF and close to D106 (III-7). Hydrogen bonding among these residues may explain why these three residues are all essential for optimal binding *(30)*. R201 (V-2) is a phenylalanine and R205 (V-6) a histidine in FPRL2, which does not exhibit appreciable binding of *f*MLF *(40)*. This observation is consistent with these residues having an important role in FPR.

F291 (VII-11) is analogous to K296 (VII-11) in rhodopsin, the residue that forms the Schiff base with retinal *(41)*. The authors' model places this phenylalanine in close contact with the formyl group of *f*MLF. In addition, L78 (II-17), which is analogous to G90 (II-17) in rhodopsin and the site of an alternative Schiff base counterion *(46,55)*, could also make close contacts with the formyl group. Together these two residues could form a tight pocket around the formyl group and impart tight binding to formylated peptides. Such a tight pocket around the formyl group is seen in both *f*MLF binding to immunoglobulin *(56)* and in *f*MYFINILTL binding to human MHC class 1b molecule H2-M3 *(57)*, and might be a general motif in binding of formylated peptides. Formylated peptides (*f*MFFINILT) that bind to the mouse MHC class 1b molecule H2-M3 have been shown to be potent chemotactic agents for neutrophils *(10)*, indicating that the MHC class 1b molecule H2-M3 molecule may bind similar peptides to those that bind to FPR. Therefore, the conformation of these peptides bound to FPR may be similar to that seen in the crystal structure of *f*MYFINILTL bound to MHC class 1b molecule H2-M3.

FPR-Mediated Signal Transduction

G Proteins Involved in FPR–G Protein Coupling

The activation of inflammatory cells by chemoattractant ligands involves the interaction of the ligand-receptor complexes with heterotrimeric ($\alpha\beta\gamma$) guanine nucleotide-binding proteins—the G proteins. Initial evidence for this interaction came from studies showing that the binding affinity of formylated peptides to FPR was affected by guanine nucleotides *(58,59)* and that ligand binding induced hydrolysis of GTP *(59,60)*. The main class of G proteins that interact with chemoattractant receptors was identified as G_i based on their sensitivity to pertussis toxin (PT) *(61)* (*Bordetella pertussis* islet-activating protein; for review, see ref. *62*). PT was shown to inhibit the chemoattractant-stimulated rise in the intracellular concentration of free calcium, polyphosphoinositide breakdown, chemotaxis, superoxide production, and release of arachidonic acid and granular enzymes *(59,61,63–66)*. G_i was also shown to associate physically with FPR in neutrophil reconstitution assays *(67,68)*. The main PT-modified G proteins in neutrophils are G proteins containing the α-subunits G_{i2} or G_{i3} *(69)*. However, G_i does not appear to be the only class of G proteins that interact with FPR, because PT-induced inhibition of the cellular activation process triggered by chemoattractant ligands is heterogeneous and differentially sensitive *(64,70–72)*. A pertussis-toxin resistant protein

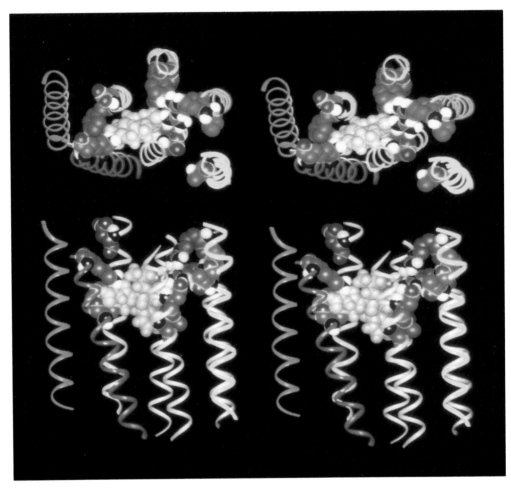

Fig. 2. A 3D model of FPR. A simplified model of the side chains of the amino acid residues that affect *f*MLF binding *(30)* are shown in atom-coded space-filling form (white: hydrogen; green: carbon; blue: nitrogen; red: oxygen). A gray space-filling model of *f*MLF was placed between the seven transmembrane helices. Transmembrane helices are colored as follows: I, blue; II, magenta; III, aqua; IV, yellow; V, orange-red; VI, light blue; and VII, orange. The sequences of the transmembrane segments of FPR were selected based on the multiple sequence alignment of GPCRs by Baldwin *(54)* except that helix II was assigned to residues 61–87 rather than 57–83 *(30)*. The basic model was generated using the automated rule-based method described by Herzyk and Hubbard *(51)* using the rhodopsin template as described in the text. The phenyl ring is positioned parallel to the helices to allow *f*MLF to fit between the helices. Adjustment based on Miettinen et al. *(30)* mutagenesis data were then made to the model as follows: Helix V was rotated 90° about its axis to position the side chains of both R201 (V-2) and R205 (V-6) on the binding pocket face of the helix. In this position, I204 (V-5) is oriented toward helix VI.

of the G_q class, $G\alpha_{16}$, is expressed in hematopoietic cells and may transduce a signal from chemoattractant receptors. Cotransfection of COS-7 cells with $G\alpha_{16}$ (but not G_q) and C5aR or FPR resulted in ligand-dependent cell activation *(73,74)*. Similarly, coexpression of C5aR or FPR with $G\alpha_{16}$ in *Xenopus* oocytes resulted in signal transduction on addition of ligand *(75)*. $G\alpha_{16}$ may thus play a role in the inflammatory response of leukocytes. In HL-60 cells, G_o has been implicated in *f*MLF-mediated cellular responses in addition to G_{i2}; transfection of antisense-oriented cDNAs encoding the α-chain of G_o into differentiated human HL-60 cells led to depressed intracellular calcium response to *f*MLF *(76)*. However, the role of G_o in FPR-mediated signal transduction is still controversial, because the major neutrophil G protein is G_{i2}. In addition, G_o mRNA was found to be below the detection level in HL-60 cells by Northern blot analysis *(69)*.

The FPR amino acid residues that contact and interact with G protein are still largely unknown. Several regions in the cytoplasmic loops and/or transmembrane regions and the cytoplasmic tail have been implicated in the binding of G_i based on mutagenesis and reconstitution studies. Regions in the putative first cytoplasmic loop, including parts of the contiguous transmembrane domains, and part of the putative third, fourth, fifth, and sixth transmembrane domains have all been implicated in G protein coupling based on in vitro reconstitution, in vivo functional, and antibody binding assays *(73,77,78)*. In many GPCRs, the amino- and carboxyterminal parts of the third cytoplasmic loop have been implicated in binding to G proteins. However, FPR has a rather short third cytoplasmic loop (13–15 amino acids), in contrast to most other GPCRs, and mutagenesis and reconstitution studies have shown that this region of FPR is not involved in G protein interaction *(77–79)*. Instead, the midregion of the putative cytoplasmic tail of FPR may participate in the interaction with G proteins, since peptides corresponding to this region (but not to other cytoplasmic tail regions) competed with FPR for binding to G proteins *(80)* and inhibited binding of anti-G_i antibody to $G_{i\alpha}$ *(78)*. Certain highly conserved transmembrane domain amino acids among the GPCRs have been implicated in G protein coupling, including asparagine (I-18), aspartic acid (II-10), aspartic acid (III-24), arginine (III-25) (DRY motif in most G protein-coupled receptors, DRC in FPR), asparagine (VII-17), and tyrosine (VII-21) (NPXXY motif). Site-specific mutagenesis of these residues in FPR has indicated that the asparagine 44 (I-18) and the

---

(Fig. 2 cont.) The side chain of R205 (V-5) was rotated so that the h1 nitrogen was within hydrogen bonding distance (2.5-3 Å) of the phenylalanine carbonyl oxygen of *f*MLF. (The oxygen chosen was one that would be present in either the free acid or amide form of the peptide in its extended chain orientation, since both bind well to FPR.) D106 (III-8) was rotated so that the carbonyl g1 oxygen was within hydrogen-bonding distance to the h2 nitrogen of R205 and so that the D106 (III-8) carbonyl g2 oxygen was oriented toward the T157 (IV-18) hydroxyl group. The nonbonding orbital of the oxygen of Y257 (VI-9) was positioned to hydrogen bond to e nitrogen of R205, and the h1 nitrogen of R201 was positioned to hydrogen bond with the other nonbonding orbital. The e amino group of K85 (II-24) was positioned to be within hydrogen bonding distance of the methionine carbonyl of *f*MLF. F306 (VII-11) and L78 (II-17) were positioned to form a tight pocket around the formyl group of *f*MLF. W254 and L109 were positioned to interact with the phenyl group of *f*MLF. **(Top)** Stereo view of FPR with bound FMLF as viewed from the extracellular space. **(Bottom)** Stereo transmembrane view with helices V–VII in the foreground. The receptor was visualized using Insight II software by Biosym on a Silicon Graphics Iris platform.

aspartic acid 122 (III-24) in the DRC sequence in the third transmembrane domain are important for proper folding of the molecule since an alanine substitution leads to retention of the protein in the endoplasmic reticulum of stably transfected Chinese hamster ovary cells (Miettinen, H. M., et al., unpublished results). The following mutations (indicated in single letter amino acid code) caused decreased G protein coupling without affecting the ligand binding affinity: D71A, D71N (II-10), and R123A (III-25) (Miettinen, H. M., et al., unpublished results). Similar results expressing FPR in L fibroblasts have been previously obtained by Prossnitz et al. *(81)*. A double mutation D71N/N297D (II-10/VII-17) resulted in reversal of the D71N mutant phenotype (Miettinen, H. M., et al., unpublished results), supporting previous evidence suggesting that a hydrogen-bonding network between these residues affects G protein coupling to various GPCRs *(82)*.

Effectors of FPR

Multiple intracellular phospholipases, protein kinases, and other proteins are involved in transducing the signal from activated G proteins to the inside of the cell. Next, the authors will discuss the major effector molecules in neutrophil signal transduction. A recent review article on signal transduction in the human neutrophil, including information about cytokine receptors, is recommended to interested readers *(83)*.

Phosphatidyl Inositol-3-Kinase as a Major Effector of FPR

The GPCR-induced production of phosphatidyl inositol (3,4,5) trisphosphate $[PI(3,4,5)P_3]$ was first observed in neutrophils by Traynor-Kaplan et al. *(84,85)* after stimulation with *f*MLF. The enzyme phosphoinositide 3-kinase (PI- 3K) phosphorylates phosphatidyl inositol (4,5) bisphosphate $[PI(4,5)P_2]$ as the major substrate in vivo and phosphatidyl inositol (PI), PI(4)P and $PI(4,5)P_2$ in vitro *(86)*. Several species of PI3K have been characterized and cloned. The PI3K isotype that can be activated in vitro by phosphatidyl inositol (4) phosphate [PI(4)P] βγ subunits of G protein without tyrosine phosphorylation *(87)* is a 110-kDa protein termed PI3Kγ *(88–90)*. The two other PI3Ks, PI3Kα and PI3Kβ, are heterodimeric molecules (p110 and p85) mainly regulated by receptors with intrinsic or associated tyrosine kinase activity *(91)*. The fungal metabolite wortmannin specifically inhibits PI3K at nanomolar concentrations, making it a useful drug for analysis of the role of PI(3,4,5)P3 in chemoattractant-mediated functions *(92)*. The most pronounced effect of wortmannin is on the neutrophil oxidative burst that can be completely inhibited at low concentrations *(93–96)*. Wortmannin does not inhibit actin polymerization *(96)*, but causes oscillatory changes *(92)*, suggesting that PI(3,4,5)P3 production may play a role in actin regulation but is not the primary event resulting in polymerization of F-actin. Signal transduction molecules directly downstream from G protein, such as phospholipases, may thus be responsible for some of the chemoattractant-induced intracellular events, including actin polymerization. Signaling molecules activated by PI(3,4,5)P3 include the mitogen-activated protein kinases (MAPKs), protein kinase C (PKC), and the small GTP-binding protein, Rac *(97–99)*.

MAPK Pathway

The MAPKs, also known as extracellular signal-regulated kinases (ERK), were first identified in transmission of extracellular signals into the cell through growth factor receptors (for review *see* ref. *100*). The initial events occur in close proximity to the

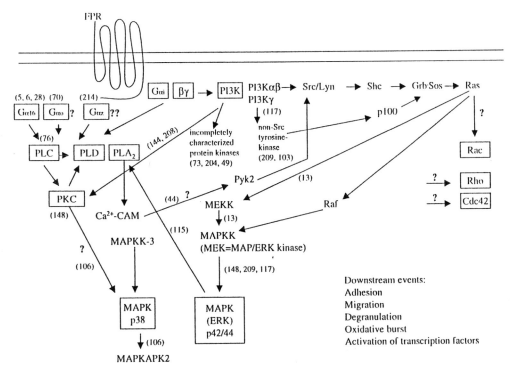

Fig. 3. Schematic diagram of signal transduction molecules thought to be involved in FPR-mediated signal transduction.

growth factor receptor and require the activation of PI3K. The following molecules have been characterized in the subsequent activation steps, as outlined in Fig. 3: An Src family tyrosine kinase, Shc and Grb2 (adaptor molecules), Sos (a guanine nucleotide exchange factor), and Ras (a small GTP-binding protein) *(101–103)*. Activated Ras binds to Raf-1 (a serine-threonine kinase), which stimulates a MAPK kinase (MEK), which in turn phosphorylates a MAPK (extracellular-signal-regulated kinase [ERK]). This phosphorylation cascade eventually activates intracellular regulatory molecules. The MAPK cascade was subsequently also found to be activated through GPCRs. *f*MLF stimulation of human neutrophils results in tyrosine phosphorylation of two distinct MAP-kinases, ERK-1 and ERK-2 (also called p42 and p44) *(104–106)*. Subsequent characterizations of the signaling pathways have found common and distinct effector molecules for growth factor receptor- and GPCR-mediated activation. In neutrophils, activation of FPR stimulates the Ras/MAPK cascade through the Src-related tyrosine kinase Lyn *(107)*. The formation of phosphorylated complexes of Lyn and the Shc adaptor protein correlates with the formation of prostacyclin3 *(107)*. An alternative to the Lyn-Shc pathway may also exist in neutrophils since FPR-transfected fibroblasts that do not express Lyn can be activated through the MAPK pathway after *f*MLF-stimulation without an increase in tyrosine phosphorylation of the adaptor protein, Shc *(108)*. Similarly, in Rat-1 fibroblasts and COS cells, G_i-mediated MAPK activation requires neither Src nor Shc *(109)*. Instead, a 100 kDa tyrosine-phosphorylated protein (p100) binds to the Src homology 3 domain of Grb2 in a ligand- and G_i-dependent fashion *(109)*. In the kinase cascade, MEKK (MAPKK kinase) and MAPKK are inhibited by wortmannin and PT, indicating a role for G_i and/or G_o and PI3Kγ in the activation cascade *(108,110,111)*. G_q also stimulates PI hydrolysis and MAPK activation. However, the MAPK activation stimulated by G_q-coupled receptors is unaffected by expression of a dominant negative mutant of p21[ras] or protein tyrosine kinase inhibitors, but is affected by cellular depletion of PKC *(76)*. Furthermore, the activation of an MAPK other than ERK, p38MAPK, is not blocked by PT *(111)* and is only partly inhibited by wortmannin or *bis*-indolylmaleimide (a PKC antagonist). These observations provide evidence that alternative pathways in addition to G$\beta\gamma$/PI3Kγ may exist to allow activation of MAPK-activated protein kinase (MAPKAPK2) *(113)*. A MAPKK inhibitor, PD98059, can block neutrophil chemotaxis but does not inhibit superoxide anion production, suggesting that the p38MAPK/MAPKAPK pathway may regulate neutrophil oxidative burst without the activation of the MEK phosphorylation cascade *(114)*.

The Role of Small GTP-Binding Proteins in fMLF-Induced Signal Transduction

Small GTP-binding signal transduction molecules of the Ras superfamily are involved in regulation of cellular events, such as cell adhesion, cell migration, superoxide generation, granule exocytosis and phagocytosis. A recent book chapter by Quinn *(115)* describes in detail the role of small GTP-binding proteins in leukocyte signal transduction. Below follows a brief summary of the most important neutrophil small GTP-binding proteins and their functions.

Ras, which defines the *ras* subfamily of small GTP-binding proteins, is required for activation of the p42/44 MAPK pathway, as outlined in the previous section, and will not be discussed further here.

The *rho* subfamily contains small GTP-binding proteins that are involved in specific cellular functions. RhoA was shown to regulate the assembly of actin stress fibers and focal adhesions in fibroblasts *(116,117)*. The role of RhoA is not equally well established in leukocytes, although it may regulate similar functions as in fibroblasts, since RhoA affects chemoattractant-activated leukocyte adhesion *(118)*. Lymphoid cells transfected with FPR or IL-8R exhibit increased $\alpha 4\beta 1$ integrin mediated cell adhesion in the presence of ligand *(118)*. The adhesion is blocked in the presence of a RhoA inhibitor, C3 exoenzyme. Similar results have been obtained using human neutrophils *(118)*. In bovine neutrophils, treatment with the RhoA inhibitor, C3 exoenzyme from *Clostridium botulinum*, led to reduced chemoattractant-induced cell motility and a disorganized actin filament network but did not affect degranulation *(189)*. It thus appears that RhoA is involved in regulation of adhesion and migration of leukocytes.

Two other small GTP-binding proteins appear to play a role in neutrophil motility. Rac, occurs as two isoforms (Rac1 and Rac2) that belong to the *rho* subfamily and are 58% homologous with Rho *(120)*. Rac2 is the more abundant isoform in neutrophils. One well known target of Rac2 is p67-*phox*, one of the components of the NADPH oxidase system *(121,122)*. Both forms of Rac can activate superoxide generation in a cell-free system *(123,124)*. In fibroblasts, Rac was first found to play a role in membrane ruffling and pinocytosis *(125)*. The role of Rac in the organization of the leukocyte cytoskeleton is now being examined more closely. A study using a macrophage cell line showed that Rac1 stimulates membrane ruffling and the assembly of adhesion sites to the extracellular matrix *(126)*. Recently, Acaro *(241)* showed that Rac promotes the dissociation of gelsolin from microfilaments in neutrophil extracts and appears to be regulated by Rho GDI and Gi but not PI3K. Finally Cdc42, another small GTP-binding protein having filopodial-inducing activity in 3T3 *(242)* cells, was shown by Zigmond et al. *(243)* to induce actin polymerization in neutrophil cytosol.

Phospholipases and PKC

Three different classes of phospholipases, phospholipases A_2 (PLA_2), C (PLC), and D (PLD) have been characterized in *f*MLF-induced neutrophil activation. The phospholipases cleave plasma membrane phospholipids at specific sites, yielding active neutrophil second messengers, the functions of which have been extensively studied by blocking or regulating their production or by adding them to permeabilized cells. PLA_2 releases from neutrophil plasma membrane arachidonic acid, which may act directly as a regulatory molecule. However, it is better known as a precursor for the biosynthesis of biologically active eicosanoids, such as LTs and PGs. The ligand-stimulated activation of PLA_2 is regulated by PKC, MAPK, and possibly other kinases *(127)*. $PLC\beta_2$, the central PLC in neutrophils, is activated by the $\beta\gamma$-subunits of G protein and catalyzes the hydrolysis of $PI(4,5)P_2$ into inositol 1,4,5-trisphosphate $I(1,4,5)P_3$ and diacylglycerol (DAG), two mediators that are involved in activation of a serine/threonine kinase, PKC *(128,129)*. PKC plays an important role in the various neutrophil activation responses. However, several cell functions are not blocked by PKC inhibitors, indicating that multiple independent pathways are involved in receptor-mediated activation. PLD catalyzes the hydrolysis of phosphatidylcholine into choline and phosphatidic acid; the latter can be further metabolized to DAG but this form of DAG (saturated/monounsaturated) does not appear to regulate PKC based on a recent finding *(130)*. PLD is a relatively newly characterized component in the neutrophil signal transduction pathway. Experiments using permeabilized cells and in vitro assays with purified protein have facilitated the identification of several proteins that regulate PLD activity. One such protein is a small GTP-binding protein, ADP-ribosylation factor (Arf), from the Ras superfamily. Arf was found to enhance GTPγS-dependent stimulation of PLD activity in HL-60 membranes, with optimal activity after addition of $PI(4,5)P_2$ *(131)*. Another family of small GTP-binding proteins, the Rho family, has also been implicated in the regulation of PLD *(132,133)*, and the regulation is synergistic with Arf *(134)*. Other work has identified roles for PKCα and PKCβ in PLD activation in HL-60 cells and neutrophils *(135,136)*. For more information on the regulation of PLA_2, PLC, and/or PLD, the reader is referred to recent review articles *(137–140)*.

Crosstalk Between FPR and Other Chemoattractant Receptors

Chemoattractant receptors, such as C5aR, IL8-R, and FPR, may blunt their own signal as well as that of the other receptors through homologous and heterologous desensitization. The hierarchy for the chemoattractant desensitization in neutrophils, as demonstrated on the levels of receptor cross-phosphorylation, intracellular calcium mobilization, and chemotaxis, is *f*MLF > C5a > IL-8 *(141–144)*: *f*MLF and C5a efficiently desensitize the IL-8R response, but C5a and IL-8 only partly desensitize FPR to stimulation with formylated peptides. C5a has also been shown to reduce *f*MLF-induced $PI(3,4,5)P_3$ formation and actin polymerization but does not affect $PI(4,5)P_2$ hydrolysis and production of superoxide *(145)*. In neutrophils, *f*MLF is the most potent chemoattractant, possibly ensuring that the cells are recruited to sites of bacterial infection even in the presence of multiple other chemoattractants in the tissue. In other types of inflammation in which formylated peptides are not involved, such as chronic allergic inflammation, one might expect a different hierarchy for receptor stimulation and desensitization. This was recently shown in eosinophils, which are the primary leukocytes involved in allergies and parasitic infections. *f*MLF or C5a at 1 and 10 n*M* enhanced, rather than inhibited, the migration toward the C-C chemokines RANTES and MCP-3, suggesting that inflammatory cells have different behavioral patterns depending on the cell type and chemoattractant *(143)*.

Regulation of FPR

FPR, like many GPCRs, appears to be regulated by phosphorylation in a ligand-dependent manner *(144,146)*. Possible sites of receptor phosphorylation were identified by using a fusion protein containing the C-terminus of FPR as a substrate for G protein receptor kinase GRK2 *(147)*. A mutant of FPR was then prepared in which these FPR phosphorylation sites (Ser or Thr) were mutated to Ala or Gly, and the effects of the loss of the phosphorylation sites on the desensitization of the Ca^{2+} response to ligand was determined *(148)*. Removal of eight possible phosphorylation sites in the C-terminal tail of FPR completely blocked ligand-induced phosphorylation of FPR in U937 cells expressing FPR. The loss of phosphorylation corresponded to a lack of desensitization of the cells' Ca^{2+} response to prior exposure to ligand, and the author concluded that phosphorylation of FPR at these sites is necessary for desensitization of FPR *(148)*.

Other studies, by Jesaitis et al. *(149–151)*, have indicated that interaction of FPR with the neutrophil cytoskeleton may be important in FPR regulation. Theses studies examined the relationship among FPR, homologous desensitization, Triton X-100 insolubility, and compartmentation in plasma membrane. Neutrophil responsiveness to FMLF was found to be inversely proportional to the number of nondissociable ligand-receptor complexes found in the Triton X-100–insoluble fraction of the cells *(152)*. It was also positively correlated with the lateral segregation of occupied FPR (in actin/fodrin-enriched high-density plasma membrane domains) from G proteins (in actin/fodrin-poor lower density domains) *(153)*. This conclusion was confirmed when these microdomains were solubilized in 1–2% octyl glucoside and examined by analytical ultracentrifugation *(154)*. Receptors from the light domain sedimented as 7S particles, whereas the desensitized receptors from the heavy domain sedimented at 4S. The 7S form could be converted to the 4S form by 100 n*M* GTPγS, and the 4S form could be reconstituted to the 7S form by exogenous G protein *(67)*. It was concluded that FPR could be regulated by physical coupling to G protein in the light domain and turned off by removing it from G protein accessibility by translocation to the heavy domain.

Subsequent experiments characterized the Triton X-100 soluble and insoluble forms of FPR. The soluble form was found to specifically associate with actin on nitrocellulose overlays and in solution and could be immunopurified or sedimented with two different anti-F–actin antibodies, suggesting that it was carrying actin in a very tight complex. Recently, A. J. Jesaitis et al. (unpublished results) have shown, by phage display analysis, that the dominant epitope recognized by these anti-F–actin antibodies, matches nearly perfectly a surface domain of rabbit β-actin revealed in its X-ray crystal structure. This result supports the argument that the antibodies recognize actin in complex with FPR. The Triton-insoluble form of FPR was also shown to arise from membrane skeleton association from protein and not an affinity for detergent-insoluble membrane lipid domains. Triton X-100 FPR insolubility was in isolated plasma membranes correlated with ligand-induced homologous desensitization *(155)* and lateral mobility studies *(156)*. FPR Triton X-100 insolubility was also shown to be sensitive to conditions that depolymerized actin (high salt, sulfhydryl inhibitors) and inversely sensitive to the energy state of the cell *(155)*.

The relationship among lateral segregation, cytoskeletal association, and phosphorylation of FPR may be closely coupled. It is clear that in the β-adrenergic system, phosphorylation of receptor does not fully inactivate receptor G protein interactions without receptor phosphorylation-dependent binding of regulatory proteins, such as arrestin, to the receptor *(157)*. Occupied FPR from *f*MLF-desensitized neutrophils complex G_i equally well as FPR from fully responsive cells *(151)*. Energy depletion of neutrophils inhibits FPR interaction with the membrane skeleton whereas okadaic acid and staurosporine have no effect *(158)*. Thus, a role for phosphorylation of FPR would be consistent with actin-FPR interactions being analogous to arrestin interaction with phosphorylated GPCRs in other systems *(159,160)*.

Conclusion

The *N*-formyl peptide receptor remains a fruitful and information rich model leukocyte receptor system whose exploitation will invariably lead to new discoveries and answers to many remaining questions about inflammation and inflammatory disease. In the next decade, it may also bring us to a new understanding of cellular chemotaxis and open the doors to augmenting host defense and controlling tissue injury.

Acknowledgments

We gratefully acknowledge Pawel Herzyk and Rod E. Hubbard for establishing the 7TM receptor modeling program at Swiss Pro on the World Wide Web. This work has been supported by PHS grants AI 22735, AI40108 to AJJ and Arthritis Foundation Investigator Award to HMM.

References

1. Gallin, J. I., Goldstein, I. M., and Snyderman, R. (1988) *Inflammation: Basic Principles and Clinical Correlates*, Raven, New York.
2. Snyderman, R. and Uhing, R. J. (1992) Phagocytic cells: Chemoattractant stimulus-response coupling, in *Inflammation: Basic principles and clinical correlates* (Gallin, J. I., Goldstein, I. M., and Snyderman, R., eds.), Raven, New York, pp. 421–439.
3. Ahuja, S. K., Gao, J. L., and Murphy, P. M. (1994) Chemokine receptors and molecular mimicry. *Immunol. Today* **15**, 281–287.
4. Murphy, P. M. (1994) The molecular biology of leukocyte chemoattractant receptors. *Ann. Rev. Immunol.* **12**, 593–633.
5. Baggiolini, M. and Dahinden, C. A. (1994) CC chemokines in allergic inflammation. *Immunol. Today* **15**, 127–133.
6. Furie, M. B. and Randolph, G. J. (1995) Chemokines and tissue injury. *Am. J. Pathol.* **146**, 1287–1301.
7. Mackay, C. R. (1997) Chemokines: What chemokine is that? *Curr. Biol.* **7**, R384–R386.
8. Schiffman, E., Corcoran, B., and Wahl, S. (1975) N-formyl methionine peptides as chemotractants for leukocytes. *Proc. Natl. Acad. Sci. USA* **72**, 1059–1062.
9. Carp, H. (1982) Mitochondrial *N*-formylmethionyl proteins as chemoattractants for neutrophils. *J. Exp. Med.* **155**, 264–275.
10. Shawar, S. M., Rich, R. R., and Becker, E. L. (1995) Peptides from the aminoterminus of mouse mitochondrially encoded NADH dehydrogenase subunit 1 are potent chemoattractants. *Biochem. Biophys. Res. Commun.* **812**, 812–818.

11. Prossnitz, E. R. and Ye, R. D. (1997) The N-formyl peptide receptor: A model for the study of chemoattractant receptor structure and function. *Pharmacol. Ther.* **74,** 73–102.

12. Ye, R. D. and Boulay, F. (1997) Structure and function of leukocyte chemoattractant receptors. *Adv. Pharmacol.* **39,** 221–289.

13. Kishimoto, T. K. and Anderson, D. C. (1992) The role of integrins in inflammation, in *Inflammation: Basic Principle and Clinical Correlates* (Gallin, J. I., Goldstein, I. M., and Snyderman, R., eds.), Raven, New York, pp. 353–406.

14. Keitoku, M., Kohzuki, M., Katoh, H., Funakoshi, M., Suzuki, S., Takeuchi, M., Karibe, A., Horiguchi, S., Watanabe, J., Satoh, S., Nose, M., Abe, K., Okayama, H., and Shirato, K. (1997) FMLP actions and its binding sites in isolated human coronary arteries. *J. Mol. Cell Cardiol.* **29,** 881–894.

15. Lacy, M., Jones J., Whittemore, S. R., Haviland, D. L., Wetsel, R. A., and Barnum, S. R. (1995) Expression of the receptors for the C5a anaphylatoxin, interleukin8 and FMLP by human astrocytes and microglia. *J. Neuroimmunol.* **61,** 718

16. Muller-Ladner, U., Jones, J., Wetsel, R. A., Gay, S., Raine, C. S., and Barnum, S. R. (1996) Enhanced expression of chemotactic receptors in multiple sclerosis lesions. *J. Neurol. Sci.* **144,** 13,541.

17. Mukhopadhyay, A., Steinberg, N., and Das, D. K. (1989) Effects of free radicals and oxidants on myocardial cellular injury. *Clin. Physiol. Biochem.* **7,** 278–285.

18. Beckman, J. S. (1991) The double-edged role of nitric oxide in brain function and superoxide-mediated injury. *J. Dev. Physiol.* **15,** 53–59.

19. Eppinger, M. J., Deeb, G. M., Bolling, S. F., and Ward, P. A. (1997) Mediators of ischemia-reperfusion injury of rat lung. *Am. J. Pathol.* **150,** 1773–1784.

20. Cook, P. J. and Lip, G. Y. (1996) Infectious agents and atherosclerotic vascular disease. *QJM* **89,** 727–735.

21. Wimmer, M. L., Sandmann-Strupp, R., Saikku, P., and Haberl, R. L. (1996) Association of chlamydial infection with cerebrovascular disease. *Stroke* **27,** 2207–2210.

22. Hurttia, H. M., Pelto, L. M., and Leino, L. (1997) Evidence of an association between functional abnormalities and defective diacylglycerol kinase activity in peripheral blood neutrophils from patients with localized juvenile periodontitis. *J. Periodont. Res.* **32,** 401–407.

23. Leino, L., Hurttia, H., and Peltonen, E. (1994) Diacylglycerol in peripheral blood neutrophils from patients with localized juvenile periodontitis. *J. Periodont. Res.* **29,** 334–338.

24. Perez, H. D., Kelly, E., Elfman, F., Armitage, G., and Winkler, J. (1991) Defective polymorpho-nuclear leukocyte formyl peptide receptor(s) in juvenile periodontitis. *J. Clin. Invest.* **87,** 971–976.

25. DeNardin, E., DeLuca, C., Levine, M. J., and Genco, R. J. (1990) Antibodies directed to the chemotactic factor receptor detect differences between chemotactically normal and defective neutrophils from LJP patients. *J. Periodontol.* **61,** 609–617.

26. Boulay, F., Tardif, M., Brouchon, L., and Vignais, P. (1990) The human N-formylpeptide receptor: Characterization of two cDNA isolates and evidence for a new subfamily of G-protein-coupled receptors. *Biochemistry* **29,** 11,123–11,133.

27. Freer, R. J., Day, A. L., Radding, J. A., Schiffmann, E., Aswanikumar, S., Showell, H. J., and Becker, E. L. (1980) Further studies on the structural requirements for synthetic peptide chemoattractants. *Biochemistry* **19,** 2404–2410.

28. Freer, R. J., Day, A. L., Muthukumaraswamy N., Pinon D., Wu A., Showell, H. J., and Becker, E. L. (1982) Formyl peptide chemoattractants: A model of the receptor on rabbit neutrophils. *Biochemistry* **21,** 257–263.

29. Marasco, W. A., Phan, S. H., Krutzsch, H., Showell, H. J., Feltner, D. E., Nairn R., Becker, E. L., and Ward, P. A. (1984) Purification and identification of formyl-methionyl-leucyl-phenylalanine as the major peptide neutrophil chemotactic factor produced by Escherichia coli. *J. Biol. Chem.* **259,** 5430–5436.

30. Miettinen, H. M., Mills, J. S., Gripentrog, J. M., Dratz, E. A., Granger, B. L., and Jesaitis, A. J. (1997) The ligand binding domain of the formyl peptide receptor maps in the transmembrane region. *J. Immunol.,* **159,** 4045–4054.

31. Perez, H. D., Vilander, L., Andrews, W. H., and Holmes, R. (1994) Human formyl peptide receptor ligand binding domain(s): Studies using an improved mutagenesis/expression vector reveal a novel mechanism for the regulation of the receptor occupancy. *J. Biol. Chem.* **269,** 22,485–22,487.

32. Ye, R. D., Quenberger, O., Thomas, K. M., Navarro, J., Cavanagh, S. L., Prossnitz, E. R., and Cochrane, C. G. (1993) The rabbit neutrophil *N*-formyl peptide receptor. *J. Immunol.* **150,** 1384–1394.

33. Gao, J.-L. and Murphy, P. M. (1993) Species and subtype variants of the N-formyl peptide chemotactic receptor reveal multiple important functional domains. *J. Biol. Chem.* **268,** 25,395–25,401.

34. Fiore, S., Maddox, J. F., Perez, H. D., and Serhan, C. N. (1994) Identification of a human cDNA encoding a functional high affinity lipoxin A4 receptor. *J. Exp. Med.* **180,** 253–260.

35. Murphy, P. M., Özçelik, T., Kenney, R. T., Tiffany, H. L., McDermott, D., and Francke, U. (1992) A structural homologue of the *N*-formyl peptide receptor: characterization and chromosome mapping of a peptide chemoattractant receptor family. *J. Biol. Chem.* **267,** 7637–7643.

36. Perez, H. D., Holmes, R., Kelly, E., McClary, J., and Andrews, W. H. (1992) Cloning of a cDNA encoding a receptor related to the formyl peptide receptor of human neutrophils. *Gene* **118,** 303,304.

37. Ye, R. D., Cavanagh, S. L., Quehenberger, O., Prossnitz, E. R., and Cochrane, C. G. (1992) Isolation of a cDNA that encodes a novel granulocyte *N*-formyl peptide receptor. *Biochem. Biophys. Res. Commun.* **184,** 582–589.

38. Fiore, S., Romano, M., Reardon, E. M., and Serhan, C. N. (1993) Induction of functional lipoxin A$_4$ receptors in HL-60 cells. *Blood* **81,** 3395–3403.

39. Fiore, S., Ryeom, S. W., Weller, P. F., and Serhan, C. N. (1992) Lipoxin recognition sites: specific binding of labeled lipoxin A$_4$ with human neutrophils. *J. Biol. Chem.* **267,** 16,168–16,176.

40. Durstin, M., Gao, J.-L., Tiffany, H. L., McDermott, D., and Murphy, P. M. (1994) Differential expression of members of the *N*-formylpeptide receptor gene cluster in human phagocytes. *Biochem. Biophys. Res. Commun.* **201,** 174–179.

41. Wang, J. K., McDowell, J. H., and Hargrave, P. A. (1980) Site of attachment of 11-*cis*-retinal in bovine rhodopsin. *Biochemistry* **19,** 5111–5117.

42. Nakanishi, S., Zhang, H., Lerro, K. A., Takekuma, S., Yamamoto, T., Lien, T. H., Sastry, L., Baek, D.-J., Moquin-Pattey, C., Boehm, M. F., Derguini, F., and Gawinowicz, M. A. (1996) Photoaffinity labeling or rhodopsin and bacteriorhodopsin. *Biophys. Chem.* **56,** 13–22.

43. Nakayama, T. A. and Khorana, H. G. (1990) Orientation of retinal in bovine rhodopsin determined by cross-linking using a photoactivatable analog of 11-cis-retinal. *J. Biol. Chem.* **265,** 15,762–15,769.

44. Sakmar, T. P., Franke, R. R., and Khorana, H. G. (1989) Glutamic acid –113 serves as the retinylidene Schiff base counterion in bovine rhodopsin. *Proc. Natl. Acad. Sci. USA* **86,** 8309–8313.

45. Han, M. and Smith, S. O. (1995) NMR constraints on the location of the retinal chromophore in rhodopsin and bathorhodopsin. *Biochemistry* 1425–1432.

46. Rao, V. R., Cohen, G. B., and Oprian, D. D. (1994) Rhodopsin mutation G90D and a molecular mechanism for congenital night blindness. *Nature* **367,** 639–642.

47. Yue, G., Sun, F. F., Dunn, C., Yin, K., and Wong, P. Y. (1996) The 21-aminosteroid tirilazad mesylate can ameliorate inflammatory bowel disease in rats. *J. Pharmacol. Exp. Ther.* **276,** 265–270.

48. Schertler, G. F. X. and Hargrave, P. A. (1995) Projection structure of frog rhodopsin in two crystal forms. *Proc. Natl. Acad. Sci. USA* **92,** 11,578–11,582.

49. Unger, V. M., Hargrave, P. A., Baldwin, J. M., and Schertler, G. F. X. (1997) Arrangement of rhodopsin transmembrane alpha helices. *Nature* **389,** 203–206.

50. Sheih, T., Han, M., Akmar, T. P., and Smith, S. O. (1997) The steric trigger in rhodopsin activation. *J. Mol. Biol.* **269,** 373–384.

51. Herzyk, P. and Hubbard, R. E. (1995) Automated method for modeling seven-helix transmembrane receptors from experimental data. *Biophys. J.* **69,** 2419–2442.

52. Nathans, J. (1992) Rhodopsin: structure, function, and genetics. *Biochemistry* **31,** 4923–4931.

53. Quehenberger, O., Prossnitz, E. R., Cavanagh, S. L., Cochrane, C. G., and Ye, R. D. (1993) Multiple domains of the N-formyl peptide receptor are required for high-affinity ligand binding. *J. Biol. Chem.* **268,** 18,167–18,175.

54. Baldwin, J. M. (1993) The probable arrangement of the helices in G protein-coupled receptors. *EMBO J.* **12,** 1693–1703.

55. Zhukovsky, E. A., Robinson, P. R., and Oprian, D. D. (1992) Changing the location of the Schiff base counterion in rhodopsin. *Biochemistry* **31,** 10,400–10,405.

56. Edmundson, A. B. and Ely, K. R. (1985) Binding of N-formylated chemotactic peptides in crystals of the Mcg light chain dimer: Similarities with neutrophil receptors. *Mol. Immunol.* **22,** 463–475.

57. Wang, C.-R., Castaño, A. R., Peterson, P. A., Slaughter, C., Fisher Lindahl, K., and Deisenhofer, J. (1995) Nonclassical binding of formylated peptide in crystal structure of the MHC class Ib molecule H2-M3. *Cell* **82,** 655–664.

58. Koo, C., Lefkowitz, R. J., and Snyderman, R. (1983) Guanine nucleotides modulate the binding affinity of the oligopeptide chemoattractant receptor on human polymorphonuclear leukocytes. *J. Clin. Invest.* **72,** 748–753.

59. Lad, P. M., Olson, C. V., and Smiley, P. A. (1985) Association of the N-formyl-Met-Leu-Phe receptor in human neutrophils with a GTP-binding protein sensitive to pertussis toxin. *Proc. Natl. Acad. Sci. USA* **82,** 869–873.

60. Hyslop, P. A., Oades, Z. G., Jesaitis, A. J., Painter, R. G., Cochrane, C. G., and Sklar, L. A. (1984) Evidence for N-formyl chemotactic peptide-stimulated GTPase activity in human neutrophil homogenates. *FEBS Lett.* **166,** 165–169.

61. Okajima, F., Katada, T., and Ui, M. (1985) Coupling of the guanine nucleotide regulatory protein to chemotactic peptide receptors in neutrophil membranes and its uncoupling by islet-activating protein, pertussis toxin: a possible role of the toxin substrate in Ca^{2+}-mobilizing receptor-mediated signal transduction. *J. Biol. Chem.* **260,** 6761–6768.

62. Ui, M. (1984) Islet-activating protein, pertussis toxin: a probe for functions of the inhibitory guanine nucleotide regulatory component of adenylate cyclase. *Trends Pharmacol. Sci.* **5,** 277–279.

63. Bokoch, G. M. and Gilman, A. G. (1984) Inhibition of receptor-mediated release of arachidonic acid by pertussis toxin. *Cell* **39,** 301–308.

64. Krause, K.-H., Schiegel, W., Wollheim, C. B., Andersson, T., Waldvogel, F. A., and Lew, P. D. (1985) Chemotactic peptide activation of human neutrophils and HL-60 cells: pertussis toxin reveals correlation between inositol trisphosphate generation, calcium ion transients, and cellular activation. *J. Clin. Invest.* **76,** 1348–1354.

65. Molski, T. F. P., Naccache, P. H., Marsh, M. L., Kermode, J., Becker, E. L., and Sha'afi, R. I. (1984) Pertussis toxin inhibits the rise in the intracellular concentration of free calcium that is induced by chemotactic factors in rabbit neutrophils: possible role of the "G proteins" in calcium mobilization. *Biochem. Biophys. Res. Commun.* **124,** 644–650.

66. Verghese, M. W., Smith, C. D., and Snyderman, R. (1985) Potential role for a guanine nucleotide regulatory protein in chemoattractant receptor mediated polyphosphoinositide metabolism, Ca^{++} mobilization and cellular responses by leukocytes. *Biochem. Biophys. Res. Commun.* **127,** 450–457.

67. Bommakanti, R. K., Bokoch, G. M., Tolley, J. O., Schreiber, R. E., Siemsen, D. W., Klotz, K.-N., and Jesaitis, A. J. (1992) Reconstitution of a physical complex between the *N*-formyl chemotactic peptide receptor and G protein: inhibition by pertussis toxin-catalyzed ADP ribosylation. *J. Biol. Chem.* **267,** 7576–7581.

68. Schreiber, R. E., Prossnitz, E. R., Ye, R. D., Cochrane, C. G., Jesaitis, A. J., and Bokoch, G. M. (1993) Reconstitution of recombinant N-formyl chemotactic peptide receptor with G protein. *J. Leukoc. Biol.* **53,** 470–474.

69. Murphy, P. M., Eide, B., Goldsmith, P., Brann, M., Gierschik, P., Spiegel, A., and Malech, H. L. (1987) Detection of multiple forms of $G_{i\alpha}$ in HL60 cells. *FEBS Lett.* **221,** 81–86.

70. McLeish, K. R., Gierschik, P., Schepers, T., Sidiropoulos, D., and Jakobs, K. H. (1989) Evidence that activation of a common G protein by receptors for leukotriene B4 and N-formylmethionyl-leucyl-phenylalanine in HL-60 cells occurs by different mechanisms. *Biochem. J.* **260,** 427–434.

71. Omann, G. M., Traynor, A. E., Harris, A. L., and Sklar, L. A. (1987) LTB4-induced activation signals and responses in neutrophils are short-lived compared to formylpeptide. *J. Immunol.* **138,** 2626–2632.

72. Verghese, M. W., Charles, L., Jakoi, L., Dillon, S. B., and Snyderman, R. (1987) Role of guanine nucleotide regulatory protein in the activation of phospholipase C by different chemoattractants. *J. Immunol.* **138,** 4374–4380.

73. Amatruda, T. T. III, Dragas-Graonic, S., Holmes, R., and Perez, H. D. (1995) Signal transduction by the formyl peptide receptor: Studies using chimeric receptors and site-directed

mutagenesis to define a novel domain for interaction with G proteins. *J. Biol. Chem.* **270**, 28,010–28,013.

74. Amatruda, T. T. III, Gerard, N. P., Gerard, C., and Simon, M. I. (1993) Specific interactions of chemoattractant factor receptors with G-proteins. *J. Biol. Chem.* **268**, 10,139–10,144.

75. Burg, M., Raffetseder, U., Grove, M., Klos, A., Köhl, J., and Bautsch, W. (1995) Gα16 comple-ments the signal transduction cascade of chemotactic receptors for complement factor C5a (C5a-R) and N-formylated peptides (fMLF-R) in *Xenopus laevis* oocytes: Gα-16 couples to chemotactic receptors in *Xenopus* oocytes. *FEBS Lett.* **377**, 426–428.

76. Goetzl, E. J., Shames, R. S., Yang, J., Birke, F. W., Liu, Y. F., Albert, P. R., and An, S. (1994) Inhibition of human HL-60 cell responses to chemotactic factors by antisense messenger RNA depletion of G proteins. *J. Biol. Chem.* **269**, 809–812.

77. Bommakanti, R. K., Dratz, E. A., Siemsen, D. W., and Jesaitis, A. J. (1995) Extensive contact between G_{i2} and *N*-formyl peptide chemoattractant receptor of human neutrophils: Mapping of binding sites using synthetic receptor-mimetic peptides. *Biochemistry* **34**, 6720–6728.

78. Schreiber, R., Prossnitz, E. R., Ye, R. D., Cochrane, C. G., and Bokoch, G. M. (1994) Domains of the human neutrophil *N*-formyl peptide receptor involved in G protein coupling. Mapping with receptor derived peptides. *J. Biol. Chem.* **269**, 326–331.

79. Prossnitz, E. R., Quehenberger, O., Cochrane, C. G., and Ye, R. D. (1993) The role of the third intracellular loop of the neutrophil N-formyl peptide receptor in G protein coupling. *Biochem. J.* **294**, 581–587.

80. Bommakanti, R. K., Klotz, K.-N., Dratz, E. A., and Jesaitis, A. J. (1993) A carboxyl-terminal tail peptide of neutrophil chemotactic receptor disrupts its physical complex with G protein. *J. Leukoc. Biol.* **54**, 572–577.

81. Prossnitz, E. R., Schreiber, R. E., Bokoch, G. M., and Ye, R. D. (1995) Binding of low affinity N-formyl peptide receptors to G protein: Characterization of a novel inactive receptor interme-diate. *J. Biol. Chem.* **270**, 10,686–10,694.

82. Sealfon, S. C., Chi, L., Ebersole, B. J., Rodic, V., Zhang, D., Ballesteros, J. A., and Weinstein, H. (1995) Related contribution of specific helix 2 and 7 residues to conformationl activation of the serotonin 5-HT2A receptor. *J. Biol. Chem.* **270**, 16,683–16,688.

83. Durstin, M. and Sha'afi, R. I. (1996) Signal transduction in the human neutrophil, in *Signal Transduction in Leukocytes: G Protein-Related and Other Pathways* (Lad, P. M., Kaptein, J. S., and Lin, C.-K. E., eds.), CRC, Boca Raton, FL, pp. 253–285.

84. Traynor-Kaplan, A. E., Harris, A. L., Thompson, B. L., Taylor, P., and Sklar, L. A. (1988) An inositol tetrakisphosphate-containing phospholipid in activated neutrophils. *Nature* **334**, 353–356.

85. Traynor-Kaplan, A. E., Thompson, B. L., Harris, A. L., Taylor, P., Omann, G. M., and Sklar, L. A. (1989) Transient increase in phosphatidylinositol 3,4-bisphosphate and phospha-tidylinositol trisphosphate during activation of human neutrophils. *J. Biol. Chem.* **264**, 15,668–15,673.

86. Stephens, L. R., Hughes, K. T., and Irvine, R. F. (1991) Pathway of phosphatidylinositol(3,4,5)-trisphosphate synthesis in activated neutrophils. *Nature* **351**, 33–39.

87. Vlahos, C. J. and Matter, W. F. (1992) Signal transduction in neutrophil activation: phosphatidylinositol 3-kinase is stimulated without tyrosine phosphorylation. *FEBS Lett.* **309**, 242–248.

88. Stephens, L., Eguinoa, A., Corey, S., Jackson, T., and Hawkins, P. T. (1993) Receptor stimulated accumulation of phosphatidylinositol (3,4,5)-trisphosphate by G protein mediated pathways in human myeloid derived cells. *EMBO J.* **12**, 2265–2273.

89. Stephens, L., Smrcka, A., Cooke, F. T., Jackson, T. R., Sternweis, P. C., and Hawkins, P. T. (1994) A novel phosphoinositide 3 kinase activity in myeloid-derived cells is activated by G protein βγ subunits. *Cell* **77**, 83–93.

90. Stoyanov, B., Volinia, S., Hhanck, T., Rubio, I., Loubtchenkov, M., Malek, D., Stoyanova, S., Vanhaesebroeck, B., Dhand, R., Nürnberg, B., Gierschik, P., Seedorf, K., Hsuan, J. J., Waterfield, M. D., and Wetzker, R. (1995) Cloning and characterization of a G protein-activated human phophoinositide-3 kinase. *Science* **269**, 690–693.

91. Kapeller, R. and Cantley, L. C. (1994) Phosphatidylinositol 3-kinase. *Bioessays* **16**, 565–576.

92. Arcaro, A. and Wymann, M. P. (1993) Wortmannin is a potent phosphatidylinositol 3-kinase inhibitor: the role of phosphatidylinositol 3,4,5-trisphosphate in neutrophil responses. *Biochem. J.* **296**, 297–301.

93. Ding, J., Vlahos, C. J., Liu, R., Brown, R. F., and Badwey, J. A. (1995) Antagonists of phosphatidylinositol 3-kinase block activation of several novel protein kinases in neutrophils. *J. Biol. Chem.* **270,** 11,684–11,691.

94. Okada, T., Sakuma, L., Fukui, Y., Hazeki, O., and Ui, M. (1994) Blockage of chemotactic peptide-induced stimulation of neutrophils by wortmannin as a result of selective inhibition of phosphatidylinositol 3-kinase. *J. Biol. Chem.* **269,** 3563–3567.

95. Sue-A-Quan, A. K., Fialkow, L., Vlahos, C. J., Schelm, J. A., Grinstein, S., Butler J., and Downey, G. P. (1997) Inhibition of neutrophil oxidative burst and granule secretion by Wortmannin: potential role of MAP kinase and renaturable kinases. *J. Cell. Physiol.* **172,** 94–108.

96. Vlahos, C. J., Matter, W. F., Brown, R. F., Traynor-Kaplan, A. E., Heyworth, P. G., Prossnitz, E. R., Ye, R. D., Marder, P., Schelm, J. A., Rothfuss, K. J., Serlin, B. S., and Simpson, P. J. (1995) Investigation of neutrophil signal transduction using a specific inhibitor of phosphatidylinositol 3-kinase. *J. Immunol.* **154,** 2413–2422.

97. Chuang, T.-H., Bohl, B. P., and Bokoch, G. M. (1993) Biologically active lipids are regulators of Rac. GDI complexation. *J. Biol. Chem.* **268,** 26,206–26,211.

98. Nakanishi, H., Brewer, K. A., and Exton, J. H. (1993) Activation of the zeta isozyme of protein kinase C by phosphatidylinositol 3,4,5-trisphosphate. *J. Biol. Chem.* **268,** 13–16.

99. Toker, A., Meyer M., Reddy, K. K., Falck, J. R., Aneja, R., Aneja, S., Parra, A., Burns, D. J., Ballas, L. M., and Cantley, L. C. (1994) Activation of protein kinase C family members by the novel polyphosphoinositides PtdIns-3,4-P2 and PtdIns-3,4,5-P3. *J. Biol. Chem.* **269,** 32,358–32,367.

100. Seger, R. and Krebs, E. G. (1995) The MAPK signaling cascade. *FASEB J.* **9,** 726–735.

101. Buday, L. and Downward, J. (1993) Epidermal growth factor regulates p21[ras] through the formation of a complex of receptor, Grb2 adapter protein, and Sos nucleotide exchange factor. *Cell* **73,** 611–620.

102. Lowenstein, E. J., Daly, R. J., Batzer, A. G., Li, W., Margolis, B., Lammers, R., Ullrich A., E. Y. Skolnik, Bar-Sagi, D., and Schlessinger, J. (1992) The SH2 and SH3 domain-containing protein GRB2 links receptor tyrosine kinases to ras signaling. *Cell* **70,** 431–442.

103. Luttrell, L. M., Hawes, B. E., van Biesen, T., Luttrell, D. K., Lansing, T. J., and Lefkowitz, R. J. (1996) Role of c-Src tyrosine kinase in G protein-coupled receptor- and G βγ subunit-mediated activation of mitogen-activated proteins kinases. *J. Biol. Chem.* **271,** 19,442–19,450.

104. Grinstein, S. and Furuya, W. (1992) Chemoattractant-induced tyrosine phosphorylation and activation of microtubule-associated protein kinase in human neutrophils. *J. Biol. Chem.* **267,** 18,122–18,125.

105. Thompson, H. L., Shiroo, M., and Saklatvala, J. (1993) The chemotactic factor N-formyl-methionyl-leucyl-phenylalanine activates microtubule-associated protein 2 (MAP) kinase and MAP kinase kinase in polymorphonuclear leucocytes. *Biochem. J.* **290,** 483–488.

106. Torres, M., Hall, F. L., and O'Neill, K. (1993) Stimulation of human neutrophils with formyl-methionyl-leucyl-phenylalanine induces tyrosine phosphorylation and activation of two distinct mitogen-activated protein-kinases. *J. Immunol.* **150,** 1563–1578.

107. Ptasznik, A., Traynor-Kaplan A., and Bokoch, G. M. (1995) G protein-coupled chemoattractant receptors regulate Lyn tyrosine kinase. Shc adapter protein signaling complexes. *J. Biol. Chem.* **270,** 19,969–19,973.

108. Torres, M. and Ye, R. D. (1996) Activation of the mitogen-activated protein kinase pathway by *f*Met-Leu-Phe in the absence of Lyn and tyrosine phosphorylation of SHC in transfected cells. *J. Biol. Chem.* **271,** 13,244–13,249.

109. Kranenburg, O., Verlaan, I., Hordijk, P. L., and Moolenaar, W. H. (1997) G$_i$ mediated activation of the Ras/MAP kinase pathway involves a 100 kDa tyrosine-phosphorylated Grb2 SH3 binding protein, but not Src nor Shc. *EMBO J.* **16,** 3097–3105.

110. Avdi, N. J., Winston, B. W., Russel, M., Young, S. K., Johnson, G. L., and Worthen, G. S. (1996) Activation of MEKK by formyl-methionyl-leucyl-phenylalanine in human neutrophils—Mapping pathways for mitogen-activated protein kinase activation. *J. Biol. Chem.* **271,** 33,598–33,606.

111. Nick, J. A., Avdi, N. J., Young, S. K., Knall, C., Gerwins, P., Johnson, G. L., and Worthen, G. S. (1997) Common and distinct intracellular signaling pathways in human neutrophils utilized by platelet activating factor and FMLP. *J. Clin. Invest.* **99,** 975–986.

112. Hawes, B. E., van Biesen, J., Koch, W., Luttrell, L. M., and Lefkowitz, R. J. (1995) Distinct pathways of G_i and G_q-mediated mitogen-activated protein kinase activation. *J. Biol. Chem.* **270,** 17,148–17,153.

113. Krump, E., Sanghera, J. S., Pelech, S. L., Furuya, W., and Grinstein, S. (1997) Chemotactic peptide *N*-formyl- Met-Leu-Phe activation of p38 mitogen-activated protein kinase (MAPK) and MAPK-activated protein kinase-2 in human neutrophils. *J. Biol. Chem.* **272,** 937–944.

114. Knall, C., Worthen, G. S., and Johnson, G. L. (1997) Interleukin 8-stimulated phosphatidylinositol-3-kinase activity regulates the migration of human neutrophils independent of extracellular signal-regulated kinase and p38 mitogen-activated protein kinases. *Proc. Natl. Acad. Sci. USA* **94,** 3052–3057.

115. Quinn, M. T. (1996) Role of small GTP-binding proteins in leukocyte signal transduction, in *Signal Transduction in Leukocytes: G Protein-Related and Other Pathways* (Lad, P. M., Kaptein, J. S., and Lin, C.-K. E., eds.), CRC, Boca Raton, FL, pp. 75–142.

116. Ridley, A. J. and Hall, A. (1992) The small GTP-binding protein rho regulates the assembly of focal adhesions and actin stress fibers in response to growth factors. *Cell* **70,** 389–399.

117. Ridley, A. J. and Hall, A. (1994) Signal transduction pathways regulating Rho-mediated stress fibre formation: requirement for a tyrosine kinase. *EMBO J.* **13,** 2600–2610.

118. Laudanna, C., Campbell, J. J., and Butcher, E. C. (1996) Role of Rho in chemoattractant-activated leukocyte adhesion through integrins. *Science* **271,** 981–983.

119. Sakane, T. and Miura, K. (1996) Research for basic and clinical aspects of Behcet's disease—recent advance and future. *Nippon. Rinsho.* **54,** 870–884.

120. Didsbury, J., Weber, R. F., Bokoch, G. M., Evans, T., and Snyderman, R. (1989) Rac, a novel ras-related family of proteins that are botulinum toxin substrates. *J. Biol. Chem.* **264,** 16,378–16,382.

121. Diekmann, D., Abo, A., Johnston, C., Segal, A. W., and Hall, A. (1994) Interaction of Rac with p67[phox] and regulation of phagocytic NADPH oxidase activity. *Science* **265,** 531–533.

122. Knaus, U. G., Heyworth, P. G., Evans, T., Curnutte, J. T., and Bokoch, G. M. (1991) Regulation of phagocyte oxygen radical production by the GTP-binding protein rac-2. *Science* **254,** 1512–1515.

123. Ando, S., Kaibuchi, K., Sasaki, T., Hiraoka, K., Nishiyama, T., Mizuno, T., Asada, M., Nunoi, H., Matsuda, I., Matsuura, Y., Polakis, P., McGormick, F., and Takai, Y. (1992) Post-translational processing of rac p21s is important both for their interaction with the GDP/GTP exchange proteins and for their activation of NADPH oxidase. *J. Biol. Chem.* **267,** 25,709–25,713.

124. Nisimoto, Y., Freeman, J. L. R., Motalebi, S. A., Hirshberg, M., and Lambeth, J. D. (1997) Rac binding to p67[phox]: structural basis for interactions of the Rac1 effector region and insert region with components of the respiratory burst oxidase. *J. Biol. Chem.* **272,** 18,834–18,841.

125. Ridley, A. J., Paterson, H. F., Johnston, C. L., Diekmann, D., and Hall, A. (1992) The small GTP-binding protein rac regulates growth factor-induced membrane ruffling. *Cell* **70,** 401–410.

126. Allen, W. E., Jones, G. E., Pollard, J. W., and Ridley, A. J. (1997) Rho, Rac and Cdc42 regulate actin organization and cell adhesion in macrophages. *J. Cell Sci.* **110,** 707–720.

127. Lin, L.-L., Wartmann, M., Lin, A. Y., Knopf, J. L., Seth, A., and Davis, R. J. (1993) cPLA2 is phosphorylated and activated by MAP kinase. *Cell* **72,** 269–278.

128. Camps, M., Carozzi, A., Schnabel, P., Scheer, A., Parker, P. J., and Gierschik, P. (1992) Isozyme-selective stimulation of phospholipase C-β2 by G protein βγ-subunits. *Nature* **360,** 684–686.

129. Katz, A., Wu, D., and Simon, M. I. (1992) Subunits of βγ of heterotrimeric G protein activate β2 isoform of phospholipase C. *Nature* **360,** 686–689.

130. Pettitt, T. R., Martin, A., Horton, T., Liossis, C., Lord, J. M., and Wakelam, M. J. O. (1997) Diacylglycerol and phosphatidate generated by phospholipases C and D, respectively, have distinct fatty acid compositions and functions—Phospholipase D-derived diacylglycerol does not activate protein kinase C in porcine aortic endothelial cells. *J. Biol. Chem.* **272,** 17,354–17,359.

131. Brown, H. A., Gutowski, S., Moomaw, C. R., Slaughter, C., and Sternweis, P. C. (1993) ADP-ribosylation factor, a small GTP-dependent regulatory protein, stimulates phospholipase D activity. *Cell* **75,** 1137–1144.

132. Malcolm, K. C., Elliott, C. M., and Exton, J. H. (1996) Evidence for Rho-mediated agonist stimulation of phospholipase D in rat1 fibroblasts. Effects of clostridium botulinum C3 exoenzyme. *J. Biol. Chem.* **271,** 13,135–13,139.

133. Malcolm, K. C., Sable, C. L., Elliott, C. M., and Exton, J. H. (1996) Enhanced phospholipase D activity and altered morphology in RhoA-overexpressing RAT1 fibroblasts. *Biochem. Biophys. Res. Commun.* **225,** 514–519.

134. Singer, W. D., Brown, H. A., Jiang, X., and Sternweis, P. C. (1996) Regulation of phospholipase D by protein kinase C is synergistic with ADP-ribosylation factor and independent of protein kinase activity. *J. Biol. Chem.* **271,** 4504–4510.

135. Lopez, I., Burns, D. J., and Lambeth, J. D. (1995) Regulation of phospholipase D by protein kinase C in human neutrophils: conventional isoforms of protein kinase C phosphorylate a phospholipase D-related component in the plasma membrane. *J. Biol. Chem.* **270,** 19,465–19,472.

136. Ohguchi, K., Banno, Y., Nakashima, S., and Nozawa, Y. (1996) Regulation of membrane-bound phospholipase D by protein kinase C in HL60 cells: synergistic action of small GTP-binding protein RhoA. *J. Biol. Chem.* **271,** 4366–4372.

137. Cockcroft, S. (1992) G protein-regulated phospholipases C, D and A_2-mediated signalling in neutrophils. *Biochim. Biophys. Acta* **1113,** 135–160.

138. Houle, M. G. and Bourgoin, S. (1996) Small GTPase-regulated phospholipase D in granulocytes. *Biochem. Cell Biol.* **74,** 459–467.

139. Reinhold, S. L., Prescott, S. M., Zimmerman, G. A., and McIntyre, T. M. (1990) Activation of human neutrophil phospholipase D by three separable mechanisms. *FASEB J.* **4,** 208–214.

140. Singer, W. D., Brown, H. A., and Sternweis, P. C. (1997) Regulation of eukaryotic phosphatidylinositol-specific phospholipase C and phospholipase D. *Ann. Rev. Biochem.* **66,** 475–509.

141. Blackwood, R. A., Hartiala, K., Kwoh, E. E., Transue, A. T., and Brower, R. C. (1996) Unidirectional heterologous receptor desensitization between both the fMLP and C5a receptor and the IL-8 receptor. *J. Leukoc. Biol.* **60,** 88–93.

142. Didsbury, J. R., Uhing, R. J., Tomhave, E., Gerard, C., Gerard, N., and Snyderman, R. (1991) Receptor class desensitization of leukocyte chemoattractant receptors. *Proc. Natl. Acad. Sci. USA* **88,** 11,564–11,568.

143. Kitayama, J., Carr, M. W., Roth, S. J., Buccola, J. M., and Springer, T. A. (1997) Contrasting responses to multiple chemotactic stimuli in transendothelial migration: heterologous desensitization in neutrophils and augmentation of migration in eosinophils. *J. Immunol.* **158,** 2340–2349.

144. Richardson, R. M., Ali, H., Tomhave, E. D., Haribabu, B., and Snyderman, R. (1995) Cross-desensitization of chemoattractant receptors occurs at multiple levels: Evidence for a role for inhibition of phospholipase C activity. *J. Biol. Chem.* **270,** 27,829–27,833.

145. Dobos, G. J., Norgauer, J., Eberle, M., Schollmeyer, P. J., and Traynor-Kaplan, A. E. (1992) C5a reduces formyl peptide-induced actin polymerization and phosphatidylinositol (3,4,5) trisphosphate formation, but not phosphatidylinositol (4,5) bisphosphate hydrolysis and superoxide production, in human neutrophils. *J. Immunol.* **149,** 609–614.

146. Tardif, M., Mery, L., Brouchon, L., and Boulay, F. (1993) Agonist-dependent phosphorylation of N-formylpeptide and activation peptide from the fifth component of (C5a) chemoattractant receptors in differentiated HL60 cells. *J. Immunol.* **150,** 3534–3545.

147. Prossnitz, E. R., Kim, C. M., Benovic, J. L., and Ye, R. D. (1995) Phosphorylation of the *N*-formyl peptide receptor carboxyl terminus by the G protein-coupled receptor kinase, GRK2. *J. Biol. Chem.* **270,** 1130–1137.

148. Prossnitz, E. R. (1997) Desensitization of N-formylpeptide receptor-mediated activation is dependent upon receptor phosphorylation. *J. Biol. Chem.* **272,** 15,213–15,219.

149. Jesaitis, A. J. and Klotz, K.-N. (1993) Cytoskeletal regulation of chemotactic receptors: Molecular complexation of N-formyl peptide receptors with G proteins and actin. *Eur. J. Haematol.* **51,** 288–293.

150. Klotz, K. N. and Jesaitis, A. J. (1994) Neutrophil chemoattractant receptors and the membrane skeleton. *Bioessays* **16,** 193–198.

151. Klotz, K. N. and Jesaitis, A. J. (1994) Physical coupling of N-formyl peptide chemoattractant receptors to G protein is unaffected by desensitization. *Biochem. Pharmacol.* **48,** 1297–1300.

152. Jesaitis, A. J., Tolley, J. O., and Allen, R. A. (1986) Receptor-cytoskeleton interactions and membrane traffic may regulate chemoattractant-induced superoxide production in human granulocytes. *J. Biol. Chem.* **261,** 13,662–13,669.

153. Jesaitis, A. J., Bokoch, G. M., Tolley, J. O., and Allen, R. A. (1988) Lateral segregation of occupied chemotactic receptors into actin and fodrin-rich plasma membrane microdomains depleted in guanyl nucleotide proteins. *J. Cell Biol.* **107,** 921–928.

154. Jesaitis, A. J., Tolley, J. O., Bokoch, G. M., and Allen, R. A. (1989) Regulation of chemoattractant receptor interaction with transducing proteins by organizational control in the plasma membrane of human neutrophils. *J. Cell Biol.* **109,** 2783–2790.

155. Klotz, K. N., Krotec, K. L., Gripentrog, J. M., and Jesaitis, A. J. (1994) Regulatory interaction of *N*-formyl peptide chemoattractant receptors with the membrane skeleton in human neutrophils. *J. Immunol.* **152,** 801–810.

156. Johansson, B., Wymann, M. P., Holmgren-Peterson, K., and Magnusson, K.-E. (1993) *N*-formyl peptide receptors in human neutrophils display distinct membrane distribution and lateral mobility when labeled with agonist and antagonist. *J. Cell Biol.* **121,** 1281–1289.

157. Lohse, M. J., Andexinger, S., Pitcher, J., Trukawinski, S., Codina, J., Faure, J.-P., Caron, M. G., and Lefkowitz, R. J. (1992) Receptor-specific desensitization with purified proteins: kinase dependence and receptor specificity of β-arrestin and arrestin in the β$_2$-adrenergic receptor and rhodopsin systems. *J. Biol. Chem.* **267,** 8558–8564.

158. Klotz, K. N. and Jesaitis, A. J. (1994) The interaction of N-formyl peptide chemoattractant receptors with the membrane skeleton is energy-dependent. *Cell Signal.* **6,** 943–947.

159. Palczewski, K., Pulvermüller, A., Buczylko, J., and Hofmann, K. P. (1991) Phosphorylated rhodopsin and heparin induce similar conformational changes in arrestin. *J. Biol. Chem.* **266,** 18,649–18,654.

160. Wilson, C. J. and Applebury, M. L. (1993) Intracellular signaling: arresting G-protein coupled receptor activity. *Curr. Biol.* **3,** 683–686.

161. Minamino, T., Kitakaze, M., Node, K., Funaya, H., Inoue, M., Hori, M., and Kamada, T. (1996) Adenosine inhibits leukocyte-induced vasoconstriction. *Am. J. Physiol.* **271,** H2622–H2628.

162. Minamino, T., Kitakaze, M., Node, K., Funaya, H., Inoue, M., Hori, M., and Kamada, T. (1996) Activated polymorphonuclear leukocytes induce constriction of canine coronary artery via Mac-1, but not LFA-1, and ICAM-1. *J. Mol. Cell Cardiol.* **28,** 1575–1581.

163. Ott, I., Neumann, F. J., and Schomig, A. (1995) Neutrophil hyper-reactivity after exercise-induced angina pectoris. *Coron. Artery Dis.* **6,** 525–532.

164. Ritter, L. S., Wilson, D. S., Williams, S. K., Copeland, J. G., and McDonagh, P. F. (1995) Early in reperfusion following myocardial ischemia, leukocyte activation is necessary for venular adhesion but not capillary retention. *Microcirculation* **2,** 315–327.

165. Pasqui, A. L., Di Renzo, M., Bova, G., Bruni, F., Saletti, M., Chiarion, C., and Auteri, A. (1995) Changes of some immune functions after percutaneous transluminal coronary angioplasty (PTCA). *Int. J. Clin. Pharmacol. Res.* **15,** 139–144.

166. Baj, Z., Kowalski, J., Kantorski, J., Pokoca, L., Kosmider, M., Pawlicki, L., and Tchorzewski, H. (1994) The effect of short-term myocardial ischemia on the expression of adhesion molecules and the oxidative burst of coronary sinus blood neutrophils. *Atherosclerosis* **106,** 159–168.

167. McDonagh, P. F. and Rauzzino, M. J. (1993) Stimulated leukocyte adhesion in coronary microcirculation is reduced by a calcium antagonist. *Am. J. Physiol.* **265,** H476–H483.

168. Raschke, P., Becker, B. F., Leipert, B., Schwartz, L. M., Zahler, S., and Gerlach, E. (1993) Postischemic dysfunction of the heart induced by small numbers of neutrophils via formation of hypochlorous acid. *Basic. Res. Cardiol.* **88,** 321–339.

169. Mugge, A., Lopez, J. A., Heistad, D. D., and Lichtlen, P. R. (1993) Vasoconstriction in response to activated leukocytes: implications for vasospasm. *Eur. Heart J.* **14(Suppl. 1),** 87–92.

170. Widermann, C. J., Niedermuhlbichler, M., and Braunsteiner, H. (1992) Priming of polymorphonuclear neutrophils by atrial natriuretic peptide in vitro. *J. Clin. Invest.* **89,** 1580–1586.

171. Bode, S. M., Kuhn, M., and Forstermann, U. (1990) Chemotactic peptide FMLP contracts human coronary arteries via cyclooxygenase products. *Am. J. Physiol.* **258,** H848–H853.

172. Sassen, L. M., Lamers, J. M., Sluiter, W., Hartog, J. M., Dekkers, D. H., Hogendoorn, A., and Verdouw, P. D. (1993) Development and regression of atherosclerosis in pigs: effects of n-3 fatty acids, their incorporation into plasma and aortic plaque lipids, and granulocyte function. *Arterioscler. Thromb.* **13,** 651–660.

173. Tanaka, H., Bradley, J. D., Baudendistel, L. J., and Dahms, T. E. (1992) Mechanisms of pulmonary vasoconstriction induced by chemotactic peptide FMLP in isolated rabbit lungs. *J. Appl. Physiol.* **72,** 1549–1556.

174. Chester, J. F., Ross, J. S., Malt, R. A., and Weitzman, S. A. (1985) Acute colitis produced by chemotactic peptides in rats and mice. *Am. J. Pathol.* **121,** 284–290.

175. Esser, E. and Loschen, G. (1991) Leukocytic O^-_2. and cardiac dysfunctions in isolated perfused rat hearts. *Arch. Toxicol.* **65,** 361–365.

176. Crouch, S. P., Crocker, I. P., and Fletcher, J. (1995) The effect of pregnancy on polymorphonuclear leukocyte function. *J. Immunol.* **155,** 5436–5443.

177. Egger, G., Klemt, C., Spendel, S., Kaulfersch, W., and Kenzian, H. (1994) Migratory activity of blood polymorphonuclear leukocytes during juvenile rheumatoid arthritis, demonstrated with a new whole- blood membrane filter assay. *Inflammation* **18,** 427–441.

178. Dularay, B., Dieppe, P. A., and Elson, C. J. (1990) Depressed degranulation response of synovial fluid polymorphonuclear leucocytes from patients with rheumatoid arthritis to IgG aggregates. *Clin. Exp. Immunol.* **79,** 195–201.

179. Dularay, B., Elson, C. J., and Dieppe, P. A. (1988) Enhanced oxidative response of polymorphonuclear leukocytes from synovial fluids of patients with rheumatoid arthritis. *Autoimmunity* **1,** 159–169.

180. Morrison, T. B., Weis, J. H., and Weis, J. J. (1997) Borrelia burgdorferi outer surface protein A (OspA) activates and primes human neutrophils. *J. Immunol.* **158,** 4838–4845.

181. De Clerck, L. S., Mertens, A. V., De, C. M., Gendt, Bridts, C. H., and Stevens, W. J. (1997) Actin polymerisation in neutrophils of rheumatoid arthritis patients in relation to treatment with nonsteroidal anti-inflammatory drugs. *Clin. Chim. Acta* **261,** 19–25.

182. Mur, E., Zabernigg, A., Hilbe, W., Eisterer, W., Halder, W., and Thaler, J. (1997) Oxidative burst of neutrophils in patients with rheumatoid arthritis: influence of various cytokines and medication. *Clin. Exp. Rheumatol.* **15,** 233–237.

183. Hashimoto, H., Yamamura, M., Nishiya, K., and Ota, Z. (1994) Impaired interleukin-8-dependent chemotaxis by synovial fluid polymorphonuclear leukocytes in rheumatoid arthritis. *Acta Med. Okayama* **48,** 181–187.

184. Rathakrishnan, C., Tiku K., Raghavan, A., and Tiku, M. L. (1992) Release of oxygen radicals by articular chondrocytes: A study of luminol-dependent chemiluminescence and hydrogen peroxide secretion. *J. Bone Miner. Res.* **7,** 1139–1148.

185. Davies, E. V., Campbell, A. K., Williams, B. D., and Hallett, M. B. (1991) Single cell imaging reveals abnormal intracellular calcium signals within rheumatoid synovial neutrophils. *Br. J. Rheumatol.* **30,** 443–448.

186. Zimmerli, W., Sansano, S., and Wiesenberg-Bottcher, I. (1991) Influence of the anti-inflammatory compound flosulide on granulocyte function. *Biochem. Pharmacol.* **42,** 1913–1919.

187. Katona, I. M., Ohura, K., Allen, J. B., Wahl, L. M., Chenoweth, D. E., and Wahl, S. M. (1991) Modulation of monocyte chemotactic function in inflammatory lesions. Role of inflammatory mediators. *J. Immunol.* **146,** 708–714.

188. Marino, I., Columbo, M., and Marone, G. (1996) The releasability of lysosomal enzymes from neutrophil leukocytes in patients with rheumatoid arthritis. *Clin. Exp. Rheumatol.* **14,** 387–394.

189. Stasia, M.-J., Jouan, A., Bourmeyster, N., Boquet, P., and Vignais, P. V. (1991) ADP-ribosylation of a small size GTP-binding protein in bovine neutrophils by the C3 exoenzyme of *Clostridium botulinum* and effect on the cell motility. *Biochem. Biophys. Res. Commun.* **180,** 615–622.

190. Egger, G., Aglas, F., and Rainer, F. (1995) Blood polymorphonuclear leukocyte migratory activities during rheumatoid arthritis. *Inflammation* **19,** 651–667.

191. Eggleton, P., Wang, L., Penhallow, J., Crawford, N., and Brown, K. A. (1995) Differences in oxidative response of subpopulations of neutrophils from healthy subjects and patients with rheumatoid arthritis. *Ann. Rheum. Dis.* **54,** 916–923.

192. Garcia-Lafuente, A., Antolin, M., Guarner, F., Vilaseca, J., and Malagelada, J. R. (1996) Bacterial peptides enhance inflammatory activity in a rat model of colitis. *Digestion* **57,** 368–373.

193. Keshavarzian, A., Haydek, J. M., Jacyno, M., Holmes, E. W., and Harford, F. (1997) Modulatory effects of the colonic milieu on neutrophil oxidative burst: a possible pathogenic mechanism of ulcerative colitis [In Process Citation]. *J. Lab. Clin. Med.* **130,** 216–225.

194. Mizuno, K., Hoshino, M., Hayakawa, T., Yamada, H., Nakazawa, T., Inagaki, T., Takeuchi, T., and Kunimatsu, M. (1996) Uncoupling of biliary lipid from bile acid secretion by formyl-methionyl-leucyl-phenylalanine in the rat. *Hepatology* **24,** 1224–1229.

195. Ledesma de Paolo, M. I., Celener Gravelle, P., De Paula, J. A., Panzita, M. T., Bandi, J. C., and Bustos Fernandez, L. (1996) Stimulation of inflammatory mediators secretion by chemotactic peptides in rat colitis model. *Acta Gastroenterol. Latinoam.* **26,** 23–30.

196. Azim, T., Islam, L. N., Halder, R. C., Hamadani, J., Khanum, N., Sarker, M. S., Salam, M. A., and Albert, M. J. (1995) Peripheral blood neutrophil responses in children with shigellosis. *Clin. Diagn. Lab. Immunol.* **2,** 616–622.

197. Griga, T., Tromm, A., Schwegler, U., and May, B. (1995) Enhanced superoxide anion release of normal neutrophil granulocytes primed with sera of patients with inactive inflammatory bowel disease. *Z. Gastroenterology* **33,** 345–348.

198. Kazi, N., Fields, J. Z., Sedghi, S., Kottapalli, V., Eiznhamer, D., Winship, D., and Keshavarzian, A. (1995) Modulation of neutrophil function by novel colonic factors: possible role in the pathophysiology of ulcerative colitis. *J. Lab. Clin. Med.* **126,** 70–80.

199. Carter, L. and Wallace, J. L. (1995) Alterations in rat peripheral blood neutrophil function as a consequence of colitis. *Dig. Dis. Sci.* **40,** 192–197.

200. Triadafilopoulos, G., Shah, M. H., and Pothoulakis, C. (1991) The chemotactic response of human granulocytes to Clostridium difficile toxin A is age dependent. *Am. J. Gastroenterol.* **86,** 1461–1465.

201. Chadwick, V. S., Schlup, M. M., Cooper, B. T., and Broom, M. F. (1990) Enzymes degrading bacterial chemotactic F-met peptides in human ileal and colonic mucosa. *J. Gastroenterol. Hepatol.* **5,** 375–381.

202. Williams, J. G., Hughes, L. E., and Hallett, M. B. (1990) Toxic oxygen metabolite production by circulating phagocytic cells in inflammatory bowel disease. *Gut* **31,** 187–193.

203. Leduc, L. E. and Zipser, R. D. (1989) Tissue origin of peptide-responsive eicosanoid production in rabbit intestine. *Am. J. Physiol.* **257,** G879–86.

204. Anton, P. A., Targan, S. R., and Shanahan, F. (1989) Increased neutrophil receptors for and response to the proinflammatory bacterial peptide formyl-methionyl-leucyl-phenylalanine in Crohn's disease. *Gastroenterology* **97,** 20–28.

205. Pedersen, M. M. (1988) Chemotactic response of neutrophil polymorphonuclear leukocytes in juvenile periodontitis measured by the Leading Front method. *Scand. J. Dent. Res.* **96,** 421–427.

206. Agarwal, S., Reynolds, M. A., Duckett, L. D., and Suzuki, J. B. (1989) Altered free cytosolic calcium changes and neutrophil chemotaxis in patients with juvenile periodontitis. *J. Periodont. Res.* **24,** 149–154.

207. Coles, R. B., Ranney, R. R., Freer, R. J., and Carchman, R. A. (1989) Thermal regulation of FMLP receptors on human neutrophils. *J. Leukoc. Biol.* **45,** 529–537.

208. Clark, R. A., Page, R. C., and Wilde, G. (1977) Defective neutrophil chemotaxis in juvenile periodontitis. *Infect. Immun.* **18,** 694–700.

209. Van Dyke, T. E. (1985) Role of the neutrophil in oral disease: receptor deficiency in leukocytes from patients with juvenile periodontitis. *Rev. Infect. Dis.* **7,** 419–425.

210. Watanabe, K., Lambert, L. A., Niederman, L. G., Punwani, I., and Andersen, B. R. (1991) Analysis of neutrophil chemotaxis and CD11b expression in pre-pubertal periodontitis. *J. Dent. Res.* **70,** 102–106.

211. Asman, B. (1988) Peripheral PMN cells in juvenile periodontitis: increased release of elastase and of oxygen radicals after stimulation with opsonized bacteria. *J. Clin. Periodont.* **15,** 360–364.

212. Van Dyke, T. E., Warbington, M., Gardner, M., and Offenbacher, S. (1990) Neutrophil surface protein markers as indicators of defective chemotaxis in LJP. *J. Periodontol.* **61,** 180–184.

213. Krause, S., Brachmann, P., Brandes, C., Losche, W., Hoffmann, T., and Gangler, P. (1990) Aggregation behaviour of blood granulocytes in patients with periodontal disease. *Arch. Oral Biol.* **35,** 75–77.

214. Van Dyke, T. E., Zinney, W., Winkel, K., Taufiq, A., Offenbacher, S., and Arnold, R. R. (1986) Neutrophil function in localized juvenile periodontitis. Phagocytosis, superoxide production and specific granule release. *J. Periodontol.* **57,** 703–708.

215. Leino, L., Hurttia, H. M., Sorvajarvi, K., and Sewon, L. A. (1994) Increased respiratory burst activity is associated with normal expression of IgG-Fc-receptors and complement receptors in peripheral neutrophils from patients with juvenile periodontitis. *J. Periodont. Res.* **29,** 179–184.

216. Agarwal, S., Suzuki, J. B., and Riccelli, A. E. (1994) Role of cytokines in the modulation of neutrophil chemotaxis in localized juvenile periodontitis. *J. Periodont. Res.* **29,** 127–137.

217. Kurihara, H., Murayama Y., Warbington, M. L., Champagne, C. M., and Van Dyke, T. E. (1993) Calcium-dependent protein kinase C activity of neutrophils in localized juvenile periodontitis. *Infect. Immun.* **61,** 3137–3142.

218. Daniel, M. A., McDonald, G., Offenbacher, S., and Van Dyke, T. E. (1993) Defective chemotaxis and calcium response in localized juvenile periodontitis neutrophils. *J. Periodontol.* **64,** 617–621.

219. Palmer, G. D., Watts, T. L., and Addison, I. E. (1993) A skin window study of neutrophil migration in subjects with localized juvenile periodontitis. *J. Clin. Periodontol.* **20,** 452–456.

220. Ashkenazi, M., White, R. R., and Dennison, D. K. (1992) Neutrophil modulation by Actinobacillus actinomycetemcomitans. II. Phagocytosis and development of respiratory burst. *J. Periodont. Res.* **27,** 457–465.

221. Ashkenazi, M., White, R. R., and Dennison, D. K. (1992) Neutrophil modulation by *Actinobacillus actinomycetemcomitans.* I. Chemotaxis, surface receptor expression and F-actin polymerization. *J. Periodont. Res.* **27,** 264–273.

222. Cogen, R. B., Roseman, J. M., Al-Joburi, W., Louv, W. C., Acton, R. T., Barger, B. O., Go, R. C., and Rasmussen, R. A. (1986) Host factors in juvenile periodontitis. *J. Dent. Res.* **65,** 394–399.

223. Mattout, C., Mege, J. L., Mattout, P., Fourel, J., and Monnet, V. (1990) Function of polynuclear neutrophils in patients with juvenile periodontitis and rapidly progressing periodontitis. *J. Periodontol.* **9,** 189–193.

224. Yang, Y. L., Hou, L. T., and Chang, W. K. (1993) Polymorphonuclear neutrophil chemotaxis in Chinese patients with post-juvenile periodontitis and rapidly progressive periodontitis. *J. Formos. Med. Assoc.* **92,** 643–648.

225. Page, R. C., Sims, T. J., Geissler, F., Altman, L. C., and Baab, D. A. (1985) Defective neutrophil and monocyte motility in patients with early onset periodontitis. *Infect. Immun.* **47,** 169–175.

226. Mouynet, P., Delamaire, M., le Goff, M. C., Kerbaol, M., Yardin, M., and Michel, J. F. (1994) Ex vivo studies of polymorphonuclear neutrophils from patients with early-onset forms of periodontitis. (I). Chemotactic assessment using the under agarose method. *J. Clin. Periodontol.* **21,** 177–183.

227. Kinane, D. F., Cullen, C. F., Johnston, F. A., and Evans, C. W. (1989) Neutrophil chemotactic behaviour in patients with early-onset forms of periodontitis (I). Leading front analysis in Boyden chambers. *J. Clin. Periodontol.* **16,** 242–246.

228. Kinane, D. F., Cullen, C. F., Johnston, F. A., and Evans, C. W. (1989) Neutrophil chemotactic behaviour in patients with early-onset forms of periodontitis (II). Assessment using the under agarose technique. *J. Clin. Periodontol.* **16,** 247–251.

229. Pippin, D. J. (1990) Increased intracellular levels of beta-glucuronidase in polymorphonuclear leucocytes from humans with rapidly progressive periodontitis. *Arch. Oral Biol.* **35,** 325–328.

230. Pippin, D. J., Cobb, C. M., and Feil, P. (1995) Increased intracellular levels of lysosomal beta-glucuronidase in peripheral blood PMNs from humans with rapidly progressive periodontitis. *J. Periodont. Res.* **30,** 42–50.

231. Shapira, L., Gordon, B., Warbington, M., and Van Dyke, T. E. (1994) Priming effect of Porphyromonas gingivalis lipopolysaccharide on superoxide production by neutrophils from healthy and rapidly progressive periodontitis subjects. *J. Periodontol.* **65,** 129–133.

232. Tufano, M. A., Ianniello, R., Sanges, M. R., and Rossano, F. (1992) Neutrophil function in rapidly progressive and adult periodontitis. *Eur. J. Epidemiol.* **8,** 67–73.

233. MacFarlane, G. D., Herzberg, M. C., Wolff, L. F., and Hardie, N. A. (1992) Refractory periodontitis associated with abnormal polymorphonuclear leukocyte phagocytosis and cigarette smoking. *J. Periodontol.* **63,** 908–913.

234. Shapira, L., Schatzker, Y., Gedalia, I., Borinski, R., and Sela, M. N. (1997) Effect of amine and stannous fluoride on human neutrophil functions in vitro. *J. Dent. Res.* **76,** 1381–1386.

235. Della Rocca, G. J., van Biesen, T., Daaka, Y., Luttrell, D. K., Luttrell, L. M., and Lefkowitz, R. J. (1997) Ras-dependent mitogen-activated protein kinase activation by G protein-coupled receptors: Convergence of G_i- and G_q-mediated pathways on calcium/calmodulin, Pyk2, and Src kinase. *J. Biol. Chem.* **272,** 19,125–19,132.

236. Grinstein, S. and Furuya, W. (1988) Receptor-mediated activation of electropermeabilized neutrophils. *J. Biol. Chem.* **263,** 1779–1783.

237. Lopez-Ilasaca, M., Crespo, P., Pellici, P. G., Gutkind, J. S., and Wetzker, R. (1997) Linkage of G protein-coupled receptors to the MAPK signaling pathway through PI 3-kinase gamma. *Science* **275,** 394–397.

238. Tsu, R. C., Lai, H. W. L., Allen, R. A., and Wong, Y. H. (1995) Differential coupling of the formyl peptide receptor to adenylate cyclase and phospholipase C by the pertussis toxin-insensitive G_z protein. *Biochem. J.* **309,** 331–339.

239. Neumann, F. J., Ott, I., Wilhelm, A., Katus, H., Tillmanns, H., and Schomig, A. (1994) Release of chemoattractants and neutrophil actuation in acute myocardial infarction immediately after successful recanalization of the infarct-related vessel by angioplasty. *Eur. Heart J.* **15,** 171–178.

240. Mills, J. S., Miettinen, H. M., Barnidge, D., Vlases, M. J., Wimer-Mackin, S., Dratz, E. A., and Jesaits, A. J. (1998) Ligand binding site of the formyl pepticle receptor by photoaffinity labeling and mass spectrometry. *J. Biol. Chem.* **273,** 10,428–10,435.

241. Acaro, A. (1998) The small GTP-binding protein Rac promotes the dissociation of gelsolin from actin filaments in neutrophils. *J. Biol. Chem.* **273,** 805–813.

242. Nobes, C. D. and Hall, A. (1995) Rho, Rac, and Cdc42 GTPases regulate the assembly of multimolecular focal complexes associated with actin stress fibers, lamellipodia, and filopodia. *Cell* **81,** 53–62.

243. Zigmond, S. H., Joyce, M., Borleis, J., Bokoch, G. M., and Devreotes, P. N. (1997) Regulation of actin polymerization in cell-free systems by GTPγS and Cdc42. *J. Cell Biol.* **138,** 363–374.

11

Pathobiology of Neutrophil Interactions with Polarized Columnar Epithelia

James L. Madara

1. Introduction

Luminal spaces in the alimentary tract, airway, and renal tubule are defined by encasing monolayers of polarized columnar epithelia. Such epithelial monolayers, which rest on a basement membrane above connective tissue through which course lymphatics and the microvasculature, serve to protect the underlying tissues from these varied, but harsh, luminal environments. This separating attribute of epithelial monolayers, termed "barrier function," is maintained in part by apical circumferential tight junctions that adjoin neighboring epithelial cells in gasketlike fashion, thus preventing free diffusion of noxious hydrophilic solutes between neighboring cells *(1)*. While maintaining barrier function, epithelial cells must simultaneously vectorially transport a host of molecules including nutrients, ions, immunoglobulin, and water across the monolayer. Tissue related variations in these transport functions of columnar epithelia largely define the specific functions assigned to various organs including the intestine, stomach, kidney, and so on. Similarly, such epithelia synthesize and secrete products including mucins and, in some areas such as the airway, have surface structures (cilia) that assist in clearing the surface of potential threats.

Given the broad menu of contributions of polarized columnar epithelia to the functions of diverse organs, it is not surprising that organ dysfunction seen as a consequence of inflammation often largely results from alterations of the delicate epithelial lining. Active (i.e., "acute") inflammation of surfaces lined by polarized columnar epithelia occurs in many diseases and is defined by the migration of neutrophils from the microvasculature and across the epithelial surfaces. This chapter will review issues related to such neutrophil-epithelial interactions. For purposes of clarity, it will primarily focus on the interactions between neutrophils and intestinal epithelial cells but will

From: *Molecular and Cellular Basis of Inflammation*
Edited by: C. N. Serhan and P. A. Ward © Humana Press Inc., Totowa, NJ

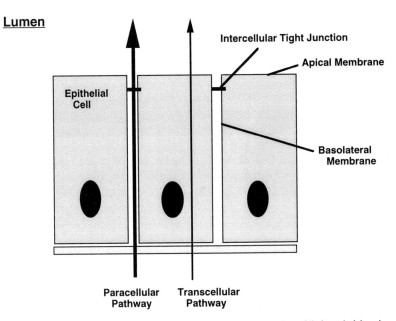

Fig. 1. Polarized columnar epithelial cells form monolayers in which neighboring cells are interconnected by a variety of junctions including a sealing circumferential apical tight junction. The tight junction also assists in maintaining the biochemically distinctive nature of the apical and basolateral membrane domains. As a result, neutrophil interactions with columnar epithelia (as modeled in this chapter by intestinal epithelia) distinctly vary depending on which surface of the epithelial cell the interaction occurs. The tight junction seals the major permeation pathway across epithelial monolayers—the paracellular pathway.

draw analogies with neutrophil interactions with other epithelia. The picture that emerges suggests that substantial crosstalk occurs between epithelia and neutrophils and additionally indicates that epithelia may serve as sensors of the external environment that can, in turn, orchestrate inflammatory responses to external threats.

Neutrophil Movement Through the Paracellular Space of Epithelia and the Nature of Neutrophil Adherence to Epithelial Surfaces

Paracellular Movement of Neutrophils

Two pathways available for passive diffusion across epithelia exist: the transcellular pathway (across cells) and the paracellular pathway (between cells) *(1)*. As shown in Fig. 1, the paracellular pathway consists of a circumferential sealing apical junction (tight or occluding junction), which is the rate-limiting barrier for movement through the paracellular space. Analyses utilizing canine renal (MDCK) or human intestinal (T84) epithelial monolayers indicate that neutrophils traverse epithelial monolayers via the paracellular route *(2,3)*. Such movement, modeled as depicted in Fig. 2, requires crossing and, thus, transient perturbation of the tight junction seal that exists between epithelial cells. At low densities of neutrophil transmigration, junctional seals between epithelial cells are able to be maintained as defined by physiological criteria *(3)*. This

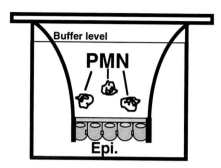

Fig. 2. In vitro assay of neutrophil polymorphec nuclear leukocyte neurophil (PMN) interaction with and transmigration across polarized monolayers of columnar epithelia. An inverted monolayer is depicted as grown on a permeable support (apical membrane facing lower chamber). Neutrophils (PMN) purified from peripheral blood can be positioned basolaterally by gravitational flow. Artificial gradients of chemoattractants can be made by adding chemoattractants to the lower well, thus stimulating basolateral to apical directed PMN movement as occurs in human disease.

finding is consistent with the ability of epithelial tight junctions to dynamically restructure under physiological perturbations, such as when individual epithelial cells are sloughed from the monolayer *(4)*. With extrusion a series of events ensure maintenance of junctional barrier function: expansion of junctional elements over the lateral membrane of neighboring cells in the vicinity of the extruding cell; establishment of new junctional contacts between basal protrusions of these neighboring cells, which extend under the extruding cell; and progressive basal to apical "zippering" of these new junctional contacts as the extruding cell lifts from the monolayer *(4)*. Similarly, as sperm cells cross testicular epithelia, dynamic restructuring of tight junctions permits low-density transmigration of this cell type without loss of barrier function *(5)*.

By contrast to low-frequency transepithelial migration by neutrophils, movement of neutrophils through epithelial monolayers at high density (flux rates approximating one neutrophil/epithelial cell/hour) result in transient, reversible loss of tight junction barrier capabilities *(3,6)*. Because neutrophils from patients with chronic granulomatous disease migrate normally in such assays, respiratory burst products are not likely to be required to break these junctional seals *(7)*. Similarly, since neutrophil migration proceeds normally in the presence of a series of inhibitors of neutrophil proteases, it is possible that either pressure associated with neutrophil lamellipodia extensions, or neutrophil-induced epithelial signals that directly control tight junction permeability serve as the basis for opening interepithelial junctions.

Transient opening of epithelial tight junctions by neutrophil migration may have additional effects on epithelial cells, which may be deleterious in nature. For example, neutrophil-induced opening of tight junctions has been shown to result in unmasking of basolaterally targeted membrane proteins to luminally positioned elements (Fig. 1) *(8)*. Thus $\beta 1$ integrins, normally sequestered basolaterally and hidden from the luminal compartment by sealing apical tight junctions, become available to luminal bacteria as a consequence of high-density neutrophil transepithelial migration *(8)*. $\beta 1$ integrins have been shown to be a ligand for the *inv* gene product of the intestinal pathogen *Yersinia enterocolitica*, and availability of basolateral ligands thus creates a window of

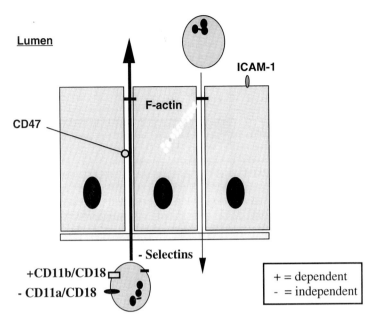

Fig. 3. Paradigm of PMN interactions with intestinal epithelia. Migration is dependent on the neutrophil β2 integrin CD11b/CD18 but independent of CD11a/CD18 and of selectins. The epithelial ligand for CD11b/CD18 is not intercellular adhesion molecule-1 (ICAM-1) because the latter, when induced, is apically expressed in most polarized columnar epithelia. Basolateral expression of epithelial CD47 assists in permitting PMN to efficiently traverse the monolayer (CD47 is also expressed on the neutrophil surface). Under any standard condition, neutrophil movement in the basolateral to apical (i.e., physiological) direction is always more efficient than in the reverse direction (dense vs light arrows between cells)— a finding owing in part to inhibition of apical to basolateral migration by epithelial F-actin. Most features of this paradigm have been shown to apply to natural as well as model mammalian intestinal epithelia. This paradigm is in contrast to that governing movement of PMN across endothelial monolayers (*see text*).

opportunity for enhanced association with particular luminal pathogens *(8)*. Such events could conceivably relate to the known enhanced risk of infection with enteric pathogens that accompanies ongoing intestinal inflammation.

Neutrophil Adherence to Columnar Epithelial Cells

To interface with the epithelial tight junction, neutrophils must first migrate along the approx 25 microns length of the epithelial paracellular space *(9)*. This distance contrasts to that of the approx 1 micron length of the endothelial paracellular space (with the neutrophil itself having an average diameter in the unspread state of 10 microns). Since the only available substrate for adhesive interactions between neutrophils and epithelial cells in this relatively long epithelial paracellular space is the lateral membrane of epithelial cells, one can assume that a series of adhesion events to epithelial counter receptor(s) must occur during transepithelial migration of neutrophils (Fig. 3). Indeed, neutrophils migrating across epithelia develop focally close membrane appositions with epithelial cells at sites at which the underlying cytoskeleton of both cell types is modified *(7)*. Recent studies indicate that remodeling of the epithelial f-actin cortical cytoskeleton during neutrophil transepithelial migration is critical for efficient migration *(10)*. Neutrophil entry into the epithelial paracellular space is dependent on the function of the neutrophil β2 integrin CD11b/CD18 whereas the other two members of this family, CD11a/CD18 and CD11c/CD18, appear to be of limited importance *(11)*. Thus, neutrophils lacking surface expression of β2 integrins fail to migrate into epithelial monolayers, subsets of monoclonal antibodies to CD11b/CD18 will block such migration, and monoclonal antibodies that prevent interactions of the other two β2 integrins with their counterreceptors do not influence neutrophil migration into and across intestinal epithelial monolayers *(11)*. The epithelial counterreceptor for CD11b/CD18 has not been identified, although it does not appear to be any of the known counterreceptors for CD11b/CD18. Important in this regard is consideration of the polarity of epithelial-neutrophil associations. For example, when epithelial expression of ICAM-1 (CD54) is induced, it is usually apically, but not basolaterally, expressed (with the possible exception of airway epithelia under selected conditions) *(12)*. Thus, although apparent CD11b/CD18-ICAM-1-mediated adherence between epithelia and neutrophils can be demonstrated under selected conditions with apical application of neutrophils, this is not the membrane domain with which neutrophils interface during physiologically directed transmigration. It remains possible that at sites at which apically polarized expression of ICAM-1 can be induced (distal airway, intestine, renal tubule), CD11b/CD18-ICAM-1-mediated interactions may occur following translocation of neutrophils into the lumen.

Recently a monoclonal antibody recognizing an epitope on CD47 has been shown to impede movement of neutrophils through the paracellular space, whereas not preventing their entry into this space (in contrast to inhibition by CD11b/CD18) *(13)*. While one element of inhibition of this response appears to be directed toward neutrophil surface CD47, it also appears that epithelial CD47 contributes to this response *(13)*. CD47 is a member of the immunoglobulin superfamily and possesses an IgV-like loop extracellular domain, and five putative membrane spanning domains *(14,15)*. Lindberg et al. *(16)* have shown that CD47 may regulate integrin function as modeled by analyses of CD47 regulation of $\alpha_v\beta_3$ binding to vitronectin. However, it is unclear how CD47 is involved mechanistically in the regulation of neutrophil movement across epithelial monolayers. Specifically, it is unknown whether CD47 might regulate either β2 integrin function on neutrophils, integrin function on epithelial cells, or have a completely different site of action during neutrophil-epithelial interactions.

The above outlined ligand-based requirements for neutrophil-epithelial interactions vary significantly from those of neutrophil-endothelial interactions. For example, ICAM-1 appears to be a major endothelial ligand supporting β2 integrin–based movement of neutrophils across endothelia *(17)*. CD31 *(18)* is likewise required for endothelial transmigration, but not for epithelial transmigration. Furthermore, both neutrophil and endothelial selectins (CD62L, CD62P, and CD62E) are crucial to neutrophil transendothelial *(19–21)* but not transepithelial *(22)* migration. Selectin independence of neutrophil-epithelial interactions is not surprising because such interactions take place in the absence of shear—the challenge for which selectin interactions appear designed to overcome *(23)*.

Neutrophil-Elicited Modifications of Epithelial Secretory Responses

Following migration of neutrophils through the epithelial paracellular space and across the intercellular tight junction, these cells interact with the biochemically dis-

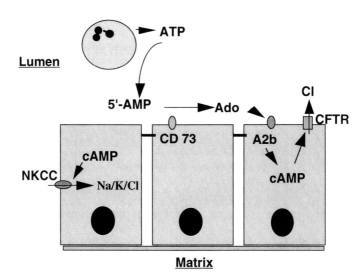

Fig. 4. Diagram of interaction of activated luminal neutrophils with epithelial apical membranes. The major direct acting neutrophil-derived secretagog is 5'-AMP, which is surface converted by epithelial CD73 to adenosine and is recognized by the A2b receptor. The resulting cAMP signal results in electrogenic Cl secretion (the basis of secretory diarrhea) via opening of apical Cl channels and activation of the Na, K, 2Cl cotransporter (NKCC) basolateral salt uptake pathway. Thus neutrophils can directly modify epithelial Cl secretion via this mechanism (in addition to the indirect influences possibly afforded by activating other subepithelial cell types that might secondarily modify Cl secretion). Most features of this paradigm have been confirmed in natural mammalian intestinal epithelia (*see text*).

tinctive epithelial apical membrane (Fig. 4) *(9)*. Evidence derived from model intestinal epithelia suggests that such interactions may exhibit important functional sequelae. For example, on entry into the luminal compartment, neutrophil derived 5'-AMP may serve as a paracrine factor for epithelial cells that possess both an ectonucleotidase activity to convert this compound to authentic adenosine and an adenosine receptor *(24)*. Model and native human intestinal epithelial cells have recently been shown to express the GPI-linked ectonucleotidase, CD73, as a preferentially apically polarized membrane protein *(25)*. Inhibition of CD73 activity also attenuates both conversion of neutrophil-derived 5'-AMP to authentic adenosine and a 5'-AMP–elicited endogenous transepithelial current *(24,25)*. Physiological analyses reveal that the current elicited by apical 5'-AMP exposure represents electrogenic Cl secretion—the basis of secretory diarrhea *(26)*. Furthermore, 5'-AMP accounts for the bulk of secretory bioactivity derived from apically positioned neutrophils *(26)*.

Adenosine released after conversion of neutrophil derived 5'-AMP by CD73 is recognized by apical adenosine receptors of the A2b subtype *(27)*. Natural human alimentary epithelia also express the A2b receptor apically (Strohmeier, G. and Madara, J. L., unpublished observations). This receptor signals via the cAMP-A kinase pathway to elicit Cl secretion by regulated gating of apical membrane Cl conductive pathways *(27)*. Through this mechanism, it appears that neutrophils can thus

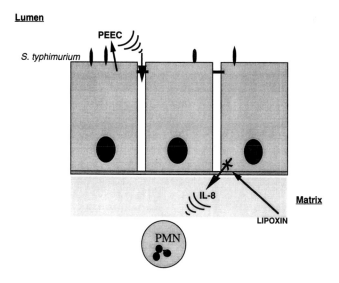

Fig. 5. Diagram of natural epithelial signaling to neutrophils by intestinal epithelia on detection of a model apical pathogen (*S. typhimurium*). Basolateral secretion of chemokines results in imprinting of underlying matrix with a gradient that resists washout and supports neutrophil movement to the immediate subepithelial space. The basis for this imprinted gradient has been shown to be owing to the C-X-C chemokine IL-8. Apical release of a pathogen elicited epithelial-derived chemokine (PEEC) then supports movement of neutrophils through the paracellular space into the lumen. Thus, epithelial cells are capable of actively orchestrating complex neutrophil migration patterns. The natural stop signal for inflammation, LXA4, downregulates neutrophil movement across the epithelium and also downregulates secretion of epithelial chemokines.

orchestrate their movement into the luminal space with a paracrine-regulated volume flush of the space they enter. Such secretory flush has been considered clinically useful, e.g., in diminishing the colonization period of luminal pathogens.

Epithelial Orchestration of the Inflammatory Response

Until recently it was largely assumed that directed neutrophil movement across columnar epithelia was likely a response to transmonolayer chemoattractant gradients. For example, bacterial contamination of spaces in contact with the external environment could readily be imagined to support lumen to tissue gradients of potent chemoattractants such as *n*-formyl peptides. One fact confounding this view, however, is that in such organs as the intestine, the normal background bacterial presence is sufficiently high that it is difficult to imagine that the addition of one virulent strain would add significantly to the basal gradient of bacterial-derived products. Moreover, in tissues such as the intestine, the organization of the subepithelial microvasculature is such that countercurrent exchange phenomena will rapidly distort gradients originating from soluble luminal factors *(28)*.

More recently it has been recognized that polarized columnar epithelia may also actively participate in the orchestration of the neutrophil inflammatory responses (Fig. 5). For example, the pathogen *Salmonella typhimurium*, by morphological criteria, elicits a host neutrophil-based inflammatory response prior to deterioration of the epithelial barrier *(29)*. Investigation of such interactions using tissue-culture models has revealed that *S. typhimurium* associates with the apical membranes of intestinal epithelial cells at high numbers (> 50/cell) without immediate deleterious sequelae on monolayer barrier function, epithelial tight junctions, or transepithelial regulation of ion transport as judged by agonist-elicited electrogenic Cl secretion *(29)*. However, as a consequence of such pathogen apical membrane interactions, neutrophils, applied basolaterally, are induced to move across the intact monolayer by a mechanism that appears independent of the *n*-formyl peptide receptor *(29)*. The in vivo ability of various strains of *S. typhimurium* to produce enteritis correlates with the ability of the same strains to produce spontaneous directed transepithelial neutrophil migration in the in vitro model *(30)*. Thus, it appears that the in vitro induction of neutrophil migration triggered by the apical association between enterocytes and bacteria appropriately models an in vivo virulence mechanism. It has recently been appreciated that attachment of *S. typhimurium* to the enterocyte apical membranes results in basolaterally directed secretion of various C-X-C and C-C chemokines *(29,31,32)*. For example, the neutrophil chemoattractant interleukin-8 (IL-8) is released basolaterally under such conditions *(29)*. However, release of basolateral IL-8 does not appear responsible for supporting neutrophil migration from the subepithelial space, across the epithelium, and into the lumen *(33)*. Basolaterally released IL-8 does bind to subepithelial matrix components and "imprints" on this matrix, a long-lived gradient that can, however, support directed neutrophil movement to the immediate subepithelial location *(33)*. Thus, it is possible that such matrix imprinting of chemoattractant gradients derived from the epithelium could assist in directing neutrophils through the subepithelial matrix—a site of high volume flow that would wash out nonfixed, soluble gradients. An unidentified chemoattractant activity that is released in a polarized apical direction in response to *S. typhimurium*-epithelial contact appears responsible for the final step in transepithelial migration *(34)*. This PEEC activity displays physical and other attributes that make it unlikely to represent a known chemoattractant, although it appears to function, like other neutrophil chemoattractants, through a signal involving a pertussis toxin–sensitive Ca^{2+} flux *(34)*.

Epithelial release of neutrophil chemoattractants has also been recognized to occur both in gastric epithelial cells as a consequence of apical interaction with the pathogen *Helicobacter pylori* and in urothelial cells interacting with pathogenic *Escherichia coli* strains *(35,36)*. Thus, it is likely that epithelia may act as early warning sensors of pathogens in the external environment and that they may actively participate in the orchestration of the inflammatory response.

Lipoxins (LXs) as Stop Signals
for Epithelial-Neutrophil Interactions

Serhan *(37,38)* has demonstrated that products of the eicosanoid pathway, LXs, may be stop signals for specific events in inflammation. Such LX-mediated stop-signal activities also apply to epithelial-neutrophil interactions. The natural LX, LXA4, potently downregulates agonist-induced transepithelial migration of neutrophils and thus prevents the deleterious sequelae of such interactions on epithelial function *(39)*. It is now known that LXA4 can directly act on model intestinal epithelia, attenuating, e.g., the pathogen-elicited proinflammatory release of basolateral IL-8 and apical PEEC activities (Gewirtz, A., Serhan, C. N., Madara, J. L., submitted).

Since LXA4 serves as a novel example of a natural receptor-mediated stop signal for inflammation, stable analogs have been prepared and analyzed with an eye toward utility in states characterized by unrestrained and/or inappropriate neutrophil-based inflammation *(40)*. It remains to be determined if such compounds will be useful in downregulating inflammatory responses at mucosal sites, although evidence in this regard at cutaneous sites has recently been published *(41)*.

Summary

Neutrophil interactions with epithelia, as occur during transepithelial migration, are complex and involve initial binding, sustaining signals that permit complete migration through the relatively long paracellular space, and paracrine signaling events that modify key aspects of epithelial transport. Ligand interactions that occur during such interactions appear to differ from those that occur during neutrophil emigration from the microvasculature. Furthermore, the epithelial cell actively participates in events that characterize neutrophil transepithelial migration and, indeed, may harbor the capacity to orchestrate neutrophil responses when intimate contact of luminally positioned pathogens is recognized. Finally, natural stop-signal pathways for inflammation may provide a useful means of downregulating the neutrophil-epithelial interactions that often lead to epithelial and, therefore, organ dysfunction.

References

1. Madara, J. L. and Trier, J. S. (1994) The functional morphology of the mucosa of the small intestine, in *Physiology of the Gastrointestinal Tract*, 3rd ed. (Johnson, L., ed.), Raven, Philadelphia, PA.
2. Milks, L., C., Conyers, G. P., and Cramer, E. B. (1986) The effect of neutrophil migration on epithelial permeability. *J. Cell Biol.* **103,** 2729–2738.
3. Nash, S., Stafford, J., and Madara, J. L. (1987) Effects of polymorphonuclear leukocyte transmigration on the barrier function of cultured intestinal epithelial monolayers. *J. Clin. Invest.* **80,** 1104–1113.
4. Madara, J. L. (1990) Maintenance of the macromolecular barrier at cell extrusion sites in intestinal epithelium: Physiological rearrangement of tight junctions. *J. Membr. Biol.* **116,** 177–184.
5. Byers, S. and Pelletier, R. M. (1991) *Tight Junctions* (Cereijido, M., ed.), CRC, Boca Raton, FL, pp. 279–302.
6. Parkos, C. A., Colgan, S. P., Delp, C., Arnaout, A., and Madara, J. L. (1992) Neutrophil migration across a cultured epithelial monolayer elicits a biphasic resistance response representing sequential effects on transcellular and paracellular pathways. *J. Cell Biol.* **117,** 757–764.
7. Nash, S., Stafford, J., and Madara, J. L. (1988) The selective and superoxide-independent disruption of intestinal epithelial tight junctions during leukocyte transmigration. *Lab. Invest.* **59,** 531–537.
8. McCormick, B. A., Nusrat, A., D'Andrea, L., Parkos, C. A., Hoffman, P., Carnes, D., and Madara, J. L. (1997) Unmasking of intestinal epithelial lateral membrane β1 integrin consequent to transepithelial neutrophil migration in vitro facilitates *inv*-mediated invasion by *Yersinia pseudotuberculosis*. *Infect. Immun.* **65,** 1414–1421.
9. Madara, J. L. (1991) The functional morphology of the epithelium of the small intestine, in *The Handbook of Physiology, Alimentary Tract Volumes* (Shultz, S., ed.), American Physiological Society.
10. Hofman, P., D'Andrea, L., Carnes, D., Colgan, S. P., and Madara, J. L. (1996) The intestinal epithelial cytoskeleton selectively constrains lumen-to-tissue migration of neutrophils. *Am. J. Physiol. (Cell)* **271,** C312–C320.

11. Parkos, C. A., Delp, C., Nash, S., Arnaout, A., Madara, J. L. (1991) Neutrophil migration across a cultured intestinal epithelium: dependence on a CD11b/CD18 mediated event and enhanced efficiency in physiological direction. *J. Clin. Invest.* **88,** 1605–1612.

12. Parkos, C. A., Colgan, S. P., Diamond, M. S., Nusrat, A., Liang, T., Springer, T. A., and Madara, J. L. (1996) Expression and polarization of ICAM-1 on intestinal epithelia: consequences for CD11b/CD18-mediated interactions with neutrophils. *Mol. Med.* **4,** 489–505.

13. Parkos, C. A., Colgan, S. P., Liang, T., Nusrat, A., Bacarra, A. E., Carnes, D. K., and Madara, J. L. (1996) CD47 mediates postadhesive events required for neutrophil migration across polarized intestinal epithelia. *J. Cell Biol.* **132,** 437–450.

14. Campbell, I. G., Freemont, P. S., Foulkes, W., and Trowsdale, J. (1992) An ovarian tumor marker with homology to vaccinia virus contains an IgV-like region and multiple transmembrane domains. *Cancer Res.* **52,** 5416–5420.

15. Lindberg, F. P., Gresham, H. D., Schwarz, C., and Brown, E. J. (1996) Molecular cloning of an integrin associated protein: An immunoglobulin family member with multiple membrane spamming domains implicated in alpha v beta 3 dependent ligand binding. *J. Cell Biol.* **123,** 485–496.

16. Lindberg, F. P., Gresham, H. D., Reinhold, M. I., and Brown, E. J. (1996) Integrin associated protein immunoglobulin domain is necessary for efficient vitronectin bead binding. *J. Cell Biol.* **134,** 1313–1322.

17. Pober, J. S. and Cotran, R. S. (1990) The role of endothelial cells in inflammation. *Transplantation* **50,** 537–544.

18. Muller, W. A., Weigl, S. A., Deng, X., and Phillips, D. M. (1993) PECAM-1 is required for transendothelial migration of leukocytes. *J. Exp. Med.* **178,** 449–460.

19. Spertini, O., Kansas, G. S., Munro, J. M., Griffin, J. D., and Tedder, T. F. (1991) Regulation of leukocyte migration by activation of the leukocyte adhesion molecule-1 (LAM-1) selectin. *Nature* **349,** 691–694.

20. Bevilacqua, M. P., Stengelin, S., Gimbrone, M. A., and Seed, B. (1989) Endothelial leukocyte adhesion molecule-1: an inducible receptor for neutrophils related to complement regulatory proteins and lectins. *Science* **243,** 1160–1165.

21. Mayadas, T. N., Johnson, R. C., Rayburn, H., Hynes, R. O., and Wagner, D. D. (1993) Leukocyte rolling and extravasation are severely compromised in P-selectin-deficient mice. *Cell* **74,** 541–544.

22. Colgan, S. P., Parkos, C. A., McGuirk, D., Brady, H. R., Papayianni, A. A., Frendl, G., and Madara, J. L. (1995) Receptors involved in carbohydrate-binding modulate intestinal epithelial-neutrophil interactions. *J. Biol. Chem.* **270,** 10,531–10,539.

23. Springer, T. A. (1990) Adhesion receptors of the immune system. *Nature* **346,** 425–434.

24. Madara, J. L., Patapoff, T. W., Gillece-Castro, B., Colgan, S., Parkos, C., Delp, C., and Mrsny, R. J. (1993) 5'-AMP is the neutrophil derived paracrine factor that elicits chloride secretion from T84 intestinal epithelial monolayers. *J. Clin. Invest.* **91,** 2320–2325.

25. Strohmeier, G. R., Lencer, W. I., Patopoff, T. W., Thompson, L. F., Carlson, S. L., Moe, S. J., Carnes, D., Mrsny, R. J., and Madara, J. L. (1997) Surface expression, polarization, and functional significance of CD 73 in human intestinal epithelia. *J. Clin. Invest.* **99,** 2588–2601.

26. Nash, S., Parkos, C., Nusrat, A., Delp, C., and Madara, J. L. (1991), in vitro model of intestinal crypt abscess: A novel neutrophil-derived secretagogue (NDS) activity. *J. Clin. Invest.* **87,** 1474–1477.

27. Strohmeier, G. R., Reppert, S. M., Lencer, W. I., and Madara, J. L. (1995) The A2b-adenosine receptor mediates cAMP responses to adenosine receptor agonists in human intestinal epithelia. *J. Biol. Chem.* **270,** 2387–2394.

28. Jodal, M. and Lundgren, O. (1986) Countercurrent mechanisms in the mammalian gastrointestinal tract. *Gastroenterology* **91,** 225–241.

29. McCormick, B. A., Colgan, S. P., Delp-Archer, C., Miller, S. I., and Madara, J. L. (1993) *Salmonella typhimurium* attachment to human intestinal epithelial monolayers: transcellular signalling to subepithelial neutrophils. *J. Cell Biol.* **123,** 895–908.

30. McCormick, B. A., Miller, S. I., Carnes, D., and Madara, J. L. (1995) Transepithelial signaling to neutrophils by *Salmonella*: a novel virulence mechanism for gastroenteritis. *Infect. Immun.* **63,** 2302–2309.

31. Eckman, L., Jung, H., Schurer-Maly, C., Panja, A., Morzycka-Wroblewska, E., and Kagnoff, M. (1993) Different cytokine expression by human intestinal epithelial cell lines: regulated expression of IL-8. *Gastroenterology* **105,** 1689–1697.

32. Eckmann, L., Kagnoff, M., and Fierer, J. (1993) Epithelial cells secrete the chemokine IL-8 in response to bacterial entry. *Infect. Immun.* **61,** 4569–4574.
33. McCormick, B., Hofman, P., Kim, J., Carnes, D., Miller, S., and Madara, J. L. (1995) Surface attachment of *Salmonella typhimurium* to intestinal epithelia imprints the subepithelial matrix with gradients chemotactic for neutrophils. *J. Cell Biol.* **131,** 1599–1608.
34. McCormick, B. A., Parkos, C. A., Colgan, S. P., Carnes, D. K., and Madara, J. L. (1998) Apical secretion of a pathogen-elicited epithelial chemokine (PEEC) activity in response to surface colonization of intestinal epithelia by Salmonella typhimurium. *Infect. Immun.,* in press.
35. Crowe, S. E. (1995) Expression of IL-8 and CD 54 by human gastric epithelium after Helicobacter pylori infection in vitro. *Gastroenterology* **108,** 65–74.
36. Agace, W. W., Patarroyo, M., Svensson, M., Carlemalm, E., and Svanborg, C. (1995) *E. coli* induces transuroepithelial neutrophil migration by an intercellular adhesion molecule 1-dependent mechanism. *Infect. Immun.* **63,** 4054–4062.
37. Serhan, C. N. (1994) Lipoxin biosynthesis and its impact in inflammatory and vascular events. *BBA* **1212,** 1–25.
38. Fiore, S., Maddox, J. F., Perez, H. D., and Serhan, C. N. (1994) Identification of a human cDNA encoding a functional high affinity lipoxin A4 receptor. *J. Exp. Med.* **180,** 253–260.
39. Colgan, S. P., Serhan, C. S., Delp, C., and Madara, J. L. (1993) Lipoxin A4 modulates transmigration of human neutrophils across intestinal epithelial monolayers. *J. Clin. Invest.* **92,** 75–82.
40. Serhan, C. N., Maddox, J. F., Petasis, N. A., Akritopoulou-Zanze, I., Papayianni, A., Brady, H. R., Colgan, S. P., and Madara, J. L. (1995) Design of lipoxin A_4 stable analogs that block transmigration and adhesion of human neutrophils. *Biochemistry* **34,** 14,609–14,615.
41. Takano, T., Fiore, S., Maddox, J. F., Brady, H. R., Petasis, N. A., and Serhan, C. N. (1997) Asprin triggered 15-epi-lipoxin A4 and LXA4 stable analogues are potent inhibitors of acute inflammation: evidence for anti-inflammatory receptors. *J. Exp. Med.* **185,** 1693–1703.

12

Adenosine and Its Receptors During Inflammation

Bruce N. Cronstein

Introduction

The number of endogenous mediators of inflammation is large and growing, but the list of endogenous inhibitors of inflammation has remained relatively small. Most investigators are familiar with glucocorticoids, and there is an increasing appreciation of lipid mediators, select cytokines, and endogenous cytokine inhibitors as anti-inflammatory mediators. Adenosine, a purine nucleoside, is another agent that has received increasing interest as an endogenous anti-inflammatory agent. In this chapter the author will discuss the generation of adenosine at inflamed sites, the cell surface receptors for adenosine, which, when occupied, affect inflammatory cell function and the functional effects of adenosine on the various inflammatory cells and the inflammatory process. Finally, the author will discuss the potential pharmacologic uses of adenosine as an anti-inflammatory agent.

Generation of Adenosine at Inflamed and Injured Sites (*see* Fig. 1)

After potassium, adenosine triphosphate (ATP) is the most abundant intracellular molecule. Its functions as an energy source, as a cofactor and substrate of a vast number of enzymatic reactions and even as a neurotransmitter are well documented. Moreover, ADP, AMP, and adenosine, the breakdown products of ATP, have also been shown to have a variety of biochemical and physiologic effects, primarily as intercellular messengers. Adenosine may be generated from adenine nucleotides intracellularly (as the product of AMP dephosphorylation) or as the result of the dephosphorylation of AMP by ecto-5' nucleotidase in the extracellular milieu (Fig. 1). Recent studies have suggested that the extracellular generation of adenosine is responsible for the greatest increase in extracellular adenosine concentration at inflamed sites when studied in vitro

From: *Molecular and Cellular Basis of Inflammation*
Edited by: C. N. Serhan and P. A. Ward © Humana Press Inc., Totowa, NJ

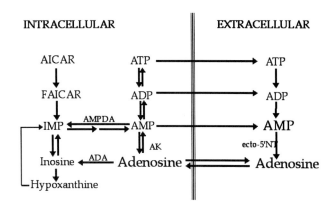

Fig. 1. Source of adenosine. AICAR, 5-aminoimidazole-4-carboxamide ribonucleotide; FAICAR, formyl-AICAR; IMP, inosine monophosphate; AMPDA, AMP deaminase; ADA, adenosine deaminase; AK, adenosine kinase; ecto-5'NT, ecto-5' nucleotidase.

and in vivo *(1–3)*. Adenosine catabolism by adenosine deaminase (ADA) and cellular uptake of adenosine may also regulate extracellular adenosine concentration *(4,5)*. Neutrophil-generated oxidants may inactivate these adenosine catabolic enzymes and thereby promote an increase in adenosine concentration at inflamed sites as well *(6)*. Thus, the regulation of adenosine concentrations at inflamed sites is complex and may vary depending on the type of cells present, the number of necrotic cells, and the generation of other inflammatory mediators. Moreover, several pharmacologic agents currently in use for the treatment of inflammatory disease may significantly affect adenosine concentrations at inflamed sites *(vide infra)*.

Cell Surface Receptors for Adenosine

The physiologic effects of adenosine were first appreciated by Drury and Szent-Gyorgi in 1929 *(7)*, but more than four decades passed before the recognition that adenosine mediated its physiologic effects via interaction with specific receptors on the cell surface *(8)*. The existence of two different adenosine receptors (A_1 and A_2) was first demonstrated on the basis of the observed differences in the pharmacologic effects of adenosine on cAMP metabolism *(9,10)*. Using the techniques of molecular biology, at least four adenosine receptors, A_1, A_{2A}, A_{2B}, and A_3, have been identified and their structure elucidated. All these receptors are members of the seven-transmembrane–spanning, heterotrimeric G-protein–associated family of cell surface receptors *(11)*.

Adenosine receptors were first differentiated on the basis of their capacity to modulate cellular cAMP concentrations, and the distinctions established using this criterion remain generally valid: adenosine A_1 receptors inhibit and adenosine A_2 receptors (both A_{2A} and A_{2B}) increase intracellular cAMP generation whereas A_3 receptors do not appear to signal by increasing or decreasing cAMP levels. Despite their documented effects on cAMP, cAMP is not the only mediator of signaling at adenosine A_2 receptors *(see refs. 12–14)*. Highly subclass-specific adenosine receptor agonists and antagonists (most of which are methylxanthine derivatives) have been developed for use in characterization of the physiologic and pharmacologic effects of adenosine, and in studies using these agents, all four adenosine receptors modulate one aspect or another of the inflammatory process.

Table 1
Adenosine Receptors Modulate Inflammatory Cell Function

	A_1 receptor	A_{2A} receptor	A_{2B} receptor	A_3 receptor
Neutrophil	↑Adhesion ↑Migration ↑Phagocytosis	↓Adhesion ↓O_2 generation ↓Degranulation ↓Phagocytosis ↓Apoptosis ↓Phlogiston release		

Monocyte/macrophage	↑Phagocytosis
	↑Giant cell
	  formation
		↓O_2^- generation
		↓Phagocytosis
		↓Cytokine
		  release?
		↓Giant cell
		  formation
		↓C2 synthesis
		↓Procoagulant
		  secretion
		↑Plasminogen
		  activator
				↓Cytokine release
				↑IL-10
				↓NOS and NO

Eosinophil		↓O_2^- generation?		
Mast cell			↑IL-8 secretion	↑Histamine release
Endothelial cell		↓Cytokine release ↑Migration ↑Proliferation ↑Angiogenesis		

Table 2
Adenosine Receptors Modulate Phlogiston Release

	A_{2A} receptor	A_{2B} receptor	A_3 receptor
Neutrophils	↓TNF-α ↓LTB_4		
Monocyte/macrophages	↓TNF-α ↓C2 ↓Procoagulant ↑Plasminogen activator		↑IL-10 ↓TNF-α ↓IL-6
Mast cells		↑IL-8	
Endothelial cells	↓IL-6 ↓IL-8		

The Effects of Adenosine on Inflammatory Cells
(*see* Tables 1 and 2)

Polymorphonuclear Leukocytes (Neutrophil)

Neutrophils are the most abundant circulating leukocytes. These cells accumulate in large numbers at sites of acute injury, bacterial invasion, and inflammation. Indeed, the most striking characteristic of acute inflammation at the microscopic level is the presence of an infiltrate of neutrophils. Neutrophils are clearly essential elements in host defense; individuals who either lack neutrophils or whose neutrophils express a variety of genetically determined functional abnormalities suffer from severe or life-threatening recurrent infections. Nonetheless, neutrophils, by virtue of their capacity to generate oxygen radicals and release a variety of proteolytic enzymes, are capable of wreaking havoc at inflamed or infected sites by injuring surrounding uninvolved tissues. Thus, it is not surprising that a variety of endogenous mechanisms have evolved for limiting neutrophil accumulation at inflamed sites and for decreasing their secretion of potentially injurious oxidants. Adenosine, acting through adenosine receptors, is quite prominent among those molecules present at acutely inflamed sites that might be involved in limiting neutrophil-mediated injury.

During the 1970s, it was increasingly appreciated that receptors for adenosine were important physiologic and pharmacologic mediators in a variety of different systems. Thus, Marone et al. *(15)* were disappointed to find that adenosine did not affect stimulated neutrophil degranulation. However, in 1983 Cronstein et al. *(16)* first demonstrated that adenosine specifically inhibits superoxide anion generation stimulated by the chemoattractant *N*-formyl-methionyl-leucyl-phenylalanine (*f*MLP), the complement component C5a, and the calcium ionophore A23187. This work further demonstrated that adenosine mediated inhibition of neutrophil function by interaction with a surface site, although the first pharmacologic characterization of adenosine receptor–mediated inhibition of stimulated neutrophil function was not reported until 1985 *(17,18)*. A large number of studies have subsequently confirmed the effects of adenosine and its receptor-specific agonists on stimulated superoxide anion generation *(19–29)*. It is clear based on a reanalysis of the relative efficacy of appropriate adenosine receptor agonists for inhibition of stimulated oxidant generation, that the adenosine receptor involved in this function is an A_{2A} receptor *(30–32)*.

In contrast to the consistent reporting of adenosine-mediated inhibition of oxidant secretion by stimulated neutrophils, the effect of adenosine, acting at its receptors, on stimulated degranulation has been more controversial. As noted, Marone et al. *(15)* were unable to demonstrate any effect of adenosine on azurophil granule release, an observation confirmed by Cronstein et al. *(16)* in their original description of the effect of adenosine on neutrophil oxidant secretion. A number of groups have reported results that generally agree with these observations *(16,27,33–35)*, although others have observed that adenosine inhibits stimulated degranulation *(36–38)*. Similar to its effects on stimulated degranulation, the effects of adenosine on neutrophil aggregation remain controversial; some laboratories report an effect whereas others do not *(16,27,33–38)*. There is, as yet, no good explanation for these experimental discrepancies.

Adenosine also modulates neutrophil chemotaxis, phagocytosis, and adhesion to vascular endothelial cells; however, the effects of adenosine on these functions are more complex and appear to be mediated by multiple receptors. In 1988 Rose et al. *(39)* reported that adenosine receptor agonists promote neutrophil migration in response to C5a and the chemoattractant *f*MLP, although the concentrations of the adenosine receptor agonists used were far lower than those required to inhibit superoxide anion generation. In a subsequent work, this same group reported that adenosine enhanced neutrophil chemotaxis via occupancy of adenosine A_1 receptors *(30)*. Similarly, adenosine acting at A_1 receptors, promotes phagocytosis of immunoglobulin-coated particles *(40)* and adhesion of neutrophils to endothelial cells and some surfaces *(41)*, but inhibits these same functions via interaction with A_2 receptors *(40–42)*. It is interesting to note that adenosine has been reported to inhibit both β2-integrin–mediated *(41)* and L-selectin–mediated adhesion to vascular endothelium *(43)*. Subsequent work has demonstrated that adenosine inhibits the stimulated upregulation of β2 integrins and shedding of L-selectin by stimulated neutrophils *(44,45)*. Although the former effect may be related to the adenosine-mediated inhibition of β2 integrin–dependent adhesion, the inhibition of L-selectin shedding does not correlate well with the documented effects of adenosine on L-selectin-mediated adhesion.

Stimulated neutrophils generate a variety of inflammatory mediators including leukotriene B4 and tumor necrosis factor-α (TNF-α), and recent studies suggest that adenosine, via its receptors, inhibits the generation and release of these phlogistons. Krump et al. *(46)* have reported that adenosine acting at A_2 receptors (most likely A_{2A} receptors, judging from the effects of various receptor-specific agonists and antagonists) inhibits the synthesis and release of LTB_4 by stimulated neutrophils. Moreover, adenosine acting at an A_2 (most likely A_{2A}) receptor inhibits the stimulated production of TNF-α as well *(47)*.

Clearly, the importance of adenosine receptor–mediated inhibition of neutrophil function is the potential to reduce tissue injury at inflamed sites. In 1986, Cronstein et al. first reported that adenosine, whether added exogenously or generated endogenously, prevents neutrophil-mediated injury to endothelial cells. This finding has subsequently been confirmed and expanded on by a number of laboratories *(48–52)*. In addition, adenosine inhibits stimulated neutrophil adhesion to and neutrophil-mediated injury of cultured cardiac myocytes *(53)*. These observations have led to the hypothesis that adenosine or agents that increase local adenosine concentrations might be useful for the prevention or treatment of ischemia-reperfusion injury. The hypothesis that adenosine might be an effective therapy for ischemia-reperfusion injury has been tested in a number of different in vivo models and, in general, has been validated (reviewed in ref. *52*).

One mechanism by which the inflammatory process is terminated and neutrophils are removed from the inflammatory site is for the neutrophils to undergo apoptosis. Apoptotic neutrophils are ingested by macrophages, thereby preventing the release of potentially injurious neutrophil granule enzymes into the site of resolving inflammation. Although the effect of adenosine on ingestion by macrophages of apoptotic neutrophils has not been studied, Walker et al. *(54)* have reported that adenosine acting at an A_2 receptor prevents neutrophils from undergoing apoptosis. The significance of this observation is not yet clear.

Signal Transduction at Neutrophil Adenosine Receptors

The intracellular signaling mechanisms responsible for transducing signals from the adenosine receptor have been extensively studied. Adenosine A_2 receptors were originally described on the basis of their capacity to stimulate cellular accumulation of cAMP *(9,10)*. Adenosine A_2 receptors on neutrophils also appear to be linked to adenylate cyclase *(33,55,56)*, but the role of cAMP as the intracellular message for inhibition of neutrophil function is less well established. Although the effect of exogenous cAMP analogs (e.g., dibutyryl cAMP) on stimulated neutrophil function parallels those of adenosine the kinetics of the adenosine-receptor–mediated increase in intracellular cAMP does not correlate with inhibition by adenosine of superoxide anion generation *(32,33,55,56)*. Moreover, downstream inhibitors of cAMP-mediated signaling (inhibitors of protein kinase A) reverse the effects of cell-soluble cAMP analogs, but not adenosine on stimulated neutrophil superoxide anion generation *(57,58)*.

Chemoattractant-stimulated neutrophils increase their turnover of phospholipids with generation of active lipid intermediates (diacylglycerol [DAG] and inositol 1,4,5-tris-phosphate). Walker et al. *(59)* have reported that adenosine does not interfere with stimulated generation of inositol 1,4,5-trisphosphate, and others have reported that adenosine does not inhibit the concomitant increase in DAG generation *(60)*. Because inositol 1,4,5-trisphosphate is thought to mediate the initial increase in intracellular free Ca^{2+} ($[Ca^{2+}]_i$), it is not surprising that no effect of adenosine on the stimulated early Ca^{2+} flux has been found *(33)*. By contrast, late fluxes in $[Ca^{2+}]_i$ are significantly altered by adenosine *(29,59)* as is the stimulated second wave in diacylglycerol generation *(60)*.

Recent studies by Revan et al. *(58)* suggest a novel mechanism of signal transduction at neutrophil adenosine receptors. Inhibitors of protein phosphatases completely reverse the effect of adenosine receptor occupancy on stimulated superoxide anion generation. Moreover, adenosine receptor occupancy stimulates a marked increase in plasma membrane-associated serine/threonine protein phosphatase activity. The increased protein phosphatase activity inhibits the association of chemoattractant receptors with the cytoskeleton, a phenomenon associated with receptor desensitization *(57,60–62)*. These observations suggest that adenosine, acting at A_2 receptors on neutrophils, desensitizes chemoattractant receptors by activating a phosphatase that dephosphorylates either the receptor itself or a signaling molecule for superoxide anion generation.

Neutrophils express at least two different adenosine receptors. which, when occupied, mediate opposing effects on stimulated neutrophil function: A_1 receptors enhance neutrophil function and appear to do so at very low concentrations of adenosine, whereas A_2 receptors inhibit neutrophil function at higher adenosine concentrations. The concentrations of adenosine that enhance neutrophil function are those that might exist in relatively acellular connective tissues, but the concentrations of adenosine that inhibit neutrophil function are those that obtain in areas that are more cellular and in which overly exuberant neutrophil activity would be detrimental.

Monocyte/Macrophages

Monocytes, like neutrophils, develop in the bone marrow and arrive at sites of inflammation or injury via the circulation. Once in the extracellular tissues, monocytes mature into macrophages and the functions taken on may vary with the tissue in which they mature. Unlike neutrophils, monocytes are long-lived cells that synthesize and release into their environment a variety of cytokines and other proteins. The cytokines released by monocyte/macrophages play a central role in the development of both acute and chronic inflammation (e.g., TNF-α and IL-1; *see* Chapter 2), and, therefore, agents that inhibit monocyte function may have a greater impact on inflammation than would be expected from any effect on their phagocytic or oxidant-releasing capacity.

The effects of adenosine and adenosine receptor agonists have been tested on human monocytes, murine macrophages, and human and murine macrophage cell lines with generally similar results. Human peripheral blood monocytes express message for all four different adenosine receptors (Li, M. and Cronstein, B. N., unpublished observation); yet A_1 receptor proteins are not detectable on monocytes fresh from the blood but only on monocytes cultured overnight *(63,64)*. Like neutrophils, monocytes phagocytose debris and immunoglobulin-coated particles; adenosine A_1 receptors, when occupied, promote phagocytosis via FcγRI and A_2 receptor occupancy inhibits phagocytosis of immunoglobulin-coated particles *(64)*. Adenosine, probably acting at A_2

receptors, inhibits stimulated generation of superoxide anion by stimulated macrophages *(65,66)*. Adenosine also inhibits the synthesis of NO synthase and NO by stimulated monocyte/macrophages *(67,68)*.

Monocytes undergo further differentiation and maturation in the tissues. Under some conditions, e.g., during infection with *Mycobacterium tuberculosis,* or in a rheumatoid nodule, macrophages will fuse into multinucleated giant cells. In a recent study Merrill et al. *(69)* reported that adenosine acting at A_1 receptors promotes multinucleated giant cell formation but that acting at A_2 receptors inhibits giant cell formation.

Adenosine modulates protein synthesis and secretion by stimulated monocyte/macrophages. Lappin and Whaley *(70)* first demonstrated that adenosine inhibits synthesis of the complement component C2. In a subsequent study, Hasday and Sitrin *(71)* and Colli and Tremoli *(72)* reported that adenosine acting at A_2 receptors inhibits synthesis and release of procoagulant but, acting at a poorly characterized (perhaps A_3) receptor, promotes the synthesis and secretion of plasminogen activator. Although Prabhakar et al. *(73)* reported that occupancy of adenosine A_2 receptors inhibits TNF-α secretion by stimulated monocyte/macrophages others have reported that A_3 receptors (or an unclassified receptor at the time) are responsible for inhibition of TNF-α synthesis *(74–79)*. The effects of adenosine A_3 receptor occupancy on TNF-α synthesis and secretion occur at the level of transcription, although effects on transcription have been reported to be mediated by an effect on either NFκB *(67,79)* or AP-1 *(74)* transcriptional regulators. Bouma et al. *(77)* also reported that adenosine A_2 receptor occupancy increased monocyte production of the inflammatory cytokines IL-6 and IL-8, an observation not confirmed by others *(76)*. IL-10 possesses a variety of anti-inflammatory properties, and its production also appears to be enhanced by adenosine receptor agonists although the receptor involved has not been well characterized *(67,80)*. Thus, adenosine acting at A_2 or A_3 receptors promotes the production of a central anti-inflammatory cytokine (IL-10) and inhibits the synthesis of the central inflammatory cytokine TNF-α. Via its effects on cytokine production, the local, receptor-mediated effects of adenosine are amplified and may lead to systemic inhibition of inflammation.

Eosinophils

Eosinophils are commonly present in the lungs of patients with asthma and at sites of parasite invasion. The role that these cells play in other inflammatory/host response settings has not been well characterized, and the difficulty in obtaining sufficient quantities of these cells for study impedes progress in this area. In the two adequately performed studies of the effects of adenosine on eosinophil function, adenosine increased stimulated fluxes in intracellular $[Ca^{2+}]_i$ and promoted chemoattractant-stimulated oxidant release *(81,82)*. These proinflammatory effects are at odds with the well-documented anti-inflammatory effects of adenosine.

Mast Cells

Mast cells play a critical role in the development of bronchoconstriction in the setting of allergic asthma. Adenosine is a potent bronchoconstrictor when inhaled, and it is believed that the effects of adenosine on bronchial smooth muscle are mediated indirectly via activation of mast cell granule release. Histamine is a potent bronchoconstrictor and vasoactive substance that is present in mast cell granules and is released after mast cell stimulation. It is quite clear, since the first report of the effect of adenosine on mast cell function *(83)*, that adenosine promotes mast cell granule release via interaction with a cell surface receptor (reviewed in ref. *84*). Although the pharmacology of the adenosine receptor involved in promotion of mast cell granule release remained unclear for a number of years, recent studies have suggested that A_3 adenosine receptors are responsible for the effects of adenosine on mast cell granule release *(85–89)*. Interestingly, Feoktistov and Biaggioni *(90)* have demonstrated that adenosine provokes IL-8 secretion by mast cells via interaction with an A_{2B} receptor. In the process of studying the effect of adenosine on IL-8 secretion, these workers also found that enprofylline, a methylxanthine not thought to antagonize adenosine receptors, was a specific adenosine A_{2B} receptor antagonist *(90)*.

Endothelial Cells

It is increasingly clear that endothelial cells play an active role in the pathogenesis of inflammation by recruiting leukocytes to injured, infected, and inflamed sites. Both by expression of adhesion molecules and by the synthesis of chemoattractants (platelet activating factor and IL-8), endothelial cells are capable of attracting leukocytes out of the circulation and stimulating them to migrate into the extravascular space (*see* Chapter 9). Moreover, angiogenesis plays a role both in resolution of inflammation (wound healing) and in the tissue destruction of chronic inflammatory states such as the synovial tissue in rheumatoid arthritis (RA).

Endothelial cells also express adenosine receptors, and the effects of adenosine on endothelial cell function are only now being explored. Adenosine induces endothelial cell migration and proliferation via interaction with specific adenosine receptors (most likely A_{2A} receptors) *(13,91–94)*. Although adenosine receptor occupancy stimulates accumulation of cAMP *(94)*, cAMP does not mediate the effects of adenosine receptor occupancy on endothelial cell proliferation *(14)*. Interestingly, adenosine A_2 receptor occupancy directly stimulates the activation of mitogen-activated protein kinase (MAPK) activity in endothelial cells *(14)*, in contrast to the effect of A_2 receptor occupancy on MAPK activity in neutrophils *(95)*. In addition to its effects on endothelial cell proliferation and migration adenosine also diminishes endothelial expression of E-selectin and intercellular adhesion module-1 (although the decrement in expression of E-selectin is probably not biologically significant) and secretion of the inflammatory cytokines IL-6 and IL-8 *(96)*. Thus, adenosine acting at A_2 receptors on endothelial cells promotes angiogenesis and inhibits the recruitment of leukocytes to inflamed sites—functions associated with resolution of inflammation and wound healing.

The In Vivo Effects of Adenosine on Inflammation

From the preceding, it is clear that adenosine, acting at one or another receptor, is capable of inhibiting the function of inflammatory cells (with the exception of eosinophils and mast cells). However, in addition to its effects on inflammation and inflammatory cells, adenosine and its analogues have a wide variety of physiologic and pharmacologic effects (e.g., bradycardia, vasodilation and hypotension, antinociceptive) that may render them difficult to use for the treatment of inflammatory conditions in experimental models or in patients. As a result, a variety of different pharmacologic agents has been developed that raise local adenosine concentrations either by increasing cellular release of adenosine or its precursors or by inhibiting cellular uptake of adenosine. Moreover, endogenously released adenosine may be an important physiologic modulator of inflammation in some tissues.

Adenosine as an Endogenous Regulator of Inflammation

Rosengren et al. *(97)* reported that an adenosine receptor antagonist, 8-phenyl theophylline, potentiates the inflammation induced by LTB_4 in the hamster cheek pouch model of inflammation. This observation suggested that endogenously released adenosine actively inhibited the LTB_4-induced inflammation. Similarly, endogenous adenosine downregulates ischemia-reperfusion injury in some systems *(49,51,52)*. Exogenous and endogenously released adenosine does not have the same effect in all experimental models; recent reports suggest that in the guinea pig heart, adenosine acting at A_1 receptors promotes neutrophil adhesion and neutrophil-mediated myocardial injury by stimulating endothelial expression of adhesive molecules *(98–101)*.

Adenosine Receptor Agonists as Anti-Inflammatory Agents

Adenosine and adenosine receptor agonists have been administered in animal models of inflammation, and, surprisingly, adenosine A_r receptor agonists appear to be potent inhibitors of inflammation *(102,103)*. One potential explanation for this observation was recently provided by Bong et al. *(104)*, who observed that there is a potent central nervous system (CNS) effect of adenosine, acting at A_1 receptors on spinal cord neurons, on inflammation in the periphery. Adenosine receptor agonists, administered into the spinal cord, markedly reduced cutaneous inflammation, in part, by increasing local adenosine release *(104)*. Although this observation is interesting and provocative, it is unlikely to lead to the development of new anti-inflammatory agents because many of the known CNS effects of adenosine, e.g., hypotension, drowsiness and coma, are undesirable side effects of drugs used to treat inflammatory diseases. Adenosine itself has been infused into the inflamed joints of animals with adjuvant arthritis resulting in marked inhibition of the joint inflammation *(105)*. It is remarkable that adenosine itself could affect inflammation in this model because the half-life of adenosine in biological fluids (e.g., plasma) is measured in seconds *(106)*.

Agents That Increase Adenosine Concentrations at Inflamed Sites (see Fig. 1)

There are several approaches to the pharmacologic elevation of extracellular adenosine at inflamed sites: (1) inhibition of adenosine uptake; (2) inhibition of adenosine utilization; and (3) modulation of adenine nucleotide metabolism. Two of these pharmacologic strategies are currently under study for the development of anti-inflammatory agents, and the last approach probably underlies the efficacy of drugs currently used to treat inflammatory disorders.

Adenosine uptake blockers can increase extracellular adenosine concentrations, and a number of studies have suggested that use of adenosine uptake blockers may prevent inflammatory injury during reperfusion or in other settings by virtue of their capacity to increase adenosine concentration at the inflamed site *(4)*. None of the adenosine uptake inhibitors are currently used to treat or diminish inflammatory injury, and testing of these agents in animal models is complicated by the insensitivity of rodent purine transporters to most adenosine uptake inhibitors.

Another approach to increasing extracellular adenosine concentrations is to inhibit adenosine utilization via inhibition of adenosine kinase. In most cell types, the adenosine generated within the cell as a result of purine nucleotide catabolism or taken up from the outside is recycled to adenine nucleotides by the enzyme adenosine kinase. Several studies have demonstrated that a specific adenosine kinase inhibitor can diminish inflammation or protect against endotoxin shock both in vitro and in vivo *(43,107–109)*. The effects of adenosine kinase inhibitors on inflammation are clearly mediated by adenosine since elimination of adenosine from the inflamed site or administration of adenosine receptor antagonists markedly or completely reverses the anti-inflammatory effects of the adenosine kinase inhibitor tested *(43,107–109)*. Interestingly, in at least one of these reports, the anti-inflammatory effects of adenosine were mediated by A_2 receptors because an A_2-specific, but not an A_1-specific, adenosine receptor antagonist reversed the anti-inflammatory effects of the adenosine kinase inhibitor *(108)*. Despite the demonstration that adenosine inhibits TNF-α secretion primarily via occupancy of A_3 receptors, the A_2-receptor–mediated inhibition of inflammation was associated with a marked reduction in TNF-α concentration in the inflammatory exudate *(108)*.

Drugs that enhance extracellular adenosine concentrations are currently in use to treat inflammatory arthritis (RA and seronegative arthritis) and inflammatory bowel disease (IBD). Both methotrexate and sulfasalazine, the two most commonly used and most effective secondline anti-inflammatory drugs for the treatment of RA and seronegative arthritis, promote adenosine release in vitro and in vivo *(110–112)*. It has been proposed that both methotrexate, which is taken up and polyglutamated by cells, and sulfasalazine inhibit the conversion of 5-aminoimidazole-4-carboxamide ribonucleotide (AICAR) to formyl-AICAR (FAICAR). The resulting intracellular AICAR accumulation leads to enhanced methotrexate release, most likely by the inhibition of AMP deaminase and release of AMP, which is converted extracellularly to adenosine *(110–113)*. The adenosine that is released by these two drugs mediates their anti-inflammatory effects in vitro and in vivo via an A_2 receptor since the anti-inflammatory effects of both methotrexate and sulfasalazine are completely reversed by an adenosine A_2 receptor–specific antagonist *(110–112)*. More recent studies also indicate that adenosine mediates the anti-inflammatory effects of adenosine in the adjuvant arthritis model because a nonspecific adenosine receptor antagonist, theophylline, markedly reverses the antirheumatic effects of methotrexate treatment *(114)*.

Conclusion

Adenosine is a potent, endogenously released autocoid with a tremendous range of physiologic and pharmacologic effects; not the least of adenosine's effects is to diminish inflammation. The recent demonstration that adenosine mediates, at least in part, the anti-inflammatory effects of two commonly used and effective anti-inflammatory drugs suggests that the development of agents that utilize adenosine receptor–mediated inhibition of inflammation may be a fruitful approach to the development of new drugs for the treatment of such illnesses as RA and IBD.

Acknowledgments

This work was supported by grants from the National Institutes of Health (AR/AI 41911 and HL1972) and Pharmacia-Upjohn. This work was also supported by the General Clinical Research Center (MOlRR00096) and the Kaplan Cancer Center (CA160877).

References

1. Pearson, J. D. and Gordon, J. L. (1979) Vascular endothelial and smooth muscle cells in culture selectively released adenine nucleotides. *Nature* **281,** 384–386.
2. Kitakaze, M., Hori, M., Morioka, T., Takashima, S:., Minamino, T., Sato, H., Inoue, M., and Kamada, T. (1993) Attenuation of ecto-5'-nucleotidase activity and adenosine release in activated human polymorphonuclear leuLocytes. *Circ. Res.* **73,** 524–533.
3. Node, K., Kitakaze, M., Minamino, T., Tasa, M., Inoue, M., Nori, M., and Kamsda, T. (1997) Activation of ecto-5'-nucleotidase by protein kinase and its role in ischaemic tolerance in the canine head. *Br. J. Pharmacol.* **120,** 273–281.
4. Van Belle, H. (1993) Nucleoside transport inhibition: a therapeutic approach to cardioprotection via adenosine? *Cardiovasc. Res.* **27,** 68–76.
5. Resta, R., Hooker, S. W., Laurent, A. B., Jamshedur, S. M., Rahman, Franklin, M., Knudsen, T. B., Nadon, N. L., and Thompson, L. F. (1997) Insights into thymic purine metabolism and adenosine deaminase deficiency revealed by transgenic mice overexpressing ecto-5'-nucleotidase (CD73) *J. Clin. Invest.* **99(4),** 676–683.
6. van Waeg, G. and Van den Berghe, G. (1991) Purine catabolism in polymorphonuclear neutrophils: Phorbol myristate acetate-induced accumulation of adenosine owing to inactivation of extracellularly released adenosine deaminase. *J. Clin. Invest.* **87,** 305–312.
7. Drury, A. N. and Szent-Gyorgi, A. (1929) *J. Physiol.* **68,** 213–237.
8. Sattin, A. and Rall, T. W. (1970) The effect of adenosine and adenine nucleotides on the cyclic adenosine-3',5'-phosphate content of guinea pig cerebral cortex slices. *Mol. Pharmacol.* **6,** 13–23.
9. van Calker, D., Muller, M., and Hamprecht, B. (1979) Adenosine regulates, via two different types of receptors, the accumulation of cyclic AMP in cultured brain cells. *J. Neurochem.* **33,** 999–1005.
10. Londos, C., Cooper, D. M. F., and Wolff, J. (1980) Subclasses of external adenosine receptors. *Proc. Natl. Acad. Sci. USA* **77,** 2551–2554.
11. Tucker, A. L. and Linden, J. (1993) Cloned receptors and cardiovascular responses to adenosine. *Cardiovasc. Res.* **27,** 62–67.
12. Revan, S., Montesinos, M. C., Naime, D., Landau, S., and Cronstein, B. N. (1996) Adenosine A2 receptor occupancy regulates stimulated neutrophil function via activation of a serine/threonine protein phosphatase. *J. Biol. Chem.* **271,** 17,114–17,118.
13. Sexl, V., Mancusi, G., Baumgartner-Parzer, S., Schutz, W., and Freissmuth, M. (1995) Stimulation of human umbilical vein endothelial cell proliferation by A2-adenosine and beta 2-adrenoceptors. *Br. J. Pharmacol.* **114,** 1577–1586.
14. Sexl, V., Mancusi, G., Holler, C., Gloria-Maercker, E., Schutz, W., and Freissmuth, M. (1997) Stimulation of the mitogen-activated protein kinase via the A_{2A}-adenosine receptor in primary human endothelial cells. *J. Biol. Chem.* **272,** 5792–5799.
15. Marone, G., Thomas, L., and Lichtenstein, L. (1980) The role of agonists that activate adenylate cyclase in the control of cAMP metabolism and enzyme release by human polymorphonuclear leukocytes. *J. Immunol.* **125,** 2277–2283.
16. Cronstein, B. N., Kramer, S. B., Weissmann, G., and Hirschhorn, R. (1983) Adenosine: a physiological modulator of superoxide anion generation by human neutrophils. *J. Exp. Med.* **58,** 1160–1177.
17. Cronstein, B. N., Rosenstein, E. D., Kramer, S. B., Weissmann, G., and Hirschhorn, R. (1985) Adenosine: a physiologic modulator of superoxide anion generation by human neutrophils. Adenosine acts via an A2 receptor on human neutrophils. *J. Immunol.* **135,** 1366–1371.
18. Roberts, P. A., Newby, A. C., Hallett, M. B., and Campbell, A. K. (1985) Inhibition by adenosine of reactive oxygen metabolite production by human polymorphonuclear leucocytes. *Biochem. J.* **227,** 669–674.
19. Burkey, T. H. and Webster, R. O. (1993) Adenosine inhibits fMLP-stimulated adherence and superoxide anion generation by human neutrophils at an early step in signal transduction. *Biochim. Biophys. Acta* **1175(3),** 312–318.

20. Axtell, R. A., Sandborg, R. R., Smolen, J. E., Ward, P. A., and Boxer, L. A. (1990) Exposure of human neutrophils to exogenous nucleotides causes elevation in intracellular calcium, transmembrane calcium fluxes, and an alteration of a cytosolic factor resulting in enhanced superoxide production in response to FMLP and arachidonic acid. *Blood* **75,** 1324–1332.

21. Basford, R. E., Clark, R. L., Stiller, R. A., Kaplan, S. S., Kuhns, D. B., and Rinaldo, J. E. (1990) Endothelial cells inhibit receptor-mediated superoxide anion production by human polymorphonuclear leukocytes via a soluble inhibitor. *Am. J. Respir. Cell Mol. Biol.* **2,** 235–243.

22. de la Harpe, J. and Nathan, C. F. (1989) Adenosine regulates the respiratory burst of cytokine-triggered human neutrophils adherent to biologic surfaces. *J. Immunol.* **143,** 596–602.

23. Currie, M. S., Rao, K. M., Padmanabhan, J., Jones, A., Crawford, J., and Cohen, H. J. (1990) Stimulus-specific effects of pentoxifylline on neutrophil CR3 expression, degranulation, and superoxide production. *J. Leukoc. Biol.* **47,** 244–250.

24. Gunther, G. R. and Herring, M. B. (1991) Inhibition of neutrophil superoxide production by adenosine released from vascular endothelial cells. *Ann. Vascular Surg.* **5,** 325–330.

25. Nielson, C. P. and Vestal, R. E. (1989) Effects of adenosine on polymorphonuclear leucocyte function, cyclic 3':5'-adenosine monophosphate, and inkacellular calcium. *Br. J. Pharmacol.* **97,** 882–888.

26. Kaneko, M., Suzuki, K., Furui, H., Takagi, K., and Satake, T. (1990) Comparison of theophylline and enprotylline effects on human neutrophil superoxide production. *Clin. Exper. Pharmacol. Physiol.* **17,** 849–859.

27. McGarrity, S. T., Stephenson, A. H., and Webster, R. O. (1989) Regulation of human neutrophil functions by adenine nucleotides. *J. Immunol.* **142,** 1986–1994.

28. Sipka, S., Szentmiklosi, A. J., Nagy, A., Taskov, V., and Szegedi, G. (1989) Inhibition of the zymosan-induced chemiluminescence of human phagocytes by adenosine, polyadenylic acid and agents influencing adenosine metabolism. *Allergol. Immunopathol.* **17,** 209–212.

29. Thiel, M. and Bardenheuer, H. (1992) Regulation of oxygen radical production of human polymorphonuclear leukocytes by adenosine: The role of calcium. *Pflugers Arch.—Eur. J. Physiol.* **420,** 522–528.

30. Cronstein, B. N., Duguma, L., Nicholls, D., Hutchison, A., and Williams, M. (1990) The adenosine/neutrophil paradox resolved: Human neutrophils possess both A1 and A2 receptors which promote chemotaxis and inhibit O_2^- generation, respectively. *J. Clin. Invest.* **85,** 1150–1157.

31. van Calker, D., Steber, R., Klotz, K. N., and Greil, W. (1991) Carbamazepine distinguishes between adenosine receptors that mediate different second messenger responses. *Eur. J. Pharmacol.* **206,** 285–290.

32. Fredholm, B. B., Zhang, Y., and van der Ploeg, I. (1996) Adenosine A2A receptors mediate the inhibitory effect of adenosine on formyl-Met-Leu-Phe-stimulated respiratory burst in neutrophil leucocytes. *Naunyn-Schmiedebergs Arch. Pharmacol.* **354(3),** 262–267.

33. Cronstein, B. N., Kramer, S. B., Rosenstein, E. D., Korchak, H. M., Weissmann, G., and Hirschhorn, R. (1988) Occupancy of adenosine receptors raises cyclic AMP alone and in synergy with occupancy of chemoattractant receptors and inhibits membrane depolarization. *Biochem. J.* **252,** 709–715.

34. Grinstein, S. and Furuya, W. (1986) Cytoplasmic pH regulation in activated human neutrophils: Effects of adenosine and pertussis toxin on Na+/H+ exchange and metabolic acidification. *Biochim. Biophys. Acta.* **889,** 301–309.

35. Walker, B. A. M., Cunningham, T. W., Freyer, D. R., Todd, R. F. III, Johnson, K. J., and Ward, P. A. (1989) Regulation of superoxide responses of human neutrophils by adenine compounds: independence of requirement for cytoplasmic granules. *Lab. Invest.* **61,** 515–521.

36. Bouma, M. G., Jeunhomme, T. M. M. A., Boyle, D. L., Dentener, M. A., Voitenok, N. N., van den Wildenberg, F. A. J. M., and Buurman, W. A. (1997) Adenosine inhibits neutrophil degranulation in activated human whole blood: Involvement of adenosine A2 and A3 receptors. *J. Immunol.* **158,** 5400–5408.

37. Richter, J. (1992) Effect of adenosine analogues and cAMP-raising agents on TNF, GM-CSF-, and chemotactic peptide-induced degranulation in single adherent neutrophils. *J. Leukoc. Biol.* **51,** 270–275.

38. Schmeichel, C. J. and Thomas, L. L. (1987) Methylxanthine bronchodilators potentiate multiple human neutrophil functions. *J. Immunol.* **138,** 1896–1903.

39. Rose, F. R., Hirschhorn, R., Weissmann, G., and Cronstein, B. N. (1988) Adenosine promotes neutrophil chemotaxis. *J. Exp. Med.* **167,** 1186–1194.
40. Salmon, J. E. and Cronstein, B. N. (1990) Fcgamma receptor-mediated functions in neutrophils are modulated by adenosine receptor occupancy: A1 receptors are stimulatory and A2 receptors are inhibitory. *J. Immunol.* **145,** 2235–2240.
41. Cronstein, B. N., Levin, R. I., Philips, M. R., Hirschhorn, R., Abramson, S. B., and Weissmann, G. (1992) Neutrophil adherence to endothelium is enhanced via adenosine A1 receptors and inhibited via adenosine A2 receptors. *J. Immunol.* **148,** 2201–2206.
42. Zalavary, S., Stendahl, O., and Bengtsson, T. (1994) The role of cyclic AMP, calcium and filamentous actin in adenosine modulation of Fc receptor-mediated phagocytosis in human neutrophils. *Biochim. Biophys. Acta* **1222,** 249–256.
43. Firestein, G. S., Bullough, D. A., Erion, M. D., Jimenez, R., Ramirez-Weinhouse, M., Barankiewicz, J., Smith, C. W., Gruber, H. E., and Mullane, K. M. (1995) Inhibition of neutrophil adhesion by adenosine and an adenosine kinase inhibitor: the role of selectins. *J. Immunol.* **154,** 326–334.
44. Wollner, A., Wollner, S., and Smith, J. B. (1993) Acting via A2 receptors, adenosine inhibits the upregulation of Mac-1 (CD11b/CD18) expression on FMLP-stimulated neutrophils. *Am. J. Resp. Cell Mol. Biol.* **9,** 179–185.
45. Thiel, M., Chambers, J. D., Chouker, A., Fischer, S., Zourelidis, C., Bardenheuer, H. J., Arfors, K. E., and Peter, K. (1996) Effect of adenosine on the expression of beta(2) integrins and L-selectin of human polymorphonuclear leukocytes in vitro. *J. Leukoc. Biol.* **59(5),** 671–682.
46. Krump, E., Lemay, G., and Borgeat, P. (1996) Adenosine A2 receptor-induced inhibition of leukotriene B4 synthesis in whole blood ex vivo. *Brit. J. Pharm.* **117,** 1639–1644.
47. Thiel, M. and Chouker, A. (1995) Acting via A2 receptors, adenosine inhibits the production of tumor necrosis factor-alpha of endotoxin-stimulated human polymorphonuclear leukocytes. *J. Lab. Clin. Med.* **126(3),** 275–282.
48. Boisseau, M. R., Pruvost, A., Renard, M., Closse, C., Belloc, F., Seigneur, M., and Maurel, A. (1996) Effect of buflomedil on the neutrophil-endothelial cell interaction under inflarnmatory and hypoxia conditions. *Haemostasis* **26(Suppl. 4),** 182–188.
49. Zhao, Z. Q., Sato, H., Williams, M. W., Fernandez, A. Z., and Vinten-Johansen, J. (1996) Adenosine A2-receptor activation inhibits neukophil-mediated injury to coronary endothelium. *Am. J. Physiol.* **271(4 Pt. 2),** H1456–H1464.
50. Minamino, T., Kitakaze, M., Node, K., Funaya, H., Inoue, M., Hori, M., and Kamada, T. (1996) Adenosine inhibits leukocyte-induced vasoconstriction. *Am. J. Physiol.* **271(6 Pt. 2),** H2622–H2628.
51. Jordan, J. E., Zhao, Z. Q., Sato, H., Taft, S., and Vinten-Johansen, J. (1997) Adenosine A2 receptor activation attenuates reperfusion injury by inhibiting neutrophil accumulation, superoxide generation and coronary endothelial adherence. *J. Pharmacol. Exp. Ther.* **280(1),** 301–309.
52. Vinten-Johansen, J., Zhao, Z. Q., and Sato, H. (1995) Reduction in surgical ischemic-reperfusion injury with adenosine and nitric oxide therapy. *Ann. Thorac. Surg.* **60(3),** 852–857.
53. Bullough, D. A., Magill, M. J., Firestein, G. S., and Mullane, K. M. (1995) Adenosine activates A2 receptors to inhibit neutrophil adhesion and injury to isolated cardiac myocytes. *J. Immunol.* **155(5),** 2579–2586.
54. Walker, B. A., Rocchini, C., Boone, R. H., Ip, S., and Jacobson, M. A. (1997) Adenosine A$_{2\alpha}$ receptor activation delays apoptosis in human neutrophils. *J. Immunol.* **158(6),** 2926–2931.
55. Iannone, M. A., Reynolds-Vaughn, R., Wolberg, G., and Zimmerman, T. P. (1985) Human neutrophils possess adenosine A2 receptors. *Fed. Proc.* **44,** 580.
56. Iannone, M. A., Wolberg, G., and Zimmerman, T. P. (1989) Chemotactic peptide induces cAMP elevation in human neutrophils by amplification of the adenylate cyclase response to endogenously produced adenosine. *J. Biol. Chem.* **264,** 20,177–20,180.
57. Cronstein, B. N., Haines, K. A., Kolasinski, S. L., and Reibman, J. (1992) Occupancy of G-alpha s-linked receptors uncouples chemoattractant receptors from their stimulus-transduction mechanisms in the neutrophil. *Blood* **80,** 1052–1057.
58. Revan, S., Montesinos, M. C., Naime, D., Landau, S., and Cronstem, B. N. (1996) Adenosine A2 receptor occupancy regulates stimulated neutrophil function via activation of a serine/threonine protein phosphatase. *J. Biol. Chem.* **271(29),** 17,114–17,118.

59. Walker, B. A. M., Hagenlocker, B. E., Douglas, V. K., and Ward, P. A. (1990) Effects of adenosine on inositol 1,4,5-trisphosphate formation and intracellular calcium changes in formyl-met-leu-phe-stimulated human neutrophils. *J. Leuk. Biol.* **48**, 281–283.

60. Cronstein, B. N. and Haines, K. A. (1992) Adenosine A2 receptor occupancy does not affect "triggering" but inhibits "activation" of human neutrophils by a mechanism independent of actin filament formation. *Biochem. J.* **281**, 631–635.

61. Cronstein, B. N., Haines, K. A., Kolasinski, S. L., and Reibman, J. (1991) Gs linked receptors (Beta-adrenergic and adenosine A2) uncouple chemoattractant receptors from G proteins. *Clin. Res.* **39**, 343A.

62. Burkey, T. H. and Webster, R. O. (1993) Adenosine inhibits fMLP-stimulated adherence and superoxide anion generation by human neutrophils at an early step in signal transduction. *Biochim. Biophys. Acta* **1175**, 312–318.

63. Eppell, B. A., Newell, A. M., and Brown, E. J. (1989) Adenosine receptors are expressed during differentiation of monocytes to macrophages in vitro. *J. Immunol.* **143**, 4141–4145.

64. Salmon, J. E., Brownlie, C., Brogle, N., Edberg, J. C., Chen, B.-X., and Erlanger, B. F. (1993) Human mononuclear phagocytes express adenosine A1 receptors: a novel mechanism for differential regulation of Fc-gamma receptor function. *J. Immunol.* **151**, 2775–2865.

65. Elliott, K. R. F., Stevenson, H. C., Miller, P. J., and Leonard, E. J. (1986) Synergistic action of adenosine and Fmet-leu-phe in raising cyclic AMP content of purified human monocytes. *Biochem. Biophys. Res. Commun.* **138**, 1376–1382.

66. Leonard, E. J., Shenai, A., and Skeel, A. (1987) Dynamics of chemotactic peptide induced superoxide generation by human monocytes. *Inflammation* **11**, 229–240.

67. Hasko, G., Szabo, C., Nemeth, Z. H., Kvetan, V., Pastores, S. M., and Vizi, E. S. (1996) Adenosine receptor agonists differentially regulate IL-10, TNF-α, and nitric oxide production in RAW 264.7 macrophages and in endotoxemic mice. *J. Immunol.* **157**, 4634–4640.

68. Hon, W. M., Moochhala, S., and Khoo, H. E. (1997) Adenosine and its receptor agonists potentiate nitric oxide synthase expression induced by lipopolysaccharide in RAW 264.7 murine macrophages. *Life Sci.* **60(16)**, 1327–1335.

69. Merrill, J. T., Shen, C., Schreibman, D., Coffey, D., Zakharenko, O., Fisher, R., Lahita, R. G., Salmon, J., and Cronstein, B. N. (1997) Adenosine A$_1$ receptor promotion of multinucleated giant cell formation by human monocytes: a mechanism for methotrexate-induced nodulosis in rheumatoid arthritis. *Arth. Rheum.* **40**, 1308–1315.

70. Lappin, D. and Whaley, K. (1984) Adenosine A2 receptors on human monocytes modulate C2 production. *Clin. Exp. Immunol.* **57**, 454–460.

71. Hasday, J. D. and Sitrin, R. G. (1987) Adenosine receptors on rabbit alveolar macrophages: binding characteristics and effects on cellular function. *J. Lab. Clin. Med.* **110**, 264–273.

72. Colli, S. and Tremoli, E. (1991) Multiple effects of dipyridamole on neutrophils and mononuclear leukocytes: adenosine-dependent and adenosine-independent mechanisms. *J. Lab. Clin. Med.* **118**, 136–145.

73. Prabhakar, U., Brooks, D. P., Lipshlitz, D., and Esser, K. M. (1995) Inhibition of LPS- induced TNF alpha production in human monocytes by adenosine (A2) receptor selective agonists. *Int. J. Immunopharmacol.* **17(3)**, 221–224.

74. Sajjadi, F. G., Takabayashi, K., Foster, A. C., Domingo, R. C., and Firestein, G. S. (1996) Inhibition of TNFα expression by adenosine: role of A3 adenosine receptors. *J. Immunol.* **156**, 3435–3442.

75. Parmely, M. J., Zhou, W.-W., Edwards, C. K. III, Borcherding, D. R., Silverstein, R., and Morrison, D. C. (1993) Adenosine and a related carbocyclic nucleoside analogue selectively inhibit tumor necrosis factor-alpha production and protect mice against endotoxin challenge. *J. Immunol.* **151**, 389–396.

76. Le Vraux, V., Chen, Y. L., Masson, I., De Sousa, M., Giroud, J. P., Florentin, I., and Chauvelot-Moachon, L. (1993) Inhibition of human monocyte TNF production by adenosine receptor agonists. *Life Sci.* **52(24)**, 1917–1924.

77. Bouma, M. G., Stad, R. K., van den Wildenberg, F. A. J. M., and Buurman, W. A. (1994) Differential regulatory effects of adenosine on cytokine release by activated human monocytes. *J. Immunol.* **153**, 4159–4168.

78. Bowlin, T. L., McWhinney, C. D., Borcherding, D. R., Edwards, C. K., Hoffman, P. F., Watts, L., and Wolos, J. A. (1995) Inhibition of NFkB nuclear translocation and TNFα gene expression by a novel adenosine A3 receptor agonist. *Arth. Rheum.* **38**, S401.

79. McWhinney, C. D., Dudley, M. W., Bowlin, T. L., Peet, N. R., Schook, L., Bradshaw, M., De, M., Borcherding, D. R., and Edwards, C. K., III (1996) Activation of adenosine A3 receptors on macrophages inhibits tumor necrosis-α. *Eur. J. Pharm.* **310,** 209–216.

80. Le Moine, O., Stordeur, P., Schandene, L., Marchant, A., de Groote, D., Goldman, M., and Deviere, J. (1996) Adenosine enhances IL-10 secretion by human monocytes. *J. Immunol.* **156,** 4408–4414.

81. Walker, B. A. (1996) Effects of adenosine on guinea pig pulmonary eosinophils. *Inflammation* **20(1),** 11–21.

82. Kohno, Y., Ji, X., Mawhorter, S. D., Koshiba, M., and Jacobson, K. A. (1996) Activation of A3 adenosine receptors on human eosinophils elevates intracellular calcium. *Blood* **88(9),** 3569–3574.

83. Marquardt, D. L., Parker, C. W., and Sullivan, T. J. (1978) Potentiation of mast cell mediator release by adenosine. *J. Immunol.* **120,** 871–878.

84. Holgate, S. T., Church, M. K., and Polosa, R. (1991) Adenosine: a positive modulator of airway inflammation in asthma. *Ann. NY Acad. Sci.* **629,** 227–236.

85. Hannon, J. P., Pfannkuche, H. J., and Fozard, J. R. (1995) A role for mast cells in adenosine A3 receptor-mediated hypotension in the rat. *Br. J. Pharmacol.* **115(6),** 945–952.

86. Ali, H., Choi, O. H., Fraundorfer, P. F., Yamada, K., Gonzaga, H. M., and Beaven, M. A. (1996) Sustained activation of phospholipase D via adenosine A3 receptors is associated with enhancement of antigen- and Ca(2+)-ionophore-induced secretion in a rat mast cell line. *J. Pharmacol. Exp. Ther.* **276(2),** 837–845.

87. Fozard, J. R., Pfannkuche, H. J., and Schuurman, H. J. (1996) Mast cell degranulation following adenosine A3 receptor activation in rats. *Eur. J. Pharmacol.* **298(3),** 293–297.

88. Shepherd, R. K., Linden, J., and Duling, B. R. (1996) Adenosine-induced vasoconstriction in vivo: role of the mast eel] and A3 adenosine receptor. *Circulation Res.* **78(4),** 627–634.

89. Meade, C. J., Mierau, J., Leon, I., and Ensinger, H. A. (1996) In vivo role of the adeno sine A3 receptor: N6-2-(4-aminophenyl)ethyladeno sine induces broncho spasm in BDE rats by a neurally mediated mechanism involving cells resembling mast cells. *J. Pharmacol. Exper. Ther.* **279(3),** 1148–1156.

90. Feoktistov, I. and Biaggioni, I. (1995) Adenosine A2b receptors evoke interleukin8 secretion in human mast cells. An enprofylline-sensitive mechanism with implications for asthma. *J. Clin. Invest.* **96(4),** 1979–1986.

91. Ethier, M. F., Chander, V., and Dobson, J. G., Jr. (1993) Adenosine stimulates proliferation of human endothelial cells in culture. *Am. J. Physiol.* **265,** H131–H138.

92. Takagi, H., King, G. L., Robinson, G. S., Ferrara, N., and Aiello, L. P. (1996) Adenosine mediates hypoxic induction of vascular endothelial growth factor in retinal pericytes and endothelial cells. *Invest. Ophthalmol. Vis. Sci.* **37,** 2165–2176.

93. Takagi, H., King, G. L., Ferrara, N., and Aiello, L. P. (1996) Hypoxia regulates vascular endothelial growth factor receptor *KDR/Flk* gene expression through adenosine A2 receptors in retinal capillary endothelial cells. *Invest. Ophthalmol. Vis. Sci.* **37,** 1311–1321.

94. Schiele, J. O. and Schwabe, U. (1994) Characterization of the adenosine receptor in microvascular coronary endothelial cells. *Eur. J. Pharm.* **269,** 51–58.

95. Pillinger, M. H., Feoktistov, A. S., Capodici, C., Solitar, B., Levy, J., Oei, T. T., and Philips, M. R. (1996) Mitogen-activated protein kinase in neutrophils and enucleate neutrophil cytoplasts: evidence for regulation of cell-cell adhesion. *J. Biol. Chem.* **271(20),** 12049-56.

96. Bouma, M. G., van den Wildenberg, F. A. J. M., and Buurman, W. A. (1996) Adenosine inhibits cytokine release and expression of adhesion molecules by activated human endothelial cells. *Am. J. Physiol.* **39,** C522–C529.

97. Rosengren, S., Arfors, K. E., and Proctor, K. G. (1991) Potentiation of leukotriene B4- mediated inflammatory response by the adenosine antagonist, 8-phenyl theophylline. *Intl. J. Microcirc. Clin. Exp.* **10,** 345–357.

98. Becker, B. F., Zahler, S., Raschke, P., Schwartz, L. M., Beblo, S., Schrodl, W., and Kiesl, D. (1992) Adenosine enhances neutrophil sticking in the coronary system: A novel mechanism contributing to cardiac reperfusion damage. *Pharm. Pharmacol. Lett.* **2,** 8–11.

99. Schwartz, L. M., Raschke, P., Becker, B. F., and Gerlach, E. (1993) Adenosine contributes to neutrophil-mediated loss of myocardial function in post-ischemic guinea-pig hearts. *J. Mol. Cell. Cardiol.* **25,** 927–938.

100. Zahler, S., Becker, B. F., Raschke, P., and Gerlach, E. (1994) Stimulation of endothelial adenosine A1 receptors enhances adhesion of neutrophils in the intact guinea pig coronary system. *Cardiovasc. Res.* **28,** 1366–1372.

101. Raschke, P. and Becker, B. F. (1995) Adenosine and PAF dependent mechanisms lead to myocardial reperfusion injury by neutrophils after brief ischemia. *Cardiovasc. Res.* **29,** 569–576.

102. Schrier, D. J., Lesch, M. E., Wright, C. D., and Gilbertsen, R. B. (1990) The antiinflammatory effects of adenosine receptor agonists on the carrageenan-induced pleural inflammatory response in rats. *J. Immunol.* **145,** 1874–1879.

103. Lesch, M. E., Ferin, M. A., Wright, C. D., and Schrier, D. J. (1991) The effects of (R)-N-(1-methyl-2-phenylethyl) adenosine (L-PIA), a standard A1-selective adenosine agonist on rat acute models of inflammation and neutrophil function. *Agents Actions* **34,** 25–27.

104. Bong, G. W., Rosengren, S., and Firestein, G. S. (1996) Spinal cord adenosine receptor stimulation in rats inhibits peripheral neutrophil accumulation: the role of N-methyl-D-aspartate receptors. *J. Clin. Invest.* **98,** 2779–2785.

105. Green, P. G., Basbaum, A. I., Helms, C., and Levine, J. D. (1991) Purinergic regulation of bradykinin-induced plasma extravasation and adjuvant-induced arthritis in the rat. *Proc. Natl. Acad. Sci. USA* **88,** 4162–4165.

106. Moser, G. H., Schrader, J., and Deussen, A. (1989) Turnover of adenosine in plasma of human and dog blood. *Am. J. Physiol.* **256,** C799–C806.

107. Rosengren, S., Bong, G. W., and Firestein, G. S. (1995) Anti-inflammatory effects of an adenosine kinase inhibitor: decreased neutrophil accumulation and vascular leakage. *J. Immunol.* **154,** 5444–5451.

108. Cronstein, B. N., Naime, D., and Firestein, G. S. (1995) The antiinflammatory effects of an adenosine kinase inhibitor are mediated by adenosine. *Arth. Rheum.* **38,** 1040–1045.

109. Firestein, G. S., Boyle, D., Bullough, D. A., Gruber, H. E., Sajjadi, F. G., Montag, A., Sambol, B., and Mullane, K. M. (1994) Protective effect of an adenosine kinase inhibitor in septic shock. *J. Immunol.* **152(12),** 5853–5859.

110. Cronstein, B. N., Eberle, M. A., Gruber, H. E., and Levin, R. I. (1991) Methotrexate inhibits neutrophil- function by stimulating adenosine release from connective tissue cells. *Proc. Natl. Acad. Sci. USA* **88,** 2441–2445.

111. Cronstein, B. N., Naime, D., and Ostad, E. (1993) The antiinflammatory mechanism of methotrexate: Increased adenosine release at inflamed sites diminishes leukocyte accumulation in an in vivo model of inflammation. *J. Clin. Invest.* **92,** 2675–2682.

112. Gadangi, P., Longaker, M., Naime, D., Levin, R. I., Recht, P. A., Montesinos, M. C., Buckley, M. T., Carlin, G., and Cronstein, B. N. (1996) The antiinflammatory mechanism of sulfasalazine is related to adenosine release at inflamed sites. *J. Immunol.* **156,** 1937–1941.

113. Morabito, L., Montesinos, M. C., Schreibman, D. M., Balter, L., Thompson, L. F., Resta, R., and Cronstein, B. N. (1997) Methotrexate and sulfasalazine promote adenosine release: the role of ecto-5' nucleotidase. *J. Invest. Med.* **45,** 241A.

114. Yap, J. S., Montesinos, M. C., McCrary, C. T., and Cronstein, B. N. (1997) Theophylline reverses the effect of methotrexate on adjuvant arthritis: evidence that adenosine mediates the anti-inflammatory effects of methotrexate. *Arth. Rheum.* **40,** 598.

13

Quantitative Studies of the Lipid Mediators of Inflammation Using Liquid Chromatography-Electrospray Mass Spectrometry

Pierre Borgeat, Serge Picard, Nancy Dallaire, Marc Pouliot, and Marc E. Surette

Introduction

Lipid Mediators of Inflammation

The lipid mediators of inflammation include diverse biologically active molecules, mainly eicosanoids, but also phospholipids that modulate functional responses of inflammatory cells, i.e., adherence, locomotion, phagocytosis, production of reactive oxygen species, release of lysosomal enzymes, and synthesis of cytokines and other mediators. Lipid mediators also regulate important events of the inflammatory process, such as leukocyte trafficking, vascular permeability and smooth muscle contractility *(1–3)*. Thus, lipid mediators play important roles in the regulation of the inflammatory process in health, in which they mediate immune response and promote tissue repair, as well as in inflammatory diseases, in which the dysregulation of their biosynthesis and/or activity results in tissue damage and other deleterious effects. Among many lipid mediators, PG E_2 (PGE$_2$), which is produced either by the constitutive cyclooxygenase (COX-1) or the inducible cyclooxygenase (COX-2), plays an important role in the regulation of phagocyte activity and acts as a potent vasodilator. Leukotriene B_4 (LTB$_4$) derived from the 5-lipoxygenase (5-LO) pathway is a potent chemoattractant for phagocytes and is likely an important component of body defense mechanisms against infection. LTB$_4$ has also been recently involved in the development of inflammation in

From: *Molecular and Cellular Basis of Inflammation*
Edited by: C. N. Serhan and P. A. Ward © Humana Press Inc., Totowa, NJ

collagen-induced arthritis in mice *(4)*, an animal model of rheumatoid arthritis. The cysteinyl-LT (LTC_4, D_4, and E_4), also derived from the 5-LO pathway, are potent stimuli of vascular permeability and have been clearly implicated as mediators of the broncho-spasm in asthma *(5)*. Lipoxin A_4 (LXA_4), synthesized through the 5-LO and the 12- or 15-LO pathways, has been shown to act as a downregulator of phagocyte migration and is therefore believed to be part of the complex network of mediators that regulate leuko-cyte trafficking in inflammation *(6)*.

Specific and sensitive assay methods for the mediators of inflammation are a prereq-uisite to the understanding of their role in immune response and in inflammatory, autoimmune, and allergic diseases. Such knowledge of the physiological and patho-physiological roles of lipid mediators is also essential for the development of novel therapeutic approaches for the treatment of inflammatory diseases. The following para-graphs briefly describe and compare the various physicochemical assay methods used for the analysis of lipid mediators, and describe the utilization of the latest technique, liquid chromatography-electrospray mass spectrometry (LC-MS), for the assay of selected eicosanoids.

Physicochemical Assay Methods for the Lipid Mediators of Inflammation

Gas Chromatography-Mass Spectrometry (GC-MS)

GC-MS, the first physicochemical assay method widely used for the analysis of lipid mediators, proved particularly useful for the assay of prostaglandins (PGs) and throm-boxanes (TXs). GC-MS provides high sensitivity (usually in the low picogram range) and a high selectivity based on the mass of analytes (or of selected fragments), and the GC retention times of analytes. GC-MS also allows high-accuracy measurements through addition of stable isotope-labeled internal standards to samples (a method named isotopic dilution). The development of GC-MS assay methods had a major impact on the current understanding of the biochemistry and pharmacology of several lipid mediators, mainly those derived from the COX pathways *(7–9)*. The availability of GC-MS assays was also critical for the validation of immunoassays. Limitations of GC-MS include instrument cost, the overall complexity of the method, and the require-ment for extensive sample purification and derivatization, resulting in low throughput. Finally, the use of GC-MS is also limited by the chemical nature of the analytes that must be amenable to GC. This latter issue constitutes a major limitation in the utiliza-tion of GC-MS; indeed, a number of LO and COX products cannot be analyzed by GC-MS because of thermal instability, particularly endoperoxide and hydroperoxide derivatives of unsaturated fatty acids. Other compounds, such as hydroxy-eicosatetraenoic acids (HETEs), some di-HETEs, and tri-HETEs (including lipoxins [LXs]) may undergo some thermal decomposition during GC analysis, depending on the conditions of the GC analysis. For example, whereas LTB_4, 20-hydroxy-LTB_4, and the 6-*trans* isomers of LTB_4 are easily amenable to GC-MS analysis following classical derivatization procedures, a geometrical isomer of LTB_4 carrying a *trans-cis-trans* con-jugated triene moiety (instead of the *cis-trans-trans* and *trans-trans-trans* geometries found in LTB_4 and 6-*trans*-LTB_4, respectively) undergoes severe thermal decomposi-tion under the same GC conditions *(10)*, indicating that the double-bond geometry is crucial for the thermal stability of polyunsaturated LO products. Similarly, HETEs car-rying a *cis-trans* conjugated diene moiety undergo thermal decomposition during GC-

MS analysis, in contrast to HETEs carrying the *trans-trans* configuration (P. Borgeat, unpublished data). Finally, compounds such as platelet-activating factor (PAF), LTC_4, LTD_4, and LTE_4 (which carry polar moieties) are not amenable to GC unless subjected to extensive chemical modifications *(11,12)*.

High-Performance Liquid Chromatography (HPLC)

The rapid development of HPLC in the 1970s provided another important tool for the measurement of the lipid mediators of inflammation, especially of LO products such as leukotrienes (LTs) and lipoxins (LXs), which carry natural chromophores (conjugated trienes and tetraenes, respectively), allowing their direct detection by ultraviolet (UV) photometry (no derivatization required) *(13–17)*. It is important to point out immediately that the utilization of HPLC as an assay method for these lipid mediators is limited by the sensitivity of the method, which is in the low nanogram range using UV detection (as opposed to low picogram sensitivity for immunoassays and GC-MS assays). This characteristic of the method precludes its utilization for the measurement of physiological levels of lipid mediators in biological samples. However, HPLC assays of lipid mediators, especially of LO products and their metabolites, was found to be convenient and useful in in vitro studies using cells or tissues. HPLC provides high selectivity based on the UV absorbance at specific wavelengths and retention times; it also provides high-accuracy measurements through the utilization of internal standards. An important feature of HPLC assays is that they require only minimal sample preparation procedures; in fact, methods have been reported that allow direct on-line extraction and analysis of biological samples denatured with organic solvents *(13–17)*. The major advantage of HPLC assays over other assays, in particular immunoassays, is the possibility to perform profiling of several LO products present in biological samples, as opposed to analysis of a single component at a time. HPLC assays of LO products have had a major impact on the current knowledge of the biosynthesis of these eicosanoids in various cells and tissues, as well as on the complex mechanisms of regulation of their synthesis in various biological systems. The absence of natural chromophores suitable for UV detection on most COX products certainly accounts for the more limited use of HPLC assays in the analysis of COX products. In fact, the HPLC assays of COX products or other eicosanoids devoid of natural chromophores requires the labeling (derivatization) of the compounds with a fluorescent or UV chromophore *(18,19)*. Such chemical modifications not only complicate the sample preparation procedures, but result in an assay method in which the selectivity is essentially based on solute retention time. HPLC assays have, however, been successfully utilized for the profiling of radiolabeled eicosanoids *(20)*. In addition, HPLC is useful as an efficient purification step for eicosanoids prior to GC-MS analysis or immunoassays.

Liquid Chromatography-Electrospray Mass Spectrometry (LC-MS)

LC-MS is the latest assay method introduced for the analysis of lipid mediators. In LC-MS, analytes present in the mobile phase eluting from an HPLC column are directly introduced into the mass spectrometer following the nebulization of the mobile phase and electrospray ionization of analytes (*see* refs. *21* and *22*). The method provides a high level of selectivity, combining the specificity of mass spectrometric analysis and the specificity provided by the retention times of the solutes on the LC column. With most eicosanoids and PAF, sensitivities in the low picogram range are easily achievable. The method also provides high-accuracy measurements through the use of internal standards, allowing isotopic dilution assays as in GC-MS analysis. As emphasized above concerning HPLC assays, LC-MS also allows profiling of products of interest present in biological samples, as opposed to quantitation of single components *(23,24)*. Other advantages of LC-MS assays include (1) the technique is directly applied to substances in solution, (2) it does not require the prior derivatization of analytes (as required in GC-MS analysis), and (3) it is of moderate complexity and provides reproducible MS data. The major limitation of the method is the cost of the instrument. Although the technology is relatively new, a number of studies already describe the use of electrospray LC-MS in the analysis of polyunsaturated fatty acids *(25)*, PGs, LTs, LXs, and other LO products *(23,24,26–29)*, fatty acid hydroperoxides *(30)*, PAF *(31–34)*, and other phospholipids *(35,36)*.

LC-MS Assay and Profiling of Eicosanoids
LC-MS Assay of Arachidonic Acid

Arachidonic acid is a fatty acid precursor of several classes of lipid mediators, including PGs, TXs, LTs, and LXs. It is well established today that arachidonic acid is found in the form of esters (phospholipids, glycerides and cholesterol esters) in cell membranes and that the concentration of free arachidonic acid is low in resting cells. Levels of free arachidonic acid in cells are tightly regulated by the activity of enzymes that promote its release, such as the phospholipases and enzymes that catalyze its acylation. Accordingly, it is recognized that the synthesis of eicosanoids is primarily regulated by the release of arachidonic acid from cellular lipids. Thus, measurement of levels of free arachidonic acid provides crucial information for the understanding of the regulation of lipid mediator synthesis.

Measurements of arachidonic acid present some specific difficulties. First, because of the presence of four methylene-interrupted double bonds, the arachidonic acid molecule is relatively unstable, being highly susceptible to autooxidation. For this reason, arachidonic acid is a good candidate for LC-MS analysis, a method which involves minimal sample manipulation. Second, in measurements of arachidonic acid in biological samples, it is important to take into consideration that the release of arachidonic acid by activated cells and tissues may be of short duration *(37)* and that released arachidonic acid is rapidly reacylated in cellular lipids. Therefore, it is advisable to investigate arachidonic acid release in kinetic studies, and although this will affect the dynamics of arachidonic acid transformation, it may be useful to carry out experiments in the presence of delipidated human or bovine serum albumin (HSA or BSA) to slow down the reuptake of arachidonic acid, allowing the detection of subtle change in the levels of free arachidonic acid *(38,39)* (as in the experiment described below). Finally, it is noteworthy that arachidonic acid is present in micromolar concentration in plasma; therefore, experiments aimed at measurement of arachidonic acid release should be carried out in absence of plasma or serum.

To illustrate the usefulness of LC-MS for measurement of arachidonic acid, the authors have investigated the kinetics of arachidonic acid accumulation in neutrophil suspensions treated with either the chemoattractant formyl-Met-Leu-Phe (*f*MLP), bacterial lipopolysaccharides (LPS, *Escherichia coli* O111-B4, Difco, Detroit, MI) or both LPS and FMLP. It is well known that circulating neutrophils show minimal reactivity (LT synthesis) toward chemoattractants and that preexposure of neutrophils to such agents as LPS, the growth factor GM-CSF, or the inflammatory cytokine tumor necrosis factor-α (TNF-α) primes neutrophils for enhanced LT synthesis to a second stimulation with such agonists as *f*MLP, C5a, or PAF *(39–43)*. Furthermore, it has been clearly established previously that such priming effects involve enhanced arachidonic acid release *(37,43)*.

Human neutrophils were isolated from the peripheral blood of normal subjects and suspended in Hank's buffered salt solution (HBSS) at the concentration of 6×10^6 cells/mL. Cells were preincubated 30 min at 37°C in HBSS containing 10% autologous plasma (required for the priming effect of LPS; *see* ref. *37*), in the presence of 1 µg/mL of LPS or its diluent (10 µL/mL of 0.9% NaCl), washed twice, and resuspended in HBSS containing 1 mg/mL of fatty acid–free BSA. Cells were then stimulated with either with 0.1 µ*M f*MLP or its diluent (1 µL/mL of dimethyl sulfoxide [DMSO]). At various times following cell stimulation, aliquots of the cell suspensions were denatured by addition of 2 vol of cold (0°C) methanol containing 10 ng/mL of octadeutero-arachidonic acid (D_8-arachidonic acid, Biomol Research Labs, Plymouth Meeting, PA) as internal standard. The denatured samples were centrifuged at 2000*g* during 15 min to remove the precipitated material, and the supernatants were diluted with water to obtain ~50% water and analyzed without further treatment by reverse phase (RP) HPLC using an on-line extraction procedure described previously *(13)*, but using mobile phases containing 0.01% acetic acid (instead of phosphoric acid). The HPLC fractions containing arachidonic acid (determined in separate HPLC analyses by using a ^{3}H-arachidonic acid standard) were collected. The samples were evaporated under reduced pressure (using a SpeedVac model SVC 100D, Savant Instruments Inc., Farmingdale, NY) and redissolved into 100 µL of acetonitrile. Arachidonic acid was assayed by LC-MS using a nebulizer-assisted electrospray (ionspray) ion source coupled to a triple-quadrupole MS (API-III, PE Sciex, Thornhill, Ont., Canada). Six microliter aliquots of the samples were injected via the 20-µL loop of a Rheodyne injector (model 7125, Rheodyne, Cotati, CA) connected to a short column (2.1 × 30 mm, packed with 5 µm C_{18} particles), using acetonitrile:water (87.5:12.5, v/v, containing 0.01% acetic acid) as solvent, at a flow rate of 150 µL/min. Samples were analyzed in the negative ion mode. The ions at *m/z* 303 and 311, representing the carboxylate anions of arachidonic acid and D_8-arachidonic acid, respectively, were monitored.

Figure 1 shows the relative intensities of peaks recorded from the successive injections of increasing amounts of arachidonic acid in the LC-MS system. The limit of detection of the method (signal-to-noise [SNR] ratio ≥10) was 10 pg/injection. The standard curve generated shows a correlation coefficient (r^2) of 1.000. Figure 2 shows the results of the above-described experiment; arachidonic acid levels were low and varied little over the 30 min incubation in unstimulated neutrophil suspensions pretreated or not with LPS (LPS/DMSO, NaCl/DMSO). In the neutrophil suspensions pretreated in the absence of LPS, stimulation with *f*MLP (NaCl/*f*MLP) caused a minor but detectable enhancement of arachidonic acid release. Finally, pretreatment with LPS strikingly enhanced the stimulatory effect of *f*MLP (LPS/*f*MLP) on arachidonic acid release in the neutrophil suspensions; the release of arachidonic acid was immediate, maximum between 1 and 5 min after addition of *f*MLP, and levels of the fatty acid progressively decreased with time. These data confirm that the priming of human neutrophils with LPS results in strikingly enhanced arachidonic acid release on a second stimulation with an agonist, and support the concept that such an effect of LPS accounts, at least in part, for the enhanced ability of neutrophils exposed to LPS to produce LT.

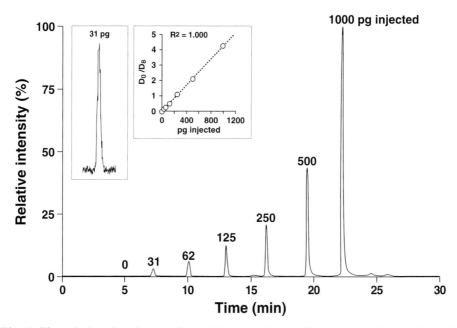

Fig. 1. The relative abundance of arachidonic acid in calibration standards. The relative abundance of the carboxylate anion of arachidonic acid (m/z 303) as determined by electrospray (Ionspray) LC-MS. Each peak results from a separate manual injection of 5 μL (acetonitrile) of a calibration standard containing 0–200 ng arachidonic acid/mL and 100 ng D_8-arachidonic acid/mL. **(Insets)** The SNR (~18) obtained on injection of 31 pg of arachidonic acid **(left)** and the calibration curve **(right)**. MS conditions were as follows: dwell time, 150 ms with a pause time of 30 ms; spray voltage, –3800 V with a nitrogen pressure of 50 psi applied to the nebulizer; orifice voltage, –70 V. Peak areas and the calibration curve were obtained using the Sciex MacQuan program.

Previous studies performed in the authors' laboratory provided similar data *(37)*; however, in these studies, LPS-primed neutrophils were stimulated with *f*MLP in the absence of BSA in the incubation media. This difference in the experimental conditions resulted in a significantly different kinetics of arachidonic acid release; indeed, in the absence of BSA, maximum levels of arachidonic acid in incubation media were lower and declined much more rapidly, reaching basal levels 10 min after *f*MLP stimulation. Such differences in the kinetics of arachidonic acid release by neutrophils incubated in the presence or absence of BSA (which binds and retains arachidonic acid in the incubation media) emphasize the importance of the reacylation process of free arachidonic acid in cell suspensions.

LC-MS-MS Assay of LTB₄

LTB_4 is a potent mediator of the inflammatory process, acting primarily as a chemoattractant for phagocytes *(1)*. LTB_4 is also an immunomodulator; it stimulates T-cell and natural killer cell cytotoxic activities *(44)*, activates B-cells, and promotes the synthesis of cytokines such as interleukin-1 (IL-1), IL-6, TNF-α, and interferon-γ *(45–47)*. Besides its capacity to promote neutrophil migration in man and animals, little is known of the ability of LTB_4 to modulate the immune response in vivo. Some knowl-

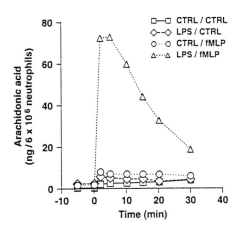

Fig. 2. Arachidonic acid release by activated neutrophils. Neutrophil suspensions were incubated under the stimulatory conditions described in LC-MS Assay of Arachidonic Acid; and arachidonic acid was measured by electrospray LC-MS using D_8-arachidonic acid as internal standard, as described in the legend to Fig. 1. The data shown are from one experiment representative of three experiments.

edge of the pharmacokinetics of LTB_4 in vivo is a prerequisite to such studies. The authors have previously shown that the half-life of LTB_4 in the rabbit circulation is ~0.5 min *(48)*; in these studies, they also showed that LTB_4 disposition in vivo is the result of rapid uptake and elimination rather than direct metabolism by blood components. Because the mouse is a more convenient model in which to investigate the in vivo effects of agents on the immune response, experiments were performed to determine the pharmacokinetics of LTB_4 on ip administration to mice. Measurements of LTB_4 concentration in mouse plasma following ip injections illustrate the usefulness of LC-MS-MS for the assay of LTB_4 in a complex biological matrix.

Eighteen Balb/C mice received an ip injection of 10 μg LTB_4 (in 100 μL of phosphate-buffered saline). At various time points, blood samples were taken by retroorbital bleeding (one blood sampling per mouse) using heparinized micropipets. The mice were sacrificed by cervical dislocation immediately after blood collection. Five hundred picograms of tetradeutero-LTB_4 (D_4-LTB_4, Biomol Research) were added to 100 μL of plasma from each animal. The plasma samples were denatured by mixing with 10 vol of acetonitrile, centrifuged to remove the precipitated material, and the supernatants were diluted with water to obtain ~50% water. LTB_4 (and D_4-LTB_4) were purified by RP-HPLC using the on-line extraction system previously described *(13)*, but using mobile phases containing 0.01% acetic acid (instead of phosphoric acid). Fractions containing LTB_4 and the internal standard were collected and evaporated using a Speed-Vac evaporator and redissolved in 20 μL of acetonitrile:water, 80:20, v/v. Measurements of LTB_4 were then performed by LC-MS-MS using a nebulizer-assisted electrospray (turbo ionspray) (API-III, PE Sciex). The samples (~15 μL) were introduced via an RP-HPLC column (2 × 150 mm, packed with 5-μm C_{18} particles), and LTB_4 was eluted using acetonitrile:water (80:20, containing 0.01% acetic acid and 1 m*M* ammonium acetate) as solvent, at a flow rate of 200 μL/min. MS-MS analyses were performed in the negative ion mode by multiple reaction monitoring (*m/z*

335/195 and *m/z* 339/195), as described previously *(24,26,29)*. Quantitation was performed by measurement of LTB_4/D_4-LTB_4 ratios using a calibration curve.

Figure 3 shows the relative intensities of LTB_4 peaks recorded by LC-MS-MS analysis from injections of increasing amounts of LTB_4. The limit of detection of the method (SNR ≥10) was 5 pg/injection. The standard curve generated shows an r^2 of 0.999. Figure 4 shows the results of the above-described experiments; although LTB_4 levels were not detectable in mouse plasma prior to the ip injection of LTB_4 (not shown), the ip administration of a 10 µg bolus resulted in the rapid appearance of LTB_4 in plasma. Plasma LTB_4 levels peaked between 2 and 5 min after ip injections and declined to undetectable levels at 30 min. The peak LTB_4 plasma concentration following ip administration of 10 µg of LTB_4/mouse was 125–150 n*M*. Each data point shows the results (mean ±SD) obtained with a group of three mice.

These data clearly indicate that on ip injection, LTB_4 is rapidly taken up into the circulation over a period of 5 min. These experiments did not allow calculation of the half-life of LTB_4 in the mouse circulation, but indicated a rapid disposition of LTB_4 in mice, as previously observed in rabbits *(48)*.

LC-MS-MS Profiling of COX-2 Products Generated by Neutrophils

The ability of monocytes and macrophages to produce COX products is well established; however, the capacity of human blood neutrophils to produce PGs or TXs has been the subject of controversy for many years. The recent observation that the inducible COX isozyme COX-2 *(49)* is expressed in neutrophils exposed to LPS *(50)* likely provides an explanation to this controversy. Furthermore, the authors have recently demonstrated that in addition to LPS, *f*MLP, TNF-α, and phorbol myristate acetate (PMA) also induced the expression of COX-2 in neutrophils as measured by Western blot analysis using a specific antiserum *(51)*. COX-2 expression was detectable 30 min after addition of the stimuli to the cell suspensions and was maximal after 4 h; levels of COX-2 remained elevated for the duration of the incubation (20 h, data not shown). The nature of the COX products generated by neutrophils exposed to inflammatory stimuli (i.e., containing COX-2) has, however, not been determined yet. In the studies described, the authors used LC-MS-MS for the profiling of COX products generated by neutrophils exposed to the inflammatory stimuli *f*MLP, TNF-α, or PMA.

Neutrophils were purified from the peripheral blood of normal subjects and suspended in HBSS at a concentration of 10×10^6/mL. The cell suspensions were incubated for 20 h at 37°C in the presence of either 0.1 µ*M f*MLP, 1000 U/mL TNF-α, or 100 n*M* PMA, in the presence or absence of the specific COX-2 inhibitor NS-398 (Biomol Research), which was used at a concentration of 1 µ*M*. After 20 h of incubation, the incubation media were freeze-thawed three times, and the cell debris was eliminated by centrifugation (5 min, 12,000*g*). Samples were acidified to pH 5.0 with acetic acid, and 5 ng of tetradeutero-PGE_2 (D_4-PGE_2, Biomol Research) were added as an internal standard. Samples were loaded on Waters Oasis HLB (60 mg) extraction cartridges (Waters, Milford, MA), and the cartridges were sequentially washed with 1 mL of acidified water (pH 4.0, acetic acid), 1 mL of water, and 1 mL of hexane to eliminate salts and neutral lipids. Eicosanoids were then eluted with 1.5 mL of methanol. Eluates were evaporated under a stream of nitrogen and reconstituted in 50 µL of methanol:water (50:50). Ten-microliter aliquots of the samples (20%) were injected into the LC-MS-MS system via an RP-HPLC column (2 × 150 mm, packed with 5-µm C_{18} particles), and the products were eluted using methanol:water (70:30, v/v, contain-

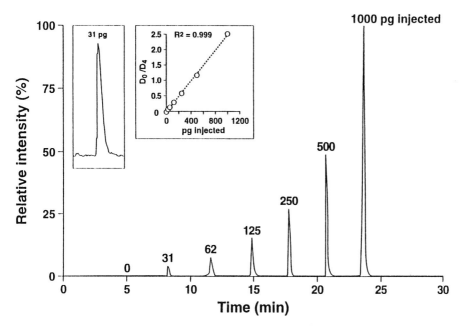

Fig. 3. The relative abundance of LTB_4 in calibration standards. The relative abundance of the daughter ion *m/z* 195 that originated from the transition m/z 335 → 195 as determined by electrospray (Turbo Ionspray) LC-MS-MS. The transition m/z 339 → 195 for D_4-LTB_4 was also monitored (not shown). Each peak results from a separate manual injection of 5 μL (acetonitrile:water, 80:20, v/v) of a calibration standard containing 0–200 ng LTB_4/mL and 100 ng D_4-LTB_4/mL. **(Insets)** The SNR (~50) obtained on injection of 31 pg of LTB_4 **(left)** and the calibration curve **(right)**. MS conditions were as follows: dwell time, 150 ms with a pause time of 30 ms; spray voltage, –3600 V with a nitrogen pressure of 60 psi on the nebulizer; orifice voltage, –55 V. Argon was used in the collision cell at a pressure equivalent to 280×10^{12} molecules/cm². Peak areas and the calibration curve were obtained using the Sciex MacQuan program.

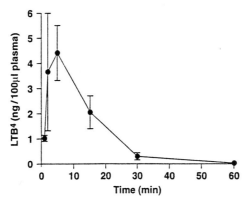

Fig. 4: Plasma levels of LTB_4 following ip injection of LTB_4 in mice. Mice received an ip injection of LTB_4 (10 mg bolus) as described in LC-MS-MS Assay of LTB_4. LTB_4 was measured in plasma by electrospray (Turbo Ionspray) LC-MS-MS using D_4-LTB_4 as internal standard, as described in the legend to Fig. 3. Each data point shows the results (mean ±SD) obtained with a group of three mice.

ing 0.01% acetic acid and 1 mM ammonium acetate) as solvent, at a flow rate of 200 µL/min. MS-MS analyses were performed in the negative ion mode by multiple reaction monitoring; the parent ion/daughter ion monitored were m/z 351/175 (PGE$_2$), 355/275 (PGE$_2$-D$_4$), 369/169 (TXB$_2$), 369/245 (6-keto-PGF$_{1\alpha}$), 351/233 (PGD$_2$), and 353/193 (PGF$_{2\alpha}$), with these daughter ions being specific markers of their respective parent ion *(23)*.

Figure 5 shows the tracings recorded for selected MS-MS analyses. The lower tracing (D$_4$-PGE$_2$) demonstrates that the internal standard was present in all samples. The top and middle tracings reveal the formation of TXB$_2$ and PGE$_2$, respectively. PMA was the most potent stimulus, followed by TNF-α and FMLP. The data also show that compound NS-398, a specific COX-2 inhibitor, blocks the formation of PGE$_2$ (~75%) and TXB$_2$ (~85%) in the three experimental conditions tested. Total amounts of TXB$_2$ and PGE$_2$ measured in the incubation media of PMA-stimulated neutrophils (Fig. 5E) were 3.8 and 1.4 ng, respectively. In these experiments, the formation of PGF$_{2\alpha}$, PGD$_2$, and 6-keto-PGF$_{1\alpha}$ was not detectable (data not shown). In several experiments, the ratio of TXB$_2$/PGE$_2$ varied between 1.5 and 2.7. Analysis of these samples using a commercial ELISA for PGE$_2$ (Cayman Chemical, Ann Arbor, MI) revealed an excellent correlation between the immunoassay and the LC-MS-MS assay (data not shown). Unstimulated neutrophils incubated for 20 h at 37°C did not produce detectable amounts of any COX product (data not shown). These data demonstrate that TXB$_2$ and PGE$_2$ are the products of the transformation of arachidonic acid through the COX-2 pathway in activated human neutrophils.

Conclusion

The development of LC-MS represents a major breakthrough in the analysis of bio-organic molecules, both for quantitation purposes and structural analysis. LC-MS provides low picogram sensitivity for the quantitative analysis of the lipid mediators of inflammation. Furthermore, MS-MS analysis allows the highly selective detection of compounds in a complex biological matrix. The greatest advantage provided by electrospray LC-MS over previously available methods is the feasibility of MS analysis of compounds directly from solutions; indeed, solutes present in the mobile phase eluting from an HPLC column are directly analyzed, minimizing sample preparation procedures. Electrospray LC-MS also makes possible the analysis of underivatized polar molecules, such as LTC$_4$ or PAF, eliminating the requirements for extensive chemical modifications of the molecules. Finally, electrospray LC-MS allows the analysis of thermally unstable molecules, such as endoperoxides, hydroperoxides, or epoxides, and of polyunsaturated and relatively fragile molecules such as LXs. It can be expected that the novel electrospray LC-MS technology will greatly facilitate and accelerate further progress in the understanding of the biological and pathophysiological significance of the lipid mediators of inflammation.

Acknowledgments

The authors thank Dr. Jacques Maclouf for his donation of antiserum and the Medical Research Council of Canada for support.

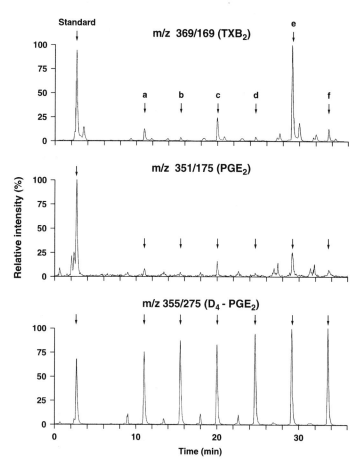

Fig. 5: LC-MS-MS analysis of COX products derived from the human neutrophil COX-2 pathway. Electrospray (turbo ionspray) LC-MS-MS analyses were performed using multiple reaction monitoring as indicated on the Fig. and as described in LC-MS-MS Profiling. D_4-PGE_2 was used as internal standard. The amount of standards (TXB_2, PGE_2, and D_4-PGE_2) injected was 1 ng. Human neutrophils were incubated with (**A**) 0.1 μ*M f*MLP, (**B**) 0.1 μ*M f*MLP and 1 μ*M* NS-398, (**C**) 1000 U TNF-α/mL, (**D**) 1000 U TNF-α/mL and 1 μ*M* NS-398, (**E**) 100 n*M* PMA, and (**F**) 100 n*M* PMA and 1 μ*M* NS-398. Samples were prepared for LC-MS analysis as described in LC-MS-MS Profiling. The other eicosanoids analyzed, $PGF_{2\alpha}$, 6-keto-$PGF_{1\alpha}$, and PGD_2, were not detectable. The data shown are from one experiment representative of three experiments. MS conditions were as follows: dwell time, 150 ms with a pause time of 30 ms; spray voltage, –3600 V with a nitrogen pressure of 60 psi on the nebulizer; orifice voltage, –55 V. Argon was used in the collision cell at a pressure equivalent to 280×10^{12} mol/cm^2. The Turbo Ionspray was operated at 450°C with the auxiliary gaz flow (nitrogen) at 5.5 L/min.

References

1. Borgeat, P. and Naccache, P. H. (1990) Biosynthesis and biological activity of leukotriene B4. *Clin. Biochem.* **23,** 459–468.
2. Serhan, C. N. and Drazen, J. M. (1997) Antiinflammatory potential of lipoxygenase-derived eicosanoids: a molecular switch at 5 and 15 positions? *J. Clin. Invest.* **99,** 1147,1148.

3. Venable, M. E., Zimmerman, G. A., Mcintyre, T. M., and Prescott, S. M. (1993) Review—platelet-activating factor—a phospholipid autacoid with diverse actions. *J. Lipid Res.* **34**, 691–702.

4. Griffiths, R. J., Pettipher, E. R., Koch, K., Farrell, C. A., Breslow, R., Conklyn, M. J., Smith, M. A., Hackman, B. C., Wimberly, D. J., Milici, A. J., Scampoli, D. N., Cheng, J. B., Pillar, J. S., Pazoles, C. J., Doherty, N. S., Melvin, L. S., Reiter, L. A., Biggars, M. S., Falkner, F. C., Mitchell, D. Y., Liston, T. E., and Showell, H. J. (1995) Leukotriene B4 plays a critical role in the progression of collagen-induced arthritis. *Proc. Natl. Acad. Sci. USA* **92**, 517–521.

5. Hay, D. W. P., Torphy, T. J., and Undem, B. J. (1995) Cysteinyl leukotrienes in asthma: old mediators up to new tricks. *Trends Pharmacol. Sci.* **16**, 304–309.

6. Takano, T., Fiore, S., Maddox, J. F., Brady, H. R., Petasis, N. A., and Serhan, C. N. (1997) Aspirin-triggered 15-epi-lipoxin A4 (LXA4) and LXA4 stable analogues are potent inhibitors of acute inflammation: evidence for anti-inflammatory receptors. *J. Exp. Med.* **185**, 1693–1704.

7. Mackert, G., Reinke, M., Schweer, H., and Seyberth, H. W. (1989) Simultaneous determination of the primary prostanoids prostaglandin E2, prostaglandin F2-alpha and 6–oxoprostaglandin-F1–alpha by immunoaffinity chromatography in combination with negative ion chemical ionization gas chromatography TANDEM mass spectrometry. *J. Chromatogr. Biomed. Appl.* **494**, 13–22.

8. Callaghan, D. H., Yergey, J. A., Rousseau, P., and Masson, P. (1994) Respiratory tract eicosanoid measurement using microdialysis sampling and GC/MS detection. *Pulmonary Pharmacol.* **7**, 35–41.

9. Murphy, R. C. (1995) Lipid mediators, leukotrienes and mass spectrometry. *J. Mass Spectrom.* **30**, 5–16.

10. Borgeat, P. and Pilote, S. (1988) Rearrangement of 5S,12S-dihydroxy-6,8,10,14-(E,Z,E,Z)-eicosatetraenoic acid during gas chromatographic analysis: formation of a cyclohexadiene derivative. *Prostaglandins* **35**, 723–732.

11. Balazy, M. and Murphy, R. C. (1986) Determination of sulfidopeptide leukotrienes in biological fluids by gas chromatography/mass spectrometry. *Anal. Chem.* **58**, 1098–1101.

12. Shindo, K. and Hashimoto, Y. (1991) Quantitative analysis of platelet activating factor treated with pentafluorobenzoyl chloride using gas chromatography/negative ion chemical ionization mass spectrometry. *Drugs Exp. Clin. Res.* **17**, 343–349.

13. Borgeat, P., Picard, S., Vallerand, P., Bourgoin, S., Odeimat, A., Sirois, P., and Poubelle, P. E. (1990) Automated on-line extraction and profiling of lipoxygenase products of arachidonic acid by high performance liquid chromatography, in *Methods in Enzymology: Arachidonate Related Lipid Mediators* (Murphy, R. C. and Fitzpatrick, F., eds.), Academic, New York, pp. 98–116.

14. Surette, M. E., Odeimat, A., Palmantier, R., Marleau, S., Poubelle, P. E., and Borgeat, P. (1994) Reverse-phase high-performance liquid chromatography analysis of arachidonic acid metabolites in plasma after stimulation of whole blood ex vivo. *Anal. Biochem.* **216**, 392–400.

15. Powell, W. S. (1987) Precolumn extraction and reversed-phase high-pressure liquid chromatography of prostaglandins and leukotrienes. *Anal. Biochem.* **164**, 117–131.

16. Ramis, I., Hotter, G., Rosellocatafau, J., Bulbena, O., Picado, C., and Gelpi, E. (1993) Application of totally automated on-line sample clean up system for extraction and high-performance liquid chromatography separation of peptide leukotrienes. *J. Pharmaceut. Biomed. Anal.* **11**, 1135–1139.

17. Fritsch, H., Molnar, I., and Wurl, M. (1994) Separation of arachidonic acid metabolites by on-line extraction and reversed-phase high-performance liquid chromatography optimized by computer simulation. *J. Chromatogr. A* **684**, 65–75.

18. McGuffin, V. L. and Zare, R. N. (1985) Femtomole analysis of prostaglandin pharmaceuticals. *Proc. Natl. Acad. Sci. USA* **82**, 8315–8319.

19. Salari, H., Yeung, M., Douglas, S., and Morozowich, W. (1987) Detection of prostaglandins by high-performance liquid chromatography after conversion to p-(9-anthroyloxy)phenacyl esters. *Anal. Biochem.* **164**, 1–10.

20. Hesse, W. H., Schweer, H., Seyberth, H. W., and Peskar, B. A. (1990) Separation and determination of prostaglandin E1 metabolites by high-performance liquid chromatography. *J. Chromatogr. Biomed. Appl.* **533**, 159–165.

21. Herderich, M., Richling, E., Roscher, R., Schneider, C., Schwab, W., Humpf, H. U., and Schreier, P. (1997) Application of atmospheric pressure ionization HPLC-MS-MS for the analysis of natural products. *Chromatographia* **45,** 127–132.
22. Kebarle, P. and Tang, L. (1993) From ions in solution to ions in the gas phase—the mechanism of electrospray mass spectrometry. *Anal. Chem.* **65,** A972–A986.
23. Margalit, A., Duffin, K. L., and Isakson, P. C. (1996) Rapid quantitation of a large scope of eicosanoids in two models of inflammation: development of an electrospray and tandem mass spectrometry method and application to biological studies. *Anal. Biochem.* **235,** 73–81.
24. Wheelan, P. and Murphy, R. C. (1997) Quantitation of 5-lipoxygenase products by electrospray mass spectrometry: effect of ethanol on zymosan-stimulated production of 5-lipoxygenase products by human neutrophils. *Anal. Biochem.* **244,** 110–115.
25. Kerwin, J. L., Wiens, A. M., and Ericsson, L. H. (1996) Identification of fatty acids by electrospray mass spectrometry and tandem mass spectrometry. *J. Mass Spectrom.* **31,** 184–192.
26. Oda, Y., Mano, N., and Asakawa, N. (1995) Simultaneous determination of thromboxane B2, prostaglandin E2 and leukotriene B4 in whole blood by liquid chromatography mass spectrometry. *J. Mass Spectrom.* **30,** 1671–1678.
27. Wu, Y. H., Li, L. Y. T., Henion, J. D., and Krol, G. J. (1996) Determination of LTE4 in human urine by liquid chromatography coupled with ionspray tandem mass spectrometry. *J. Mass Spectrom.* **31,** 987–993.
28. Kerwin, J. L. and Torvik, J. J. (1996) Identification of monohydroxy fatty acids by electrospray mass spectrometry and tandem mass spectrometry. *Anal. Biochem.* **237,** 56–64.
29. Griffiths, W. J., Yang, Y., Sjövall, J., and Lindgren, J. A. (1996) Electrospray/collision-induced dissociation mass spectrometry of mono-, di- and tri-hydroxylated lipoxygenase products, including leukotrienes of the B-series and lipoxins. *Rapid Commun. Mass Spectrom.* **10,** 183–196.
30. Schneider, C., Schreier, P., and Herderich, M. (1997) Analysis of lipoxygenase-derived fatty acid hydroperoxides by electrospray ionization tandem mass spectrometry. *Lipids* **32,** 331–336.
31. Silvestro, L., Dacol, R., Scappaticci, E., Libertucci, D., Biancone, L., and Camussi, G. (1993) Development of a high-performance liquid chromatographic mass spectrometric technique, with an ionspray interface, for the determination of platelet-activating factor (PAF) and lyso-PAF in biological samples. *J. Chromatogr.* **647,** 261–269.
32. Borgeat, P., Picard, S., Braquet, P., Allen, M., and Shushan, B. (1994) LC-MS-MS with ion spray: A promising approach for analysis of underivatized platelet activating factor (PAF). *J. Lipid Media. Cell Signal.* **10,** 11,12.
33. Savu, S. R., Silvestro, L., Sorgel, F., Montrucchio, G., Lupia, E., and Camussi, G. (1996) Determination of 1-o-acyl-2–acetyl-sn-glyceryl-3-phosphorylcholine, platelet-activating factor and related phospholipids in biological samples by high-performance liquid chromatography tandem mass spectrometry. *J. Chromatogr. B* **682,** 35–45.
34. Weintraub, S. T. and Pinckard, N. R. (1991) Electrospray ionization for analysis of platelet-activating factor. *Rapid Commun. Mass Spectrom.* **5,** 309–311.
35. Olsson, N. U. and Salem, N. (1997) Molecular species analysis of phospholipids. *J. Chromatogr. B* **692,** 245–256.
36. Han, X. L. and Gross, R. W. (1996) Structural determination of lysophospholipid regioisomers by electrospray ionization tandem mass spectrometry. *J. Am. Chem. Soc.* **118,** 451–457.
37. Surette, M. E., Palmantier, R., Gosselin, J., and Borgeat, P. (1993) Lipopolysaccharides prime whole human blood and isolated neutrophils for the increased synthesis of 5-lipoxygenase products by enhancing arachidonic acid availability—involvement of the CD14 antigen. *J. Exp. Med.* **178,** 1347–1355.
38. Palmantier, R., Rocheleau, H., Laviolette, M., Mancini, J., and Borgeat, P. (1998) Characteristics of leukotriene synthesis by human granulocytes in presence of plasma. *Biochim. Biophys. Acta* **1389,** 187–196.
39. Dieter, P. (1994) Arachidonic acid and eicosanoid release. *J. Immunol. Methods* **174,** 223–229.
40. Dahinden, C. A., Zingg, J., Maly, F. E., and DeWeck, A. L. (1988) Leukotriene production in human neutrophils primed by recombinant human granulocyte/macrophage colony-stimulating factor and stimulated with the complement component C5a and FMLP as second signals. *J. Exp. Med.* **167,** 1281–1295.

41. DiPersio, J. F., Naccache, P. H., Borgeat, P., Gasson, J. C., Nguyen, M.-H., and McColl, S. R. (1988) Characterization of the priming effects of human granulocyte-macrophage colony-stimulating factor on human neutrophil leukotriene synthesis. *Prostaglandins* **36,** 673–691.
42. Palmantier, R., Surette, M. E., Sanchez, A., Braquet, P., and Borgeat, P. (1994) Priming for the synthesis of 5-lipoxygenase products in human blood ex vivo by human granulocyte-macrophage colony-stimulating factor and tumor necrosis factor-alpha. *Lab. Invest.* **70,** 696–704.
43. McColl, S. R., Krump, E., Naccache, P. H., Poubelle, P. E., Braquet, P., Braquet, M., and Borgeat, P. (1991) Granulocyte-macrophage colony-stimulating factor increases the synthesis of leukotriene B4 by human neutrophils in response to platelet-activating factor—enhancement of both arachidonic acid availability and 5-lipoxygenase activation. *J. Immunol.* **146,** 1204–1211.
44. Rola-Pleszczynski, M. (1985) Immunoregulation by leukotrienes and other lipoxygenase metabolites. *Immunol. Today* **6,** 302–307.
45. Yamaoka, K. A., Claesson, H. E., and Rosen, A. (1989) Leukotriene B4 enhances activation, proliferation, and differentiation of human lymphocytes B. *J. Immunol.* **143,** 1996–2000.
46. Claesson, H. E., Odlander, B., and Jakobsson, P. J. (1992) Leukotriene B4 in the immune system. *Int. J. Immunopharmacol.* **14,** 441–449.
47. Rola-Pleszczynski, M. and Stankova, J. (1992) Leukotriene B4 enhances interleukin-6 (IL-6) production and IL-6 messenger RNA accumulation in human monocytes in vitro—transcriptional and posttranscriptional mechanisms. *Blood* **80,** 1004–1011.
48. Marleau, S., Dallaire, N., Poubelle, P. E., and Borgeat, P. (1994) Metabolic disposition of leukotriene B4 (LTB4) and oxidation-resistant analogues of LTB4 in conscious rabbits. *Br. J. Pharmacol.* **112,** 654–658.
49. Smith, W. L., Garavito, R. M., and Dewitt, D. L. (1996) Prostaglandin endoperoxide h synthases (cyclooxygenases)-1 and -2. *J. Biol. Chem.* **271,** 33,157–33,160.
50. Niiro, H., Otsuka, T., Izuhara, K., Yamaoka, K., Ohshima, K., Tanabe, T., Hara, S., Nemoto, Y., Tanaka, Y., Nakashima, H., and Niho, Y. (1997) Regulation by interleukin-10 and interleukin-4 of cyclooxygenase-2 expression in human neutrophils. *Blood* **89,** 1621–1628.
51. Pailiot, M., Gilbert, C., Bongeat, P., Poubelle, P. E., Bourgoin, S., Ghassi, J., Maclouf, J., McColl, S. R., and Naccache, P. H. (1998) Expression and activity of mastaglandin endoperoxide synthase-2 in agonist-actuated human neutrophils. *FASEB J.*, in press.

14

Molecular Biology of Autoimmune Arthritis

Edward F. Rosloniec, Leslie R. Ballou, Rajendra Raghow,
Karen A. Hasty, and Andrew H. Kang

Introduction

Rheumatoid arthritis is one of the most common autoimmune diseases of humans. Although this crippling, debilitating disease is generally characterized as a localized inflammation of synovial tissue that often results in the loss of joint function, systemic effects of the autoimmune disease are also clearly present. Despite advances in the understanding of the pathological processes involved in rheumatoid arthritis, its etiology remains a mystery. In this chapter, the authors will consider the current hypotheses put forth to explain the molecular basis for susceptibility to rheumatoid arthritis, and discuss recent information concerning the role of cytokines in modulating the inflammatory response and mechanisms of induction of matrix metalloproteinase (MMP) gene expression, and the role of these enzymes in tissue degradation. In addition, they will examine the role animal models of experimental autoimmune arthritis have played in advancing the authors' understanding of the autoimmunity of rheumatoid arthritis and its associated pathology. Finally, they will highlight the significance of ongoing studies toward the development of promising therapies for the treatment of rheumatoid arthritis.

General Characterization of Rheumatoid Arthritis

Pathogenesis of Rheumatoid Arthritis

Rheumatoid arthritis is an inflammatory disease of the joints that is considered to be autoimmune in origin. Etiologically, rheumatoid arthritis appears to be the result of a combination of factors that includes genetic predisposition and an antigenic stimulus, perhaps as the result of infection by microbial organisms. Immunological processes play a central role in the pathogenesis of rheumatoid arthritis as evident from (1) the presence of T-cells, B-cells, and macrophages in the inflamed joint and the cytokines that these cells produce; (2) the presence of autoantibodies (rheumatoid

From: *Molecular and Cellular Basis of Inflammation*
Edited by: C. N. Serhan and P. A. Ward © Humana Press Inc., Totowa, NJ

factor); (3) the identification of complement activation products at the site of inflammation; and (4) the association between rheumatoid arthritis susceptibility and the expression of specific major histocompatibility complex (MHC) class II alleles, the molecular recognition elements used by CD4+ T-cells. All these observations are consistent with the paradigm of rheumatoid arthritis as an autoimmune, antigen-driven disease in which T-cells are directly involved. Yet, despite intense efforts, the antigen(s) driving the underlying autoimmunity of rheumatoid arthritis remain unknown.

The hypothesis that rheumatoid arthritis is a T-cell–mediated disease is strongly supported by the presence of T-cells in the arthritic lesions and the association of this disease with MHC class II molecules. Histopathologic and ultrastructural studies of rheumatoid synovial tissues show synovial lining cell hyperplasia along with chronic inflammatory infiltrates containing T- and B-lymphocytes, and macrophages that are reminiscent of classic delayed type hypersensitivity reactions. Staining of cells with fluorescein-tagged monoclonal antibodies indicates that the majority of the cells in the synovial tissues are activated T-cells expressing MHC class II molecules. It is postulated that the presumably antigen-specific T-cells preferentially expand in the synovium and produce potent lymphokines (e.g., interleukin-2 [IL-2], IL-4, IL-5, IL-6, IFN-γ, and so on) that initiate inflammation. These cytokines lead to the activation of B-cells and the local production of antibodies resulting in the formation of immune complexes. These complexes in turn activate the complement cascade, generating a number of biologically active complement proteins such as C3a and C5a that further amplify the inflammatory reaction. Immune complexes are also phagocytized by polymorphonuclear leukocytes, macrophages, and synovial lining cells, and in the process a wide variety of mediators is released, including lysosomal enzymes, oxygen-free radicals, oxidation products of arachidonic acid, and MMPs that degrade the cartilage matrix. In parallel, inflammation is perpetuated by mediators derived from activated macrophages and synovial fibroblast-like cells that produce IL-1, tumor necrosis factor-α (TNF-α), IL-6, GM-CSF, prostaglandins (PGs) and other arachidonate metabolites, and oxygen-free radicals. Some of these extracellularly released mediators in turn stimulate macrophages and synovial cells to produce various MMPs that readily degrade the extracellular matrix of joint tissues. Thus, complex interactions of cells and mediators are involved in the chronic inflammation and destruction of cartilage, bone, and surrounding connective tissues in rheumatoid arthritis.

Despite the difficulties in identifying the etiologic agents of rheumatoid arthritis, substantial progress in understanding the pathological processes of rheumatoid arthritis has opened up novel therapeutic opportunities. For example, the molecular basis for MHC-based susceptibility to rheumatoid arthritis has been defined in detail, identifying critical amino acids within the MHC class II sequences. A number of the inflammatory mediators of rheumatoid arthritis have been identified, and some have become the focus of experimental anti-inflammatory therapies. In addition, a wealth of information pertinent to the mechanism of the chronic degradation of cartilage has emerged from identification and functional analysis of the MMPs. Structure-function specificities of MMPs are being exploited to design novel therapeutic modalities to intervene in the erosive destruction of cartilage in the joints.

Molecular Basis for Susceptibility to Rheumatoid Arthritis

One of the strongest pieces of evidence indicating that rheumatoid arthritis is an autoimmune disease is that susceptibility is closely linked to the expression of specific alleles of MHC class II molecules. Many years ago it was noted that a strong correlation exists between the expression of MHC class II molecules HLA-DR1 or DR4 and an increased risk of developing rheumatoid arthritis *(1–3)*. These findings were significant because we now know that the class II molecules of the MHC serve as a focal control point in antigen-specific CD4⁺ T-cell stimulation. Antigen specific stimulation of CD4⁺ T-cells is completely dependent on the ability of class II molecules to bind and present peptides, and the allelic polymorphisms within these class II molecules control their peptide-binding function. Thus, the capacity of a protein to be immunogenic (or autoimmunogenic) varies with the allele of class II molecule in question. Although specificity in peptide binding is a hallmark function of class II molecules, discrimination between self and nonself peptides is not. Class II molecules bind with equal efficiency peptides derived from "self" or foreign proteins *(4–7)*. Given the milieu of the class II-expressing cells, they are exposed to self proteins at a frequency orders of magnitude higher than foreign proteins. Indeed, the vast majority of peptides eluted from class II molecules are derived from self proteins *(8–10)*. Consequently, from the point of view of the class II molecule, the risk of developing an autoimmune response is ever present, but tight controls on T-cell development and stimulation appear to keep this risk to a minimum.

It is now known that in most cases, increased susceptibility to rheumatoid arthritis is directly associated with the DRB1 locus, with the majority of patients with rheumatoid arthritis possessing the DRB1*0101, DRB1*0401, DRB1*0404, or DRB1*0405 genetic allotypes *(11)*. Individuals possessing these allotypes have a fourfold greater risk of developing rheumatoid arthritis compared to that of the general population. In addition, there is some evidence that combined expression of susceptibility alleles leads to a greater risk and increased severity of rheumatoid arthritis *(12–15)*. The relationship between the expression of specific DR alleles and the predisposition to develop rheumatoid-arthritis has been the subject of intense study. Structural analysis of both rheumatoid-arthritis–associated and nonassociated DRB1 alleles has revealed a conserved sequence within the amino acid residues 67–74 of the alpha helical portion of DRB1 chains associated with rheumatoid arthritis. This polypeptide sequence, termed the shared epitope *(16–18)*, has become the focus of several hypotheses aimed at defining the mechanism(s) by which class II alleles predispose the risk of developing rheumatoid arthritis; conceivably this information will identify disease specific antigens and eventually the etiological mechanism of the disease *(19–23)*. One hypothesis proposes that the shared epitope acts as a recognition structure for the T-cell receptor (TCR) involved in the selection of pathogenic T-cells that promote the autoimmune response *(21)*. Stimulation of such pathogenic T-cells would still be dependent on the presence of an antigenic peptide, of unknown origin, bound and presented by the DR molecule. Others have suggested that the shared epitope contributes specificity to the binding pocket located in the same region of the DR molecule *(24,25)*, thus potentially allowing for the selection of pathogenic peptides by the susceptibility alleles. Specifically, the amino acid residue 71, which is located within the shared epitope of the DRB1 chain, has been found to contribute to the peptide-binding specificity of the DR4 molecule *(26,27)*.

The shared epitope has also received considerable attention as the potential source of a peptide that alters either the function of other MHC class II molecules or T-cell selection, rather than a structural element in the function of the DRB1 molecule. Zanelli et al. *(22)* proposed that the shared epitope sequence is the source of an antigenic peptide that influences the function of the HLA-DQ8 class II molecule. This MHC molecule is closely linked to the expression of DR alleles associated with rheumatoid arthritis *(28,29)*; thus, an extended DQ/DR haplotype is proposed to confer susceptibility to rheumatoid arthritis, and the shared epitope as a peptide, derived from the DRB1 chain, is proposed to control this susceptibility *(23)*. According to this hypothesis, if this DRB1 peptide is derived from a nonsusceptible DR allele, it will bind tightly to an HLA-DQ8 molecule and this DQ8-peptide complex will alter the T-cell repertoire, resulting in protection from rheumatoid arthritis *(23)*. However, when the analogous peptide is derived from DRB1 alleles associated with susceptibility to rheumatoid arthritis, it binds poorly to the DQ molecule, thus allowing the potentially autoreactive T-cells to survive. By contrast to the shared epitope hypotheses just described, this hypothetical scheme predicts that the DQ molecule, and not the DR molecule, mediates the autoimmune response in rheumatoid arthritis. Indeed, experimental support for this hypothesis has been demonstrated recently; transgenic HLA-DQ8 mice are susceptible to collagen-induced arthritis (CIA) elicited by immunization with a candidate rheumatoid arthritis antigen, type II collagen (CII) *(30)*.

If an antigen-specific response drives the autoimmunity of rheumatoid arthritis, then what is the antigen? This question has puzzled investigators since the recognition of rheumatoid arthritis as an autoimmune disease. Certainly there has been no shortage of candidate antigens, and new ones are destined to emerge. The difficulty has been in convincingly demonstrating immunity or autoimmunity to the proposed antigens in the majority of rheumatoid arthritis patients. A number of plausible explanations can be offered for this difficulty including (1) rheumatoid arthritis is actually a collection of autoimmune diseases in which the initiating antigen/event differs among different forms of the disease; (2) perhaps rheumatoid arthritis is not an autoimmune disease *per se*, but rather a manifestation of unregulated inflammatory responses brought on by such factors as microbial infections or superantigen stimulation; or (3) by the time rheumatoid arthritis is diagnosed, the antigenic repertoire of the autoimmune response is obfuscated by the overwhelming inflammatory response. Immunity to a number of different antigens has been detected in rheumatoid arthritis patients, and candidate antigens for the autoimmune response in rheumatoid arthritis have included gp39 (a component of articular cartilage) *(31)*, mycobacterium and heat shock proteins *(32)*, CII *(33–36)*, Epstein-Barr virus *(37)*, cytomegalovirus *(38)*, and proteoglycan *(39)*. Because it is not possible to fully test Koch's postulate for any of these antigens, it will be difficult to determine if any of these actually induces the autoimmunity responsible for rheumatoid arthritis. Indeed, it has been suggested that a combination of antigenic stimuli in concert with genetic risk factors is required *(40)*.

An important approach to study the role of the potential antigens in rheumatoid arthritis has been to use them to establish animal models of experimental autoimmune arthritis (Table 1; for a review of animal models, *see* ref. *41*). Because rheumatoid arthritis is an autoimmune disease of articular joints, the focus of most animal models has been to use constituents of cartilage, such as gp39, proteoglycan (aggrecan), or CII as antigen. For each of these model antigens, immunization of specific strains of rodents leads to the development of a polyarticular autoimmune arthritis that resembles rheumatoid arthritis. The animals develop an inflammatory polyarticular arthritis with prominent synovitis and erosion of cartilage and bone, and the susceptibility is linked to the expression of specific class II molecules of the murine MHC. Of these model antigens, CII, a major component of articular cartilage, has received

Table 1
Animal Models of Autoimmune Arthritis

Antigen	Animal model	Genetic susceptibility	Reference
Type II collagen	Mouse	MHC I-A^q and I-A^r	*144*
Type II collagen	Transgenic mouse	MHC DRB1*0101 and DRB1*0401	*57,58*
Type II collagen	Rat	MHC RT-1^a, RT-1^{av1}, RT-1^b, RT-1^l, RT-1^u	*145,146*
Type XI collagen	Mouse	MHC I-A^q	*147*
Proteoglycan (aggrecan)	Mouse	MHC I-Ad	*148*
Mycobacterium (adjuvant)	Rat	MHC and non-MHC^a	*149*
Pristane	rat and mouse	MHC and non-MHC	*150–153*
Streptococcal cell wall	Rat and mouse	MHC and non-MHC	*154*
None (spontaneous)	Transgenic mouse	MHC with TCR transgene	*155*

^{a}Genetic susceptibility not fully defined, but clearly is a mix of MHC genes and non-MHC genes.

considerable attention as a potential autoantigen in rheumatoid arthritis for several reasons. First, CIA can be elicited in several species including mouse *(42)*, rat *(43)*, and monkey *(44,45)*. Second, several studies have demonstrated the existence of T-cell *(36)* or B-cell *(46–49)* immunity to CII in rheumatoid arthritis patients, and anti-CII antibodies have been eluted from a high percentage of joint cartilages of rheumatoid arthritis patients *(50)*. The autoimmune response in the murine CIA model is typified by both a strong T- and B-cell response, capable of recognizing the autoantigen murine CII *(51)*. Like the studies in rheumatoid arthritis *(50)*, antibody specific for homologous CII can be readily detected in the arthritic joints of mice. Based on experiments of passive transfer of disease with sera or CII-specific monoclonal antibodies *(52–54)*, it appears that antibody is the major immunological mechanism of pathogenesis in the CIA model. Although, for obvious ethical reasons, it is yet to be demonstrated that the CII-specific antibody found in rheumatoid arthritis patients is pathogenic, passive transfer of such antibodies into mice induces a destructive arthritis *(55)*.

Although these data do not indicate that autoimmunity to CII is the initiating event in rheumatoid arthritis, it does seem clear that at least some of the autoimmunity in rheumatoid arthritis is directed toward CII. The difficulty, however, has been in determining the relationship between immunity to CII and the role of the HLA-DR alleles that confer susceptibility to rheumatoid arthritis. Recently, transgenic mice expressing the HLA-DR1 (DRB1*0101) or DR4 (DRB1*0401) rheumatoid arthritis susceptibility alleles were produced to address this relationship *(56)*. Both of these DR alleles were found to bind and present antigenic peptides derived from human CII, and immunization of the DR transgenic mice with human CII elicited an autoimmune arthritis identical to that seen in the nontransgenic CIA model described above *(57,58)*. Thus the autoimmunity to CII observed in rheumatoid arthritis patients is likely mediated by the DR1 and DR4 alleles that confer susceptibility to rheumatoid arthritis. If this proves true, this autoimmune response could be targeted therapeutically, in an immunospecific manner, to create a noninflammatory environment within the diseased joint. It is interesting to note that both of these rheumatoid arthritis-associated alleles, DR1 and DR4, bound and presented the same antigenic determinants derived from human CII *(57–59)*, yet the CII-specific T-cells are clearly DR1 or DR4 restricted. Consequently, it may be possible to design an immunospecific therapy based on the antigenic determinant that will affect both DR-mediated responses.

Most of the dominant T-cell determinants that have been described for CII, regardless of their MHC restriction, are clustered within a small region of the CII molecule. The dominant determinant, CII(260–267), for I-A^q, one of the natural murine susceptibility alleles, partially overlaps with the HLA-DR1 and DR4 determinant, CII(263–270), although they clearly utilize different class II binding motifs *(59,60)*. Why this should be is not clear, and may be more representative of the primary structure of the collagen molecule itself. Since these determinants are all derived from the alpha helical portion of CII, they all have a repetitive primary amino acid sequence of Gly-X-Y, in which X and Y are frequently proline and hydroxyproline, respectively. Since Gly has no side chain with which to interact with a binding pocket within the class II molecules, the number of potential antigenic peptides contained in a Gly-rich protein would likely be lower than the number of antigenic peptides in a noncollagenous protein. Indeed, given its size (>1000 amino acids), very few antigenic peptides have been identified in CII, regardless of the specificity of the class II molecule *(57,58,61)*. Structural analysis of the CII molecule indicates that the region that contains these antigenic determinants is indeed unique to the CII molecule.

Inflammatory Component of Autoimmune Arthritis
Mediators of Inflammation

Although rheumatoid arthritis is classified as an autoimmune disease, the hallmark of its pathology is an intense, severe, and chronic inflammation. The process of inflammation in general is initiated and perpetuated through a complex network of immunological and biochemical reactions elicited in response to physical or immunological insults. At the cellular level, the inflammatory response is characterized by the mobilization and infiltration of neutrophils, mononuclear leukocytes, and macrophages to the site of inflammation. The infiltrating cells produce an array of biologically active molecules that initiate a cascade of intracellular and intercellular signaling events capable of affecting both lymphoid and nonlymphoid cells; thus, macrophages, lymphocytes, synovial fibroblasts, and endothelial cells are activated to produce additional mediators that further perpetuate the inflammatory response. The two major components of the rheumatoid arthritis susceptibility phenotype that the authors will consider here are the generation of proinflammatory cytokines (e.g., IL-1 and TNF-α) and their ability to stimulate lymphoid and nonlymphoid cells to produce eicosanoid inflammatory mediators. Although many other potent biological agents participate in the pathology of rheumatoid arthritis, such as the vaso- and neuroactive peptides, growth factors, pro- and anti-inflammatory cytokines, and a variety of noneicosanoid, lipid-derived mediators, such as diacylglycerol, phosphatidic acid, ceramide, platelet-activating factor, and other lysophospholipids, a comprehensive discussion of these is well outside the scope of this chapter.

The eicosanoids are oxygenated metabolites of arachidonic acid that are divided into the prostanoids (PGs, thromboxanes, and prostacyclins) and the leukotrienes (LTs). Functionally they may act as paracrine and/or autocrine hormones *(62)*. Because the expression and engagement of specific cell surface receptors stimulate varied biochemical signaling pathways that modulate immune and inflammatory responses *(63)*, the relationship between enhanced PG synthesis and inflammation is complex. However, the importance of prostanoids in arthritis may be best exemplified by the prevalent use of nonsteroidal anti-inflammatory drugs (NSAIDs), which inhibit prostanoid production, as a primary mode of treatment for diseases characterized by acute and/or chronic inflammation *(64–70)*. The perpetuation of downstream inflammatory signals via the generation of prostanoids and other inflammatory mediators is largely regulated by cytokines produced by activated T-cells. Again, in addition to induction of prostanoid synthesis, cytokines induce the production of an array of other multifunctional, lipid- and nonlipid-derived, intra- and extracellular signaling molecules including other cytokines, which modulate the inflammatory response; many have feedback regulatory effects on the cells involved in mediating the immune response themselves. Indeed, the multifunctional properties of cytokines adds to the overall complexity of this signaling network, and although cytokine-induced prostanoid synthesis represents a major inflammatory pathway, it is but one of many critical pathways stimulated by cytokines.

Proinflammatory Cytokines

Two prototypic proinflammatory cytokines that are potent inducers of prostanoid synthesis are IL-1β and TNF-α; both are produced and secreted by lymphocytes and monocytes as well as some nonlymphoid tissues in response to a variety of stimuli *(71)*. Monoclonal antibodies directed against IL-1β and TNF-α or disruption of cytokine-receptor binding by specific receptor antagonists appear to abrogate at least some of the inflammatory responses seen in animal models of disease *(72–74)* and in rheumatoid arthritis *(75,76)*. IL-1β induces synovitis after intra-articular injection and anti-IL-1β antibodies prevent the spontaneous arthritis seen in TNF-α transgenic rats, suggesting that the effect of TNF-α may be mediated by IL-1β *(72)*. The systemic administration of IL-1β, like TNF-α, increases the incidence and severity of CIA in mice, and it also accelerates the time of arthritis onset *(77)*. TNF-α not only accelerates arthritis in passively immunized rats when administered intra-articularly, but also when given systemically to actively immunized animals *(78)*.

Regulation of Prostanoid Synthesis

Prostanoids, such as prostaglandin E_2 (PGE$_2$), are pivotal modulators of tissue homeostasis, and their aberrant regulation is known to cause serious pathophysiological consequences *(62,63,79,80)*. The pathways summarizing the regulation of prostanoid biosynthesis and their involvement as modulators of immune and/or inflammatory responses are shown in Fig. 1. Synthesis of PGE$_2$ is regulated by successive metabolic steps involving the release and conversion of arachidonic acid to PGE$_2$ *(62,79–82)*. Although cytosolic phospholipase A_2 is primarily responsible for agonist-induced arachidonic acid release from membrane phospholipids *(83,84)*, secretory PLA$_2$ may also regulate arachidonic acid availability via a transcellular mechanism *(85)*. The LTs are formed from the conversion of arachidonic acid by the 5-lipoxygenase pathway (for review, *see* ref. *62*). Conversion of arachidonic acid to prostanoids is mediated by the rate-limiting reactions catalyzed by cyclooxygenases (COX), COX-1 and COX-2, which are encoded by two unique genes, located on different chromosomes *(79)*. Whereas COX-1 is generally constitutively expressed, the expression of COX-2 is highly inducible *(62,79)*. Based on their respective modes of expression, it is believed that COX-1 is primarily involved in cellular homeostasis whereas COX-2 plays a major role in inflammation and mitogenesis. The COX isoenzymes are the primary target enzymes for NSAIDs, which act by inhibiting the COX activity of COX-1 and

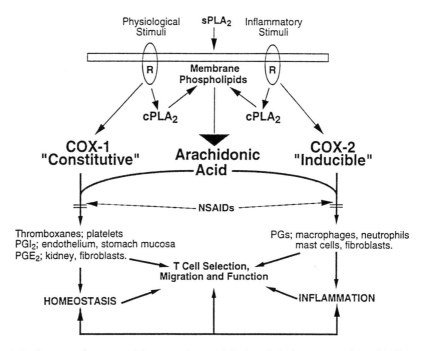

Fig. 1. Pathways of prostanoid generation and their role in homeostasis and inflammation. Ligated specific cell-surface receptors couple the mobilization of arachidonic acid as well as its conversion to PGs by activating phospholipase A_2 (PLA_2) and COX. Depending on the type of cell and stimuli, COX-1 and/or COX-2 catalyze the conversion of arachidonic acid to PGH_2, the common precursor for all PGs. PG generation is cell-type specific, and PGs ultimately become part of a complex signal transduction system that modulates the immune response, inflammation, and homeostasis. NSAIDs inhibit COX-1 and COX-2, thereby blocking the generation of PGs and providing a mechanism for therapeutic intervention.

COX-2, thereby blocking their ability to convert arachidonic acid to PGG_2 *(86,87)*. In addition to the use of NSAIDs as analgesics and for alleviation of acute and chronic inflammation, these agents have proven effective in decreasing the frequency of heart attacks and strokes *(64,67,88)*, and in reducing the incidence of colon cancer *(89, 90)*. While these observations suggest a complete functional separation of COX-1 and COX-2 derived prostanoids, there is undoubtedly crosstalk between the two COX enzymes and their products in terms of their respective contributions to homeostasis, inflammation, and the modulation of the immune response via direct effects on T-cell selection, migration, and function.

Prostanoids and LTs as Feedback Modulators of the Immune Response

In addition to the direct role of prostanoids as mediators of inflammation, PGs and the LTs also modulate downstream lymphocyte functions (for review, *see* ref. *63*). For example, eicosanoids are involved in the negative and positive selection of $CD4^+$ and $CD8^+$ thymocytes and thereby influence the balance between CD4/CD8 positive T-cells. Both PGE_2 and LTs inhibit thymocyte apoptosis whereas thromboxane A_2 promotes apoptosis via a PGE_2-inhibitable pathway, thus influencing the selection process *(91)*. B-cell function is also affected by eicosanoids by means of differential selection of immature vs mature B-lymphocytes; PGE_2 inhibits mature B-lymphocyte function *(92)* whereas it induces apoptosis in immature B-cells. Eicosanoids enhance the ability of T-cells to migrate across the basement membrane by stimulating chemotaxis and by enhancing their production of metalloproteinases which are involved in basement membrane degeneration *(93)*. Furthermore, eicosanoids modulate T-cell effector specificity by affecting the types of cytokines they produce via effects on the proliferation of antagonistic T helper and T suppressor cells *(94)*. Thus, both prostanoids and LTs play central roles in the mechanisms involved in the induction and perpetuation of the inflammatory reactions characteristically associated with autoimmune arthritis.

MMPs in Autoimmune Arthritis

The degradation of articular cartilage is a central feature in the pathology of rheumatoid arthritis, and the MMPs derived from synovial cells, infiltrating inflammatory cells, and resident chondrocytes play a key role in this process. The MMP family of enzymes consists of at least 16 distinct entities including collagenases, gelatinases, stromelysins, matrilysin, and the membrane type MMPs *(95)*. All the known extracellular matrix components including collagens, proteoglycans, elastins, and matrix glycoproteins can be degraded by the various MMPs elaborated *in situ*. Because the production of most MMPs is upregulated by inflammatory cytokines, it is widely accepted that in rheumatoid arthritis, increased expression of these enzymes plays a major role in the degradation of cartilage and subchondral bone. Articular cartilage is truly a unique tissue because its constituent cells exist in single lacunae without direct contact with other cells. Cartilage is avascular and is highly resistant to invasion by blood vessels and tumor cells. The extracellular matrix of articular cartilage is also unique in its composition. The collagens found in cartilage are specific to cartilage and to the vitreous of the eye. The architectural framework of cartilage extracellular matrix is made up of type II, IX, and XI collagens, the majority of which is type II, and is assembled into highly ordered, wide, cross-banded collagen fibril structure *(96,97)*. Although much of the work to date has focused on the degradation of proteoglycan by the stromelysins, it is the MMP-mediated disruption of the collagenous scaffold that leads to irreversible joint dysfunction in rheumatoid arthritis *(98)*.

The collagenase subfamily of the MMPs is composed of three different enzymes: (1) fibroblast collagenase (MMP-1 or collagenase-1) *(99)*; (2) neutrophil collagenase (MMP-8 or collagenase-2) *(100)*; and, (3) collagenase-3 (MMP-13) *(101)*. All three collagenases are upregulated by major inflammatory cytokines (e.g., IL-1 and TNF-α) implicated in the pathophysiology of rheumatoid arthritis. Although investigation of cartilage degradation has historically concentrated on collagenase-1, evidence to date supports that both collagenase-2 and -3 are upregulated in rheumatoid arthritis *(102)*. Collerganse-3, the newest member of the family, degrades soluble CII at a rate 20-fold higher than collagenase-1, suggesting a major role for this enzyme in cartilage destruction *(103)*. Messenger RNAs encoding collagenase-1, -2, and -3 are readily detected in cartilage stimulated with inflammatory mediators *(104,105)*. Normal porcine chondrocytes constitutively express collagenase-1 and -3, but only express collagenase-2 after stimulation with inflammatory mediators *(106)*. Thus, the upregulation of the three collagenases by a wide spectrum of agents supports the notion that collagenolytic activity in cartilage is the collective summation of at least three distinct collagenases that degrade the interstitial collagens and cartilage proteoglycans. It will be critical to determine the origin and contribution of each of the collagenases before effective therapeutic strategies to protect cartilage collagens can be designed.

One of the earliest lesions in rheumatoid arthritis is synovial hypertrophy owing to proliferation of the synovial lining cells, giving rise to villi of tissue that project into the synovial cavity adjacent to the articular surface. In rheumatoid arthritis, this interface is characteristically the vanguard of the eroded cartilage. It is not surprising that increased levels of several different MMPs are present in the synovial pannus because MMP production is characteristic of a proliferative response of many different cell types, including activated macrophages *(107)*. Inflammatory cell infiltrates also contribute to the upregulated expression of MMPs. Although high numbers of neutrophils for short periods of time, such as seen in gout, may not be associated with significant cartilage degradation, the resulting moderate excess of collagenase-2 produced by theses neutrophils over months or years in the rheumatoid patient may significantly contribute to the overall pathology. Lymphocytes and monocytes also infiltrate the joint and secrete a variety of inflammatory cytokines that stimulate MMP production. Increased MMP expression occurs in response to a number of growth factors and cytokines, such as TNF-α and -β, IL-1α and -β, platelet-derived growth factor, and basic fibroblast growth factor. Many of these pathways converge commonly at the AP-1 binding site present on many MMP genes *(108–110)* (for review, *see* ref. *111*), which has been defined as the phorbol ester response element *(112,113)*. Significantly, increased AP-1 activity can be detected in nuclear extracts from synovial cells and macrophages isolated from rheumatoid synovium as compared to those isolated from osteoarthritis synovium *(114)*.

Although many of the growth factors and cytokines stimulate MMP production, very few have been shown to directly downregulate MMP synthesis. Retinoic acid has been shown to downregulate the expression of rat stromelysin *(115)*, but by contrast it upregulates collagenase-3 expression, similar to its effect on human chondrocytes *(116)*. These differential effects likely contributed to the lack of effective treatment of rheumatoid arthritis with retinamide *(117)*. IFN-γ also differentially affects MMP expression, dependent on cell type, downregulating collagenase-1 and stromelysin-1 in fibroblasts *(118)* and macrophages *(119)* but upregulating their expression in keratinocytes *(120)*. The cytokine-induced upregulation of most MMPs is prevented by transforming growth factor-β (TGF-β) treatment (for review *see* ref. *121*); downregulation of MMPs by TGF-β1 is of considerable interest because high levels of TGF-β are produced in synovial tissues of rheumatoid arthritis *(122)*. The negative regulation by TGF-β on rat stromelysin transcription is mediated by the TGF-β inhibitory element localized in the rat stromelysin-1 promoter *(123)*, and requires induction of c-fos expression. This is somewhat paradoxical, because c-*fos* expression is necessary for induction of stromelysin by a number of growth factors, tumor promoters, and oncogenes through an AP-1–dependent mechanism *(124)*.

Therapeutic Prospects in Autoimmune Arthritis

The pathogenesis of rheumatoid arthritis is multifaceted, and virtually every mechanistic aspect of the disease is amenable to being exploited for therapeutic intervention. These approaches have included antibodies to cytokines and cellular antigens, anti-inflammatory cytokines, soluble cytokine receptors, vaccinations, oral tolerance, and, more recently, gene therapy. Unfortunately the lack of identification of infectious agents or antigens capable of inducing rheumatoid arthritis has limited most of the therapeutic approaches in rheumatoid arthritis to nonspecifically controlling the immune response or blocking the action of the proinflammatory cytokines or the MMPs responsible for cartilage degradation. Although two approaches to specific immunotherapy have been tried in patients, TCR vaccinations *(125)* and oral tolerance with CII *(126,127)*, neither has been very successful at reducing the overall pathology of the disease. However, it is not clear if the basic approaches were flawed or whether their application was not sufficiently defined for rheumatoid arthritis. In the case of TCR vaccination for rheumatoid arthritis, a specific TCR Vβ element was selected as the vaccinogen based on its expression by T-cells in the synovium of a majority of rheumatoid arthritis patients analyzed. Since the antigen specificity of this receptor is unknown, it is not clear what the role of this receptor is in the disease process. Both oral tolerance and TCR vaccination approaches have been used successfully in the CIA model of rheumatoid arthritis *(128–131)* and the experimental autoimmune encephalitis (EAE) model of another autoimmune disease, multiple sclerosis *(132–136)*, but in both cases the antigens responsible for inducing the experimental autoimmune disease were known, and the TCRs utilized were specific for these antigens. Once again these data indicate how much the therapeutic approaches to rheumatoid arthritis are hindered by the lack of knowledge of its etiology.

Biological therapies for rheumatoid arthritis, the use of molecules produced by cells of the immune system or those that participate in the inflammatory reactions, have been used in several different clinical studies. Of all the therapeutic regimens tested, including antibodies to CD antigens, intercellular adhesion molecules, cytokines, and others, the best results to date have been achieved by treatment with a chimeric antibody specific for TNF-α. In a double-blind, controlled clinical trial, in vivo infusion of a TNF-α antibody was found to be highly effective in the treatment of rheumatoid arthritis *(137,138)*. Similarly, soluble TNF-α receptor has also been shown to be an effective means of inhibiting TNF-α function *(75)*. The inactivation or removal of TNF-α from rheumatoid arthritis joints affected the inflammatory response in several ways. Both MMP-1 and, especially, MMP-3 levels were significantly reduced following treatment with anti–TNF-α *(139)*. In addition, decreases in cell influx into the synovium were also observed, apparently as a result of decreased expression of cellular adhesion molecules *(140)*. Studies in the CIA model of rheumatoid arthritis indicate that the anti-inflammatory effect of anti–TNF-α may actually be enhanced by cotreatment with an antibody specific for IL-1α/β. Although several questions remain unanswered concerning potential host immune responses to the mouse/human chimeric antibody and the effectiveness of repeat administration, in all, these studies with TNF-α are quite promising. Similarly, approaches to prevent IL-1 function have also been found to be effective in reducing inflammatory responses, and the combination of anti–TNF-α and anti–IL-1α/β proved to be even more efficient in preventing autoimmune arthritis in the CIA model *(141)*.

The pace of discovery to devise gene-based therapies for rheumatoid arthritis has accelerated tremendously in recent years. The present gene therapy research is aimed at efficiently delivering genes encoding anti-inflammatory cytokines (e.g., TGF-β1 or IL-1 receptor antagonist [IL-1 Ra]) to the inflamed synovium. In the CIA animal model, DNA encoding TGF-β1 packaged in a retrovirus was used successfully to reduce the inflammation of active disease and to prevent spreading to unaffected joints *(142)*.

Similarly, coimplantation of human IL-1 Ra expressing synovial fibroblasts with normal human cartilage in immunodeficient mice completely prevented cartilage degradation *(143)*. Although expectations based on these studies are high for current clinical trials, there remain a number of problems that must be addressed before gene therapy for rheumatoid arthritis becomes a reality. The selection of a safe and efficient vector for transmitting the gene to the targeted tissue is critical; better means by which desirable levels of expression can be achieved for suitable durations need to be devised. If the therapy is to be in vivo based, tissue specificity of the vector is important, although this can be overcome somewhat by ex vivo infection of cells and subsequent transplantation. The investigators also must be mindful of the possible systemic effects of generalized inhibition of these cytokines that play important roles in other desirable immune and inflammatory responses. Finally, very few, if any, of these therapeutic approaches represent an attempt to cure the disease, a problem largely owing to the unknown etiology of rheumatoid arthritis. Regardless, several investigators appear to be on the verge of new biological therapies that will significantly reduce the inflammation with perhaps fewer side effects than current pharmaceutical treatments.

References

1. Stastny, P., Ball, E. J., Dry, P. J., and Nunez, G. (1983) The human immune response region (HLA-D) and disease susceptibility. *Immunol. Rev.* **70**, 113–154.
2. Stastny, P., Ball, E., Kahn, M., Olsen, N., Pincus, T., and Gao, X. (1988) HLA-DR4 and other genetic markers in rheumatoid arthritis. *Br. J. Rheumatol.* **27**, 132–138.
3. Nepom, G. T., Byers, P., Seyfried, C., Healey, L. A., Wilske, K. R., Stage, D., and Nepom, B. S. (1989) HLA genes associated with rheumatoid arthritis: Iidentification of susceptibility alleles using specific oligonucleotide probes. *Arthritis Rheum.* **32**, 15–21.
4. Babbit, B., Allen, P. M., Matsueda, G., Haber, E., and Unanue, E. R. (1985) Binding of immunogenic peptides to Ia histocompatibility molecules. *Nature* **317**, 359–361.
5. Allen, P. M., Matsueda, G. R., Evans, R. J., Dunbar, J. B. J., Marshall, G. R., and Unanue, E. R. (1987) Identification of the T-cell and Ia contact residues of a T-cell antigenic epitope. *Nature* **327**, 713–715.
6. Rosloniec, E. F., Vitez, L. J., Buus, S., and Freed, J. H. (1990) MHC class II-derived peptides can bind to class II molecules, including self molecules, and prevent antigen presentation. *J. Exp. Med.* **171**, 1419–1430.
7. Benichou, G., Takizawa, P. A., Ho, P. T., Killiow, C. C., Olson, C. A., McMillan, M., and Sercarz, E. E. (1990) Immunogenicity and tolerogenicity of self-MHC peptides. *J. Exp. Med.* **172**, 1341–1346.
8. Vogt, A. B., Kropshofer, H., Kalbacher, H., Kalbus, M., Rammensee, H. G., Coligan, J. E., and Martin, R. (1994) Ligand motifs of HLA-DRB5*0101 and DRB1*1501 molecules delineated from self-peptides. *J. Immunol.* **153**, 1665–1673.
9. Rudensky, A. Y., Preston-Hurlburt, P., Hong, S., Barlow, A., and Janeway, C. A. (1991) Sequence analysis of peptides bound to MHC class II molecules. *Nature* **353**, 622–627.
10. Chicz, R. M., Urban, R. G., Gorga, J., Vignali, D. A. A., Lane, W. S., and Strominger, J. L. (1993) Specificity and promiscuity among naturally processed peptides bound to HLA-DR alleles. *J. Exp. Med.* **178**, 27–47.
11. Wordsworth, B. P., Lanchbury, J. S., Sakkas, L. I., Welsh, K. I., Panayi, G. S., and Bell, J. I. (1989) HLA-DR4 subtype frequencies in rheumatoid arthritis indicate that DRB1 is the major susceptibility locus within the HLA class II region. *Proc. Natl. Acad. Sci. USA* **86**, 10,049–10,053.
12. Moreno, I., Valenzula, A., García, A., Yélamos, J., Sánchez, B., and Hernánz, W. (1996) Association of the shared epitope with radiological severity of rheumatoid arthritis. *J. Rheumatol.* **23**, 6–9.
13. Evans, T. I., Han, J., Singh, R., and Moxley, G. (1995) The genotypic distribution of shared-epitope DRB1 alleles suggests a recessive mode of inheritance of the rheumatoid arthritis disease-susceptibility gene. *Arthritis Rheum.* **38**, 1754–1761.

14. Weyand, C. M., Xie, C., and Goronzy, J. J. (1992) Homozygosity for the HLA-DRB1 allele selects for extraarticular manifestations in rheumatoid arthritis. *J. Clin. Invest.* **89,** 2033–2039.
15. Weyand, C. M., Hicok, K. C., Conn, D. L., and Goronzy, J. J. (1992) The influence of HLA-DRB1 genes on disease severity in rheumatoid arthritis. *Ann. Intern. Med.* **117,** 801–806.
16. Gregersen, P., Silver, J., and Winchester, R. (1987) The shared epitope hypothesis: an approach to understanding the molecular genetics of susceptibility to rheumatoid arthritis. *Arthritis Rheum.* **30,** 1205–1213.
17. Winchester, R., Dwyer, E., and Rose, S. (1992) The genetic basis of rheumatoid arthritis. The shared epitope hypothesis. *Rheum. Dis. Clin. North. Am.* **18,** 761–783.
18. Winchester, R., and Dwyer, E. (1991) MHC and autoimmune diseases: Susceptibility to rheumatoid arthritis associated with a hydrophobic strip of alpha helix encoded by several MHC alleles. *Immunol. Ser.* **55,** 203–219.
19. Albani, S., Tuckwell, J. E., Esparza, L., Carson, D. A., and Roudier, J. (1992) The susceptibility sequence to rheumatoid arthritis is a cross-reactive B cell epitope shared by the Escherichia coli heat shock protein dnaJ and the histocompatibility leukocyte antigen DRB10401 molecule. *J. Clin. Invest.* **89,** 327–331.
20. Albani, S., Carson, D. A., and Roudier, J. (1992) Genetic and environmental factors in the immune pathogenesis of rheumatoid arthritis. *Rheum. Dis. Clin. North. Am.* **18,** 729–740.
21. Penzotti, J. E., Doherty, D., Lybrand, T. P., and Nepom, G. T. (1996) A structural model for TCR recognition of the HLA class II shared epitope sequence implicated in susceptibility to rheumatoid arthritis. *J. Autoimmunity* **9,** 287–293.
22. Zanelli, E., Gonzalez-Gay, M. A., and David, C. S. (1995) Could HLA-DRB1 be the protective locus in rheumatoid arthritis? *Immunol. Today* **16,** 274–278.
23. Zanelli, E., Krco, C. J., Baisch, J. M., Cheng, S., and David, C. S. (1996) Immune response of HLA-DQ8 transgenic mice to peptides from the third hypervariable region of HLA-DRB1 correlates with predisposition to rheumatoid arthritis. *Proc. Natl. Acad. Sci. USA* **93,** 1814–1819.
24. Woulfe, S. L., Bono, C. P., Zacheis, M. L., Kirschmann, D. A., Baudino, T. A., Swearingen, C., Karr, R. W., and Schwartz, B. D. (1995) Negatively charged residues interacting with the p4 pocket confer binding specificity to DRB1*0401. *Arthritis Rheum.* **38,** 1744–1753.
25. Kirschmann, D. A., Duffin, K. L., Smith, C. E., Welply, J. K., Howard, S. C., Schwartz, B. D., and Woulfe, S. L. (1995) Naturally processed peptides from rheumatoid arthritis associated and nonassociated HLA-DR alleles. *J. Immunol.* **155,** 5655–5662.
26. Hammer, J., Gallazi, F., Bono, E., Karr, R. W., Guenot, J., Valsasnini, P., Nagy, Z. A., and Sinigaglia, F. (1995) Peptide binding specificity of HLA-DR4 molecules: correlation with rheumatoid arthritis association. *J. Exp. Med.* **181,** 1847–1855.
27. Weyand, C. M., McCarthy, T. G., and Goronzy, J. J. (1995) Correlation between disease phenotype and genetic heterogeneity in rheumatoid arthritis. *J. Clin. Invest.* **95,** 2120–2126.
28. Lanchbury, J. S., Sakkas, L. I., Marsh, S. G., Bodmer, J. G., Welsh, K. I., and Panayi, G. S. (1989) HLA-DQ beta 3.1 allele is a determinant of susceptibility to DR4-associated rheumatoid arthritis. *Hum. Immunol.* **26,** 59–71.
29. Singal, D. P., D'Souza, M., Reid, B., Bensen, W. G., Kassam, Y. B., and Adachi, J. D. (1987) HLA-DQ beta-chain polymorphism in HLA-DR4 haplotypes associated with rheumatoid arthritis. *Lancet* **2,** 1118–1120.
30. Nabozny, G. H., Baisch, J. M., Cheng, S., Cosgrove, D., Griffiths, M. M., Luthra, H. S., and David, C. S. (1996) HLA-DQ8 transgenic mice are highly susceptible to collagen-induced arthritis: A novel model for human polyarthritis. *J. Exp. Med.* **183,** 27–37.
31. Verheijden, G. F., Rijnders, A. W., Bos, E., Coenen-de Roo, C. J., van Staveren, C. J., Miltenburg, A. M., Meijerink, J. H., Elewaut, D., de Keyser, F., Veys, E., and Boots, A. M. (1997) Human cartilage glycoprotein-39 as a candidate autoantigen in rheumatoid arthritis. *Arthritis Rheum.* **40,** 1115–1125.
32. Hogervorst, E. J., Boog, C. J., Wagenaar, J. P., Wauben, M. H., Van der Zee, R., and Van Eden, W. (1991) T cell reactivity to an epitope of the mycobacterial 65-kDa heat-shock protein (hsp 65) corresponds with arthritis susceptibility in rats and is regulated by hsp 65–specific cellular responses. *Eur. J. Immunol.* **21,** 1289–1296.
33. Steffan, C. and Timpl, R. (1963) Antigenicity of collagen and its application in the serologic investigation of rheumatoid arthritis sera. *Int. Arch. Allergy Appl. Immunol.* **22,** 333–340.

34. Stuart, J. M., Postlethwaite, A. E., Townes, A. S., and Kang, A. H. (1980) *Cell*-mediated immunity to collagen and collagen α chains in rheumatoid arthritis and other rheumatic diseases. *Am. J. Med.* **69,** 13–18.

35. Stuart, J. M., Watson, W. C., and Kang, A. H. (1988) Collagen autoimmunity and arthritis. *FASEB J.* **2,** 2950–2956.

36. Londei, M., Savill, C. M., Verhoef, A., Brennan, F., Leech, Z. A., Duance, V., Maini, R. N., and Feldman, M. (1989) Persistence of collagen type II-specific T-cell clones in the synovial membrane of a patient with rheumatoid arthritis. *Proc. Natl. Acad. Sci. USA* **86,** 636–640.

37. Roudier, J., Rhodes, G., Petersen, J., Vaughan, J. H., and Carson, D. A. (1988) The Epstein-Barr virus glycoprotein gp110, a molecular link between HLA DR4, HLA DR1, and rheumatoid arthritis. *Scand. J. Immunol.* **27,** 367–371.

38. Fujinami, R. S., Nelson, J. A., Walker, L., and Oldstone, M. B. (1988) Sequence homology and immunologic cross-reactivity of human cytomegalovirus with HLA-DR beta chain: a means for graft rejection and immunosuppression. *J. Virol.* **62,** 100–105.

39. Banerjee, S. and Poole, A. R. (1992) Immunity to cartilage proteoglycans. *J. Rheumatol.* **19,** 36–39.

40. Weyand, C. M. and Goronzy, J. J. (1997) Pathogenesis of rheumatoid arthritis. *Med. Clin. North Am.* **81,** 29–55.

41. Brahn, E. (1991) Animal models of rheumatoid arthritis. Clues to etiology and treatment. *Clin. Orthop.* **265,** 42–53.

42. Courtenay, J. S., Dallman, M. J., Dayan, A. D., Martin, A., and Mosedale, B. (1980) Immunisation against heterologous type II collagen induces arthritis in mice. *Nature* **283,** 666–668.

43. Trentham, D. E., Townes, A. S., and Kang, A. H. (1977) Autoimmunity to type II collagen: an experimental model of arthritis. *J. Exp. Med.* **146,** 857–868.

44. Terato, K., Arai, H., Shimozuru, Y., Fukuda, T., Tanaka, H., Watanabe, H., Nagai, Y., Fujimoto, K., Okubo, F., Cho, F., Honjo, S., and Cremer, M. A. (1989) Sex-linked differences in susceptibility of cynomolgus monkeys to type II collagen-induced arthritis: evidence that epitope-specific immune suppression is involved in the regulation of type II collagen autoantibody formation. *Arthritis Rheum.* **6,** 748–758.

45. Yoo, T. J., Kim, S. Y., Stuart, J. M., Floyd, R. A., Olson, G. A., Cremer, M. A., and Kang, A. H. (1988) Induction of arthritis in monkeys by immunization with type II collagen. *J. Exp. Med.* **168,** 777–782.

46. Jasin, H. E. (1985) Autoantibody specificities of immune complexes sequestered in articular cartilage of patients with rheumatoid arthritis and osteoarthritis. *Arthritis Rheum.* **28,** 241–248.

47. Watson, W., Cremer, M., Wooley, P., and Townes, A. (1986) Assessment of the potential pathogenicity of type II collagen autoantibodies in patients with rheumatoid arthritis. *Arthritis Rheum.* **29,** 1316–1321.

48. Terato, K., Shimozuru, Y., Katayama, K., Takemitsu, Y., Yamashita, I., Miyatsu, M., Fujii, K., Sagara, M., Kobayashi, S., Goto, M., Nishioka, K., Miyasaka, N., and Nagai, Y. (1990) Specificity of antibodies to type II collagen in rheumatoid arthritis. *Arthritis Rheum.* **33,** 1493–1500.

49. Stuart, J. M., Huffstutter, E. H., Townes, A. S., and Kang, A. H. (1983) Incidence and specificity of antibodies to type I, II, III, IV, and V collagen in rheumatoid arthiritis and other rheumatic diseases as measured by 125I-radioimmunoassay. *Arthritis Rheum.* **26,** 832–840.

50. Watson, W. C., Tooms, R. E., Carnesale, P. G., and Dutkowsky, J. P. (1994) A case of germinal center formation by CD45RO T and CD20 B lymphocytes in rheumatoid arthritic subchondral bone: proposal for a two-compartment model of immune-mediated disease with implications for immunotherapeutic strategies. *Clin. Immunol. Immunopathol.* **73,** 27–37.

51. Brand, D. D., Marion, T. N., Myers, L. K., Rosloniec, E. F., Watson, W. C., Stuart, J. M., and Kang, A. H. (1996) Autoantibodies to murine type II collagen in collagen induced arthritis: a comparison of susceptible and non susceptible strains. *J. Immunol.* **157,** 5178–5184.

52. Terato, K., Hasty, K. A., Reife, R. A., Cremer, M. A., Kang, A. H., and Stuart, J. M. (1992) Induction of arthritis with monoclonal antibodies to collagen. *J. Immunol.* **148,** 2103–2108.

53. Stuart, J. M., Tomoda, K., Townes, A. S., and Kang, A. H. (1983) Serum transfer of collagen induced arthritis. II. Identification and localization of autoantibody to type II collagen in donor and recipient rats. *Arthritis Rheum.* **26,** 1237–1244.

54. Stuart, J. M. and Dixon, F. J. (1983) Serum transfer of collagen induced arthritis in mice. *J. Exp. Med.* **158,** 378–392.

55. Wooley, P. H., Luthra, S. H., Singh, S., Huse, A., Stuart, J. M., and David, C. S. (1984) Passive transfer of arthritis in mice by human anti-type II collagen antibody. *Mayo Clinic Proc.* **59**, 737–743.

56. Woods, A., Chen, H. Y., Trumbauer, M. E., Sirotina, A., Cummings, R., and Zaller, D. M. (1994) Human major histocompatibility complex class II-restricted T cell responses in transgenic mice. *J. Exp. Med.* **180**, 173–181.

57. Rosloniec, E. F., Brand, D. D., Myers, L. K., Esaki, Y., Whittington, K. B., Zaller, D. M., Wood, A., Stuart, J. M., and Kang, A. H. (1998) Induction of auotimmune arthritis in HLA-DR4 (DRB1*0401) transgenic mice by immunization with human and bovine type II collagen. *J. Immunol.*, **160**, 2573–2578.

58. Rosloniec, E. F., Brand, D. D., Myers, L. K., Whittington, K. B., Gumanovskaya, M., Zaller, D. M., Woods, A., Altmann, D. M., Stuart, J. M., and Kang, A. H. (1997) An HLA-DR1 transgene confers susceptibility to collagen-induced arthritis elicited with human type II collagen. *J. Exp. Med.* **185**, 1113–1122.

59. Fugger, L., Rothbard, J. B., and Sonderstrup-McDevitt, G. (1996) Specificity of an HLA-DRB1*0401-restricted T cell response to type II collagen. *Eur. J. Immunol.* **26**, 928–933.

60. Rosloniec, E. F., Whittington, K. B., Brand, D. D., Myers, L. K., and Stuart, J. M. (1996) Identification of MHC class II and TCR binding residues in the type II collagen immunodominant determinant mediating collagen induced arthritis. *Cell. Immunol.* **172**, 21–28.

61. Brand, D. D., Myers, L. K., Whittington, K. B., Stuart, J. M., Kang, A. H., and Rosloniec, E. F. (1994) Characterization of the T cell determinants in the induction of autoimmune arthritis by bovine α1(II)-CB11 in H-2^q mice. *J. Immunol.* **152**, 3088–3097.

62. Herschman, H. (1996) Prostaglandin synthase 2. *Biochim. Biophys. Acta* **1299**, 125–140.

63. Goetzl, E. J., An, S., and Smith, W. L. (1995) Specificity of expression and effects of eicosanoid mediators in normal physiology and human diseases. *FASEB J.* **9**, 1051–1058.

64. Vane, J. R. and Botting, R. M. (1995) New insights into the mode of action of anti-inflammatory drugs. *Inflamm. Res.* **44**, 1–10.

65. Smith, W. L., Meade, E. A., and De Witt, D. L. (1994) Pharmacology of prostaglandin endo-peroxide synthase isozymes-1 and -2. *Ann. NY Acad. Sci.* **714**, 136–142.

66. Barnett, J., Chow, J., Ives, D., Chiou, M., Mackenzie, R., Osen, E., Nguyen, B., Tsing, S., Bach, C., Freire, J., et al. (1994) Purification, characterization and selective inhibition of human prostaglandin G/H synthase 1 and 2 expressed in the baculovirus system. *Biochim. Biophys. Acta* **1209**, 130–139.

67. Vane, J. R. and Botting, R. M. (1994) Regulatory mechanisms of the vascular endothelium: an update. *Pol. J. Pharmacol.* **46**, 499–421.

68. Seibert, K. and Masferrer, J. L. (1994) Role of inducible cyclooxygenase (COX-2) in inflammation. *Receptor* **4**, 17–23.

69. Seibert, K., Zhang, Y., Leahy, K., Hauser, S., Masferrer, J., Perkins, W., Lee, L., and Isakson, P. (1994) Pharmacological and biochemical demonstration of the role of cyclooxygenase 2 in inflammation and pain. *Proc. Natl. Acad. Sci. USA* **91**, 12,013–12,017.

70. Seibert, K., Masferrer, J., Zhang, Y., Gregory, S., Olson, G., Hauser, S., Leahy, K., Perkins, W., and Isakson, P. (1995) Mediation of inflammation by cyclooxygenase-2. *Agents Actions Suppl.* **46**, 41–50.

71. Dinarello, C. A. (1994) Inflammatory cytokines: interleukin-1 and tumor necrosis factor as effector molecules in autoimmune disease. *Curr. Opin. Immunol.* **3**, 941–948.

72. Keffer, J., Probert, L., Cazlaris, H., Georgopoulos, S., Kaslaris, E., Kioussis, D., and Kollias, G. (1991) Transgenic mice expressing human tumour necrosis factor: a predictive genetic model of arthritis. *EMBO J.* **10**, 4025–4031.

73. Piguet, P. F., Grau, G. E., Vesin, C., Loetscher, H., Gentz, R., and Lesslauer, W. (1992) Evolution of collagen arthritis in mice is arrested by treatment with anti-tumour necrosis factor (TNF) antibody or a recombinant soluble TNF receptor. *Immunology* **77**, 510–514.

74. Williams, R. O., Feldmann, M., and Maini, R. N. (1992) Anti-tumor necrosis factor ameliorates joint disease in murine collagen-induced arthritis. *Proc. Natl. Acad. Sci. USA* **89**, 9784–9788.

75. Moreland, L. W., Baumgartner, S. W., Schiff, M. H., Tindall, E. A., Fleischmann, R. M., Weaver, A. L., Ettlinger, R. E., Cohen, S., Koopman, W. J., Mohler, K., Widmer, M. B., and Blosch, C. M. (1997) Treatment of RA with a recombinant human tumor necrosis factor receptor(p75)-Fc fusion protein. *N. Engl. J. Med.* **337**, 141–147.

76. Moreland, L. W., Heck, L. W., and Koopman, W. J. (1997) Biologic agents for treating rheumatoid arthritis. *Arthritis Rheum.* **40,** 397–409.

77. Hom, J. T., Cole, H., Estridge, T., and Gliszczynski, V. L. (1992) Interleukin-1 enhances the development of type II collagen-induced arthritis only in susceptible and not in resistant mice. *Clin. Immunol. Immunopathol.* **62,** 56–65.

78. Cooper, W. O., Fava, R. A., Gates, C. A., Cremer, M. A., and Townes, A. S. (1992) Acceleration of onset of collagen-induced arthritis by intra-articular injection of tumour necrosis factor or transforming growth factor-beta. *Clin. Exp. Immunol.* **89,** 244–250.

79. Smith, W. L., Garavito, R. M., and DeWitt, D. L. (1996) Prostaglandin endoperoxide H synthase (cyclooxygenases)-1 and -2. *J. Biol. Chem.* **271,** 33,157–33,160.

80. Herschman, H. R., Gilbert, R. S., Xie, W., Luner, S., and Reddy, S. T. (1995) The regulation and role of TIS10 prostaglandin synthase-2. *Adv. Prostaglandin Thromboxane Leukotriene Res.* **23,** 23–28.

81. Herschman, H. R. (1994) Regulation of prostaglandin synthase–1 and prostaglandin synthase-2. *Cancer Metastasis Rev.* **13,** 241–256.

82. Smith, W. L. and De Witt, D. L. (1995) *Biochemistry* of prostaglandin endoperoxide H synthase-1 and synthase-2 and their differential susceptibility to nonsteroidal anti-inflammatory drugs. *Semin. Nephrol.* **15,** 179–194.

83. Lin, L. L., Lin, A. Y., and Knopf, J. L. (1992) Cytosolic phospholipase A_2 is coupled to hormonally regulated release of arachidonic acid. *Proc. Natl. Acad. Sci. USA* **89,** 6147–6151.

84. Clark, J. D., Lin, L. L., Kriz, R. W., Ramesha, C. S., Sultzman, L. A., Lin, A. Y., Milona, N., and Knopf, J. L. (1991) A novel arachidonic acid-selective cytosolic PLA_2 contains a $Ca^{(2+)}$-dependent translocation domain with homology to PKC and GAP. *Cell* **65,** 1043–1051.

85. Reddy, S. T. and Herschman, H. R. (1996) Transcellular prostaglandin production following mast cell activation is mediated by proximal secretory phospholipase A_2 and distal prostaglandin synthase 1. *J. Biol. Chem.* **271,** 186–191.

86. Vane, J. R. and Botting, R. M. (1995) A better understanding of anti-inflammatory drugs based on isoforms of cyclooxygenase (COX-1 and COX-2) *Adv. Prostaglandin Thromboxane Leukotriene Res.* **23,** 41–48.

87. DeWitt, D. L., Meade, E. A., and Smith, W. L. (1993) PGH synthase isozyme selectivity: potential safer nonsteroidal antiinflammatory drugs. *Am. J. Med.* **95,** 40s–44s.

88. Vane, J. R. (1995) NSAIDs, Cox-2 inhibitors, and the gut. *Lancet* **346,** 1105,1106 (letter).

89. Kargman, S. L., O'Neill, G. P., Vickers, P. J., Evans, J. F., Mancini, J. A., and Jothy, S. (1995) Expression of prostaglandin G/H synthase-1 and -2 protein in human colon cancer. *Cancer Res.* **55,** 2556–2559.

90. Rigas, B., Goldman, I. S., and Levine, L. (1993) Altered eicosanoid levels in human colon cancer. *J. Lab. Clin. Med.* **122,** 518–523.

91. Goetzl, E. J., An, S., and Zeng, L. (1995) Specific suppression by prostaglandin E2 of activation-induced apoptosis of human CD4+8+ T lymphocytes. *J. Immunol.* **154,** 1041–1047.

92. Roper, R. L. and Phipps, R. P. (1992) Prostaglandin E2 and cyclic AMP inhibit B lymphocyte activation and simultaneously promote IgE and IgG1 synthesis. *J. Immunol.* **149,** 2984–2991.

93. Leppert, D., Hauser, S. L., Kishiyama, J. L., An, S., Zeng, L., and Goetzl, E. (1995) Prostaglandin E2 and leukotriene B4 stimulation of matrix metalloproteinase-dependent migration of human T cells across a model basement membrane. *FASEB J.* **9,** A853.

94. Betz, M. and Fox, B. S. (1984) Prostaglandin E2 inhibits production of Th1 but not Th2 lymphokines. *J. Immunol.* **146,** 1719–1726.

95. Sato, H., Tanaka, M., Takino, T., Inoue, M., and Seiki, M. (1997) Assignment of the human genes for membrane-type–1, -2, and -3 matrix metalloproteinases (MMP14, MMP15, and MMP16) to 14q12.2, 16q12.2–q21, and 8q21, respectively, by in situ hybridization. *Genomics* **39,** 412,413.

96. Muller, G. W., Humbel, B., Glatt, M., Strauli, P., Winterhalter, K. H., and Bruckner, P. (1986) On the role of type IX collagen in the extracellular matrix of cartilage: type IX collagen is localized to intersections of collagen fibrils. *J. Cell Biol.* **102,** 1931–1939.

97. Morris, N. P. and Bachinger, H. P. (1987) Type XI collagen is a heterotrimer with the composition (1 alpha, 2 alpha, 3 alpha) retaining nontriple-helical domains. *J. Biol. Chem.* **262,** 11,345–11,350.

98. Harris, E. D., Jr., ed. (1985) *Pathogenesis of Rheumatoid Arthritis.* Saunders, Philadelphia, PA.

99. Goldberg, G. I., Wilhelm, S. M., Kronberger, A., Bauer, E. A., Grant, G. A., and Eisen, A. Z. (1986) Human fibroblast collagenase: complete primary structure and homology to an oncogene transformation-induced rat protein. *J. Biol. Chem.* **261,** 6600–6605.

100. Hasty, K. A., Pourmotabbed, F., Goldberg, G. I., Thompson, J. P., Nelson, R. L., Spinella, D., and Mainardi, C. L. (1990) Human neutrophil collagenase: a distinct gene product with homology to other matrix metalloproteinases. *J. Biol. Chem.* **265,** 11,421–11,424.

101. Freije, J. M., Diez, I. I., Balbin, M., Sanchez, L. M., Blasco, R., Tolivia, J., and Lopez, O. C. (1994) Molecular cloning and expression of collagenase-3, a novel human matrix metalloproteinase produced by breast carcinomas. *J. Biol. Chem.* **269,** 16,766–16,773.

102. Stahle-Backdahl, M., Sandstedt, B., Bruce, K., Lindahl, A., Jimenez, M. G., Vega, J. A., and Lopez, O. C. (1997) Collagenase-3 (MMP-13) is expressed during human fetal ossification and re-expressed in postnatal bone remodeling and in rheumatoid arthritis. *Lab. Invest.* **76,** 717–728.

103. Mitchell, P. G., Magna, H. A., Reeves, L. M., Lopresti-Morrow, L. L., Yocum, S. A., Rosner, P. J., Geoghegan, K. F., and Hambor, J. E. (1996) Cloning, expression and type II collagenolytic activity of matrix metalloproteinase-13 from human osteoarthritic cartilage. *J. Clin. Invest.* **97,** 761–768.

104. Chubinskaya, S., Huch, K., Mikecz, K., Cs-Szabo, G., Hasty, K. A., Kuettner, K. E., and Cole, A. A. (1996) Chondrocyte matrix metalloproteinase-8, Upregulation of neutrophil collagenase by interleukin-1B in human cartilage from knee and ankle joints. *Lab. Invest.* **74,** 232–240.

105. Borden, P., Solymar, D., Sucharczuk, A., Lindman, B., Cannon, P., and Heller, R. A. (1996) Cytokine control of interstitial collagenase and collagenase-3 gene expression in human chondrocytes. *J. Biol. Chem.* **271,** 23,577–23,581.

106. Shlopov, B. V., Lie, W., Mainardi, C. L., Cole, A. A., Chubinskaya, S., and Hasty, K. A. (1997) Osteoarthritic lesions: involvement of three different collagenases. *Arth. Rheum.,* **40,** 2065–2074.

107. Crawford, H. C. and Matrisian, L. M. (1996) Mechanisms controlling the transcription of matrix metalloproteinase genes in normal and neoplastic cells. *Enzyme Protein* **49,** 20–37.

108. Kirstein, M., Sanz, L., Quinones, S., Moscat, J., Diaz, M. M., and Saus, J. (1996) Cross-talk between different enhancer elements during mitogenic induction of the human stromelysin–1 gene. *J. Biol. Chem.* **271,** 18,231–18,236.

109. Kerr, L. D., Holt, J. T., and Matrisian, L. M. (1988) Growth factors regulate transin gene expression by c-fos-dependent and c-fos-independent pathways. *Science* **242,** 1424–1427.

110. Schonthal, A., Herrlich, P., Rahmsdorf, H. J., and Ponta, H. (1988) Requirement for fos gene expression in the transcriptional activation of collagenase by other oncogenes and phorbol esters. *Cell* **54,** 325–334.

111. Benbow, U. and Brinckerhoff, C. E. (1997) The AP–1 site and MMP gene regulation: what is all the fuss about? *Matrix Biol.* **15,** 519–526.

112. Angel, P., Imagawa, M., Chiu, R., Stein, B., Imbra, R. J., Rahmsdorf, H. J., Jonat, C., Herrlich, P., and Karin, M. (1987) Phorbol ester-inducible genes contain a common cis element recognized by a TPA-modulated trans-acting factor. *Cell* **49,** 729–739.

113. Angel, P., Baumann, I., Stein, B., Delius, H., Rahmsdorf, H. J., and Herrlich, P. (1987) 12-O-tetradecanoyl-phorbol-13-acetate induction of the human collagenase gene is mediated by an inducible enhancer element located in the 5'-flanking region. *Mol. Cell. Biol.* **7,** 2256–2266.

114. Asahara, H., Fujisawa, K., Kobata, T., Hasunuma, T., Maeda, T., Asanuma, M., Ogawa, N., Inoue, H., Sumida, T., and Nishioka, K. (1997) Direct evidence of high DNA binding activity of transcription factor AP-1 in rheumatoid arthritis synovium. *Arthritis Rheum.* **40,** 912–918.

115. Nicholson, R. C., Mader, S., Nagpal, S., Leid, M., Rochette, E. C., and Chambon, P. (1990) Negative regulation of the rat stromelysin gene promoter by retinoic acid is mediated by an AP1 binding site. *EMBO J.* **9,** 4443–4454.

116. Ballock, R. T., Heydemann, A., Wakefield, L. M., Flanders, K. C., Roberts, A. B., and Sporn, M. B. (1994) Inhibition of the chondrocyte phenotype by retinoic acid involves upregulation of metalloprotease genes independent of TGF-beta. *J. Cell. Physiol.* **159,** 340–346.

117. Gravallese, E. M., Handel, M. L., Coblyn, J., Anderson, R. J., Sperling, R. I., Karlson, E. W., Maier, A., Ruderman, E. M., Formelli, F., and Weinblatt, M. E. (1996) N-[4-hydroxyphenyl] retinamide in rheumatoid arthritis: A pilot study. *Arthritis Rheum.* **39,** 1021–1026.

118. Varga, J., Yufit, T., and Brown, R. R. (1995) Inhibition of collagenase and stromelysin gene expression by interferon-gamma in human dermal fibroblasts is mediated in part via induction of tryptophan degradation. *J. Clin. Invest.* **96,** 475–481.

119. Shapiro, S. D., Campbell, E. J., Kobayashi, D. K., and Welgus, H. G. (1990) Immune modulation of metalloproteinase production in human macrophages: selective pretranslational suppression of interstitial collagenase and stromelysin biosynthesis by interferon-gamma. *J. Clin. Invest.* **86,** 1204–1210.

120. Tamai, K., Ishikawa, H., Mauviel, A., and Uitto, J. (1995) Interferon-gamma coordinately upregulates matrix metalloprotease (MMP)-1 and MMP-3, but not tissue inhibitor of metalloproteases (TIMP), expression in cultured keratinocytes. *J. Invest. Dermatol.* **104,** 384–390.

121. Matrisian, L. M., Ganser, G. L., Kerr, L. D., Pelton, R. W., and Wood, L. D. (1992) Negative regulation of gene expression by TGF-beta. *Mol. Reprod. Dev.* **32,** 111–120.

122. Lafyatis, R., Thompson, N., Remmers, E., Flanders, K., Roberts, A., Sporn, M., and Wilder, R. (1988) Demonstration of local production of PDGF and TGF-beta by synovial tissue from patients with rheumatoid arthritis. *Arthritis Rheum.* **31,** S62.

123. Kerr, L. D., Miller, D. B., and Matrisian, L. M. (1990) TGF-beta 1 inhibition of transin/stromelysin gene expression is mediated through a Fos binding sequence. *Cell* **61,** 267–278.

124. Kerr, L. D., Magun, B. E., and Matrisian, L. M. (1992) The role of C-Fos in growth factor regulation of stromelysin/transin gene expression. *Matrix Suppl.* **1,** 176–183.

125. Moreland, L. W., Heck, L. W., Jr., Koopman, W. J., Saway, P. A., Adamson, T. C., Fronek, Z., O'Connor, R. D., Morgan, E. E., Diveley, J. P., Richieri, S. P., Carlo, D. J., and Brostoff, S. W. (1996) V beta 17 T cell receptor peptide vaccination in rheumatoid arthritis: results of phase I dose escalation study. *J. Rheumatol.* **23,** 1353–1362.

126. Sieper, J., Kary, S., Sorensen, H., Alten, R., Eggens, U., Huge, W., Hiepe, F., Kuhne, A., Listing, J., Ulbrich, N., Braun, J., Zink, A., and Mitchison, N. A. (1996) Oral type II collagen treatment in early rheumatoid arthritis: a double-blind, placebo-controlled, randomized trial. *Arthritis Rheum.* **39,** 41–51.

127. Trentham, D. E., Dynesius-Trentham, R. A., Orav, E. J., Combitchi, D., Lorenzo, C., Sewell, K. L., Hafler, D. A., and Weiner, H. L. (1993) Effects of oral administration of type II collagen on rheumatoid arthritis. *Science* **261,** 1727–1730.

128. Rosloniec, E. F., Brand, D. D., Whittington, K. B., Stuart, J. M., Ciubotaru, M., and Ward, E. S. (1995) Vaccination with a recombinant V alpha domain of a TCR prevents the development of collagen-induced arthritis. *J. Immunol.* **155,** 4504–4511.

129. Staines, N. A. (1991) Oral tolerance and collagen arthritis. *Br. J. Rheumatol.* **30,** 40–43.

130. Khare, S. D., Krco, C. J., Griffiths, M. M., Luthra, H. S., and David, C. S. (1995) Oral administration of an immunodominant human collagen peptide modulates collagen-induced arthritis. *J. Immunol.* **155,** 3653–3659.

131. Nagler, A. C., Bober, L. A., Robinson, M. E., Siskind, G. W., and Thorbecke, G. J. (1986) Suppression of type II collagen-induced arthritis by intragastric administration of soluble type II collagen. *Proc. Natl. Acad. Sci. USA* **83,** 7443–7446.

132. Weinberg, A. D., Celnik, B., Vainiene, M., Buenafe, A. C., Vandenbark, A. A., and Offner, H. (1994) The effect of TCR V beta 8 peptide protection and therapy on T cell populations isolated from the spinal cords of Lewis rats with experimental autoimmune encephalomyelitis. *J. Neuroimmunol.* **49,** 161–170.

133. Vandenbark, A. A., Hashim, G., and Offner, H. (1989) Immunization with a synthetic T cell receptor V-region peptide protects against experimental autoimmune encephalomyelitis. *Nature* **341,** 541–543.

134. Offner, H., Hashim, G. A., and Vandenbark, A. A. (1991) T cell receptor peptide therapy triggers autoregulation of experimental encephalomyelitis. *Science* **251,** 430–432.

135. Miller, A., Lider, O., Roberts, A. B., Sporn, M. B., and Weiner, H. L. (1992) Suppressor T cells generated by oral tolerization to myelin basic protein suppress both in vitro and in vivo immune responses by the release of transforming growth factor beta after antigen-specific triggering. *Proc. Natl. Acad. Sci. USA* **89,** 421–425.

136. Miller, A., Lider, O., Al, S. A., and Weiner, H. L. (1992) Suppression of experimental autoimmune encephalomyelitis by oral administration of myelin basic protein. V. Hierarchy of suppression by myelin basic protein from different species. *J. Neuroimmunol.* **39,** 243–250.

137. Elliott, M. J., Maini, R. N., Feldmann, M., Kalden, J. R., Antoni, C., Smolen, J. S., Leeb, B., Breedveld, F. C., Macfarlane, J. D., Bijl, H., et al. (1994) Randomised double-blind comparison of chimeric monoclonal antibody to tumour necrosis factor alpha (cA2) versus placebo in rheumatoid arthritis. *Lancet* **344,** 1105–1110.

138. Maini, R. N., Elliott, M. J., Brennan, F. M., and Feldmann, M. (1995) Beneficial effects of tumour necrosis factor-alpha (TNF-alpha) blockade in rheumatoid arthritis (RA). *Clin. Exp. Immunol.* **101,** 207–212.

139. Brennan, F. M., Browne, K. A., Green, P. A., Jaspar, J. M., Maini, R. N., and Feldmann, M. (1997) Reduction of serum matrix metalloproteinase 1 and matrix metalloproteinase 3 in rheumatoid arthritis patients following anti-tumour necrosis factor-alpha (cA2) therapy. *Br. J. Rheumatol.* **36,** 643–650.

140. Tak, P. P., Taylor, P. C., Breedveld, F. C., Smeets, T. J., Daha, M. R., Kluin, P. M., Meinders, A. E., and Maini, R. N. (1996) Decrease in cellularity and expression of adhesion molecules by anti-tumor necrosis factor alpha monoclonal antibody treatment in patients with rheumatoid arthritis. *Arthritis Rheum.* **39,** 1077–1081 (see comments).

141. Joosten, L. A., Helsen, M. M., van de Loo, F. A., and van den Berg, W. B. (1996) Anticytokine treatment of established type II collagen-induced arthritis in DBA/1 mice. A comparative study using anti-TNFalpha, anti-IL-1 alpha/beta, and IL-1Ra. *Arthritis Rheum.* **39,** 797–809.

142. Chernajovsky, Y., Adams, G., Triantaphyllopoulos, K., Ledda, M. F., and Podhajcer, O. L. (1997) Pathogenic lymphoid cells engineered to express TGF beta 1 ameliorate disease in a collagen-induced arthritis model. *Gene Ther.* **4,** 553–559.

143. Muller-Ladner, U., Roberts, C. R., Franklin, B. N., Gay, R. E., Robbins, P. D., Evans, C. H., and Gay, S. (1997) Human IL–1Ra gene transfer into human synovial fibroblasts is chondroprotective. *J. Immunol.* **158,** 3492–3498.

144. Wooley, P. H., Luthra, H. S., Stuart, J. M., and David, C. S. (1981) Type II collagen induced arthritis in mice. I. Major histocompatibility complex (I region) linkage and antibody correlates. *J. Exp. Med.* **154,** 688–700.

145. Griffiths, M. M. and DeWitt, C. W. (1984) Genetic control of collagen-induced arthritis in rats: the immune response to type II collagen among susceptible and resistant strains and evidence for multiple gene control. *J. Immunol.* **132,** 2830–2836.

146. Griffiths, M. M. and DeWitt, C. W. (1981) Immunogenetic control of experimental collagen induced arthritis in rats. II. ECIA susceptibility and immune response to type II collagen (CALF) are linked to RT1. *J. Immunogenet.* **8,** 63–70.

147. Cremer, M., Terato, K., Seyer, J., Watson, W., O'Hagan, G., Townes, A., and Kang, A. (1991) Immunity to type XI collagen in mice. Evidence that alpha3(XI) chain of type XI collagen and the alpha1(II) chain of type II collagen share arthritogenic determinants and induce arthritis in DBA/1 mice. **146,** 4130–4137.

148. Banerjee, S., Webber, C., and Poole, A. R. (1992) The induction of arthritis in mice by the cartilage proteoglycan aggrecan. *Cell Immunol.* **144,** 347–357.

149. Pearson, C. M. (1956) Development of arthritis, periarthritis and periostitis in rats given adjuvant. *Proc. Soc. Exp. Biol. Med.* **91,** 101–107.

150. Hopkins, S. J., Freemont, A. J., and Jayson, M. I. (1984) Pristane-induced arthritis in Balb/c mice. I. Clinical and histological features of the arthropathy. *Rheumatol. Int.* **5,** 21–28.

151. Wooley, P. H., Seibold, J. R., Whalen, J. D., and Chapdelaine, J. M. (1989) Pristane-induced arthritis: the immunologic and genetic features of an experimental murine model of autoimmune disease. *Arthritis Rheum.* **32,** 1022–1030.

152. Bedwell, A. E., Elson, C. J., and Hinton, C. E. (1987) Immunological involvement in the pathogenesis of pristane-induced arthritis. *Scand. J. Immunol.* **25,** 393–398.

153. Vingsbo, C., Sahlstrand, P., Brun, J. G., Jonsson, R., Saxne, T., and Holmdahl, R. (1996) Pristane induced arthritis in rats: a new model for rheumatoid arthritis with a chronic course influenced by both major histocompatibility complex and nonmajor histocompatibility complex genes. *Am. J. Pathol.* **149,** 1675–1683.

154. Cromartie, W. J., Craddock, J. C., Schwab, J. H., Anderle, S. K., and Yang, C. H. (1977) Arthritis in rats after systemic injection of streptococcal cells or cell walls. *J. Exp. Med.* **146,** 1585–1602.

155. Kouskoff, V., Korganow, A. S., Duchatelle, V., Degott, C., Benoist, C., and Mathis, D. (1996) Organ-specific disease provoked by systemic autoimmunity. *Cell* **87,** 811–822.

15

Lupus Erythematosus

The Role of Adhesion Molecules and Local Mediators

H. Michael Belmont and Steven B. Abramson

Introduction

Inflammation in systemic lupus erythematosus (SLE) is mediated by a complex interaction of the cellular and humoral components of the immune system. Central to the development of tissue injury is an interaction between inflammatory cells and vascular endothelium, which requires the recruitment, activation, and ligation of surface adhesion molecules. These events, induced by immune complexes, cytokines, and complement components are prerequisite for leukocyte egress and local mediator production. This chapter will review mediators that act on inflammatory and endothelial cells to promote vascular injury in SLE.

Activation of the Complement System

In most instances, inflammatory disease of blood vessels and tissues in SLE involves complement activation in the presence or absence of immune complex deposition. Complement cleavage products, particularly C3a, C5a, and C5b-9, are key mediators in the promotion of local tissue injury.

Complement System

The complement system is comprised of at least 20 plasma proteins that participate in a variety of host defense and immunological reactions. Each complement component is cleaved via a limited proteolytic reaction that proceeds by either the classical or alternative pathway. The alternative pathway is more primitive and may be activated by contact with a variety of substances including polysaccharides (such as endotoxin) found in the cell walls of microorganisms. The activation of the classical pathway by

From: *Molecular and Cellular Basis of Inflammation*
Edited by: C. N. Serhan and P. A. Ward © Humana Press Inc., Totowa, NJ

immune complexes requires binding of the first complement component, C1, to sites on the Fc portions of immunoglobulins, particularly of the IgG-1, IgG-3, and IgM isotypes.

Activation of C3

Activation of the third component of complement is central to both the classical and alternative pathways. C3 is cleaved by convertases to two active products, C3a and C3b. C3a, released into the fluid phase, provokes the release of histamine from mast cells and basophils, causes smooth muscle contraction and induces platelet aggregation. C3b has two functions: It is part of the C5 convertase that continues the complement cascade and it is the major opsonin of the complement system. C3b binds to immune complexes and to a variety of activators such as microbial organisms. The binding of C3b to these particles facilitates the attachment of the particle to the C3b receptor on cells—complement receptor 1 (CR1), which is present on erythrocytes, neutrophils, monocytes, B-lymphocytes, and glomerular podocytes. CR1 on phagocytes potentiates phagocytosis. CR1 on erythrocytes, which accounts for approx 90% of CR1 in blood, facilitates the clearance of immune complexes from the circulation by transporting erythrocyte-bound complexes to the liver and spleen for removal. Recently, a new biological role for C3a and C3a desArg has been described in the regulation of tumor necrosis factor-α (TNF-α) and interleukin-1β (IL-1β) synthesis in nonadherent peripheral blood mononuclear cells (PBMC) *(1)*. C3a and C3a desArg suppressed endotoxin-induced synthesis of TNF-α and IL-1β. By contrast, in adherent PBMC, C3a and C3a desArg enhanced endotoxin-induced production of these cytokines. Thus, both C3a and C3a desArg may enhance cytokine synthesis by adherent monocytes at local inflammatory sites, whereas inhibiting the systemic synthesis of proinflammatory cytokines by circulating cells.

Activation of C5

In addition to its role as an opsonin, C3b also forms part of the C5 convertase that leads to the generation of C5a and C5b. C5a, like C3a, is an anaphylatoxin, capable of activating basophils and mast cells. C5a is also among the most potent biological chemoattractants for neutrophils. C5b, which will attach to the surface of cells and microorganisms, is the first component in the assembly of the membrane attack complex (MAC), C5b-9.

Membrane Attack Complex

The MAC, or the terminal complement assembly of C5b-9, has long been known to lytic bacteria. However, assembly of MAC on homologous leukocytes is not a cytotoxic event. After insertion of MAC into a leukocyte membrane, the cell sheds a small membrane vesicle containing the MAC complex. What is less appreciated is that insertion of MAC into the cell membrane triggers cell activation before it is shed *(2,3)*. MAC acts as an ionophore, provoking increases in cytosolic calcium and consequently triggering cell functions (reviewed in ref. *4*). These include generation of toxic oxygen products as well as activation of both the cyclooxygenase (COX) (platelets, monocyte/macrophages, synoviocytes) and lipoxygenase (LO) pathways of arachidonate metabolism. Furthermore, the deposition of MAC increases the surface expression of P-selectin on the endothelial cell surface, promoting adhesion to circulating neutrophils *(5)*. In vivo evidence that vascular endothelium represents a site of C5b-9 deposition has been demonstrated in immune vasculitis *(6–8)* and infarcted myocardium *(9)*. Mechanisms by which

C5b-9 activates vascular endothelium and promotes the upregulation of surface adhesion molecules is discussed below.

Complement Activation During Exacerbations of SLE

A major consequence of immune complex deposition in SLE is the activation of complement. The consumption of complement components and their deposition in tissue is reflected by a decrease in serum levels of C3 and C4 in most patients with active disease *(10)*. However, because the synthesis of both C3 and C4 increases during periods of disease activity, the serum levels of these proteins may be normal despite accelerated consumption *(11)*. Conversely, chronically depressed levels of individual complement components owing to decreased synthesis, hereditary deficiencies, or increased extravascular distribution of complement proteins has been reported in SLE *(12)*. The decreased serum complement levels in these patients may lead to the mistaken conclusion that excessive complement activation is ongoing. To define more precisely the role of complement activation with respect to clinical disease activity of SLE, circulating levels of complement degradation products during periods of active and inactive disease have been measured *(13–18)*. Levels of plasma C3a, Ba, and the serum complement attack complex, SC5b-9, were each shown to be more sensitive indicators of disease activity than either total C3 or C4 level *(13–16,18)*. Elevations of plasma C3a levels may precede other serologic or clinical evidence of an impending disease flare *(18)*.

Receptors for Complement and Intercellular Adhesion in Inflammation

Complement Receptors and Surface Integrins

Neutrophils

The first event in an inflammatory process initiated by complement activation and the generation of potent chemoattractants, such as C5a, requires the margination, attachment, and egress of activated neutrophils from the circulation. Neutrophils express receptors for the complement fragment C3b (receptor designated CR1) and its inactivated cleavage product iC3b (receptor designated CR3, or CD11b/CD18) *(19)*. On the surface of phagocytes, both CR1 and CD11b/CD18 play important roles in the clearance of particles, such as opsonized bacteria, to which C3b or iC3b are bound. This clearance mechanism is also essential for the removal of immune complexes containing C3b and iC3b *(20)*. In addition to its role as a receptor for iC3b, CD11b/CD18 is the major neutrophil adhesion molecule responsible for the capacity of the neutrophil to adhere to vascular endothelium and to other neutrophils *(21)*. CD11b/CD18 is a member of a family of surface glycoproteins known as β2 integrins, which are heterodimers consisting of a common β-subunit (CD18) and distinct α-subunits (CD11a, CD11b, CD11c). In the neutrophil, the most important β2 integrin appears to be CD11b/CD18 (CD11B/CD18), required for normal phagocytosis, aggregation, adhesion, and chemotaxis. Intercellular adhesion molecule-1 (ICAM-1), expressed on resting and activated endothelial cells, has been identified as a ligand for the CD18 integrins *(22)*. Interaction between CD18 and ICAM-1 modulates both the adhesion of neutrophils to vascular endothelium and their egress to the extravascular space. The initial rolling of activated neutrophils on endothelium, a prerequisite for CD18-dependent adhesion under conditions of flow, is mediated by a separate molecular interaction: that between the selectins

(E-selectin and P-selectin) on the endothelial cell and a carbohydrate ligand (sialyl-Le^x) on the neutrophil *(22–24)*. In addition, the neutrophil expresses L-selectin on its surface, which also promotes rolling, and is shed from the plasma membrane on cell activation. The redundancy with regard to selectin function may in part be explained by the different kinetics of their participation in the events of intracellular adhesion: (1) L-selectin is shed within seconds of neutrophil activation; (2) P-selectin is stored in the Weibel-Palade bodies in endothelial cells and is expressed on the surface within minutes following exposure of the cells to acute stimuli, such as thrombin; and (3) E-selectin is upregulated over several hours following cytokine exposure in a process that requires transcription and translation of new protein.

Macrophages/Monocytes

Macrophages/monocytes play an important role in immune-mediated tissue injury, particularly in nephritis *(25)*. These cells express the three major classes of Fc receptors as well as β1, β2, and β3 integrins, which facilitate phagocytosis of opsonized particles, intercellular adhesion, and adhesion to extracellular matrix proteins. Monocytes are recruited into tissues from the circulation in response to chemotactic factors (e.g., C5a, IL-8, transforming growth factor-β [TGF-β], fragments of collagen, and fibronectin) produced at inflammatory sites. Recruitment requires the expression of adhesion molecules on activated vascular endothelium (e.g., ICAM-1, vascular cell adhesion molecule-1 [VCAM-1]) that are recognized by counterligands of the circulating monocyte (e.g., LFA-1, VLA-4). When monocytes emigrate into tissues, they can be transformed into activated macrophages following exposure to cytokines such as interferon-γ (IFN-γ), IL-1, and TNF. Macrophage activation results in an increase in cell size, increased synthesis of proteolytic enzymes, and the secretion of a variety of inflammatory products (Table 1).

Platelets

Platelets express two surface adhesion-promoting molecules, and P-selection. gpIIb/IIIa expression increases with platelet activation by ADP and binds fibrinogen, fibronectin, vitronectin, and von Willeband factor. P-selectin (GMP-140, PADGEM), a member of the selectin family of adhesion molecules, is a membrane glycoprotein located in the alpha granules of platelets and Weibel-Palade bodies of endothelium. When these cells are activated by such agents as thrombin, P-selectin is rapidly translocated to the plasma membrane where it functions as a receptor for neutrophils and monocytes. Expression of P-selectin on activated platelets may therefore facilitate recruitment of neutrophils and monocytes to sites of thrombosis or inflammation *(23)*.

Platelets have been identified in the glomeruli of patients with SLE nephritis in which they are believed to play a particularly important role *(27)*. Urinary TX levels are elevated in patients with active lupus nephritis, a finding that has several implications: first, it is a sign of abnormal platelet aggregation in the microvasculature with the potential for thrombosis and endothelial injury; second, the vasoconstrictive properties of TXA$_2$ would be expected to decrease glomerular filtration rate (GFR) and renal blood flow (RBF); and, third, the release of growth factors and other mediators by activated platelets could aggravate the proliferative glomerular lesion. Recent studies of the administration of specific TXA$_2$ antagonists have shown promise in the improvement of both GFR and RBF in SLE nephritis *(28)*.

Platelet activation in lupus glomerulonephritis has been attributed to a variety of substances, including immune complexes, activated complement components (includ-

Table 1
Local Mediators Released by Neutrophils, Macrophages, and Platelets

I. Secretory products produced by neutrophils and macrophages
    1. Reactive oxygen intermediates (e.g., superoxide anion)
    2. Proteolytic enzymes
    3. Reactive nitrogen intermediates (e.g., nitric oxide)
    4. Bioactive lipids
       a. COX products: prostaglandin E_2 (PGE_2), PG $F_{2\alpha}$, prostacyclin, thromboxane (TX)
       b. LO products: monohydroxyeicosatetraenoic acids, dihydroxyeicosatetraenoic acids, leukotrienes, lipoxins
       c. PAFs (1 O-alkyl-2-acetyl-*sn*-glyceryl-3-phosphorylcholine)
    5. Chemokines (e.g., IL-8)
II. Secretory products produced by macrophages
    1. Polypeptide hormones
       a. IL-1α and IL-1β (collectively, IL-1)
       b. TNF-α (cachectin, TNF)
       c. IFN-α
       d. IFN-γ (confirmation needed)
       e. Platelet-derived growth factor(s) (PDGF)
       f. TGF-β
       g. b-Endorphin
    2. Complement (C) components
       a. Classical path: C1, C4, C2, C3, C5
       b. Alternative path: factor B, factor D, properdin
    3. Coagulation factors
       a. Intrinsic path: IX, X, V, prothrombin
       b. Extrinsic path: VII
       c. Surface activities: tissue factor, prothrombinase
       d. Prothrombolytic activity: plasminogen activator inhibitors, plasmin inhibitors
III. Secretory products produced by platelets
    1. Plasminogen
    2. α2-Plasmin inhibitor
    3. PDGF
    4. Platelet factor 4
    5. TGF-α and TGF-β
    6. Serotonin
    7. Adenosine diphosphate
    8. Thromboxane A_2
    9. 12-hydroxytetraenoic acid

ing C3a and the MAC, C5b-9), platelet-activating factor (PAF), and vasopressin. In addition, neutrophils may also be able to activate platelets via the release of oxidants and proteases. Platelets may aggravate immune injury in glomerulonephritis via several mechanisms, which include (1) promoting thrombosis; (2) reducing GFR through the production of TX and other vasoactive substances; and (3) release of products that activate macrophages, neutrophils, and glomerular mesangial cells *(29)*.

Adhesion Molecules and Local Mediators Promote Vascular Injury in SLE

SLE is the autoimmune disease that best exemplifies the consequences of the generation of inflammatory mediators and the activation of the cellular constituents of inflammation as outlined above. Immune complex formation, episodic complement activation, the recruitment of stimulated leukocytes and platelets into tissues, and endothelial cell activation produce vascular injury during SLE exacerbations. Vascular disease in SLE can be classified into two broad categories: inflammatory and thrombotic. The former may be associated with local deposition of immune complexes or result from leukocyte–endothelial cell interactions in the absence of immune complex deposition, and the latter is almost invariably associated with circulating antiphospholipid antibodies.

Inflammatory Vasculitis

Vasculitis in SLE is most commonly owing to the local deposition of immune complexes, particularly those containing antibodies to DNA (anti-DNA), in blood vessel walls (30,31). This lesion is best modeled by the Arthus reaction and experimental serum sickness. Maurice Arthus reported in 1903 that the repeated cutaneous injection of horse serum into a group of rabbits produced inflammatory reactions characterized by intense polymorphonuclear leukocyte infiltration, hemorrhage, and sometimes necrosis (32). It is now known that this reaction is owing to the formation of antigen-antibody complexes in the vicinity of blood vessel walls, complement activation, and the generation of anaphylatoxins (e.g., C4a, C3a, C5a) and chemotaxins (C5a) (33,34). The resulting infiltration of vessel walls by polymorphonuclear leukocytes leads histologically to leukocytoclastic vasculitis and the release of lysosomal enzymes and oxygen radicals to tissue injury (31).

Modifications of the classic active Arthus reaction include immunization by iv, rather than cutaneous, injection of the antigen as well as the local passive Arthus reaction (e.g., simultaneous cutaneous injection of antigen and antibody), direct passive Arthus reaction (e.g., passive transfer of preformed antibody by the iv injection of serum from another immunized rabbit), and the reverse passive Arthus reaction (e.g., antibody injected cutaneously and antigen injected intravenously) (35). The necessary elements of these reactions have been examined and require antigen, precipitating antibody, intact complement pathway, and neutrophils (36). A recent study suggests that the inflammatory response to immune complexes also requires cell-bound Fc receptors with subsequent amplification by cellular mediators and complement (37).

Shwartzman-Like Inflammatory Vascular Injury

Some patients with SLE have small vessel disease and inflammatory vasculopathy in the absence of local immune complex deposition, particularly those patients with central nervous system (CNS) involvement (15,38,39). Several lines of investigation now suggest yet another mechanism for this complement-mediated vascular injury in SLE, one not dependent on immune complex deposition (40–45). This mechanism is best modeled experimentally by the Shwartzman phenomenon. The local Shwartzman lesion requires a preparatory intradermal injection of endotoxin, which is followed in 4–18 h by the iv injection of endotoxin (46,47). This results in the intravascular activation of complement triggering the release of anaphylatoxins, such as C3a and C5a, into the circulation (48). The split products attract and activate inflammatory cells, such as neutrophils and platelets, causing them to aggregate, to adhere to vascular endothelium, to occlude small vessels, and to release toxic mediators. Activation of complement thus leads to an occlusive vasculopathy that may also result in widespread ischemic injury (48).

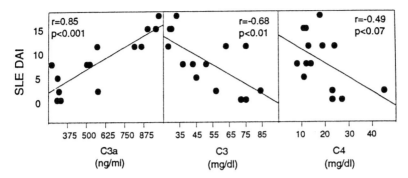

Fig. 1. Correlation between complement levels (C3a desArg, C3, and C4) and the Systemic Lupus Erythematosus Activity Index (SLEDAI) score. There is a positive correlation between the SLEDAI and C3a and a negative correlation of a lesser magnitude between SLEDAI and C3 and C4.

The Shwartzman phenomenon was originally described as a model of meningococcal sepsis, but it is now recognized that cytokines such as IL-1β and TNF-α can substitute for endotoxin *(49)*. Such agents stimulate the up-regulation on the endothelial cell surface of ICAM-1 and E-selectin, which are the counterreceptors for the neutrophil adhesion molecule CD11b/CD18 and sialyl-Le^X, respectively *(50)*. It had long been established that complement activation in plasma stimulates circulating neutrophils to produce the local Shwartzman lesion, but it was recently recognized that the preparatory phase represents a time of ICAM-1 and E-selectin upregulation *(47)*. The importance of this local endothelial cell activation is supported by the capacity of antibodies to ICAM-1 administered intravenously to prevent the development of the experimental lesion *(47)*.

The episodic, uncontrolled activation of complement proteins is a characteristic feature of SLE. Disease exacerbations are typically accompanied by decreases in total C3 and C4 values in association with elevations in plasma of the biologically active complement split products, C3a desArg and C5a desArg *(15,16,51,52; Fig. 1)*. During periods of disease flare, circulating neutrophils are activated to increase their adhesiveness to vascular endothelium, as indicated by the upregulation of the surface B2 integrin CD11b/CD18 (complement receptor 3) *(21,53)*. A recent study demonstrated that the surface expression of three distinct endothelial cell adhesion molecules, E-selectin, VCAM-1, and ICAM-1, is also upregulated in patients with SLE (Fig. 2) *(39)*. Endothelial cell activation was most marked in patients with disease exacerbations characterized by significant elevations of plasma C3a desArg, and the activation reversed with improvement in disease activity *(39)*. In these studies, endothelial cell adhesion molecule upregulation was observed in otherwise histologically normal skin and was notable for the absence of local immune complex deposition *(39)*. These data suggest that excessive complement activation in association with primed endothelial cells can induce neutrophil–endothelial cell adhesion and predispose to leuko-occlusive vasculopathy during SLE disease flares. This pathogenic mechanism may be of particular relevance to vascular beds that lack the fenestrations that permit the trapping of circulating immune complexes. Such an example is the CNS in which the blood–brain barrier can prevent the access of circulating immune complexes to the perivascular

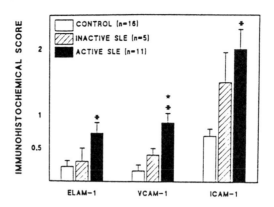

Fig. 2. Endothelial cell adhesion molecule expression in patients with active vs inactive SLE, and in healthy control subjects. The mean expression of all three adhesion molecules was significantly greater in patients with active SLE vs controls. Adhesion molecule expression was also greater in patients with active vs those with inactive SLE. Bars show the mean and SEM. (Note: ELAM-1 is now designated as E-selectin).

tissues. But in the setting of widespread endothelial cell activation, exuberant systemic complement activation can promote diffuse microvascular injury in the absence of immune complex deposition and produce the most common pathologic finding of CNS lupus, microinfarction *(51,54–57)*.

Similar pathologic events may also be present in the mesenteric circulation and produce features of SLE enteritis *(38)* or produce pulmonary leukosequestration and acute, reversible hypoxemia during disease exacerbations *(58)*.

Thrombotic Noninflammatory Vascular Injury in SLE

Antiphospholipid Antibody Syndrome (APS)

The presence of antibodies to negatively charged phospholipids is associated with recurrent arterial and venous thrombosis, thrombocytopenia, and fetal wastage *(59,60)*. APS requires the demonstration of an antiphospholipid antibody (e.g., biologic false positive venereal disease research laboratory (VDRL), lupus anticoagulant, anticardiolipin antibodies) and thrombotic phenomena. It is known that the presence in serum of this family of autoantibodies, perhaps operating through cofactors (e.g., $\beta2$ glycoprotein-1 or prothrombin), can generate a thrombotic diathesis *(61–65)*. The mechanism(s) for this hypercoagulable state has not yet been fully understood, although it appears to involve interactions between the antibodies to anionic phospholipid-protein complexes and antigen targets on platelets *(66,67)*, endothelial cells *(68–71)*, or components of the coagulation cascade *(72,73)*. Experimental evidence exists suggesting that increased platelet aggregation, altered endothelial cell function (e.g., decreased prostacyclin or increased thrombomodulin production), or disturbed function of clotting factors (e.g., decreased protein C activation by thrombomodulin, decreased protein S function, as well as decreased prekallikrein and fibrinolytic activity) may explain the predisposition to thrombosis. The role of cytokines in the primary APS or in APS secondary to SLE requires clarification *(74)*. Evidence that antiphospholipid antibodies can activate endothelial cells and increase expression of adhesion molecules suggests another mechanism for the thrombosis, described in greater detail next *(75)*.

Thrombotic Thrombocytopenia Purpura (TTP)

SLE exacerbations are infrequently accompanied by secondary TTP with complete or incomplete features of the clinical pentad: fever, microangiopathic hemolytic anemia, thrombocytopenia, renal disease, and neurologic dysfunction *(76)*. In the absence of antiphospholipid antibodies, the characteristic pathology of TTP, eosinophilic hyaline microthrombi, has been identified in patients with SLE. Large multimers of von Willebrand factor (vWF) capable of mediating disseminated intravascular platelet aggregation have been demonstrated in patients with chronic, relapsing TTP as well as SLE *(77,78)*. A consequence of the endothelial cell activation or injury observed in SLE may be the release of vWF multimers or other mediators of platelet aggregation capable of initiating a TTP-like illness *(79)*.

Role of Endothelial Cell Activation

Upregulation of Endothelial Adhesion Molecules

Recent in vitro and in vivo investigations have indicated that the perturbation of endothelial cells in SLE is an important accompaniment of active disease. It is increasingly clear that the endothelium is not just a passive target of injury, but plays an active role in accounting for the localization and propagation of the leukocyte- and autoantibody-mediated inflammation *(80)*. The potential importance of endothelial adhesion molecule expression in SLE was recently illustrated by a report from Elkon et al. These investigators demonstrated in MRL/MpJ-Fas^{lpr} (Fas^{lpr}) mice that ICAM-1 deficiency resulted in a striking improvement in survival *(81)*. Histological examination of ICAM-1–deficient mice revealed a significant reduction in glomerulonephritis and vasculitis of kidney, lung, and skin.

In human disease, Jones et al. *(82)* examined lesional skin in patients with SLE and scored the intensity of adhesion molecule expression immunohistochemically. They demonstrated increased expression of ICAM-1, VCAM-1, and E-selectin in lesional skin vs normal controls. The authors have examined endothelial cell adhesion molecule expression immunohistochemically in biopsy specimens from nonlesional, non-sun exposed skin from SLE patients. Their findings demonstrated upregulation of the surface expression of all three adhesion molecules, E-selectin, VCAM-1, and ICAM-1, in patients with active SLE *(39,50)*. The abnormal expression of these endothelial cell adhesion molecules in histologically normal appearing skin was most marked in patients with active disease characterized by significant elevations of the complement split product C3a desArg. In related studies, the authors could also demonstrate that endothelial cells in these same biopsy specimens overexpressed the inducible form of nitric oxide synthase (NOS-2) *(83)*. The activation of endothelial cells of nonlesional skin is a striking reminder of the systemic nature of immune stimulation in SLE and is likely owing to the circulation of a variety of stimuli capable of activating endothelium, as will be discussed below.

Consistent with activation and perturbation of vascular endothelium, elevations of soluble adhesion molecules (E-selectin, sICAM-1, sVCAM-1) have been reported in active SLE *(80,84)*. Although levels of soluble adhesion molecules reflect immune stimulation and tend to correlate with disease activity, their utility as monitors of disease activity remains to be established.

Immune Stimuli That Activate Endothelial Cells

Cytokines

Cytokines are likely to be important mediators of endothelial cell activation and injury in SLE vasculitides. TNF-α, INF-γ, and IL-1 each stimulate adhesion molecule expression. Different studies have variably reported increased levels of TNF-α, IL-1β, IL-6, IFN-γ, and IL-8 in the circulation during vasculitis *(80)*, but the specific role of a specific cytokine remains to be determined. It should also be noted that although endothelial cells may be acted on by cytokines produced by other inflammatory cells, they also can be stimulated to produce cytokines, such as IL-1, IL-6, IL-8, and TNF-α, which can act as autacoids to upregulate adhesion molecule expression *(85)*.

Complement Components

Several products of the activated complement system (e.g., C3b, iC3b, and C5a) are known to activate endothelial cells in vitro. More recently, the role of the MAC in endothelial cell activation has emerged. Kilgore et al. *(86)* demonstrated that by using human umbilical vein endothelial cells (HUVECs), assembly of the MAC resulted in a marked increase in neutrophil binding as compared to that observed in cells treated with TNF-α alone. Enhanced neutrophil binding was attributable to upregulation of E-selectin and ICAM-1.

The MAC has also recently been shown, in a study by Saadi et al. *(87)*, to participate in the upregulation of endothelial cell tissue factor activity. The expression of tissue factor by the endothelium promotes a procoagulant state that is likely to be of major importance in the pathogenesis of the vascular injury. Using the interaction of antiendothelial cell antibodies and complement with cultured endothelium as a model, these authors studied the expression and function of tissue factor, a cofactor for factor VIIa–mediated conversion of factor X to Xa. Cell surface expression of tissue factor activity required activation of complement and assembly of the MAC. Expression of tissue factor was not a direct consequence of the action of the MAC on the endothelial cell but was a secondary response that required as an intermediate step the release of IL-1α, an early product of the endothelial cell response to complement activation.

Finally, there is recent evidence that C1q is a cofactor required for immune complexes to stimulate endothelial expression of E-selectin, ICAM-1, and VCAM-1 *(88)*. In these studies, immune complexes caused the upregulation of HUVEC adhesion molecules and stimulated endothelial cell adhesiveness for added leukocytes in the presence of complement-sufficient normal human serum. The dependency on serum could be shown to be owing to a requirement for complement activation and the generation of C1q. HUVECs expressed a 100- to 126-kDa C1q-binding protein. However, soluble C1q alone, unbound to immune complexes, did not induce adhesion molecule upregulation.

Autoantibodies

Autoantibodies to phospholipids, endothelial cells, and DNA have each been demonstrated to react with endothelial cells in vitro and promote the upregulation of adhesion molecules or tissue factor. The capacity of antiendothelial cell antibodies, e.g., to increase tissue factor expression in the presence of complement was noted above *(87)*. Neng et al. *(89)* have reported that anti-DNA autoantibodies stimulate the release of IL-1 and IL-6 from human endothelial cells. In these studies, the incubation of endothelial

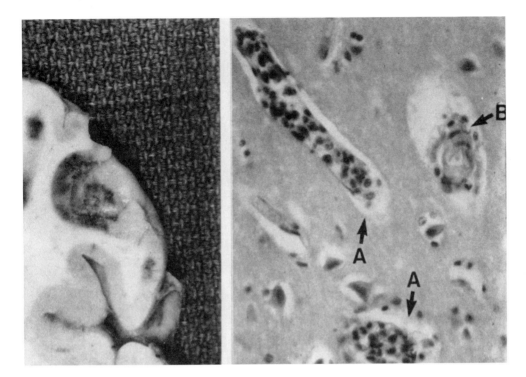

Fig. 3. Specimen of brain obtained postmortem from a patient with fatal exacerbation of neuropsychiatric lupus without antiphospholipid antibodies. **(Left)** The frontal lobe reveals multiple small cortical infarcts. **(Right)** High magnification reveals leukothrombosis, with occlusion of small blood vessels by leukocyte aggregates **(A)**, as well as fibrin thrombi **(B)**.

cells with purified IgG containing anti-dsDNA (compared to those incubated with anti-dsDNA–depleted IgG) caused a significant increase of supernatant IL-1 and IL-6 in association with increased mRNA expression for these cytokines. These investigators, using a similar strategy, also demonstrated the upregulation of adhesion molecule expression on endothelial cells by anti-DNA autoantibodies in patients with SLE *(90)*. In these studies, the expression of ICAM-1 and VCAM-1 on HUVECs cultured with either control IgG or anti-dsDNA were compared by flow cytometry. Compared with either control IgG or anti-dsDNA–depleted IgG, HUVEC incubated with anti-dsDNA expressed a significantly higher mean fluorescence intensity of ICAM-1 and VCAM-1. At the same time, ICAM-1 mRNA was also raised.

Summary

The upregulation and activation of adhesion molecules are pivotal to the development of tissue injury in SLE. This is particularly true in the case of vascular injury in which a collaboration of cytokines, activated complement components and autoantibodies act on the endothelial cell to increase its adhesiveness and procoagulant activity (Fig. 4). These same mediators act locally on leukocytes and platelets to increase their adhesion to vascular endothelium and to stimulate the local release of toxic inflammatory mediators, including proteases and oxygen-derived free radicals. This cascad-

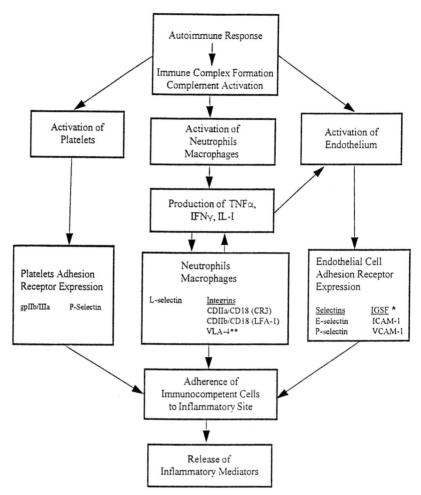

Fig. 4. Adhesion molecules play an important role in the inflammatory response but do not represent all of the adhesion molecules expressed by these cells. *IGSF = Immunoglobulin Superfamily; **macrophages only.

ing response requires further clarification with respect to the specific roles of the selectins, integrins, and immunoglobulin superfamily of adhesion molecules. Blockade of the interaction between inflammatory cells and adhesion molecules could provide a useful therapeutic strategy in the future.

References

1. Takabayashi, T., Vannier, E., Clark, B. D., Margolis, N. H., Dinarello, C. A., Burke, F., and Gelfand, J. A. (1996) A new biologic role for C3a and C3a desArg: regulation of TNF-alpha and IL-1 beta synthesis. *J. Immunol.* **156,** 3455–3460.
2. Stein, J. M. and Luzio, J. P. (1989) Membrane sorting during vesicle shedding from neutrophils during sublytic complement attack. *Biochem. Soc. Trans.* **16,** 1082,1083.
3. Morgan, B. P., Dankert, J. R., and Esser, A. F. (1987) Recovery of human neutrophils from complement attack: Removal of the membrane attack complex by endocytosis and exocytosis. *J. Immunol.* **138,** 246–253.

4. Morgan, B. P. (1989) Complement membrane attack on nucleated cells: resistance, recovery and nonlethal effects. *Biochem. J.* **264,** 1–14.

5. Hattori, R., Hamilton, K. K., McEver, R. P., and Sims, P. J. (1989) Complement proteins C5b-9 induce secretion of high molecular weight multimers of endothelial von Willebrand factor and translocation of granule membrane. *J. Biol. Chem.* **264,** 9053–9060.

6. Biesecker, G., Katz, S., and Koffler, D. (1981) Renal localization of the membrane attack complex in systemic lupus erythematosus nephritis. *J. Exp. Med.* **154,** 1779–1794.

7. Biesecker, G., Lavin, L., Zisking, M., and Koffler, D. (1982) Cutaneous localization of the membrane attack complex in discoid and systemic lupus erythematosus. *N. Engl. J. Med.* **306,** 264–270.

8. Kissel, J. T., Mendell, J. R., and Rammohan, K. W. (1986) Microvascular deposition of complement membrane attack complex in dermatomyositis. *N. Engl. J. Med.* **314,** 329–334.

9. Schafer, H., Mathey, D., Hugo, F., and Bhakdi, S. (1986) Deposition of the terminal C5b-9 complement complex in infarcted areas of human myocardium. *J. Immunol.*, **137,** 1945–1949.

10. Ruddy, S., Carpenter, C. B., Chin, K. W., Knostman, J. N., Soter, N. A., Gotze, O., Muller-Eberhard, H. J., and Austen, K. F. (1975) Human complement metabolism: an analysis of 144 studies. *Medicine (Baltimore)* **54,** 165–178.

11. Charlesworth, J. A., Williams, D. G., Sherington, E., Lachmann, P. J., and Peters, D. K. (1974) Metabolic studies of the third component of complement and the glycine rich glycoprotein in patients with hypocomplementemia. *J. Clin. Invest.* **53,** 1578–1587.

12. Sliwinski, A. J. and Zvaifler, N. J. (1972) Decreased synthesis of the third component (C3) in hypocomplementemic systemic lupus erythematosus. *Clin. Exp. Immunol.* **11,** 21–29.

13. Kerr, L., Adelsberg, B. R., Schulman, P., and Spiera, H. (1989) Factor B activation products in patients with systemic lupus erythematosus: a marker of severe disease activity. *Arthritis Rheum.* **32,** 1406–1413.

14. Falk, R. J., Dalmasso, A. P., Kim, Y., Lam, S., and Michael, A. (1985) Radioimmunoassay of the attack complex of complement in serum from patients with systemic lupus erythematosus. *N. Engl. J. Med.* **312,** 1594–1599.

15. Belmont, H. M., Hopkins, P., Edelson, H. S., Kaplan, H. B., Ludewig, R., Weissmann, G., and Abramson, S. (1986) Complement activation during systemic lupus erythematosus: C3a and C5a anaphylatoxins circulate during exacerbations of disease. *Arthritis Rheum.* **29,** 1085–1089.

16. Buyon, J., Tamerius, J., Belmont, H. M., and Abramson, S. (1992) Assessment of disease activity and impending flare in patients with systemic lupus erythematosus: comparison of the use of complement split products and conventional measurements of complement. *Arthritis Rheum.* **35,** 1028–1037.

17. Buyon, J., Tamerius, J., Ordica, S., Young, B., and Abramson, S. (1992) Activation of the alternative complement pathway accompanies disease flares in systemic lupus erythematosus during pregnancy. *Arthritis Rheum.* **35,** 55–61.

18. Hopkins, P. T., Belmont, H. M., Buyon, J., Philips, M. R., Weissmann, G., and Abramson, S. B. (1988) Increased levels of plasma anaphylatoxins in systemic lupus erythematosus predict flares of the disease and may elicit vascular injury in lupus cerebritis. *Arthritis Rheum.* **31,** 632–641.

19. Ross, G. D. and Medof, M. E. (1985) Membrane complement receptors specific for bound fragments of C3. *Adv. Immunol.* **37,** 217–267.

20. Schifferli, J. A., Ng, Y. C., and Peters, D. K. (1986) The role of complement and its receptor in the elimination of immune complexes. *N. Engl. J. Med.* **315,** 488–495.

21. Philips, M. R., Abramson, S. B., and Weissmann, G. (1989) Neutrophil adhesion and autoimmune vascular injury. *Clin. Aspects Autoimmunity* **3,** 6–15.

22. Yong, K. and Khwaja, A. (1990) Leukocyte cellular adhesion molecules. *Blood Rev.* **4,** 211–225.

23. McEver, R. P. (1991) Selectins: novel receptors that mediate leukocyte adhesion during inflammation. *Thromb. Haemostasis* **65,** 223–228.

24. Lawrence, M. B. and Springer, T. A. (1991) Leukocytes role on a selection of physiologic flow rates: distinction from and prerequisite for adhesion through integrins. *Cell* **65,** 859–873.

25. Nikolic-Paterson, D. J., Lan, H. Y., Hill, P. A., and Atkins, R. C. (1994) Macrophages in renal injury. *Kidney Int.* **45,** S79–S82.

26. Pytela, R., Pierschbacher, M., Ginsberg, M., Plow, E., and Rouslahti, E. (1986) Platelet membrane glycoprotein IIb/IIIa: member of a family of Arg-Gly-Asp-specific adhesion receptors. *Science* **231,** 1559–1562.

27. Johnson, R. J. (1991) Platelets in inflammatory glomerular injury. *Semin. Nephrol.* **11,** 276–284.
28. Pierucci, A., Simonetti, B. M., and Pecci, G. (1989) Improvement in renal function with selective thromboxane antagonism in lupus nephritis. *N. Engl. J. Med.* **320,** 421–425.
29. Johnson, R. J., Lovett, D., Lehrer, R. I., Couser, W. G., and Klebanoff, S. J. (1994) Role of oxidants and proteases in glomerular injury. *Kidney Int.* **45,** 352–359.
30. Koeffler, P., Schur, P., and Kunkel, H. (1967) Immunological studies concerning the nephritis of systemic lupus erythematosus. *J. Exp. Med.* **126,** 607–624.
31. Fauci, T. Y., Haynes, B. F., and Katz, P. (1978) The spectrum of vasculitis. *Ann. Int. Med.* **89,** 660–676.
32. Arthus, M. (1903) Injections repetees de serum de cheval chez la lapin. *Soc. Biol.* 847–850.
33. Ishizaka, K. (1963) Gamma globulin and molecular mechanisms in hypersensitivity reations, in *Progress in Allergy,* vol. 7 (Kallos, P. and Waksman, B. H., eds.), Karger, New York, pp. 32–106.
34. Frank, M. M., Ellman, L., Green, I., and Cochrane, C. (1973) Site of deposition of C3 in arthus reactions of C4 deficient guinea pigs. *J. Immunol.* **110,** 11,447–11,451.
35. Lawley, T. J. and Frank, M. M. (1980) Immune complexes and immune complex diseases, in *Clinical Immunology* (Parker, C. W., ed.) Saunders, Philadelphia, pp. 143.
36. Cochrane, C. G. (1965) The Arthus reaction, in *The Inflammatory Process* (Zweifach, B. W., Grant, L., and McCluskey, R. T., eds.), Academic, New York, pp. 613–648.
37. Sylvestre, D. L. and Ravetch, J. V. (1994) Fc receptors initiate the Arthus reaction: Redefining the inflammatory cascade. *Science* **265,** 1095–1098.
38. Hopkins, P., Belmont, M., Buyon, J., Philips, M. R., Weissmann, G., and Abramson, S. B. (1988) Increased plasma anaphylotoxins in systemic lupus erythematosus predict flares of the disease and may elicit the adult cerebral distress syndrome. *Arthritis Rheum.* **31,** 632–641.
39. Belmont, H. M., Buyon, J., Giorno, R., and Abramson, S. B. (1994) Upregulation of endothelial cell adhesion molecules characterizes disease activity in systemic lupus erythematosus: the Shwartzman Phenomenon revisited. *Arthritis Rheum.* **37,** 376–383.
40. Jacob, H. S., Craddock, P. R., Hammerschmidt, D. E., and Moldow, C. F. (1980) Complement-induced granulocyte aggregation: an unsuspected mechanism of disease. *N. Engl. J. Med.* **302,** 789–794.
41. Hammerschmidt, D. E., Weaver, L. J., Hudson, L. D., Craddock, P. R., and Jacob, H. S. (1980) Association of complement activation and elevated plasma-C5a with adult respiratory distress syndrome. *Lancet* **1,** 947–949.
42. Hakim, R., Breillatt, J., Lazarus, M., and Prt, K. (1984) Complement activation and hypersensitivity reactions to hemodialysis membranes. *N. Engl. J. Med.* **311,** 878–882.
43. Craddock, P., Fehr, J., Dalmasso, A., Brigham, K., and Jacob, H. (1977) Hemodialysis leukopenia. *J. Clin. Invest.* **59,** 879–888.
44. Chenoweth, D. E., Cooper, S. W., Hugli, T. E., Stewart, R. W., Balckstone, E. H., and Kirklin, S. W. (1981) Complement activation during cardiopulmonary bypass. *N. Engl. J. Med.* **304,** 497–505.
45. Perez, H. D., Horn, J. K., Ong, R., and Goldstein, I. (1983) Complement (C5)-derived chemotactic activity in serum from patients with pancreatitis. *J. Lab. Clin. Med.* **101,** 123–129.
46. Shwartzman, G. (1937) *Phenomenon of Local Tissue Reactivity.* Paul Hoeber, New York.
47. Argenbright, L. and Barton, R. (1992) Interactions of leukocyte integrins with intercellular adhesion molecule 1 in the production of inflammatory vascular injury in vivo: the Shwartzman Phenomenon revisited. *J. Clin. Invest.* **89,** 259–273.
48. Abramson, S. B. and Weissmann, G. (1988) Complement split products and the pathogenesis of SLE. *Hosp. Pract.* **23(12),** 45–55.
49. Pohlman, T. M., Stanness, K. A., Beatty, P. G., Ochs, H. D., and and Harlan, J. M. (1986) *J. Immunol.* **136,** 4548–4553.
50. Pober, J. S., Gimbrone, M., Lapierre, D., Mendrick, L., Fiers, W., Rothlein, R., and Springer, T. (1986) Overlapping patterns of activation of human endothelial cells by interleukin-1, tumor necrosis factor and immune interferon. *J. Immunol.* **137,** 1893–1896.
51. Fletcher, M. P., Seligmann, B. E., and Gallin, J. I. (1982) Correlation of human neutrophil secretion, chemoattractant receptor mobilization and enhanced functional capacity. *J. Immunol.* **128,** 941.
52. Schur, P. H. and Sandson, J. (1968) Immunologic factors and clinical activity in systemic lupus erythematosus. *N. Engl. J. Med.* **278,** 533–538.

53. Buyon, J. P., Shadick, N., Berkman, R., Hopkins, P., Dalton, J., Weissmann, G., Winchester, R., and Abramson, S. B. (1988) Surface expression of gp165/95, the complement receptor CR3, as a marker of disease activity in systemic lupus erythematosus. *Clin. Immunol. Immunopathol.* **46,** 141–149.
54. Johnson, R. T. and Richardson, E. P. (1968) The neurological manifestations of systemic lupus erythematosus: a clinical pathological study of 24 cases and a review of the literature. *Medicine (Baltimore)* **47,** 337–369.
55. Ellis, S. G. and Verity, M. A. (1979) Central nervous system involvement in systemic lupus erythematosus: a review of the neuropathologic findings in 57 cases, 1955–1977. *Semin. Arthritis Rheum.* **8,** 212–233.
56. Hammad, A., Tsukada, Y., and Torre, N. (1992) Cerebral occlusive vasculopathy in systemic lupus erythematosus and speculation on the part played by complement. *Ann. Rheum. Dis.* **51,** 550–552.
57. Devinsky, O., Petito, C. K., and Alonso, D. R. (1988) Clinical and neuropathological findings in systemic lupus erythematosus: the role of vasculitis heart emboli and thrombotic thrombocytopenic purpura. *Ann. Neurol.* **23,** 380.
58. Abramson, S. B., Dobro, J., Eberle, M. A., Benton, M., Reibman, J., Epstein, H., Belmont, H. M., Rapoport, D. M., and Goldring, R. M. (1991) The syndrome of acute reversible hypoxemia of systemic lupus erythematosus. *Ann. Int. Med.* **114,** 941–947.
59. Hughes, G. R. and Khamashta, M. A. (1994) The antiphospholipid syndrome. *J. Royal Coll. Phys. London* **28,** 301–304.
60. Ordi-Ros, J., Perez-Peman, P., and Monasterio, J. (1994) Clinical and therapeutic aspects associated to phospholipid binding antibodies (lupus anticoagulant and anticardiolipin antibodies). *Haemostasis* **24,** 165–174.
61. Bevers, E. M. and Galli, M. (1992) Cofactors involved in the antiphospholipid syndrome. *Lupus* **1,** 51–53.
62. Ozawa, N., Makino, T., Matsubayashi, H., Hosokawa, T., Someya, K., Nozawa, S., and Matsuura, E. (1994) Beta 2-GPI-dependent and independent binding of anticardiolipin antibodies in patients with recurrent spontaneous abortions. *J. Clin. Lab. Analysis* **8,** 255–259.
63. Aron, A. L., Gharavi, A. E., and Shoenfeld, Y. (1995) Mechanisms of action of antiphospholipid antibodies in the antiphospholipid syndrome. *Int. Arch. Allergy Immunol.* **106,** 8–12.
64. Pierangeli, S. S. and Harris, E. N. (1994) Antiphospholipid antibodies in an in vivo thrombosis model in mice. *Lupus* **3,** 247–251.
65. Triplett, D. A. (1992) Antiphospholipid antibodies: proposed mechanisms of action. *Am. J. Reprod. Immunol.* **28,** 211–215.
66. Wiener, H. M., Vardinon, N., and Yust, I. (1991) Platelet antibody binding and spontaneous aggregation in 21 lupus anticoagulant patients. *Vox Sanguinis* **61,** 111–121.
67. Vazquez-Mellado, J., Llorente, L., Richaud-Patin, Y., and Alarcon-Segovia, D. (1994) Exposure of anionic phospholipids upon platelet activation permits binding of beta 2 glycoprotein I and through it that of IgG antiphospholipid antibodies: studies in platelets from patients with antiphospholipid syndrome and normal subjects. *J. Autoimmunity* **7,** 335–348.
68. Lindsey, N. J., Henderson, F. I., Malia, R., Milford-Ward, M. A., Greaves, M., and Hughes, P. (1994) Inhibition of prostacyclin release by endothelial binding anticardiolipin antibodies in thrombosis-prone patients with systemic lupus erythematosus and the antiphospholipid syndrome. *Br. J. Rheumatol.* **33,** 20–26.
69. Westerman, E. M., Miles, J. M., Backonja, M., and Sundstrom, W. R. (1992) Neuropathologic findings in multiinfarct dementia associated with anticardiolipin antibody: evidence for endothelial injury as the primary event. *Arthritis Rheum.* **35,** 1038–1041.
70. McCraw, K. R., DeMichele, A., Samuels, P., Roth, D., Kuo, A., Meng, Q. H., Rauch, J., and Cines, D. B. (1991) Detection of endothelial cell-reactive immunoglobulin in patients with antiphospholipid antibodies. *Br. J. Haematol.* **79,** 595–605.
71. Silver, R. K., Adler, L., Hickman, A. R., and Hageman, J. R. (1991) Anticardiolipin antibody-positive serum enhances endothelial cell platelet-activating factor production. *Am. J. Obst. Gyn.* **165,** 1748–1752.
72. Freyssinet, J. M., Toti-Orfanoudakis, F., Ravanat, C., Grunebaum, L., Gauchy, J., Cazenave, J. P., and Wiesel, M. L. (1991) The catalytic role of anionic phospholipids in the activation of

protein C by factor Xa and expression of its anticoagulant function in human plasma. *Blood Coagul. Fibrin* **2**, 691–698.

73. Joseph, J. and Scopelitis, E. (1994) Seronegative antiphospholipid syndrome associated with plasminogen activator inhibitor. *Lupus* **3**, 201–203.

74. Ahmed, K., Vianna, J., Khamashta, M., and Hughes, G. (1992) IL-2, IL-6, and TNF levels in primary antiphospholilip antibody syndrome. *Clin. Exp. Rheumatol.* **10**, 503 (letter).

75. Simantov, R., LaSala, J. M., Lo, S. K., Gharavi, E., Sammaritano, L. R., Salmon, J. E., and Silverstein, R. L. (1996) Activation of cultured vascular endothelial cells by antiphospholipid antibodies. *J. Clin. Invest.* **96**, 2211–2219.

76. Stricker, R. B., Davis, J. A., Gershow, J., Yamamoto, K. S., and Kiprov, D. D. (1992) Thrombotic thrombocytopenic purpura complicating systemic lupus erythematosus: case report and literature review from the plasmapheresis era. *J. Rheumatol.* **19**, 1469–1473.

77. Cockerell, C. J. and Lewis, J. E. (1993) Systemic lupus erythematosus-like illness associated with syndrome of abnormally large von Willebrand's factor multimers. *South. Med. J.* **86**, 951–953.

78. Moake, J. L., Rudy, C. K., Troll, J. H., Weinstein, M. J., Colannino, N. M., Azocar, J., Seder, R. H., Hong, S. L., and Deykin, D. (1982) Unusually large plasma factor VIII: von Willebrand factor multimers in chronic relapsing thrombotic thrombocytopenic purpura. *N. Engl. J. Med.* **303**, 1432–1435.

79. Takahashi, H., Hanano, M., Wada, K., Tatewaki, W., Niwano, H., Tsubouchi, J., Nakano, M., Nakamura, T., and Shibata, A. (1991) Circulating thrombomodulin in thrombotic thrombocytopenic purpura. *Am. J. Hematol.* **38**, 174–177.

80. Arnaout, M. A. and Colten, H. R. (1984) Complement C3 receptors: structure and function. *Molec. Immun.* **21**, 1191–1199.

81. Bullard, D. C., King, P. D., Hicks, M. J., Dupont, B., Beaudet, A. L., and Eldon, K. B. (1997) Intercellular adnesion molecule-1 deficiency protects MRL/MpJ-Fas (1pr) mice from early lethality. *J. Immunol.* **159**, 2057–2067.

82. Springer, T. Z., Teplow, D. B., and Dreyer, W. J. (1985) [Article title]. *Nature* **314**, 540–542.

83. Belmont, H. M., Amin, A. R., Giorno, R., and Abramson, S. B. (1995) Inducible nitric oxide synthase expression by endothelial cells characterizes systemic lupus erythematosus disease exacerbation, submitted.

84. Nyberg, F., Acevedo, F., and Stephansson, E. (1997) Different patterns of soluble adhesion molecules in systemic and cutaneous lupus erythematosus. *J. Immunol.* **65**, 230–235.

85. Berger, M. D., Birx, L., Wetzler, E. M., O'Shea, J. J., Brown, E. J., and Cross, A. S. (1985) Increased expression of C3b receptors or polymarphonuclear leukocytes induced by chemotactic factors and by purification procedures. *J. Immunol.* **135**, 1342–1348.

86. Kilgore, K. S., Shen, J. P., Miller, B. F., Ward, P. A., and Warren, J. S. (1995) Enhancement by the complement membrane attack complex of tumor necrosis factor-alpha-induced endothelial cell expression of E-selectin abd ICAM–1. *J. Immunol.* **155**, 1434–1441.

87. Jones, S. M., Mathew, C. M., Dixey, J., Lovell, C. R., and McHugh, N. J. (1996) VCAM-1 expression on endothelium in lesions from cutaneous lupus erythematosus is increased compared with systemic and localized scleroderma. *J. Exp. Med.* **135**, 678–686.

88. Lozada, C., Levin, R. I., Huie, M., Hirschhorn, R., Naime, D., Whitlow, M., Recht, P. A., Golden, B., and Cronstein, B. N. (1995) Identification of C1q as the heat-labile serum cofactor required for immune complexes to stimulate endothelial expression of the adhesion molecules E-selectin and intercellular and vascular cell adhesion molecules. *Proc. Natl. Acad. Sci. USA* **92**, 8378–8382.

89. Neng Lai, L. K., Leung, J. C., Bil Lai, K., Li, P. K., and Lai, C. K. (1996) Anti-DNA autoantibodies stimulate the release of interleukin–1 and interleukin-6 from human endothelial cells. *J. Pathol.* **178**, 451–458.

90. Lai, K. N., Leung, J. C., Lai, K. B., Wong, K. C., and Lai, C. K. (1996) Upregulation of adhesion molecule expression on endothelial cells by anti-DNA autoantibodies in systemic lupus erythematosus. *Clin. Immunol. Immunopathol.* **81**, 229–238.

Index